Image Based MCQs
in
Dermatology, Venereology and Leprology

Image Based MCQs in Dermatology, Venereology and Leprology

Ramesh Bansal MD (Skin VD and leprosy)
Ex Registrar
Department of Skin VD and Leprosy
Pt. BDS PGIMS, Rohtak, Haryana, India
Skin VD and Allergy Clinic (Estd. 1990)
Jhajjar Road, Rohtak, Haryana, India

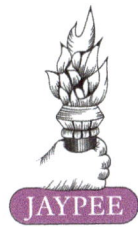

JAYPEE BROTHERS MEDICAL PUBLISHERS
The Health Sciences Publisher
New Delhi | London

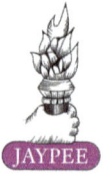

Jaypee Brothers Medical Publishers (P) Ltd.

Headquarters
Jaypee Brothers Medical Publishers (P) Ltd.
EMCA House, 23/23-B
Ansari Road, Daryaganj
New Delhi 110 002, India
Landline: +91-11-23272143, +91-11-23272703
+91-11-23282021, +91-11-23245672
Email: jaypee@jaypeebrothers.com

Overseas Office
J.P. Medical Ltd.
83 Victoria Street, London
SW1H 0HW (UK)
Phone: +44 20 3170 8910
Email: info@jpmedpub.com

Corporate Office
Jaypee Brothers Medical Publishers (P) Ltd.
4838/24, Ansari Road, Daryaganj
New Delhi 110 002, India
Phone: +91-11-43574357
Fax: +91-11-43574314
Email: jaypee@jaypeebrothers.com

EU GPSR Authorised Representative
Logos Europe, 9 rue Nicolas Poussin
17000, La Rochelle, France
Phone: +33 (0) 6 67 93 73 78
E-mail: Contact@logoseurope.eu

Website: www.jaypeebrothers.com
Website: www.jaypeedigital.com

© 2024, Jaypee Brothers Medical Publishers

The views and opinions expressed in this book are solely those of the original contributor(s)/author(s) and do not necessarily represent those of editor(s) and publisher of the book.

All rights reserved. No part of this publication may be reproduced, stored or transmitted in any form or by any means, electronic, mechanical, photocopying, recording or otherwise, without the prior permission in writing of the publishers.

All brand names and product names used in this book are trade names, service marks, trademarks or registered trademarks of their respective owners. The publisher is not associated with any product or vendor mentioned in this book.

Medical knowledge and practice change constantly. This book is designed to provide accurate, authoritative information about the subject matter in question. However, readers are advised to check the most current information available on procedures included and check information from the manufacturer of each product to be administered, to verify the recommended dose, formula, method and duration of administration, adverse effects and contraindications. It is the responsibility of the practitioner to take all appropriate safety precautions. Neither the publisher nor the author(s)/editor(s) assume any liability for any injury and/or damage to persons or property arising from or related to use of material in this book.

This book is sold on the understanding that the publisher is not engaged in providing professional medical services. If such advice or services are required, the services of a competent medical professional should be sought.

Every effort has been made where necessary to contact holders of copyright to obtain permission to reproduce copyright material. If any have been inadvertently overlooked, the publisher will be pleased to make the necessary arrangements at the first opportunity.

Inquiries for bulk sales may be solicited at: jaypee@jaypeebrothers.com

Image Based MCQs in Dermatology, Venereology and Leprology

First Edition: 2024

ISBN: 978-93-5696-807-3

Preface

In medical science including dermatology, making a correct diagnosis is a cornerstone in correct management of any disease. Otherwise, whole management including investigations and treatment will be distracted from right path.

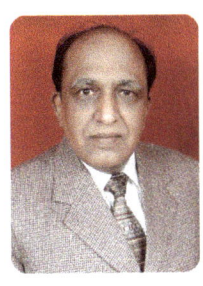

Most of the time, the diagnosis can easily be made in dermatology on the morphological clinical features of the disease. Sometimes, even without taking history, spot diagnosis can easily be made at the first glance of morphology of the lesions. A skin disease can manifest in many clinical forms. So, every clinician must be well exposed to diverse clinical manifestations of various dermatological disorders.

In this book, 1,123 image-based multiple choice questions (MCQs) have been framed based on diagnosis, structure of skin, hair and nail, histopathology, investigations, treatment, and side effects of treatment. I have tried to incorporate all types of clinical presentations of various skin diseases which one can come across in day-to-day practice.

The answers have been well explained with supporting features of correct option. Features of incorrect options are also mentioned along with their reference MCQ.

I am sure this unique book will be very helpful to undergraduates, junior residents, senior residents, and all practitioners who have interest in dermatology. One can get oneself exposed to all types of possible patients in a very short time. This book is especially helpful for students seeking PG entrance examination in which students have to answer some MCQs based on clinical photograph.

Ramesh Bansal

Acknowledgments

I thank almighty God and dedicate this book to my parents who have blessed me this noble profession for taking care of human ailments.

I express my sincere thanks and regards to all my worthy teachers Dr SD Chaudhary, Dr VK Jain, and Dr KK Bhatia who have trained me in this superspeciality.

Thanks to all my friends Dr Sunil Gupta, Dr Surabhi Dayal, Dr US Pahwa, Dr VB Dixit, Dr RA Mittle, Dr SN Bansal, and Dr Sushil Bathla for showering their best wishes.

My IMA friends Dr SL Verma, Dr RK Chaudhary, Dr DK Puri, Dr PS Mann, and Dr VK Govila had been a source of inspiration for me.

I thank my very close relatives Dr Rakesh Gupta (Ortho), Dr (Mrs) Shashi Kiran Gupta (Anesth), Shri Naresh Singla, and Shri Kewal Singhal who always encouraged me for this work.

My real younger brothers Jaiprakash and Rajnish are my pillars.

My sisters are my real well wishers.

I will fail in my duty, if I do not appreciate my wife Nishi Bansal who always supported me.

The biggest contribution is of my son-in-law Dr Vijay Singhal who is a Senior Consultant Dermatologist in Sri Balaji Action Medical Institute, Paschim Vihar, New Delhi. He gave very useful suggestions and provided many photographs. He did a tough job of proofreading of whole book for the needful corrections.

My family young generations, Dr Aparna Singhal (MDS Prosthodontics), Raja, Sachi, Prashant, Seema, Keshav, Madhur, Pranshu, and Mohit helped me in solving technical problems.

I am grateful to all my patients for their kind cooperation.

Special acknowledgments to M/s Jaypee Brothers Medical Publishers (P) Ltd, New Delhi, India:
My gratitude to Shri Jitendar P Vij (Group Chairman), Mr Ankit Vij (Managing Director), Mr MS Mani (Group President), Dr Madhu Choudhary (Director–Educational Publishing), Ms Pooja Bhandari [Director–Production (Books and Journals)], Ms Sunita Katla (Executive Assistant to Group Chairman and Publishing Manager), Mr Ajay Kumar Sharma [Deputy General Manager (Books and Journals)].

I would also like to thank Dr Upma Tomar (Development Editor) and her entire team who brought the book to its present shape.

Thanks are due to production team-members for speedy completion of this mega task.
- Mr Rajesh Sharma (Production Coordinator)
- Mr Jagvir Singh Tomar (DTP Typesetter)
- Mr Vakil Khan (Proofreader)
- Ms Neha (Cover Designer)
- Mr Nitesh Jain (Graphic Designer)

Contents

1. Structure of Human Skin 1
2. Approach to Diagnosis in Dermatology 5
3. Availability of Commonly Used Drugs in Dermatology, Venereology and Leprology 12
4. MCQs of Dermatology, Venereology and Leprology 27
5. Answers of MCQs in Dermatology, Venereology and Leprology 308

CHAPTER 1

Structure of Human Skin

INTRODUCTION

Skin is the largest organ in human body and has a surface area of about two square meters. A human body has two main kinds of skin:
1. **Nonhairy skin (glabrous skin):**
    - It is seen on palms and soles.
    - It has thick epidermis with an additional layer of stratum lucidum below stratum corneum.
    - This part is devoid of hair follicles and sebaceous glands but is rich in encapsulated sense organs in the dermis.
2. **Hair-bearing skin:**
    - It covers the larger part of our body and has both hair follicles and sebaceous glands.
    - It is devoid of encapsulated sense organs.

STRUCTURE

- Human skin consists of continuously renewing stratified squamous epithelium known as *epidermis*.
- Epidermis is about 0.05-0.1 mm thick (total thickness of skin, 1.5-4 mm).
- Beneath the epidermis there is underlying dermal connective tissue. The ratio between epidermis and dermis is about 1:20.
- Between dermis and epidermis there is a dermal-epidermal junction (DEJ) which provides mechanical support and resistance against external shearing forces.
- Below the dermis, there is a subcutaneous fatty tissue.

Epidermis

Embryology

- Epidermis originates from surface area of early gastrula.
- Dermis is derived from mesoderm.
- Neural crest contributes pigment cells.

Structurally

Epidermis is largely composed of keratinocytes which are formed by division of basal layer cells. After division, cells move outwardly toward skin surface and get differentiated to form well defined different layers of epidermis **(Fig. 1.1)**. Following layers have been recognized in the epidermis.

Stratum Basale or Germinativum (Basal cell layer)

Generally, it is one cell thick continuous layer. Cells are small, columnar having dark staining nuclei and dense cytoplasm. These cells are mitotically active and give rise to cells of epidermal layers.
- **Melanocytes:** Among the basal cells, there are pigment synthesizing, dendritic cells known as *melanocytes*. They transfer pigment to the associated keratinocytes. Melanocytes are derived from neural crest.
- **Merkel cells:** They are also present among basal keratinocytes of the skin of certain regions of body having high tactile sensitivity. They are found in hairy skin, glabrous skin of digits, lips, oral cavity and outer root sheath of hair follicle. These cells function as *mechanoreceptors*. They are also pale staining and have lobulated nuclei.

Stratum Spinosum (Prickle Cell Layer)

- This layer lies immediately above the basal cell layer and is 8-10 layers thick.
- Its cells are polyhedral, larger, more flattened and contain **lamellar granules**.
- It is named as spinous after the spine-like appearance of cell margins in histological sections. Spines are due to abundant desmosomes which provide mechanical coupling between keratinocytes.
- Sometimes, the term **"malpighian layer"** is used to include both the basal and spinous cells.

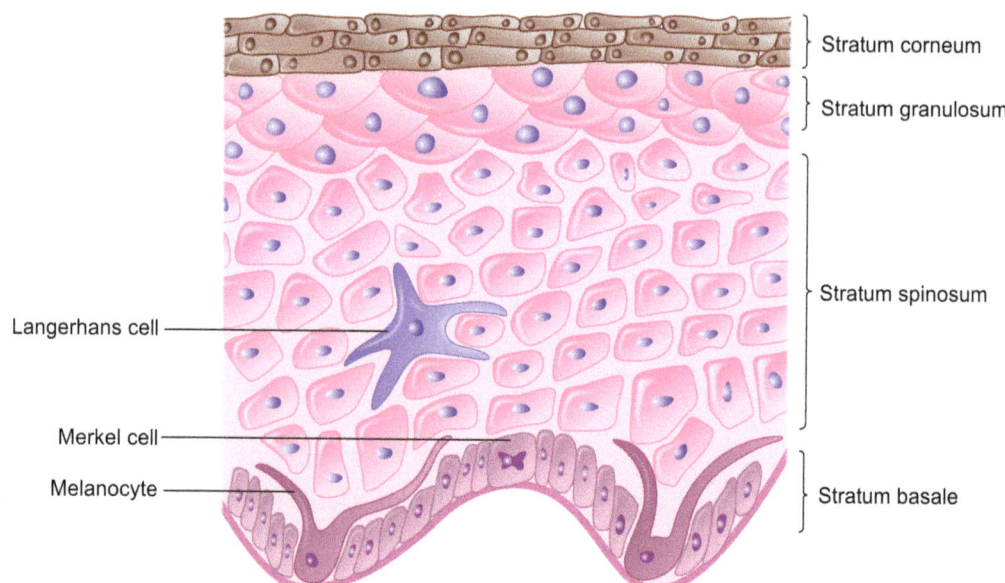

Fig. 1.1: Diagrammatic representation of epidermal cell layers.

Stratum Granulosum (Granular Cell Layer)

- Cells of spinous cell layer get differentiated into cells of granular cell layer which is 2–5 layers thick.
- These cells consist of basophilic keratohyalin granules.

Langerhans cells:
- These are other dendritic cells seen in epidermis.
- They are found in basal, spinous and granular cell layers, preferentially at suprabasal position.
- Microscopically, they are pale staining and have convoluted nuclei.
- Electron microscopically, rod and racket-shaped Birbeck granules are seen in the cytoplasm.
- These cells are derived from bone marrow and have involvement in T-cell responses.

Stratum Lucidum (Transitional Cell Layer)

- It is seen only in the skin of palms and soles.
- The cells in this layer still have nucleus and are called as *transitional cells*.

Stratum Corneum (Horny Cell Layer)

- During transition from granular cell layer, these cells normally lose their nuclei, cytoplasmic organelles and desmosomal connections and get flattened and polyhedral in shape.
- This layer provides mechanical protection and allows permeation of soluble substances and acts as a barrier to water loss.

Epidermal Cell Kinetics

The basal layer cells have proliferative capacity. After division, the daughter cells gradually move toward surface.

Epidermal Turnover Time

The amount of time taken by whole epidermal cell population to replace itself is called **turnover time** or **epidermal turnover time**. It is also called as **regeneration time** or **replacement time**. The mean turnover time of normal skin is 47–48 days. It is reduced to 6–8 days in psoriasis.

Epidermal Cell Cycle

The cell cycle (Tc) refers to the interval between two successive mitoses (M). A dividing cell passes through following four stages **(Fig. 1.2)**:
1. Mitosis (M)
2. Postmitotic growth phase or interphase (G1)
3. A period of active deoxyribonucleic acid (DNA) synthesis (S)
4. Premitotic growth or resting phase (G2)

Postmitotic growth phase is quite longer, while premitotic growth phase is short. After division, cells may become quiescent (G0 phase), but can reenter the cell cycle again when they are required to do so. After division, cells have another option to get differentiated (D).

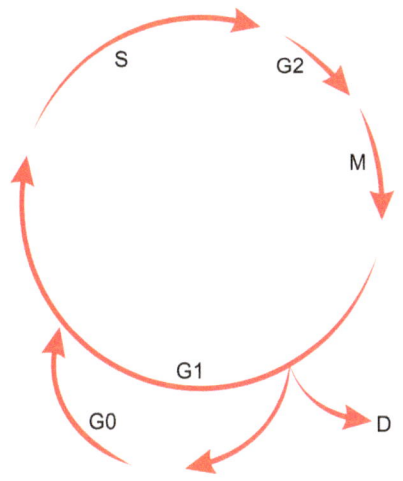

Fig. 1.2: Cell cycle.
(G0: quiescent phase; G1: interphase; G2: resting phase;
M: mitosis; S: active DNA synthesis period; D: differentiated)

Dermal-Epidermal Junction

It forms an interface between dermis and epidermis and is continuous around epidermal appendages also. Its structure is highly complex **(Fig. 1.3)**. Electron microscopically from epidermis to dermis, DEJ can be subdivided into following various components.

Hemidesmosomes

These are electron dense focal thickenings which stud the trilaminar plasma membrane of basal keratinocytes at frequent intervals. Tonofilaments are associated perpendicularly with the cytoplasmic portion of hemidesmosomes.

Inner to plasma membrane is the **basement membrane**, which is comprised of three layers, i.e., lamina lucida, lamina densa and lamina fibroreticularis.

Lamina Lucida

It is an electron lucent intermembranous space which separates plasma membrane from lamina densa. In areas of lamina lucida, there are linear densities beneath each hemidesmosome. These densities are termed as sub-basal dense plaques (SBDP). Fine anchoring filaments traverse the SBDP and extend perpendicularly from plasma membrane to mesh with lamina densa. Lamina lucida is considered as the **weakest zone** of DEJ.

Lamina Densa (Basal Lamina)

It is an electron dense layer lying next to lamina lucida and is parallel to the lower border of plasma membrane. Type IV collagen is its primary component.

Lamina Fibroreticularis

It is a fibroreticular layer which is composed of three major structures, namely anchoring fibrils, type III collagen and dermal bundle of microfibrils.
1. Anchoring fibrils are major constituent and are irregularly spaced cross banded fibers. Their epidermal

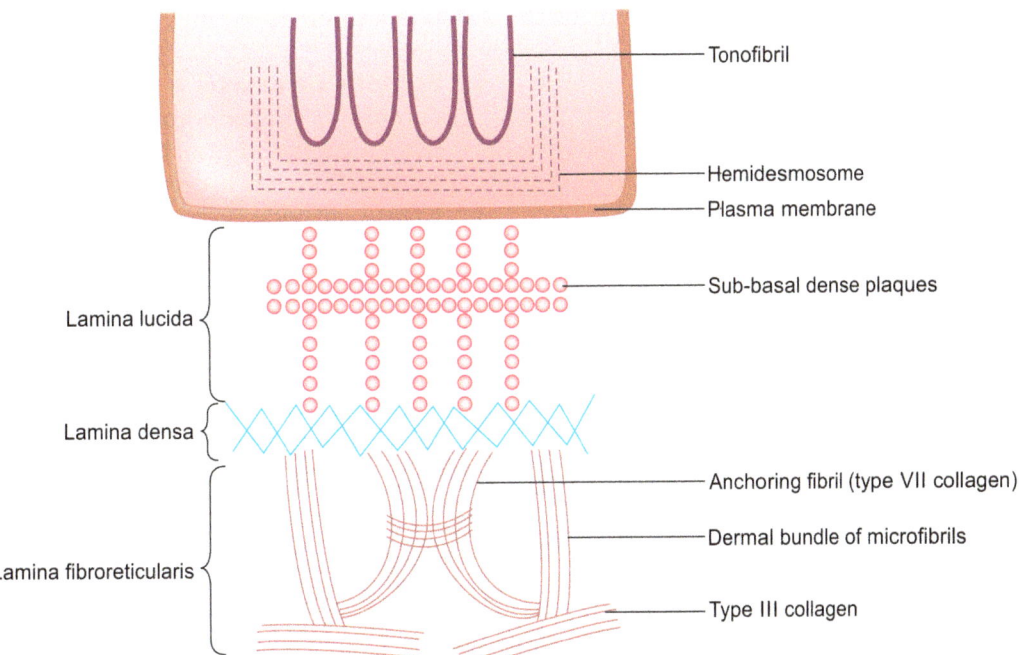

Fig. 1.3: Diagrammatic representation of dermal-epidermal junction.

ends mesh with lamina densa and dermal end with papillary dermis. Type VII collagen is the major component of anchoring fibrils.
2. Type III fibers are randomly oriented type fibers.
3. Dermal microfibrils extend perpendicularly from basal lamina to papillary dermis.

Dermis

The dermis is bounded externally by DEJ and internally by hypodermis. It constitutes the major part of skin but varies in thickness. It is about 1 mm thick on eyelids and 5 mm on the back.

Hypodermis

- Also known as **subcutaneous fat** or **subcutis**. It is present almost in all regions of body surface between skin and deep fascia except in the regions of eyelids and male genitalia.
- The main constituent is adipocytes which are organized into lobules that are separated by fibrous connective tissue septa. Histologically, the adipocytes appear as **signet-ring** due to the peripherally displaced oval nucleus by a large single intracellular vacuole containing fat.
- The projections of epidermis into dermis are called **rete ridges**. Simultaneously, dermis also projects into epidermis as **dermal papillae** alternating with rete ridges.

Cutaneous Receptors of Skin

Receptors

Sensory receptors can be either sensory fibers itself (free nerve endings) or specialized structures (corpuscular structures).

Various receptors **(Fig. 1.4)** are as under:
- **Free nerve endings:** These are rapidly adapting receptors that are present subepidermally in the papillary dermis.

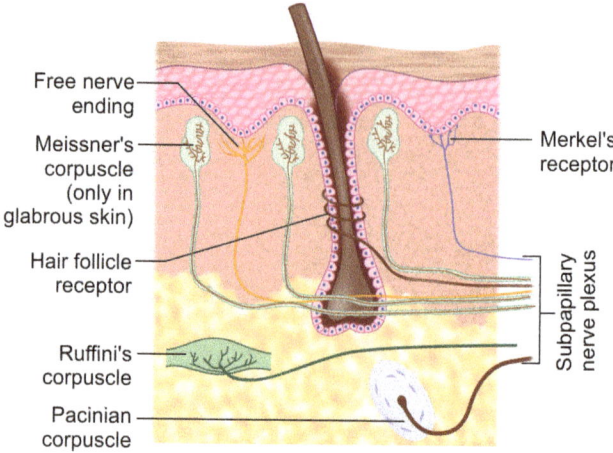

Fig. 1.4: Cutaneous receptors.

They perceive stimuli of touch, temperature, pain and itch.
- **Merkel's receptors or discs:** These are formed by association of Merkel cells with free nerve endings. The Merkel cell-nerve complexes are also called as touch domes or Merkel's touch spots.
- **Meissner's corpuscle:** It is found only in glabrous skin and is located superficially in the dermal papillae of digital skin. They are oriented vertically to epidermal surface. It responds to light touch and slow vibrations.
- **Pacinian corpuscle:** These are located deeply in dermis and subcutaneous tissue. Structurally, it consists of a characteristic perineural capsule made up of concentric layers (onion-like) of cells and fibrous connective tissue.
- **Ruffini's corpuscle:** It is also known as bulbous corpuscle. They are present in deeper dermis in human digits and respond to sustained pressure by maintaining stress in dermal collagen.
- **Krause end bulb:** These receptors respond to sensation of cold. It is an encapsulated swelling on myelinated fibers located in superficial layers of dermis.
- **Golgi-Mazzoni corpuscle:** These are located in subcutaneous tissue of human fingers.

Approach to Diagnosis in Dermatology

INTRODUCTION

In dermatological clinical practice, many a times an instant diagnosis can be easily made by a trained and experienced dermatologist by a mere look at the skin lesions. But it is always necessary to assess the extent of disease, severity, complications and predisposing, and aggravating factors. As in other medical specialties, evaluation of a patient consists of three main steps—medical history, physical examination and investigations.

MEDICAL HISTORY

A brief initial examination before obtaining medical history will avoid unnecessary details and will give more fruitful results. Following points should be given due consideration while taking history:

- **Onset, progression, remission, relapses and duration of the disease, e.g.**
  - *Site of first involvement and progression:* In pityriasis rosea, first lesion herald patch is noticed on trunk, later secondary eruption appears.
  - Overnight changing of color in a lesion to black is most likely due to intralesional bleeding and not due to melanoma.
  - The disappearance of individual urticarial lesion within 24 hours is a characteristic feature of urticaria.
- **Diurnal variation:** Nocturnal itching is a characteristic feature of scabies.
- **Seasonal variation:**
  - Xerosis, ichthyotic disorders, senile eczema, psoriasis, chilblains and systemic sclerosis get worsen during winter season.
  - Miliaria rubra and fungal infections are more common in summer season.
- **Precipitating factors:**
  - Exercise aggravates cholinergic urticaria.
  - Photodermatoses are aggravated by sun exposure.
  - Drug may be found to be responsible for inducing urticaria, fixed drug eruption, Stevens-Johnson syndrome or toxic epidermal necrolysis, etc.
- **Inquiry about itching, burning or asymptomatic nature of lesions.**
  - Syphilitic rash is usually asymptomatic.
  - Pain in herpes zoster is of burning type.
- **Nature of previous treatments taken:** Application of topical steroids should be enquired for the diagnosis of—steroid dermatitis, perioral dermatitis, tinea incognito.
- **Presence of underlying medical conditions:** For example, diabetes, hypertension, tuberculosis, hypothyroidism, seizures, etc.
- **Personal history:** Of smoking, alcohol intake, tobacco chewing, etc., has its own importance.
- **Family history of similar disorders:**
  - *Infectious diseases:* Scabies and pediculosis
  - *Genetic disorders:* Neurofibromatosis, epidermolysis bullosa, ichthyosis, Hailey-Hailey disease, etc.
- **Occupation:** May enlighten the aggravating factors in patients suffering from hand eczema, chronic paronychia, intertrigo, etc.

With experience, one automatically learns to ignore unnecessary details and enquires only essential information.

PHYSICAL EXAMINATION

- It should always be made in good light.
- A magnifying glass should be used for more morphological details of small lesions.
- If possible entire skin should be examined especially when diagnosis is in doubt.

Dermatological Examination

It consists of examination of skin,[1] mucous membranes, palms and soles, nails, scalp and hair. Examination of skin should take into consideration of:

- **Morphology of individual lesion:** It includes color, consistency, margins, shape, surface and scaling **(Table 2.1)**.
- **Arrangement of lesions:** It can be in various patterns, e.g., grouped (herpes group of diseases), linear (linear epidermal nevus) and unilateral in a dermatomal pattern (segmental vitiligo and herpes zoster).
- **Site of involvement:** It is characteristic for some disorders as follows:
  - Acne involves face, chest, back and upper arm.
  - Seborrheic dermatitis involves scalp, nasolabial folds, eye lashes, chest, interscapular region, etc.
  - Papular lesions of scabies are seen on genitalia, finger webs, thighs and suprapubic region but spares face.
  - Chronic discoid lupus erythematosus lesions are common on sun-exposed sites.
- **General physical examination:** It should also be carried out as per need based on medical history and dermatological assessment with special attention to lymph node enlargement, splenomegaly and hepatomegaly.

Descriptive Terms

These are commonly used for various morphologic cutaneous lesions in order to convey the details of lesions among each other. The initial characteristic lesions of a disease are called *primary lesions*. These lesions can get modified by scratching, ulceration or other events. These modified lesions are called *secondary lesions, e.g., erosion, ulcer, excoriation, etc.*

Primary Skin Lesions

Eruption or a lesion that appears in normal skin without any prior eruption is called a *primary skin lesion*.

Papule

A solid, circumscribed and elevated lesion <0.5 cm in diameter is called as *papule* **(Figs. 2.1A and B)**.

- When papule is surmounted with scale, it is referred as *papulosquamous*. In addition, surface of papule **(Table 2.1)** may be flat topped (plane warts), verrucous (common warts), dome shaped (trichoepithelioma), umbilicated (molluscum contagiosum), acuminated (condyloma acuminatum) or sometimes pedunculated (skin tags).

Nodule

It differs from papule in having size >0.5 cm.

Tumor

It is a general term used for any swelling **(Fig. 2.1C)** composed of pathological material. It may be inflammatory, benign or malignant.

Table 2.1: Different types of shapes and surfaces of lesions.

Shape and configuration	Example
Flat topped	Plane warts
Verrucous	Common warts
Dome shaped	Trichoepithelioma
Umbilicated	Molluscum contagiosum
Acuminated	Condyloma acuminata
Pedunculated	Skin tags
Digitate type	Genital warts
Polygonal	Lichen planus
Punctate	Petechiae
Serpentine	Larva migrans
Annular	Leprosy
Gyrate	Gyrate erythema (erythema annular centrifugum)
Arcuate	Granuloma annulare
Oval	Psoriasis
Moniliform	Moniliform blepharosis (lipoid proteinosis)
Polycyclic	Herpes simplex
Iris shaped or target shaped	Erythema multiforme
Reticulate (Retiform)	Reticulate pigmentation (Dyskeratosis congenita)

---

[1] In a patient complaining of pruritus, examination is not complete if genitals, groins and buttocks are not examined.

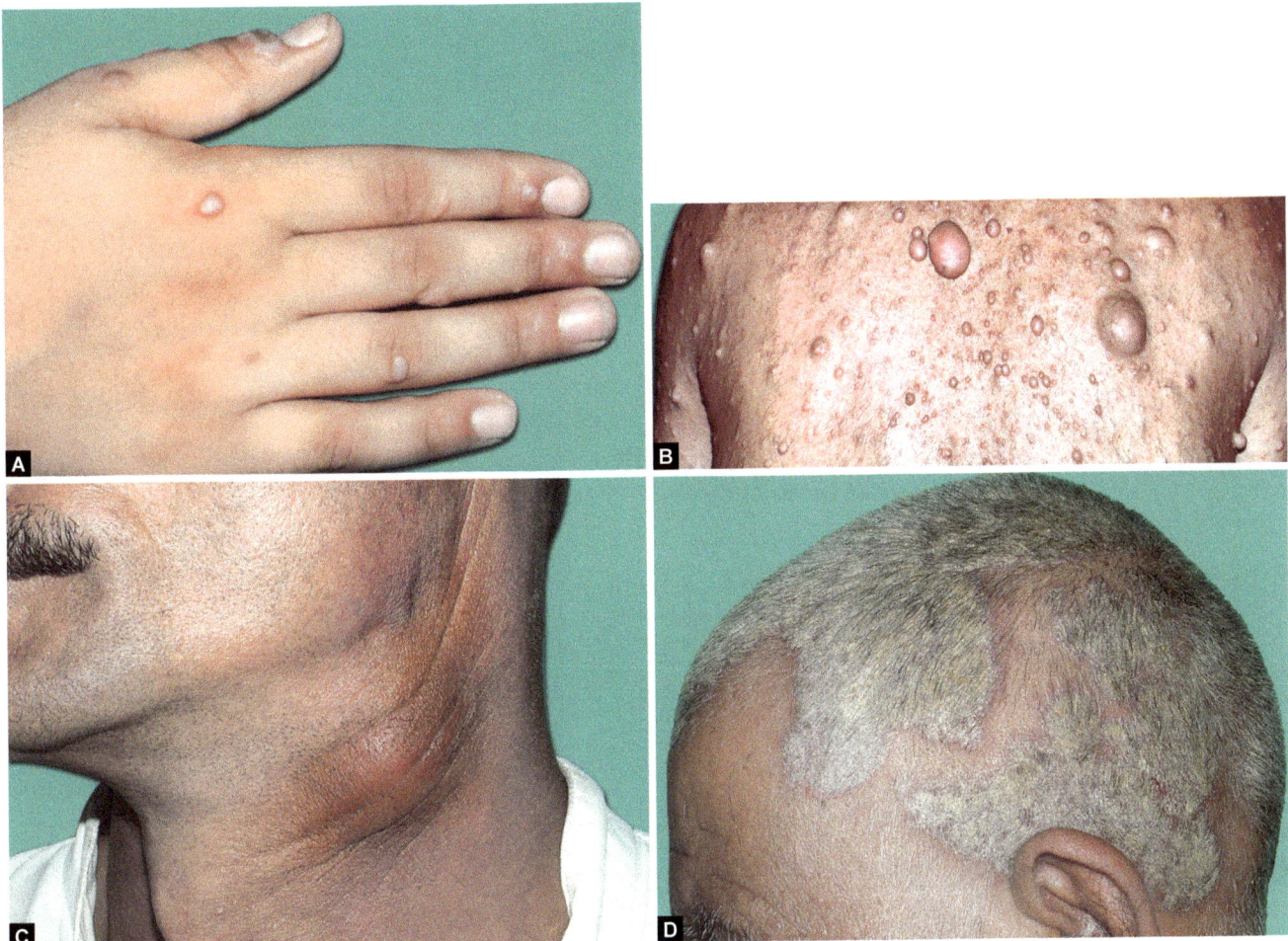

Figs. 2.1A to D: Solid elevations. (A) Papules; (B) Papules and nodules on back; (C) Tumor on neck; (D) Psoriatic plaques on scalp.

Plaque

An elevated or depressed solid, plateau like area 2 or >2 cm in diameter with larger surface area than height is called as *plaque* (Fig. 2.1D).
- A plaque may form by extension or confluence of papules. A psoriatic lesion is a classic example.
- A plaque may be discoid, annular or irregular shaped.

Macule

Nonpalpable discoloration (with no texture change) of skin <0.5 cm is called as *macule* (Fig. 2.2A).
Color change may be described as:
- **Hyperpigmented:** It may be of following types:
  - *Brown:* It is due to excessive melanin in epidermis as in café au lait spots.
  - *Slate gray:* It is due to dermal melanocytosis as in Mongolian spots.
- **Hypopigmented:** As seen in pityriasis alba.
- **Depigmented:** When there is complete absence of pigment, e.g., in vitiligo, piebaldism, etc.
- **Erythematous:** It can be due dilatation of capillaries or extravasation of RBC (purpura). Diascopy (Fig. 2.6) will make the differentiation between the two.

Patch

It differs from macule in having size >0.5 cm. Very large patches (Fig. 2.2B) are seen in patients of vitiligo.

Vesicles and Bullae

A visible fluid filled elevation <0.5 cm in size within or beneath epidermis is called a *vesicle* (Fig. 2.3A).
- Vesicles may be grouped (herpes zoster) or widespread individual lesions with surrounding erythema (chickenpox).

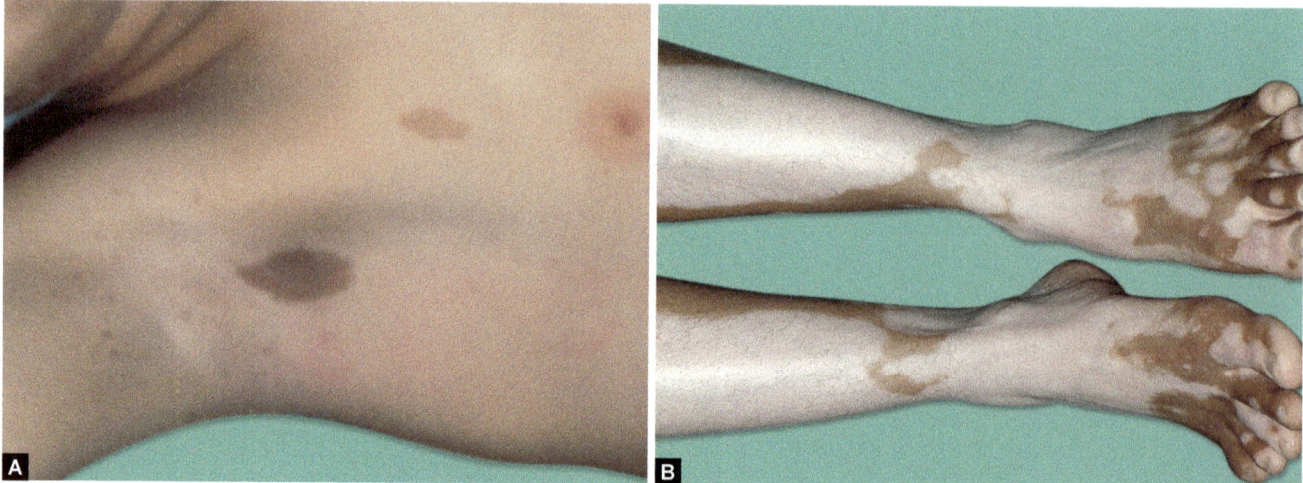

Figs. 2.2A and B: (A) Macule; (B) Very large patches of vitiligo.

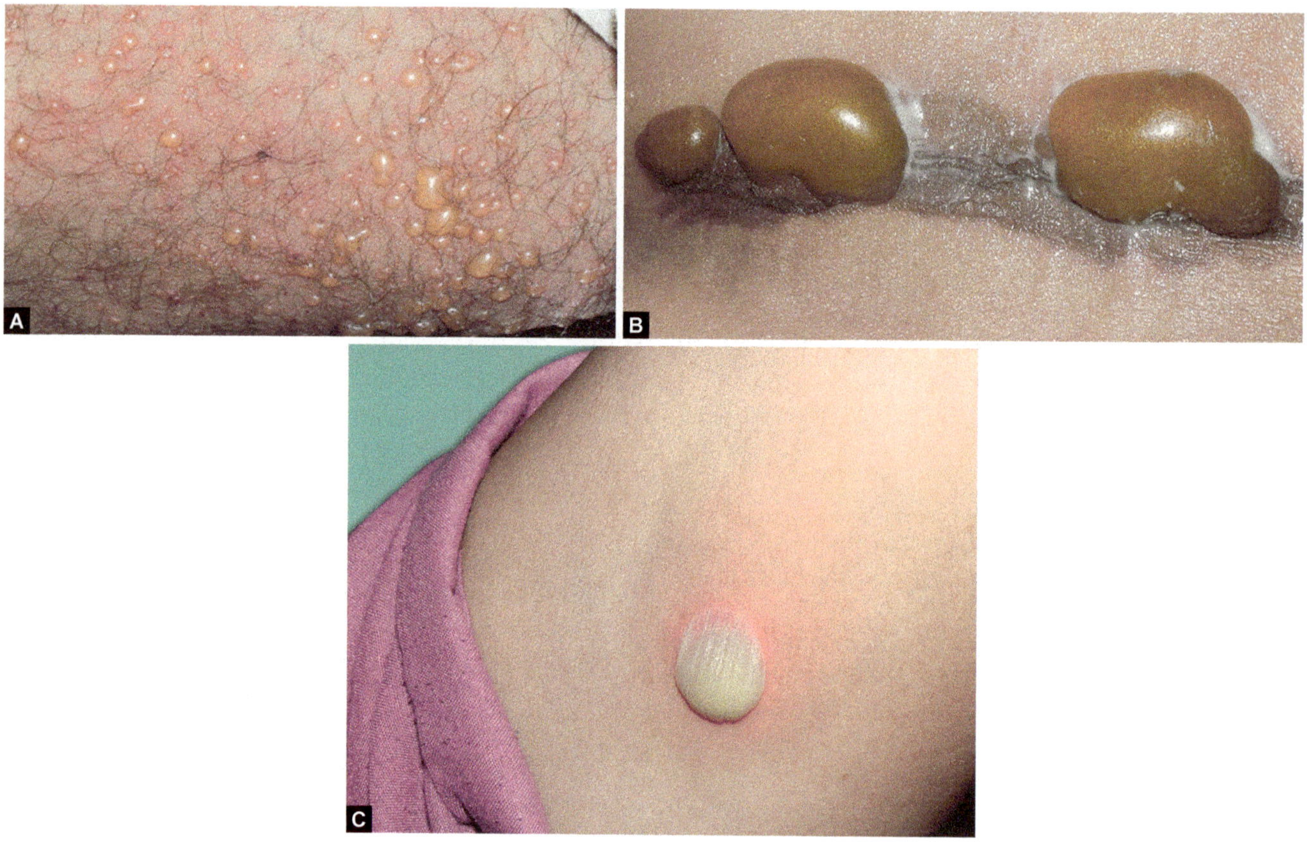

Figs. 2.3A to C: Fluid-filled elevations. (A) Vesicles; (B) Bullae on abdomen; (C) Large pustule.

- When size is >0.5 cm, it is termed as ***bulla*** (**Fig. 2.3B**).
- Vesicles may form due to cleavage at intraepidermal site as seen in pemphigus group of diseases. Cleavage can be at dermoepidermal site as seen in bullous pemphigoid.

Lesions Due to Pus Collection

Pustule

When vesicle is filled with visible purulent material, it is termed as ***pustule*** (**Fig. 2.3C**).

Abscess

It is a localized collection of pus. In subcutaneous tissue, it is localized by surrounding inflammatory tissue. It is characterized by redness, swelling and tenderness.

Lesions Due to Extravasation of Blood

Purpura

It is defined as nonblanchable (on diascopy) red macule due to extravasation of blood. It can be called as:

- **Petechiae:** It refers to 1–2 mm sized punctate hemorrhagic spots **(Fig. 2.4A)** with extravasation of RBCs.
- **Ecchymosis:** When macular hemorrhagic area is >2 mm size, it is labeled as ecchymosis **(Fig. 2.4B)**.
- **Hematoma:** It refers to swelling caused by extravasation of blood in large amount. Usually, it needs no active intervention. It subsides by spontaneous reabsorption.

Lesions Due to Dilatation of Blood Vessels

Telangiectasia

It refers to fine red lines or net-like pattern of permanently dilated small capillaries of superficial dermis **(Fig. 2.4C)**.

Telangiectasia may/may not blanch on diascopy. It is typically seen:

- On face of an elderly man due to chronic exposure to sun, mat-like telangiectasia (in systemic sclerosis), rosacea, etc.
- In periungual area, is patients of lupus erythematosus (LE) and dermatomyositis.

Poikiloderma

This term comprises telangiectasia, reticulate hyperpigmentation and atrophy of skin. It is seen in dermatomyositis and mycosis fungoides.

Erythema

It is a cutaneous redness **(Fig. 2.4D)** produced by increased perfusion due to vascular dilatation or congestion. Unlike ecchymosis, it blanches on diascopy.

Lesions Due to Edema

Wheal

It is a transient elevated lesion due to dermal edema. It is characteristically seen in urticaria patients. The lesions

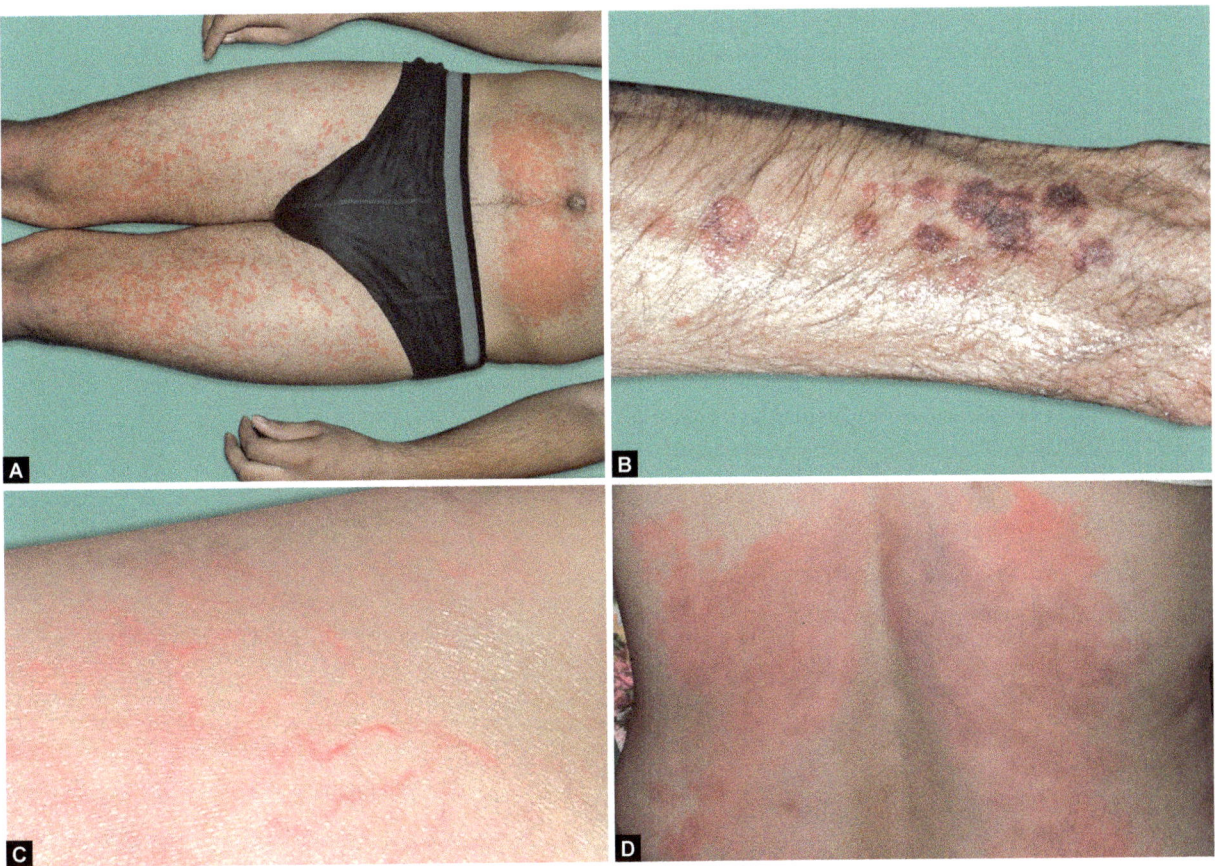

Figs. 2.4A to D: Erythematous lesions. (A) Petechiae on thighs and ecchymosis on abdomen; (B) Ecchymosis on forearm due to senile purpura; (C) Telangiectasia; (D) Erythema on back.

are usually accompanied by itching and are surrounded by erythema.

Angioedema

It is due to deep dermal or subcutaneous edema. It is painful rather than itchy. It most frequently affects face, eyelids and lips.

Miscellaneous Lesions

Comedones

These are typical lesions seen in acne. They form due to inspissation of keratin and sebum in pilosebaceous orifices. Two types of comedones are seen:

Open Comedones (Black Heads)

They are seen as flat or slightly raised lesions with dark colored keratotic follicular impaction in center.

Closed Comedones (White Heads)

They appear as slightly elevated pale papules with no clinically visible opening.

Cyst

Any closed encapsulated cavity or sac lined by membranous lining containing fluid or semisolid material is called cyst.

Burrow

It is a characteristic lesion of scabies. It can be seen as few millimeters sized superficial, serpentine, thread like and gray or dark tunnel harboring mite. The open end of burrow usually has a papule. Interdigital webs and shaft of penis are common sites. A magnifying lens should be used to identify burrow.

Secondary Skin Lesions

A secondary skin lesion is an eruption that appears secondarily after a primary skin lesion, *e.g., erosion, ulcer, excoriation, etc*.

Lesions Due to Exudates or Cells

Crusts

Dried serum or exudates are called **crusts**.

Scale

A scale is a flat plate or flake of stratum corneum.

Other Changes

Atrophy

Decrease in thickness of epidermis, dermis and subcutaneous tissue in various proportions is called **atrophy**.

- ❖ Atrophic epidermis becomes glossy, papery thin, translucent and wrinkled with loss of normal skin lines, e.g., leprosy.
- ❖ Dermal atrophy manifests as depression.
- ❖ Injudicious application of topical steroid on a skin lesion can lead to cutaneous atrophy which is particularly common in flexures (**Fig. 2.5**). It is termed as **striae atrophicans**.
- ❖ Depressed scars on face are quite common after healing of chickenpox vesicles.

Lichenification

It is seen as cutaneous response to repeated scratching and rubbing. It is typically seen in patients of lichen simplex chronicus and atopic dermatitis. It comprises of:
- ❖ Skin thickening
- ❖ Hyperpigmentation
- ❖ Increased cutaneous markings

DERMATOLOGICAL INVESTIGATIVE PROCEDURES

Apart from routine general investigations, there are certain diagnostic procedures which can help the dermatologist in making a correct diagnosis. Some of them are as under.

Examination by Magnifying Glass

Hand held magnifying lens with magnification 2-10 fold can be utilized for identification of subtle morphological features of skin lesions in more detail.

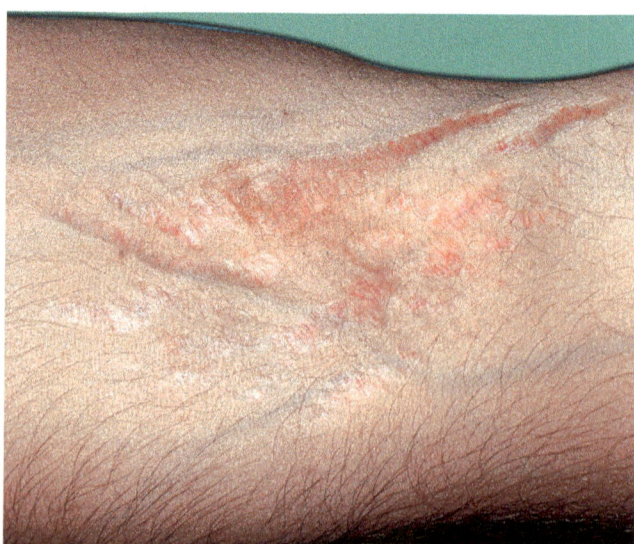

Fig. 2.5: Striae atrophicans. Cutaneous atrophy after topical application of steroid in cubital fossa.

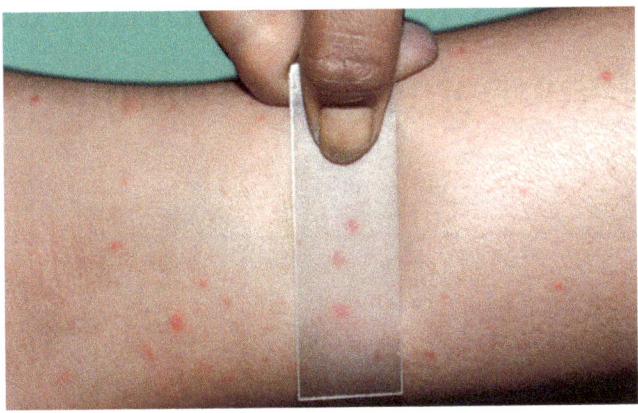

Fig. 2.6: Diascopy. Absence of blanching in purpuric lesions.

Diascopy

It is performed by firmly pressing two microscopic glass slides **(Fig. 2.6)** or any other firm transparent hard flat object over the skin. It will evacuate the blood from small vessels and will allow the evaluation of other colors.

- Nevus anemicus is a localized area of vasoconstriction. Diascopy of its adjacent normal skin will make the margins unapparent. It will distinguish it from vitiligo.
- Unlike purpura, erythema due to vasodilation is blanchable on diascopy and makes distinction between the two.
- With diascopy, yellowish brown apple-jelly nodules in certain granulomatous plaques can be detected, e.g., lupus vulgaris, sarcoidosis, etc.

KOH Smear Examination

This is a simple, easy and the most common bedside investigation performed by dermatologists. Besides diagnosis of dermatophytosis, it is also helpful in diagnosis of pityriasis versicolor, candidiasis and chromomycosis. In the latter, it reveals large rounded structures (copper pennies) in groups.

- Scales are collected with the help of edge of a surgical blade from the peripheral margins of scaly lesion or roof of the blister. Sample may be taken as remnants of broken off hair or scales from the scalp. Nail clippings have to be kept in potassium hydroxide (KOH) solution for many hours before microscopic examination.
- A drop of 20% KOH solution is put on a clean glass slide and sample is transferred on it.
- A cover slip is put on the specimen and kept for some time. KOH solution causes separation and destruction of stratum corneum cells. This clearing of sample can be accelerated by slight heating of underside of slide. But, over heating leads to precipitation of KOH and should be avoided. Clearing of sample allows identification of hyphae, spores, etc.
- The specimen is then examined under low power (10X) of microscope keeping substage condenser at lower position. Gentle tapping of cover slip with a pencil point time to time during examination is helpful.
- Findings under low magnification can be confirmed under high power (40X) magnification **(Fig. 2.7)**.
- When specimen is in sufficient amount, an experienced person can be confident enough for the positive or negative results of examination.

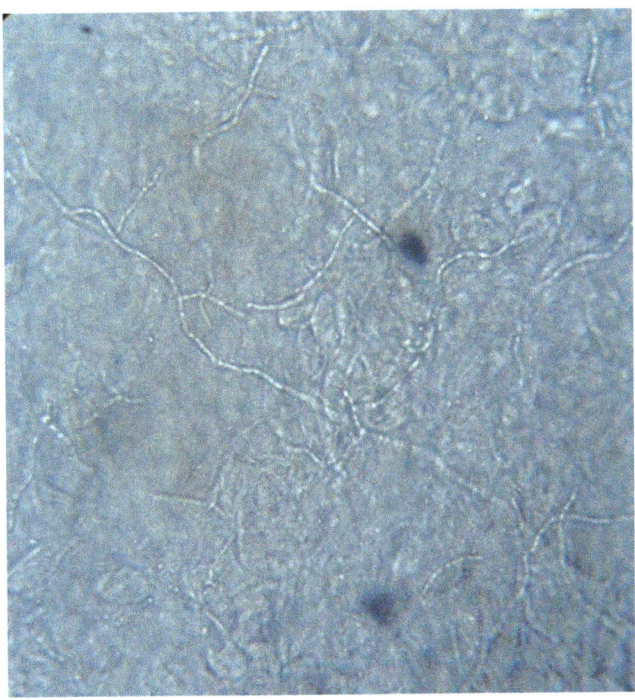

Fig. 2.7: KOH smear under high power magnification showing branching of septate hyphae.

CHAPTER 3

Availability of Commonly Used Drugs in Dermatology, Venereology and Leprology

AGENTS FOR TOPICAL THERAPY (TABLE 3.1)

Table 3.1: Agents for topical therapy.

Pharmacological ingredients	Trade names	Comments
Emollients or moisturizing agents		
White soft paraffin and light liquid paraffin	Emoderm, Cutimax, Dermoys, Logisoft	• Urea containing emollients can cause irritation • Preferably applied on moist skin surface along the direction of hair follicles about 30 minutes before going outside and effect lasts for 4 hours
Glycerine 15%	Aquasoft, Adonia, Secalia	
Squalene, Aloe vera, vitamin E and others	Venusia, NMF-e cream, Alonurish, Dewderm	
Propylene glycol	Emolene	
Urea (7%), aloe vera 10%	NMF-e urea cream	
Glycolic acid, urea	Xerina	
Arachis oil	Olemessa oil	
Ammonium lactate 12%	Lacsoft	It increases the moisture of skin
Ceramide, cholesterol, free fatty acids	Oryza, Moisawave	
Face cleansing lotions		
Cetyl alcohol stearyl alcohol	Cetaphil	They emulsify desquamated cells, dust particles and other leftover substances. These are eliminated and give the skin a healthy appearance
Salicylic acid 2%	Saslic, Saliwash	
Aloe vera, glycolic acid, vitamin E	Ahaglow	
Multiple ingredients	Derclean, Alonurish	
Mandelic acid 2%, salicylic acid 1%	Mandisha, Acnelak	
Sunscreens		
Octinoxate (UVB filter), oxybenzone avobenzone (UVA filter), zinc oxide (inorganic filter)	Suncros 50, Melagard 50, UV AVO, Ultraguard, Rivela, Sunheal 50, Photoban gel, etc.	• Apply 30 minutes before going outdoors • Effect lasts for 3 hours • Repeat application if get washed off
Zinc oxide + Titanium dioxide	Zoray CPS	These are physical sun screens
Zinc oxide 20% gel	Zoray APS, La Shield Fisico	
Depigmenting agents		
Hydroquinone 2%	Ibglow ultra	• It takes many weeks to be effective • Avoid sun exposure • If redness or irritation is there, can be applied intermittently
Hydroquinone + tretinoin + allantoin	Skinlite ever, Melalong, Melapik Ever	

Contd...

Contd...

Pharmacological ingredients	Trade names	Comments
Hydroquinone	Lumacip, Hyde cream/lotion	
Hydroquinone + Glycolic acid	Glyaha HQ	
Hydroquinone + sunscreens	Brite, Eslite-15, Melanorm-2, Melanorm-4	
Kojic acid + vitamin C cream	Clearz Plus	
Kojic acid + arbutin + octinoxate	Clearz Ultra, Carofit, Kojivit Plus	
Kojic acid + glycolic acid	Britelite, Glyaha-koj	
Glycolic acid 10%	Glyaha lotion, Glyco-A, Demelan	
Cysteamine 5% cream	Cystec	
Hydroquinone 2% + tretinoin + mometasone or hydrocortisone or flucinolone 0.01%	Cosmelite, Aret-HC, Melanorm MS, Lumacip Plus, Clears max	Avoid depigmenting agents containing steroids
Tranexamic acid once a day (significant effect in 2–3 months)	FixglowTx 500	Promising therapy with long-term benefits for stubborn melasma and other hyperpigmentation conditions
Antiacne agents		
Isotretinoin 0.05% gel	Sotret gel	Dryness and irritation are common. If it is there, it should be applied intermittently
Tretinoin 0.025%, 0.05%, 0.1%	Retino-A, Aret, Nexret, Nioret	
Tretinoin + clindamycin	Retino AC, Supatret C	
Adapalene 0.1%	Adiff, Adaret, Adaferin	
Adapalene + clindamycin	Faceclin-A	
Adapalene + Benzoyl peroxide	Epiduo, Peroduo, Oxidoben,	
Benzoyl peroxide	Benzac AC, Pernex AC Microbenz, Persol, Brevoxyl	Safe during pregnancy
Clindamycin	Clin-3	
Azithromycin or erythromycin	Azifast gel, Erytop	
Minocycline gel 4%	Minym gel	Avoided during pregnancy
Anti-rosacea agents		
Brimonidine tartrate 0.33%	Rosabril gel, Erythego (Once a day)	It is safe, effective with rapid onset for facial erythema of rosacea
Metronidazole 0.75% gel	Metrogyl gel 2%	
Topical Steroids		
Superpotent		
Clobetasol propionate ointment 0.05%	Tenovate, Topinate, Lozivate	• Topical steroids on face should be avoided • If applied, discontinue as early as possible

Contd...

Contd...

Pharmacological ingredients	Trade names	Comments
Clobetasol propionate cream 0.05%	Clop, Topinate, Cosvate, Lobate	Ointments are more potent than creams
Halobetasol propionate ointment 0.05%	Ultravex, Halox, Halotop	
Potent		
Mometasone furoate 0.1% ointment	Elocon, Topcort	
Potent (upper-mid strength)		
Fluticasone propionate ointment (0.005%)	Flutopic, Flutivate, Lutiderm	
Clobetasone butyrate	Eumosone	
Potent (mid strength)		
Mometasone furoate 0.1% cream	Topcort, Momtas, MMS, Momate	
Fluocinolone acetonide 0.025%	Flucort	
Triamcinolone acetonide 0.1%	Ledercort	
Potent (lower mid strength)		
Fluticasone propionate cream 0.05%	Flutivate	
Hydrocortisone	Cutisoft, Lutica	
Desonide lotion 0.05%	Desowen lotion	
Least potent		
Desonide	Desowen cream	
Methylprednisolone aceponate 0.1% cream	Advantan, PH-MPA	
Topical steroids + SA		
Clobetasol propionate + SA	Topisal, Clop-S	These are useful for hyperkeratotic lesions
Halobetasol propionate + SA	Ultravex S6	
Beclomethasone dipropionate + SA	Lupiderm SA	
Keratolytic creams		
Salicylic acid 6% and 12%	Salicylix	
Antifungal creams		
Luliconazole 1	Lulifin, Ludura	Avoid use of antifungal cream containing steroids even in the initial phase of treatment. Net result of steroid creams is flare-up of infections
Clotrimazole 1%	Canesten, Candid, Kansel	
Miconazole 2%	Daktarin, Zole, Candistat, Dk gel	
Eberconazole 1%	Ebernet	
Sulconazole 1%	Exelderm	
Sertaconazole 2%	Sertacide, Sercos	

Contd...

Contd...

Pharmacological ingredients	Trade names	Comments
Fluconazole 0.5%	Flucos gel	
Bifonazole 1%	Mycospor	
Oxiconazole 1%	Auxerg	
Ketoconazole	Nizral, Zykt	
Itraconazole cream 1%	Itrafen, Itratrox, Itrawel	
Terbinafine 1%	Terbest, Terbicip, Zimig, Tyza	
Butenafine 1%	Butenaskin, Fintop	
Amorolfine 0.25% cream	Amrobrut, Livafin, Fintop-AF	
Naftifine HCL 2% cream	Naftifast	
Ciclopirox Olamine 1%	8X, Batrafan, Candidox, Civaderm, Onabet	
Lipid-based amphotericin B gel 0.1%	Amfy Gel	
Antifungal lotions		
Luliconazole 1%	Lulifin, Ludura, Lulican	Lotions are useful for hairy areas and patients of chronic paronychia
Tolnaftate	Tinaderm	
Clotrimazole	Canesten, Surfaz, Candid	
Miconazole	Zole	
Selenium sulfide 2.5%	Selsun, Seldan	Apply once weekly at bed time for pityriasis versicolor
Amorolfine 5% nail lacquer	Loceryl (2.5 mL), Fintop NL	Apply at bed time with applicator brush on entire nail and 5 mm surrounding skin
Ciclopirox olamine 8% topical lotion	Penlac, Nail on	
Antifungal vaginal preparations		
Clotrimazole 100 mg	Canesten V6, Candid-V, Imidil vaginal, Surfaz	Inserted into vagina at bedtime and it get dissolves overnight
Clotrimazole + clindamycin	Candid CL, VH3	
Sertaconazole 500 mg	Sercos VT, Onabet V1	
Povidone iodine	Betadine vaginal	
Fenticonazole ovule 600 mg	Fenza	It is pregnancy category 'C" drug
Topical antifungal for oral cavity		
Clotrimazole mouth paint 1%	BNC, Candid	Used for oral candidiasis
Itraconazole oral solution 10 mg/mL (for oral and/or esophageal candidiasis)	Itratuf (100 mL bottle)	Swish the liquid around the oral cavity for 20 seconds and swallow. Do not rinse after swallowing. Dose: 200 mg (20 mL) per day in two intakes for 1 week

Contd...

Contd...

Pharmacological ingredients	Trade names	Comments
Antibiotic creams		
Fusidic acid 2%	Fusibest, Fucidin, Futop	Antibiotic creams in combination with steroids give better results for the treatment of pyodermas
Mupirocin 2%	Bactroban, Supirocin, T-bact	
Nadifloxacin 1%	Nadibact,	
Povidone iodine	Betadine cream	
Framycetin sulfate 1%	Soframycin	
Sisomicin sulfate 0.1%	Ensamycin	
Silver sulfadiazine 1% cream	Silverex, Dibact	Commonly used for cutaneous burns
Ozenoxacin 1% cream	Ozefit, S-clear, Tigotreat	It is used for impetigo and is a novel, non-fluorinated quinolone that is safe and effective
Anti-scabies agents		
Permethrin 5%, 1%	Perlice, Scabper, Permite	Commonly used safe, effective and can be used during pregnancy (category B). Avoid below 2 months of age
Gama benzene hexachloride 1%	GAB, GBHC	Do not use during pregnancy and lactation
Benzyl benzoate 25%	Ascabiol	Not used nowadays
Crotamiton 10%	Crotorax	Weak anti-scabietic
Ivermectin cream 1%	Ivernol, Ivrea	Also used for the treatment of rosacea
Anti-psoriasis agents		
Coal tar 6% + SA 3%	Salytar-WS	Irritation is common side effect. Use of these agents should be avoided in unstable psoriasis
Dithranol 1.15%	Derobin ointment	
Calcipotriol 0.005% ointment	Daivonex, Heximar, Pasitrex, Calpsor	
Calcipotriol + Clobetasol	Sorifix, Heximar-B, Calpsor C	
Tazarotene 0.05% and 0.1%	Tazret, Tazet Forte	
Tacalcitol ointment 4 µg/g	Tacalsis	Wash hands well after use. It is vitamin D analogue
Methotrexate gel 1%	Folitrax LP gel	Clean and dry the affected area. Gently and thoroughly massage it into the skin. Be careful not to get the medication in your eyes or mouth
Immunomodulators (Calcineurin inhibitors)		
Tacrolimus (0.03% and 0.1%)	TBIS, Tacrotopic, Tacrel, Crolim, Tacroz	Do not use below 2 years of age
Pimecrolimus 1% cream	Pacroma, Picon	Should not be used below 3 months of age
Antipruritic or soothing agents		
Calamine 15% + ZnO 5%	Caladryl, Calak	Undesirably, it has drying effect on skin
Calamine + Aloe vera + light liquid paraffin	Calosoft, Allsuth, Calak-A Linical, Efatop-C	

Contd...

Chapter 3 ♦ Availability of Commonly Used Drugs in Dermatology, Venereology and Leprology

Contd...

Pharmacological ingredients	Trade names	Comments
Shampoos		
Clotrimazole 1% + selenium sulfide 2.5%	Candid TV	Also used as a once-a-week overnight application on trunk to treat pityriasis versicolor
Ketoconazole 2%	Nizral, Arcolane, Novale	To be applied 5–10 minutes before bath twice or thrice a week
Ketoconazole + zinc pyrithione (ZPTO)	Danclear, Nuforce, Scalpe	
Ketoconazole + Coal tar + SA	Protar-k, Seboclear	
Ciclopirox 1% + ZPTO	8X shampoo	
Cetrimide solution 5%, 20%	Cetrilak	
Fluocinolone acetonide 0.01% (shampoo)	Sebowash	
Coal tar 1% + SA 3%	Salytar scalp lotion	
Clobetasol 0.05%	Powercort shampoo	
Antiviral agents		
Podophyllum resin paint	Podowart	Effective for genital warts
SA + lactic acid	Salex-L, Duofilm, Salactin	Effective for common warts, but not for genital warts
Imiquimod 5% cream (Imiquimod is an immune response enhancer that induces production of interferon and several other cytokines)	Imiquad, Nilwart, Zyclara	• Less efficacious for cutaneous warts • Used 3 times a week for 16 weeks
Acyclovir 5% cream	Herpex cream, Acivir, Ocuvir	Use only for patients of primary herpes genitalis. Not effective for recurrent herpes genitalis and herpes zoster
Topical anesthetics for oral application		
Triamcinolone acetonide oral paste 0.1%	Kenacort, Cinort, Triora	Apply after meals, in patients having lichen planus or mouth ulcers
Benzalkonium chloride 0.01%, choline salicylate 8.7%	Zytee	These are analgesic, antiseptic and apply them before meals
Choline salicylate 8.7% and lignocaine hcl 2%	Orasore	
Choline salicylate 8.7%, Tannic acid 5%	Orasep	
Benzalkonium chloride 0.01%, choline salicylate 8.7% and lignocaine HCl 2%	Dologel, Dentogel, Biosore	
Polidocanol 1%	Solcoseryl Dental Adhesive Paste	
Benzocaine 20%	Mucopain gel	
Benzocaine and cetylpyridinium	Cepacol Anesthetic, Protac, Bucalsep Solution	
Chlorhexidine 1%, metronidazole 1%, lignocaine 2%	Rexidine-M forte gel	
Topical antiseptics and anti-inflammatory agents for oral application		
Chlorhexidine gluconate 0.2%	Hexigel, Hexidine, Xedine	Take 15 mL of mouthwash, rinse thoroughly and expel after 30 seconds. These are used for removing and reducing the bacteria in the mouth
Chlorhexidine gluconate 0.2% Sodium fluoride 0.05% Zinc chloride 0.09%	Clohex ADS, Orahex plus	

Contd...

Contd...

Pharmacological ingredients	Trade names	Comments
Miscellaneous		
Lidocaine + tetracaine	Viveta	Need to be applied for 30–40 minutes for anesthesia
Lidocaine + prilocaine	Prilox, Toplap	
5-fluorouracil 1%, 5%	Flonida cream	May cause irritation
20% aluminum chloride in alcohol	Noswet, Aldry	Used for hyperhidrosis. Applied over dry axilla at night
Formaldehyde	Formalin	1% soaks advised for soles (not suitable for palms and axillae)
Benzyl nicotinate, vitamin K, salicylic acid hair tincture	Folica, Folifast	It is effective in the treatment of alopecia areata
Decapeptide	Melgain, Melbild, Glendep, MHG	It is a basic fibroblast growth factor (bFGF) derivative used for inducing repigmentation
Estradiol	Evalon, Evolon, Vagimoist cream	Used to treat symptoms of menopause, e.g., vaginal burning, dryness and itching due to lack of estrogen

(SA: salicylic acid; UVB: ultraviolet B; UVA: ultraviolet; ZPTO: zinc pyrithion)

AGENTS FOR SYSTEMIC THERAPY (TABLE 3.2)

Table 3.2: Agents for systemic therapy.

Pharmacological ingredients	Trade names	Comments
Steroids		
Tablets		
Prednisolone 5, 10, 20, 30, 40 mg	Wysolone, Delsone, Deltacortril, Omnacortil	Low-dose or short-term period systemic steroids do not have significant side effect
Methyl prednisolone 2, 4, 8, 16 mg	Zempred, Predace, Macpred, Nicort, Nidcort-M	
Betamethasone 0.5 mg tablet	Betnelan, Celestone	
Triamcinolone 4 mg tablet	Kenacort, Tricort	
Deflazacort 1, 6, 12, 18, 24, 30 mg	Defza, Cortimax, Orthocort	
Dispersible tablets		
Prednisolone	Omnacortil 2.5, 5, 10, 20 mg	
Betamethasone 0.5 mg tablet	Betnesol	
Deflazacort	Defsco-6	
Syrups		
Prednisolone 5 mg/TSF	Kidpred, Omnacortil	
Prednisolone 15 mg/TSF	Omnacortil forte solution	
Deflazacort 6 mg/TSF	Defcort, Intracort, Dezo	

Contd...

Contd...

Pharmacological ingredients	Trade names	Comments
Injections		
Dexamethasone 8 mg/2 mL/vial	Decadron, Dexona	
Hydrocortisone 100 mg/vial	Efcorlin, Wycort	
Triamcinolone acetonide 10, 40 mg vials	Kenacort, Tricort, Decort, Injicort	Very commonly used intralesional steroid
Methyl prednisolone 40 mg/mL	Depo-medrol (2 mL vial)	
Drops		
Betamethasone drops 0.5 mg/mL	Betnesol, Stemin, Celestone	
Prednisolone drops 5 mg/mL	Omnacortil	
Antiacne agents		
Isotretinoin 5, 10, 20, 30 mg	Isotroin, Iso-Aret, Acutret	Very effective especially for severe acne. It is teratogenic
Tetracycline	Resteclin, Hostacycline	Do not take with milk or milk products
Doxycycline HCl 100 mg	Doxitab, Doxt, Nixidox	Take once a day with/without food
Minocycline 50, 100 mg	CNN, Minolox, Cynomycin, Nidcyclin 50	
Azithromycin 500 mg	Azifast, Azee, Azithral	Can be used during pregnancy
Erythromycin 250, 500 mg	Althrocin	
Other antibacterial agents		
Benzathine penicillin 1.2, 2.4 megaunits	Penidure LA	First drug of choice for syphilis, but less commonly used because of risk of anaphylaxis
Levofloxacin 500, 750 mg	Lek, Levoflox, L-flox	Frequently used to treat urinary tract infections
Ofloxacin 200, 400 mg	Oflex, Ofbact	
Nitrofurantoin 100 mg tablet/cap	Furadantin, Urifast, Sysnit	
Cephalexin 125, 250, 500 mg	Ceff, Sporidex, Phexin	Very effective in treating pyoderma and soft tissue infections
Ceftriaxone injection 250, 1 g	Cefast, Cefaxone, Alof	Very effective in gonorrhea
Cefixime 400 mg	Cefi, Ceftas, Secef	Single tablet is a very effective oral treatment for gonorrhea as a part of syndromic management
Metronidazole tablet 200, 400 mg	Flagyl, Aldezole	Used to treat *Trichomonas vaginalis* and anaerobic infections
Secnidazole 1 g	Secnil Forte	
Ornidazole	Entamizole plus, Orni, Zil	
Antifungal agents		
Terbinafine 125, 250, 500 mg tablets (pregnancy category 'C')	Terbicip, Zimig, Terbest, Fintrix, Ifin	In spite of being fungicidal, terbinafine is not effective in all patients and recurrences are also common
Ketoconazole 200 mg tablet	Nizral, Hyphoral, Fungizole	
Itraconazole capsule 100, 200, 400 mg	Canditral, Onitraz, Syntran, Candiforce, Itaspor, Itralase	In adults: Usual dose is 100 mg BD
Voriconazole 50, 200 mg tablet	Voriva, Vfend, Vorizole, Vorifast	Serious side effects: Sudden behavioral changes, hepatitis, uneven heart rate, severe skin rash, fall in urine output

Contd...

Contd...

Pharmacological ingredients	Trade names	Comments
Fluconazole tablet 50, 150, 200, 300, 400 mg	Zocon, AF150, Fusys, Forcan	Considered safe during breastfeeding
Griseofulvin 250, 500 mg	Grisovin, Dermonorm, Grisure, Zorbax, Ecovin	Drug of choice for tinea capitis
Griseofulvin syrup 125 mg/5 mL	Zorbax	Not recommended to use in children younger than 2 years
Amphotericin-B 50 mg injection	Phosome, Ambisome, Ampholip, Amfight, Abhope, Anolip	Reserved for severe infections/immunocompromised patients mucormycosis, cryptococcal meningitis, visceral leishmaniasis, primary amoebic meningoencephalitis
Posaconazole 100 mg Tab	Posoxil GR	Used for aspergillosis, mucormycosis, candidiasis
Antileprotic and antitubercular drugs		
DDS	Dapsone 100 mg	Stop immediately if there is methemoglobinemia (blue coloration of lips) or hemolysis
Clofazimine cap 50, 100 mg	Hansepran, Lamprene, Clofros	Make aware the patient regarding coloration of skin and body secretions
Rifampicin 450, 600 mg	Rimactane, Rcin, Zucox	Patient passes red color urine
INH 300 mg	Tubernex Forte	Always supplement with pyridoxine
Rifampicin + INH	Rifacin, Rimactazid	
Ethambutol 200, 400, 600, 800 mg	Mycobutol, Myambutol, Combutol	Avoid in children, as it reduces visual acuity
Pyrazinamide 250, 500, 750 mg	Pza-Ciba	Common cause of exfoliative rash (1–2 weeks after initiation of therapy)
Pyridoxine	10, 40 mg tablet	Always supplement during ATT for prevention of peripheral neuritis
Thalidomide 50, 100, 200 mg cap	Thalix, Thyocad, Onchothal, Thaangio	Thalidomide is a potent teratogen. Use 2 forms of effective birth control together 4 weeks before, during, and for at least 4 weeks after your last dose. Other adverse effects are somnolence, paresthesia, constipation, peripheral neuropathy, bone marrow depression, blood clots, gynecomastia and weight gain
Drugs for hair disorders		
Ethinyl estradiol 0.035 mg Cyproterone acetate 2 mg	Diane 35,	Drospirenone is a preferred option for use in the treatment of PCOS
Ethinyl estradiol 30 µg drospirenone 3 µg	Yasmin, Crisanta	
Spironolactone 50 mg	Aldactone	Can be combined with OCPs
Finasteride 1 mg	Finpecia, Finax	Side effects of dutasteride and finasteride are similar include impotence, decreased sex drive, testicle swelling or pain. Dutasteride may also cause ejaculation disorder, breast enlargement, and breast tenderness. Both should be avoided during pregnancy. Both are used for prostate enlargement. Dutasteride hasn't received FDA approval for hair loss.

Contd...

Contd...

Pharmacological ingredients	Trade names	Comments
Dutasteride 0.5 mg	Duprost, Dutastron, Duteron	
Flutamide 250 mg tablet	Drogenil	
Bromocriptine: Initially 1.25–2.5 mg PO (usual 2.5–15 mg)	Tab Parlodel, Sicriptin 2.5 mg, Cap Parlodel 5 mg	Indicated for treatment of dysfunctions associated with hyperprolactinemia including amenorrhea with or without galactorrhea, infertility or hypogonadism, prolactin-secreting adenomas, PCOS
Dutasteride lotion 0.025%	Dutamax	Dutasteride has been shown to treat and prevent hair loss. But, FDA has yet to approve it for this specific purpose
Minoxidil (2%, 5%, 10%)	Mintop, Coverit, Tugain, Morr	5% is not recommended in females
Vitamin K, Benzyl nicotinate, salicylic acid (hair tincture)	Folifast, Folica	
Minoxidil Tab 2.5 mg	Loniten, Lonitab	0.625 mg/d for women and 1.25 mg/d for men are common starting dosages
Eflornithine HCl cream (13.9%)	Elyn, Eflora	It slows the growth of facial hair and takes 4–8 weeks to show response
Antiviral agents		
Aciclovir 200, 400, 800 mg	Herpex, Ocuvir	Should be given at the earliest to prevent PHN
Aciclovir injection	Acivir IV 25/mL (10 mL amp)	
Famciclovir 250 mg	Famtrex, Microvir, Penvir	
Valaciclovir 500 mg, 1g	Valcivir, Zimivir, Valtoval, Valanext	
First generation antihistamines		
Hydroxyzine*	Atarax, Prugo, Hicope, Hyzine, HXZ, Zeerax	Tablet 10, 25 mg; syrup 10 mg/5 mL; drops 6 mg/mL; injection 25 mg/mL
Dexchlorpheniramine*	Polaramine	Tablet 2 mg, syrup 0.5 mg/5 mL
Promethazine**	Phenergan	Tablet 10 mg, 25 mg, elixir 5 mg/5 mL
Cyproheptadine*	Peritol, Trisolene, Cypolene	Tablet 4 mg, syrup 2 mg/5 mL, drops 1.5 mg/mL
Pheniramine	Avil	Tablet 25, 50 mg; syrup 15 mg/5 mL; injection 22.5 mg/mL
Second generation antihistamines		
Cetrizine*	Alerid	Tablet 10 mg, syrup 5 mg/5 mL
Levocetirizine*	Zyncet, Zipcet	Tablet 5, 10 mg; syrup 2.5 mg/5 mL
Loratadine*	Lorfast, Lorinol	Tablet 10 mg, suspension 1 mg/mL
Desloratadine**	Deslor	Tab 5 mg
Fexofenadine**	Allegra, Air	Tab 120, 180
Mizolastine	Elina	Tab 10 mg
Ebastine*	Ebast	Tab 10 mg
Bilastine*	Bilanix, Histabil, B-sys	Tablet 20 mg, Syp 2.5 mg/mL (not for below 6 years/20 kg body wt) 4 mL syrup/d in children.

Contd...

Contd...

Pharmacological ingredients	Trade names	Comments
Some other drugs used for uremic and hepatic pruritus		
Ketotifen 1 mg tablet	Zaditen, ketasma	
Paroxetine	Pari 10, 20, 30, 40, mg Pari CR 12.5, 25, 37.5 mg	These are a selective serotonin reuptake inhibitors (SSRIs). Besides their use as antidepressant, they are used for palliative care of itching due to various causes. Also used for menopausal flushing
Sertraline 50 mg tablet	Zosert, Serta	
Mirtazapine 7.5, 15, 30 mg tablet	Mirat, Mirtaneo, Mitocent	It is also used as an antidepressant
Naltrexone 50 mg tablet (an µ-opioid antagonist)	Nalcon, Naltima, Naltrex, Nodict	Used (50 mg/d) for cholestatic pruritus
Nalfurafine HCl (selective κ-opioid receptor agonist) 2.5 µg Cap	Remitch	Used for the treatment of hemodialysis-related uremic pruritus
Butorphanol 1 or 2 mg/mL 5 mL ampoules	Butodol, Butrum	It is also a κ-opioid receptor agonist. Can directly inhibit itch, especially opiate-induced itch
Ondansetron Tab: 4, 8 mg Syp: 2 mg/5 mL Inj: 2 mg/mL	Emeset, Emetron, Ondern, Osetron	It is a 5-HT$_3$ antagonist and is frequently used as an antiemetic
Doxepin 10, 25, 75 mg cap	Spectra, Oxipin, Doxin, Doxitar, Doxbrin	It is a tricyclic antidepressant. It can be used in an anxious urticarial patient
Doxepin cream 5%	Zonalon, Goldopin	Used in atopic dermatitis patients
Menthol 1% aqueous cream	Dermacool	Used for localized neuropathic itch
Pramoxine	Nevlon anti-itch, Atarax anti-itch lotion	Helpful for neuropathic pruritus
Ursodeoxycholic acid (UDCA)	Tab 300 (Udiliv, Ursocol), Tab 250, 500 (Ursodil, Ursofalk)	Promotes excretion of bile acids, starting dose 500 mg BD (max 10–15 mg/kg/d)
Cholestyramine (bile acid binding resin which forms an insoluble complex)	Prevalite, Questran (mix the powder with 60–180 mL of liquid)	Removes bile acids from body. Liver will make more bile acids from cholesterol. So, lowers cholesterol levels also. Take 1 pkt 1–2 times/d. Maintenance dose: 2–4 pkt (8–16 g)/d
Erythropoietin injection (single dose prefilled syringe)	Zyrop 4000 IU, Renocel 4000, 10000 IU/1.0 mL	Given S/C or I/V only
Oral activated charcoal	Acticoal 250 mg tablet	It is effective in the treatment of uremic pruritus (6 g/d)
Aluminum hydroxide Tab	Allumcare, Asinil-T	Aluminum hydroxide is used as antacid. It is also used to reduce phosphate levels to treat uremic pruritus
Topical capsaicin 0.025% cream	Kapsi gel 0.025%, Capsitop 0.025%, Zostrix 0.033%, Capsin 0.025%	When applied 4 times/d for 4 weeks gives marked relief in uremic pruritus and localized neuropathic itch
Omega-3 fatty acids	Osmega 300 mg, Omega-3, Ultra Seacod, Salmon Omega-3	It is helpful in treating nephrogenic pruritus. Fish oil, Cod liver oil, Walnuts, Soybean are natural resources

Contd...

Contd...

Pharmacological ingredients	Trade names	Comments
Immunosuppressive drugs		
Tab methotrexate 2.5, 7.5 mg	Neotrexate, Folitrax Oncotrexate, Nidtrex-2.5	**Monitoring** • Complete blood count (CBC) every week • If patient develops leucopenia, give injection (S/C or I/M)) **filgrastim** (Neukine, Neupogen, Granix and Zarxio). It is also called as **granulocyte-colony stimulating factor (G-CSF)**. It stimulates the production of granulocytes. Neupogen injection is a sterile, clear, colorless, preservative-free liquid containing filgrastim. The product is available in single-use vials and prefilled syringes. The single-use vials contain either 300 µg/mL or 480 µg/1.6 mL of filgrastim. Filgrastim should be refrigerated. Remove from refrigerator 30 minutes before injection. Do not shake the medication. Protect from light • LFT and kidney function test every month
Inj methotrexate 25 mg/mL	Folitrax, Biotrexate (2 mL vial)	
Cyclophosphamide Tab 50 mg	Endoxan, Bdcyclo, Adcyclo	
Inj cyclophosphamide 200, 500 mg, 1 g vials	Cycloxan, Cyphos, Oncomide	
Tablet azathioprine 50 mg	Azoran, Imuran	
Cap cyclosporine 25, 50,100 mg	Psorid, Imusporin, Immusol, Pasilow, Arpimune, Zymmune	
Cyclosporine solution 50 mL	Neooral 100 mg/mL	
Mycophenolate mofetil 200, 500 mg tablet/cap	MMF, Baxmune, Cellmune, Mycept, Mycofit, Mycophen	
Tofacitinib (JAK1 and JAK3 inhibitor) 5, 11 mg tablet	Novanib-T, TFCT-NIB, Tofe, Tnib, Jantib-5	Used to treat rheumatoid arthritis, psoriatic arthritis and ulcerative colitis (diarrhea, headache and high blood pressure are common side effects. Infections, cancer and pulmonary embolism are serious ones)
Tofacitinib Oint 2%.	TFCT-NIB	It is used for atopic dermatitis, vitiligo, alopecia areata patients
Intralesional immunotherapy/cytotoxic agents for warts		
MMR vaccine	Tresivac, Priorix	Injected I/L 0.25 mL in per lesion
Inj. Bleomycin 15, 30 units	Metbleo, Bleocel	Can be injected I/L in the conc. of 1 mg/mL
Tuberculin purified protein derivative (PPD)		10 TU of tuberculin PPD (0.1 mL) intralesional in the largest wart at 2 weekly intervals for maximum of 6 sessions
Systemic immunotherapy		
Intravenous immunoglobulin (IVIG) 5% 100 mL (5 g)	ImmunoRel, PlasmaGlob, Plasmagen Gammagard, carimune, Gammplex	400 mg/kg/d for 2–5 d. Contraindicated in patients having IgA deficiency
Zinc sulfate	Z-life, Zitcare forte, Roczin	10 mg/kg (2.5 mg/kg/d elemental zinc) is used for recalcitrant warts
Biological agents		
Rituximab	Rituxipca 500 mg/50 mL vial (MRP: ₹ 39,000/-)	Used in pemphigus 375 mg/m² body surface IV slowly in 5–7 hours
Adalimumab	Adalipca given S/C 40 mg/0.4 mL in prefilled syringe, MRP: Rs 25000/	Used in moderate to severe plaque psoriasis, 80 mg on day 1, 40 mg on day 8, then 40 mg/week
Vitamins, calcium, potassium and zinc		
Tablet vitamin D3 (cholecalciferol 60,000 IU)	Kalzin 60K, Tayo, Calcirol	Patients on systemic steroids and old patients should be supplemented
Drops vitamin D3 (400 IU/mL)	Kalzin, Wal-D3 DS	It is recommended (1 mL/day) for all fully or partially breastfed newborns up to 1 year of age
Tablet vitamin D3 + calcium citrate malate	GCS, Milical, Revocal	Calcium alone does not prevent bone loss in patients receiving systemic steroids

Contd...

Contd...

Pharmacological ingredients	Trade names	Comments
Suspension vitamin D3 + calcium citrate malate	Calday Susp	
Vitamin E cap 200, 400, 600 mg	Ephynal, Evion	It has nonspecific role in the treatment of epidermolysis bullosa, cutaneous ulcers and yellow nail syndrome
Vitamin E drops 50 mg/mL	Evion drops	
Biotin	H-Vit Forte, BTN, Essvit	Used for thin brittle fingernails
Vitamin C 500 mg tablet	Celin, Chewee, Limcee	Used to treat photoaging, hyperpigmentation and promotes tissue healing
Vitamin A (50,000 IU)	Arocap, Arovit drops (150,000 IU/mL)	Used to treat phrynoderma, Darier-White disease and PRP
Folic acid	Sysfol, Folvite	Supplement patient receiving methotrexate
Vit B-3 Niacin 1000 mg tablet	Niacin-NF Initial dose: 500 mg HS Maintenance: 1000–2000 mg HS	Used for intermittent claudication, stasis dermatitis. It might slow blood clotting and increases the risk of bleeding
Nicotinamide 500 mg	Nialip tablet	500 mg/d for several weeks to treat pellagra
Multivitamin drops	Abdec, Becadex	
Zinc syrup	5 mg/Tsf: Syrup Zemin, 20 mg/TSF: Syrup Zemin 20, Zincris, Ascazin	Excessive intake of calcium can interfere with normal absorption of zinc
Zinc drops	Zevit drops	
Potassium chloride oral solution 0.5 g/5 mL	Potchlor, Keylyte (Take Potklor with a full glass of water just after a meal)	Used to treat hypokalemia resulting from: diuretics, steroid therapy, diarrhea, vomiting, etc.
Analgesics		
Tramadol Hydrochloride 37.5 mg+ Acetaminophen 325 mg Tab	Ultracet, Ultram	Preferred drug for renal disease patients
Agents for PHN		
Carbamazepine 100, 200, 300, 400 mg tablet	Mazetol, Tegretol, Zen	• They are used for many weeks • Patient may complain sedation
Amitriptyline 10, 25, 50, 75 mg tablet	Tryptomer, Sarotena	
Gabapentin 100, 300 mg	Cap Gabapin	
Pregabalin 75, 150 mg	Pregab, Gabanext	
Pregabalin 75 mg + Nortriptiline 10 mg	Pregagsis NT	
Pregabalin 75 mg + Methylcobalamin	ME-PR, Revlin M, Pregab-M	
Pregabalin 75 mg + Methylcobalamin 1500 µg + Nortriptyline 10 mg Tab	Pregabid MNT, Nervite plus, Dubinor	
For vascular disorders/ digital ischemia		
Pentoxifylline 400 mg tablet	Trental	It is given for at least 8 weeks. Ineffective for peripheral arterial disease
Oxerutins 250, 500 caps	Paroven	It reduces capillary leakage and helps in reducing pedal edema

Contd...

Contd...

Pharmacological ingredients	Trade names	Comments
Cilostazol 50, 100 mg caps	Stiloz, Cilodoc, Cilotab	Used in treatment of intermittent claudication. Avoided in CHF patients
Acetylsalicylic acid	Aspirin, Colsprin 100 mg, Ecosprin 75, 150, 325 mg	Helpful in both venous and arterial peripheral vascular diseases
Acetylsalicylic acid + Clopidogrel	Cap (Myogrel AP-75, Combiplet, Plagril A 75), Tab (Ecosprin C75, Clodrel plus)	It is antiplatelet (antithrombotic)
Sildenafil 50 mg tablet	Bigfun, Caverta	These agents relax vascular smooth muscle and have vasodilator effect which treat digital ischemia
Captopril tablet 12.5, 25 mg (ACE inhibitor)	Aceten, Angiopril, Captril	
Nifedipine 5, 10, 20 mg (10–20 mg QID)-Short acting Ca channel blocker	Depin	
Amlodipine-long acting Ca channel blocker	Amcard, Amdepin, Amlip 2.5, 5, 10 mg	
Bosentan 62.5 mg (endothelial receptor antagonist)	Bosentas, Bozetan, Bosenat, Lupibose	Prevents new digital ulcer formation
Drugs for Psoriasis and vitiligo		
Acitretin 10, 25 cap	Aceret, Acetec, Acrotac, Sorid, Acitrin, Acetroin-25	It is a retinoid and does not suppress immune system. Drug of choice for generalized pustular psoriasis
Apremilast 30 mg tablet	Aprezo, Apraise, Aprimila	• Do not crush, split or chew the tablet before taking it • Concomitant intake of phenytoin, rifampicin, Carbamazepine decreases its efficacy
8-MOP 10 mg tablet	Melanocyl, Octamop	First-line systemic drug for extensive psoriasis especially young patient
Methoxsalen 1%	Melanocyl solution, Octamop solution	Dilute with eau de cologne/spirit/water. Then apply 30 min before sun exposure for 2 min. Increase by 1 min every day
TMP 5, 25 mg tablet	Neosoralen, Soralen Desoralen, Trimop, Sensitex	Very good systemic drug for vitiligo. Avoid below 12 years age
Monobenzone 20%	Benoquin	Used for depigmentation of remaining pigmented skin in patients of universal vitiligo
Miscellaneous		
Ivermectin 3, 6, 12 mg tablet	Ivecop, Iverpil	Used in combination with topical therapy for scabies and pediculosis
Levamisole 50, 150 mg tablet	Decaris, Vemisol, Dewormis, Vapal	Potent immunomodulatory action: utilized for warts, leprosy, Behcet's disease, aphthous ulcers, etc. Skin rash, nausea, vomiting, headache and agranulocytosis are its side effects
Miltefosine 50 mg cap	Impavido	Do not crush or chew. Take with food. It is used for leishmaniasis
Adrenaline/epinephrine	1 mL (1 mg) ampule	Give 0.5 mg/0.5 mL IM as lifesaving drug for anaphylaxis or angioedema

Contd...

Contd...

Pharmacological ingredients	Trade names	Comments
Chloroquine 250 mg	Lariago, Emquin, Resochin Nivaquine	They are safe and long-term side effects are very minimal
Hydroxychloroquine tablet 200, 400 mg	Hydrocad, HCQS, Nid-Q 200	
Sulfasalazine 500 mg, 1 g Initially 500 mg/d, increase by 500 mg/week to 1,500–3,000 mg/d	Saaz, Sazo Avoid use with Azathioprine, Digoxin, Warfarin, Hypoglycemic drugs	It is useful in dermatology when standard therapy does not work or contraindicated, e.g., in Ps, LP, AA, pemphigus, etc.
Colchicine 0.5 mg tablet Adverse effects are the most frequent and include diarrhea, nausea, vomiting, and abdominal pain, Bone marrow suppression, myopathy	Zycolchin, Colchicindon, Goutnil, Colchicine Do not use with ketoconazole, Itraconazole, azithromycin, Digoxin, Anti-HIV drugs, Simvastatin, Cyclosporine, Verapamil	Effective in erythema nodosum leprosum, pyoderma gangrenosum, severe cystic acne, keloids, sarcoid, condyloma acuminata, erythema nodosum, scleroderma, and actinic keratosis
Pimozide	Larap 2, 4; Mozep 2; Orap 4, 10; Pimodac 4 mg	Useful for delusion of parasitosis
D-penicillamine 150, 250 mg Caps	Cilamin	Used in the treatment of Wilson's disease, rheumatoid arthritis, Scleroderma
Injection botox (100 units)	Neuronox (Ranbaxy)	

Food and Drug administration (FDA) Pharmaceutical Pregnancy Categories
*Category B: Animal reproduction studies have failed to demonstrate a risk to the fetus, and there are no adequate and well-controlled studies in pregnant women.
**Category C: Animal reproduction studies have shown an adverse effect on the fetus, and there are no adequate and well-controlled studies in humans.

(DDS: 4,4' diamino diphenyl sulphone; INH: Isonicotinic acid hydrazide; ATT: antitubercular treatment; OCPs: oral contraceptive pills; PHN: post-herpetic neuralgia; CBC: complete blood count; LFT: liver function test; 8-MOP: 8-methoxy psoralen; TMP: trimethoxy psoralen; IM: intramuscular)

MCQs of Dermatology, Venereology and Leprology

CHAPTER 4

1. Which one of the followings is the clinical diagnosis of this patient presenting with skin colored, slightly elevated, smooth, plane topped, multiple lesions with no itching?

   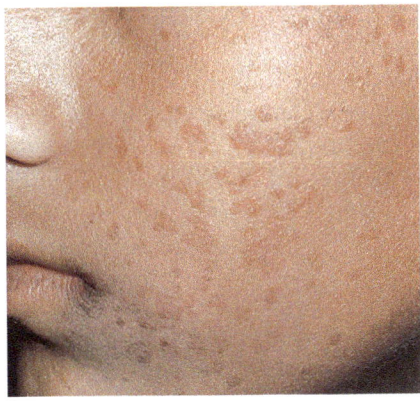

   a. Acne vulgaris
   b. Plane warts
   c. Post chickenpox scars
   d. Seborrheic dermatitis (SD)

2. This patient presents with recurrent, ill defined itchy plaques on both hands. What is the clinical diagnosis?

   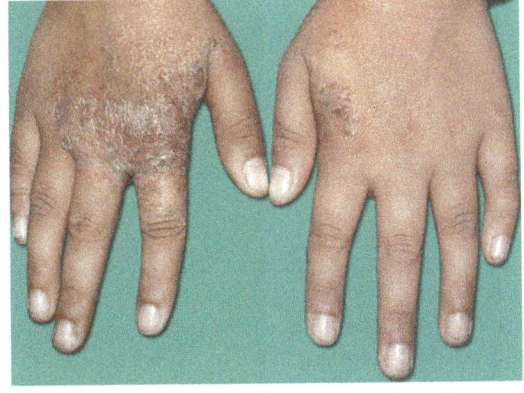

   a. Tinea manuum
   b. Eczema hands
   c. Psoriasis
   d. Lichen planus

3. This acne patient developed cheilitis during treatment. Which one of the following drugs is he taking?

   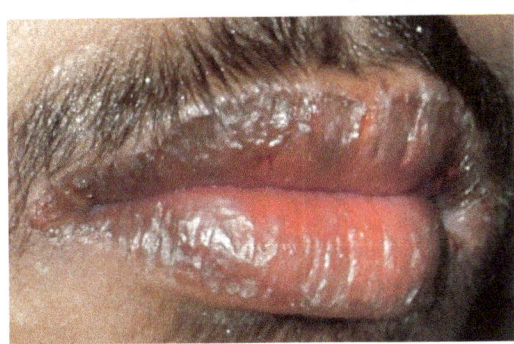

   a. Tetracycline
   b. Minocycline
   c. Azithromycin
   d. Isotretinoin
   e. Doxycycline

4. What is appropriate management for this patient?

   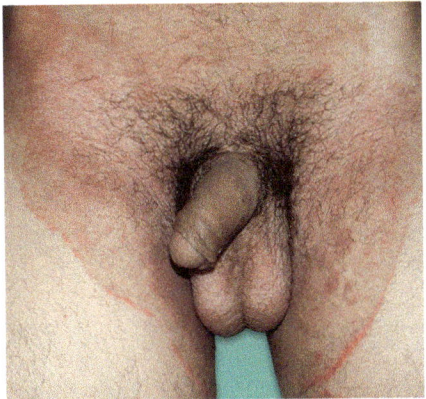

   a. Only topical antifungal creams
   b. Systemic antifungal + topical antifungal cream
   c. Systemic antifungal only
   d. Systemic antifungal + topical steroids

5. A 45-year-old female applied a cream on face for more than 1 year. She complained of erythema, burning, papules, pustules and growth of fine hair on her face. Which one of the followings is most probable clinical diagnosis?

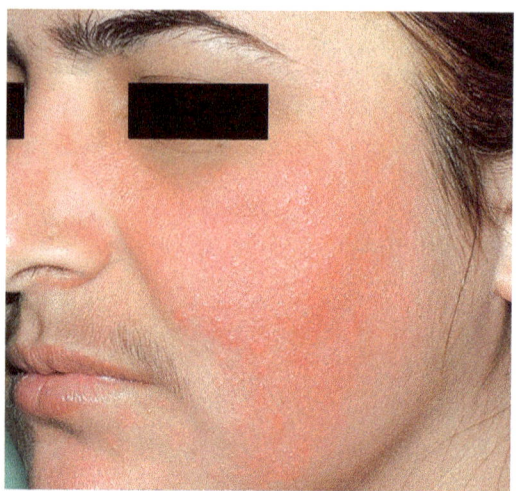

a. Contact dermatitis due to topical cream
b. Photo dermatitis
c. Adult or hormonal acne
d. Topical steroid damaged face (TSDF)

6. This patient has a single, well-defined plaque with loss of sensations, loss of hair and absence of sweating. What is the clinical diagnosis?

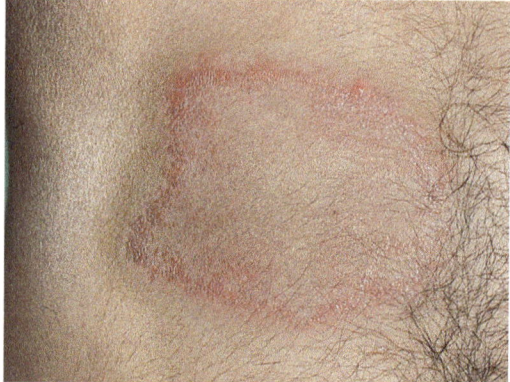

a. Indeterminate leprosy
b. Lepromatous leprosy
c. Tuberculoid leprosy
d. Histoid leprosy

7. This patient has an itchy, round patch in axilla with fine scaling, active margins and central clearing with no loss of sensations. What is the clinical diagnosis?

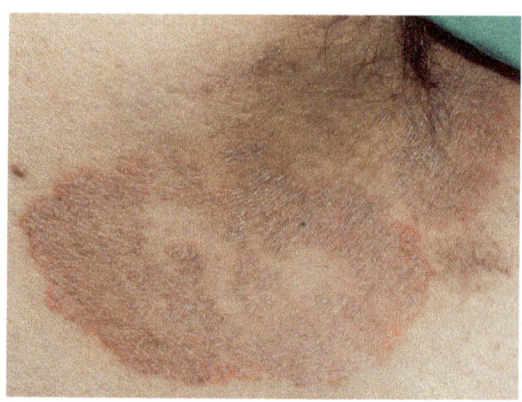

a. Psoriasis
b. Discoid eczema
c. Mother patch of pityriasis rosea
d. Tinea corporis
e. Hansen's disease

8. This child has multiple small patches having partial hair loss with minimal inflammation. What is the closest clinical diagnosis?

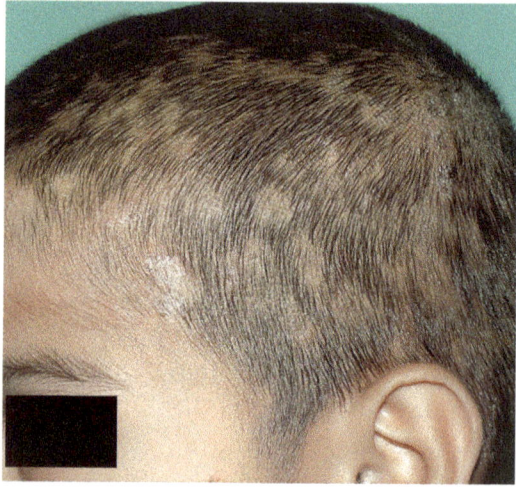

a. Seborrheic dermatitis (SD)
b. Tinea capitis
c. Trichotillomania
d. Alopecia areata

9. Which one of the followings is not true about this disease?

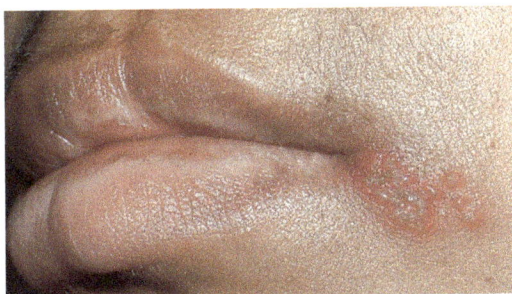

a. It may precipitate erythema multiforme
b. It results from reactivation of HSV-1 in trigeminal ganglion
c. Require systemic antiviral therapy for 5 days
d. Topical acyclovir is not beneficial

10. This child presents on knee with single, hyperkeratotic, purplish, asymptomatic indurated plaque with finger like projections. What is the closest clinical diagnosis?

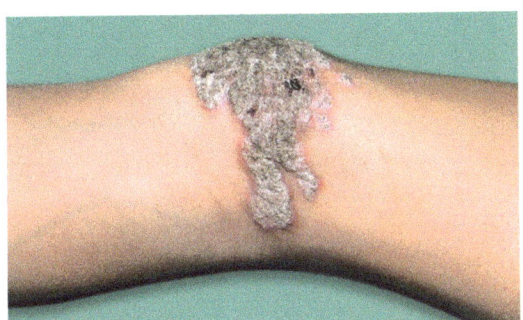

a. Psoriasis
b. Tuberculosis verrucosa cutis (TVC)
c. Common wart
d. Hypertrophic lichen planus

11. This child presents with an inflammatory boggy swelling having easily pluckable hairs and pus discharging follicles. It is accompanied by cervical lymphadenopathy and mild fever. What is the clinical diagnosis?

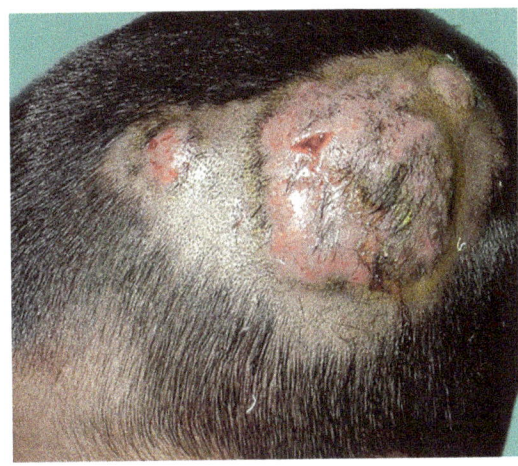

a. Abscess
b. Infected sebaceous cyst
c. Kerion
d. Carbuncle

12. An 18-year-old male presents with following rash. It was preceded by fever. Rash is centripetal in distribution and consists of small vesicles surrounded by irregular area of erythema giving a 'dew drop on rose petal' appearance. What is the clinical diagnosis?

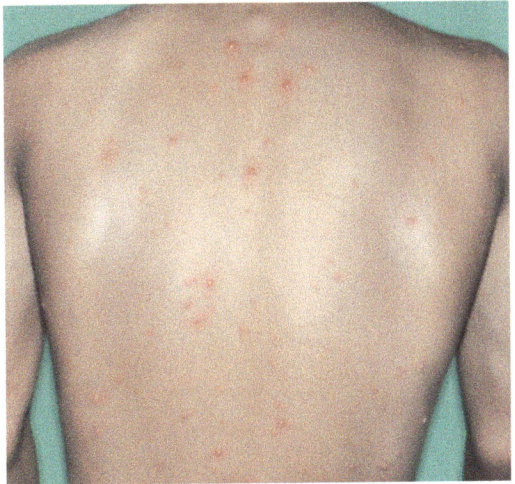

a. Multiple boils
b. Measles
c. Acne vulgaris
d. Chickenpox

13. This figure shows striae atrophicans in cubital fossa. Which one of the following topical agents this patient must have used?

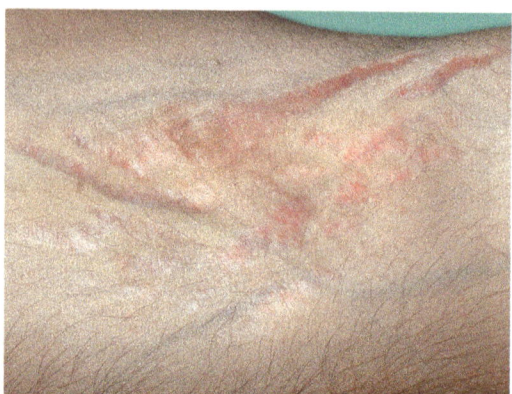

   a. Nadifloxacin cream
   b. Dithranol ointment
   c. Calcipotriol ointment
   d. Potent topical corticosteroid cream for long periods.
   e. Tacrolimus ointment

14. This lady complained of Raynaud's phenomenon. She has developed insidiously expressionless face, smooth and shiny forehead skin, pinched nose and constricted mouth opening. What is the clinical diagnosis?

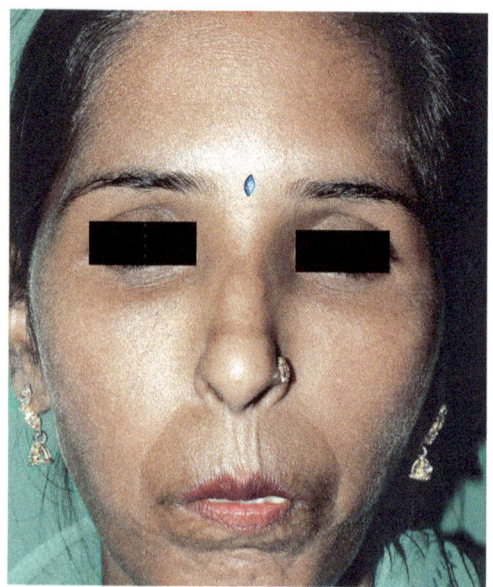

   a. Systemic lupus erythematosus
   b. Systemic sclerosis (SS)
   c. Scleredema
   d. Generalized morphea

15. This patient complained of purplish papules on glans and undersurface of prepuce. What is the clinical diagnosis?

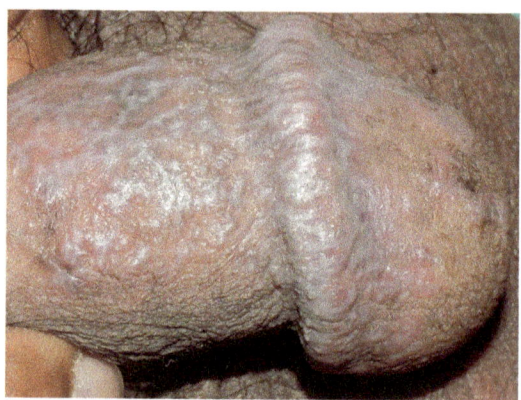

   a. Lichen planus
   b. Fixed drug eruption (FDE)
   c. Psoriasis
   d. Lichen sclerosus et atrophicus

16. An young adult complained of asymptomatic shiny flat topped discrete, pinpoint to pinhead sized flesh colored papules on his penile skin. What is the clinical diagnosis?

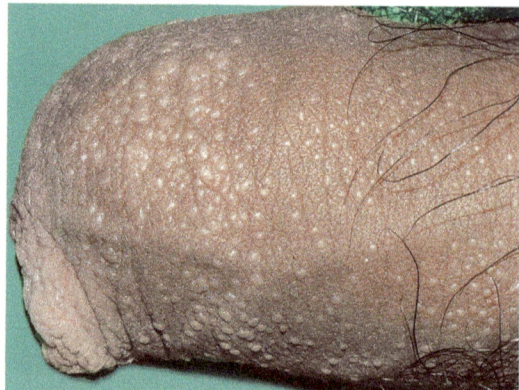

   a. Lichen planus
   b. Scabies
   c. Warts
   d. Lichen nitidus

17. A 10-year-old child presented with acute onset of polymorphic eruption in crops which consisted of red papules, vesicles, pustules, erosions and crusts. Lesions are concentrated on trunk and extremities sparing face, scalp, palms and soles. What is the clinical diagnosis?

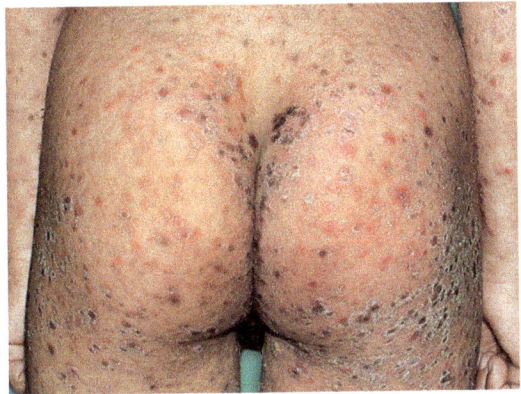

   a. Pityriasis lichenoides chronica (PLC)
   b. Pityriasis rosea
   c. Chickenpox
   d. Pityriasis lichenoides et varioliformis acuta (PLEVA)

18. A 12-year-old child is having herpes zoster ophthalmicus. Which one of the following statements is true?

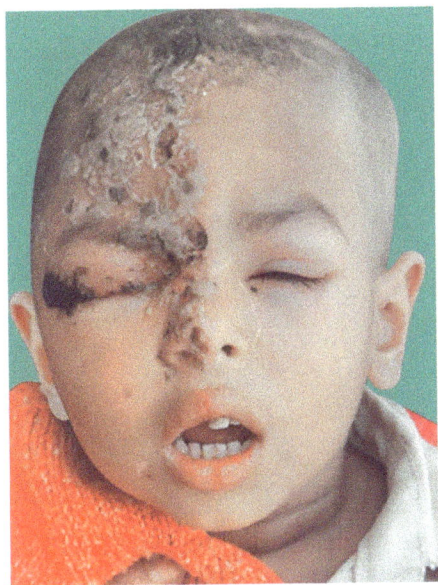

   a. In children, antiviral therapy is not required
   b. Herpes zoster ophthalmicus requires systemic antiviral therapy and NSAIDs irrespective of age
   c. It requires no treatment. It is a self-limiting condition
   d. It requires topical calamine lotion only

19. For nodulocystic acne in this patient which one of the following systemic drugs is the drug of choice?

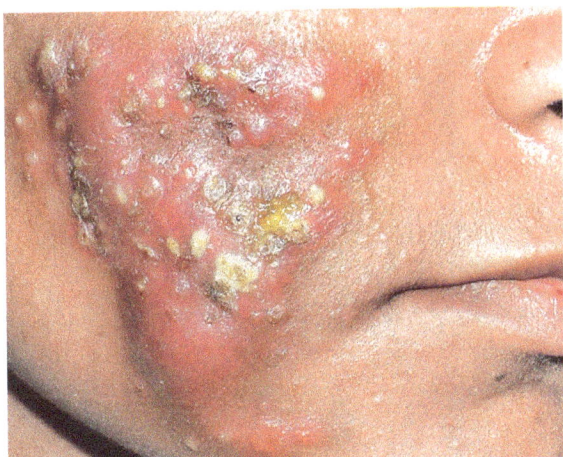

   a. Tetracycline
   b. Isotretinoin
   c. Azithromycin
   d. Minocycline
   e. Cephalexin

20. This patient presented with itchy, purplish, thick elevated papules on ankle. He also had lacy network of white streaks inside cheeks. What is the clinical diagnosis?

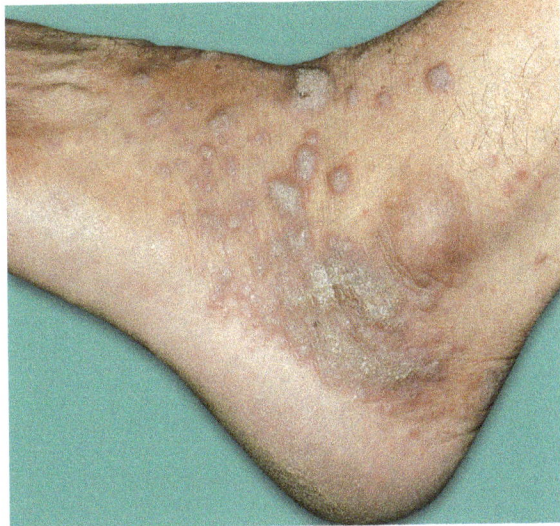

   a. Common warts
   b. Lichen simplex chronicus (LSC)
   c. Prurigo nodularis (PN)
   d. Hypertrophic lichen planus

21. This patient presented with purplish, plane topped, pruritic, polygonal papules on peripheral parts with mild scaling. What is the clinical diagnosis?

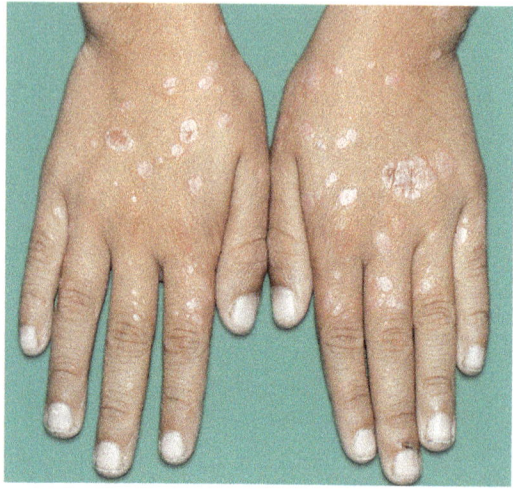

a. Psoriasis
b. Pityriasis rosea
c. Common warts
d. Lichen planus
e. Parapsoriasis

22. What is the clinical diagnosis for following nail changes?

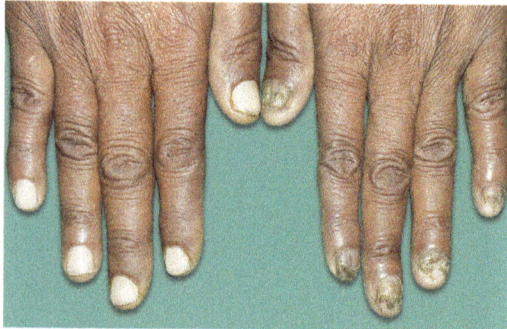

a. Psoriasis
b. Tinea unguium
c. Alopecia areata
d. Lichen planus

23. Which topical cream this patient has applied that has lead to hypopigmentation, cutaneous thinning and telangiectasia?

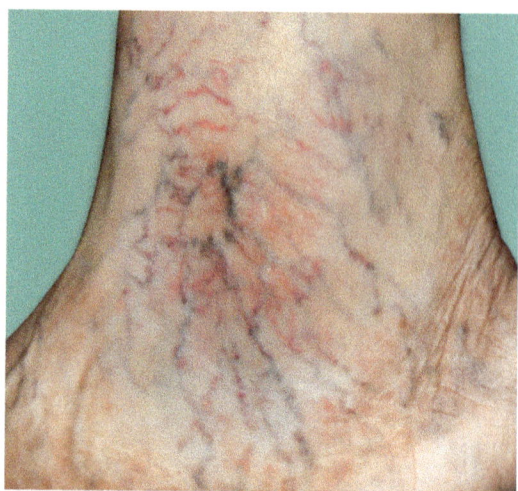

a. Nadifloxacin cream
b. Potent topical corticosteroid cream
c. Tacrolimus ointment
d. Calcipotriol ointment
e. Dithranol ointment

24. This patient of alopecia is also having purplish papular plane topped itchy papules on peripheral parts of body. What is the clinical diagnosis?

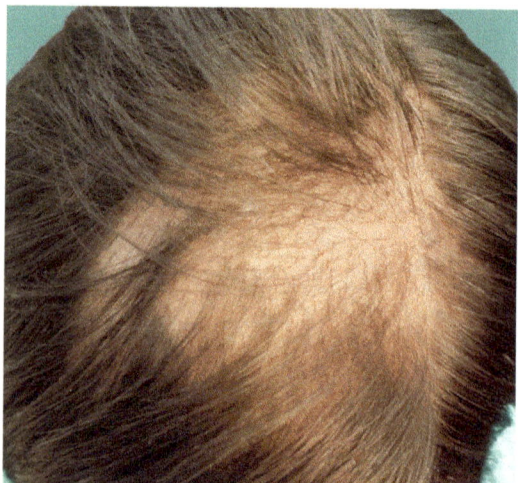

a. Cicatricial alopecia due to lichen planus.
b. Alopecia areata
c. Trichotillomania
d. Cicatricial alopecia due to chronic cutaneous lupus erythematosus (CCLE)

25. This female has symmetrically distributed erythema and edema on nose and malar eminences characteristically sparing the nasolabial folds. Rash is accompanied by mild fever for the last 2 months. What is the clinical diagnosis?

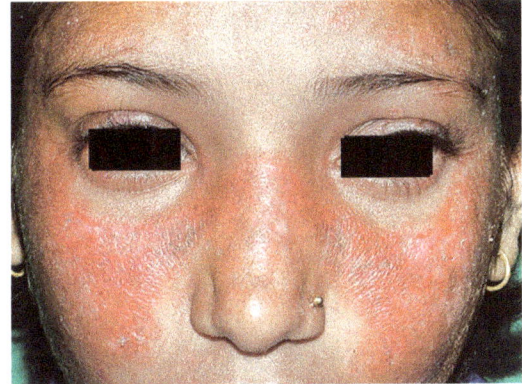

a. Melasma
b. 'Malar' or 'butterfly rash' in lupus erythematosus
c. Polymorphous light eruption (PLE)
d. Systemic sclerosis (SS)

26. She presented with a chronic plaque on face with psoriasiform scaling, reddish brown color, advancing active margins peripherally with trailing scar towards centre. Apple jelly nodules are seen on diascopy at active edge. Which one of the followings is correct clinical diagnosis?

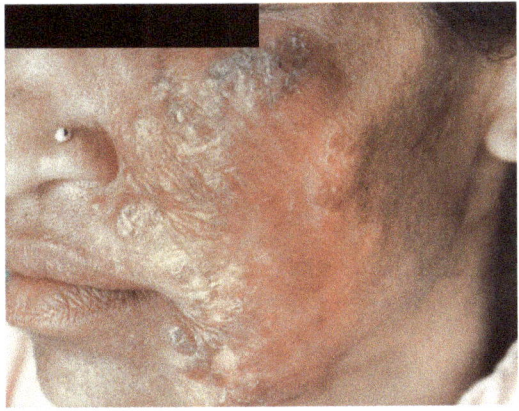

a. Chronic cutaneous lupus erythematosus (CCLE)
b. Basal cell carcinoma (BCC)
c. Psoriasis
d. Plaque type lupus vulgaris

27. An adult presented with widespread eruption of monomorphic, small red papules on trunk, upper arms and shoulders for the last two months. What is the clinical diagnosis?

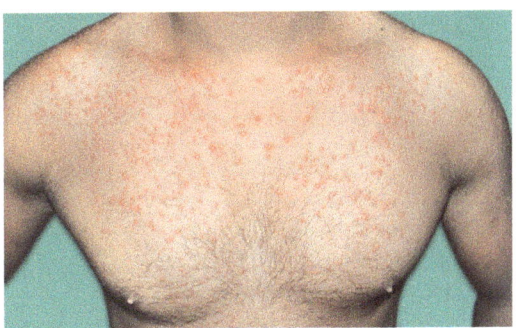

a. Acne vulgaris
b. Chickenpox
c. Measles
d. Acneiform eruption (drug induced acne)

28. Which one of the following statements is not correct about this patient having senile comedones?

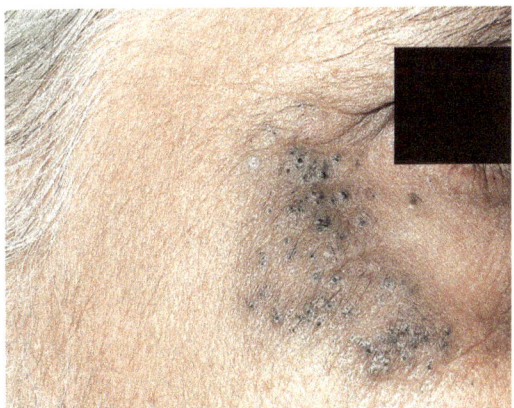

a. Senile comedones have same etiopathogenesis as acne
b. They are seen in middle aged or elderly person on sun exposed areas
c. Patient should apply oil free sunscreens
d. Express them with comedo expressor and advise retinoid cream for bed time
e. Usually, they do not get inflamed and are very persistent

29. What is the diagnosis of this patient?

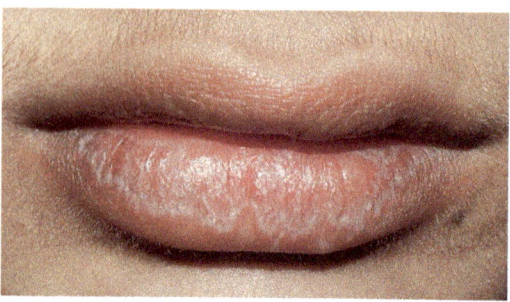

a. Lip stick cheilitis
b. Fixed drug eruption (FDE) lower lip
c. Lichen planus of lower lip
d. Chronic cutaneous lupus erythematosus (CCLE) of lower lip
e. Lip-lick cheilitis

30. A patient presented with herpes zoster on the right side of his chest and left arm simultaneously. Which one of the following interpretations is correct?

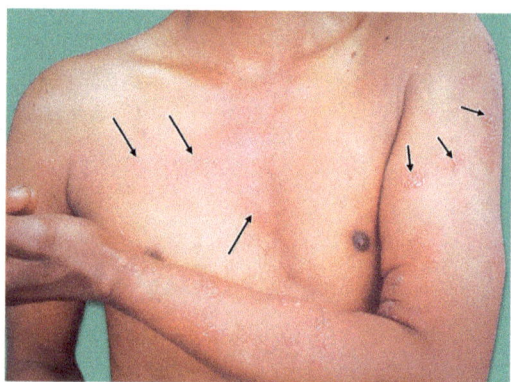

a. Nothing alarming, it can rarely involve more than one site
b. It is alarming, HIV infection must be ruled out
c. It can occur in a diabetic patient
d. It can occur in a patient receiving systemic steroids

31. In which of the following conditions following nail change is considered as a classic nail change?

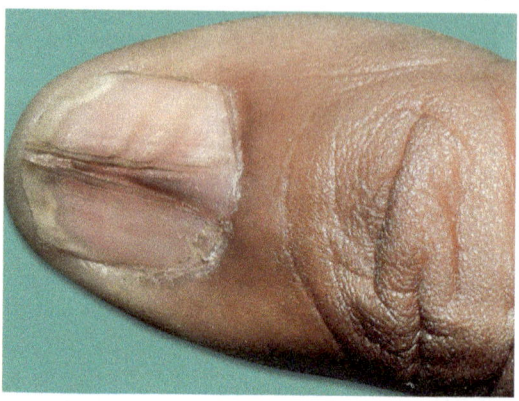

a. Lichen planus
b. Psoriasis
c. Alopecia areata
d. Onychomycosis

32. What is the clinical diagnosis?

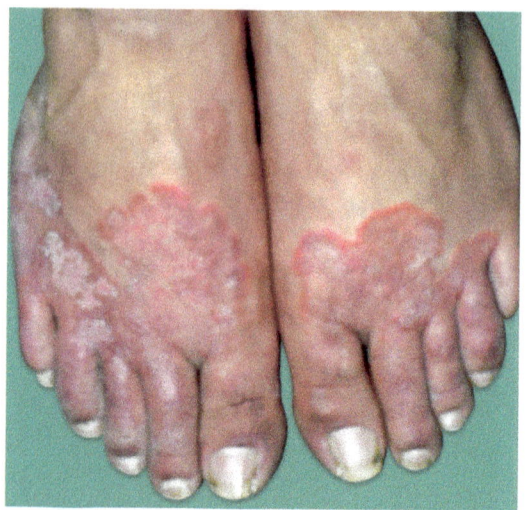

a. Tinea pedis
b. Contact dermatitis due to shoes
c. Candidiasis feet
d. Eczema feet

33. Due to the prolonged systemic use of which one of the following drugs this patient has developed widespread striae atrophicans?

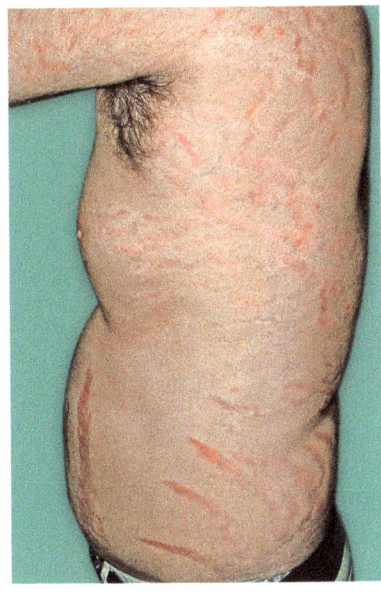

a. Phenytoin
b. Antituberculosis treatment (ATT)
c. Repeated corticosteroid injections at short intervals
d. Anticancer therapy

34. An adult presented with these polymorphic lesions on his back without significant itching. Similar lesions are also seen on face and chest. What is the clinical diagnosis?

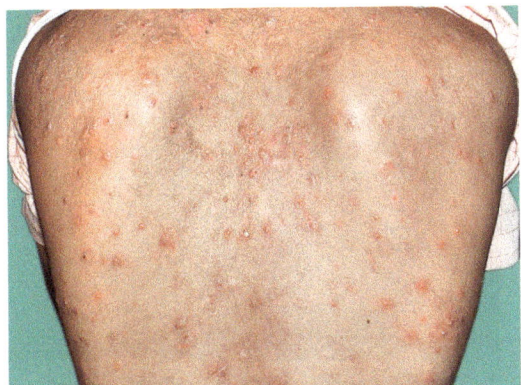

a. Dermatitis herpetiformis (DH)
b. Drugs induced acne
c. Acne vulgaris
d. Chickenpox

35. This acne patient during treatment develops redness, dryness, itching and burning on face. Which one of the following actions is incorrect for immediate relief?

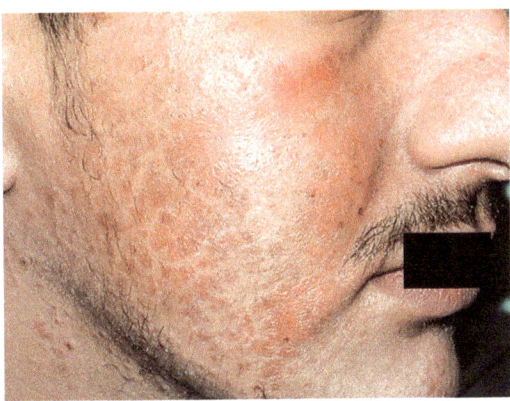

a. Advise frequent use of face wash
b. Stop systemic isotretinoin till relief
c. Stop topical antiacne creams
d. Apply emollients and/or mild topical steroid cream
e. Low dose systemic steroid for few days

36. An adult male presented with irregular linear groups of persistent firm papules forming hairless keloidal plaques on the nape of neck just below hairline. There is no history of any injury at this site. What is the clinical diagnosis?

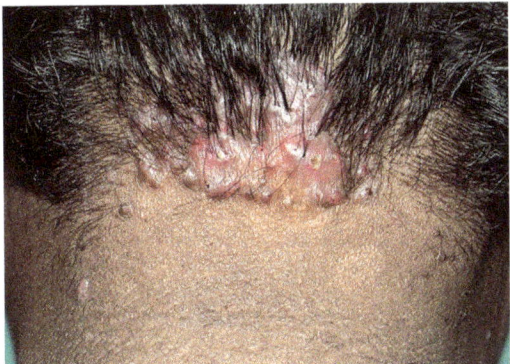

a. Hypertrophic scar
b. Squamous cell carcinoma (SCC)
c. Kerion
d. Acne keloidalis nuchae

37. Following patient develops expanding erythema following the tick bite. What is the closest clinical diagnosis?

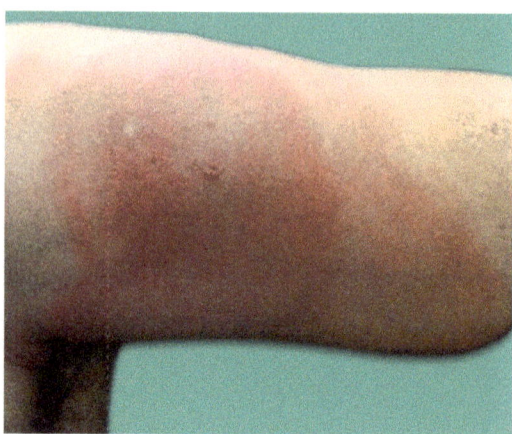

(*Courtesy:* Dr Mayanka batra)

a. Tinea corporis
b. Urticaria
c. Erythema multiforme (EM)
d. Lyme disease

38. This patient complains of soreness, irritation, redness, difficulty in retraction of prepuce. What is the closest clinical diagnosis?

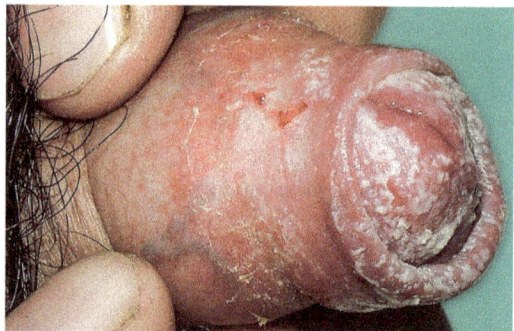

a. Candidiasis due to underlying diabetes
b. Secondary syphilis (SS)
c. Fixed drug eruption (FDE)
d. Poor hygiene

39. Upper part of back shows following asymptomatic hypopigmented macules with fine scaling. What is the clinical diagnosis?

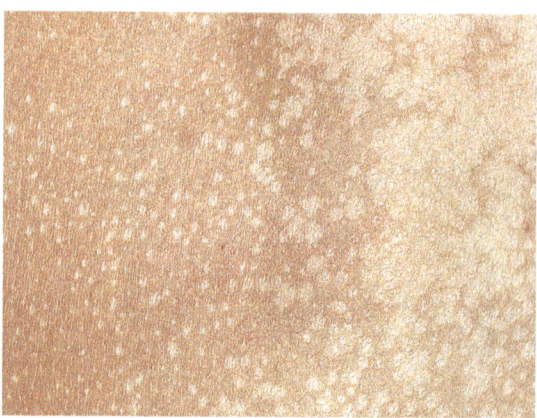

a. Pityriasis versicolor
b. Vitiligo
c. Pityriasis rosea
d. Pityriasis alba

40. This patient presented with an itchy lesion on glabrous skin of trunk with well defined margins with formation of concentric rings. Which of the following diagnoses is correct?

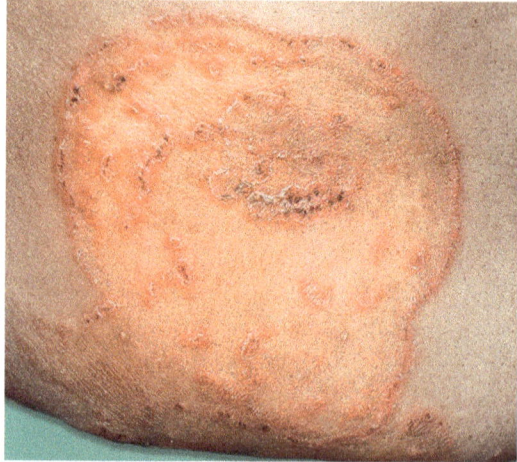

a. Annular lesion of mid borderline leprosy
b. Granuloma annulare
c. Discoid eczema
d. *T. imbricata* caused by *T. concentricum*

41. This patient shows lacy network of white streaks on the inner side of both cheeks. In which one of the following conditions, it is seen characteristically?

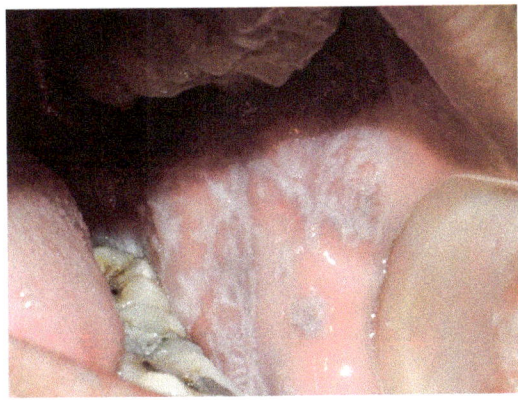

a. Oral leucoplakia (OL)
b. Chronic cutaneous lupus erythematosus (CCLE)
c. Lichen planus
d. Pemphigus vulgaris

42. This patient is presenting with bilateral herpes zoster. Which one of the following interpretations is correct?

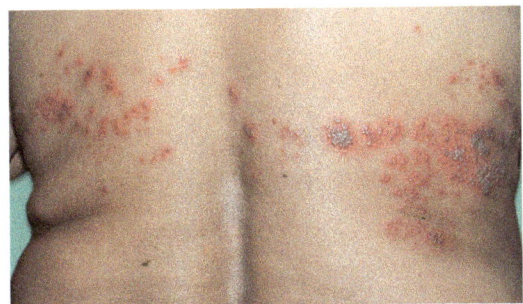

a. It is not alarming. Rarely, it can occur
b. It can occur in a diabetic patient
c. It is alarming. HIV infection must be ruled out
d. It can occur in patient receiving systemic corticosteroids

43. Which one of the following drugs cannot cause 'drug induced acne' in this patient?

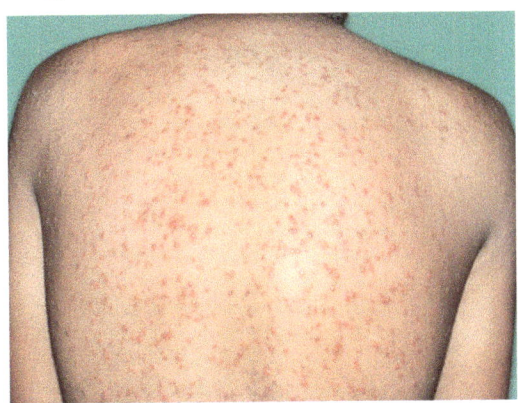

a. Systemic corticosteroids
b. Antihistamines for long periods
c. Antitubercular drugs
d. Antiepileptics

44. Within few hours of taking certain drug this patient developed ulceration on palate and glans penis only. What is the clinical diagnosis?

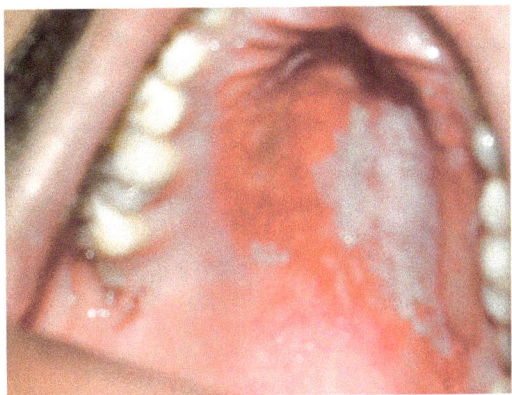

a. Erythema multiforme (EM)
b. Stevens-Johnson syndrome (SJS)
c. Toxic epidermal necrolysis (TEN)
d. Fixed drug eruption (FDE)

45. Which one of the followings is most probable clinical diagnosis of this patient having hyperkeratosis and scaling of right palm?

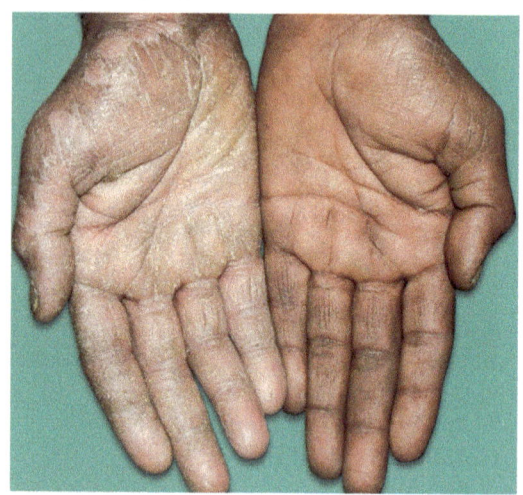

a. Contact dermatitis
b. Tinea manuum
c. Cutaneous tuberculosis of right palm
d. Psoriasis of right palm

46. Which one of the followings is not true about this patient?

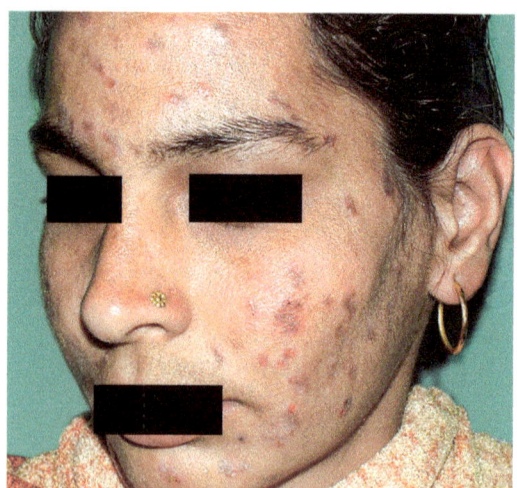

a. It is acne excoriee and she is in habit of picking her skin
b. In acne excoriee extensive excoriations accompanies mild acne lesions
c. It is treated with antiacne agents, antidepressants and psychotherapy
d. Only antiacne therapy is sufficient

47. This patient presented with crop of asymptomatic, multiple, smooth, glistening, firm and non-tender papules on apparently normal looking skin of trunk. Both pinnae showed thickening and infiltration. What is the clinical diagnosis?

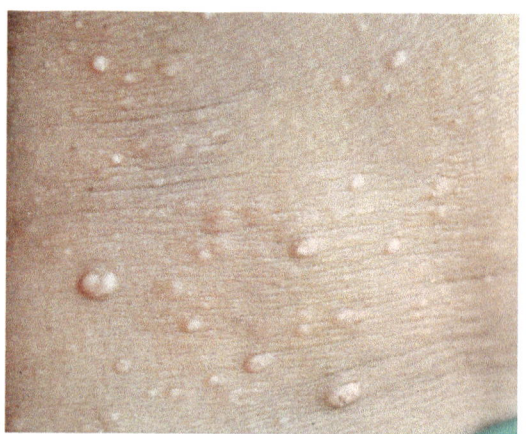

a. Molluscum contagiosum
b. Guttate psoriasis
c. Histoid leprosy
d. Acne on the back

48. This patient presented with 1-2 sized mm sized uniform dome-shaped papules with smooth non umbilicated top. There is no family history of such disease. What is the clinical diagnosis?

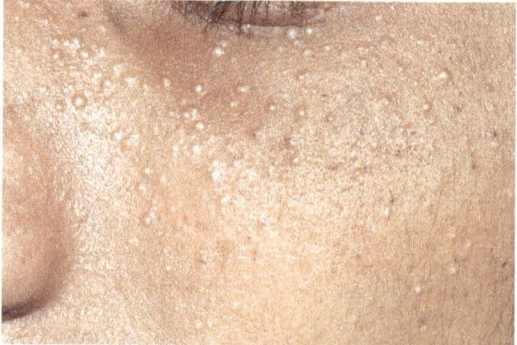

a. Acne vulgaris
b. Milia
c. Molluscum contagiosum
d. Syringoma
e. Trichoepithelioma

Chapter 4 ✦ MCQs of Dermatology, Venereology and Leprology

49. What is with appropriate topical treatment among the following options for this psoriasis patient having widespread involvement?

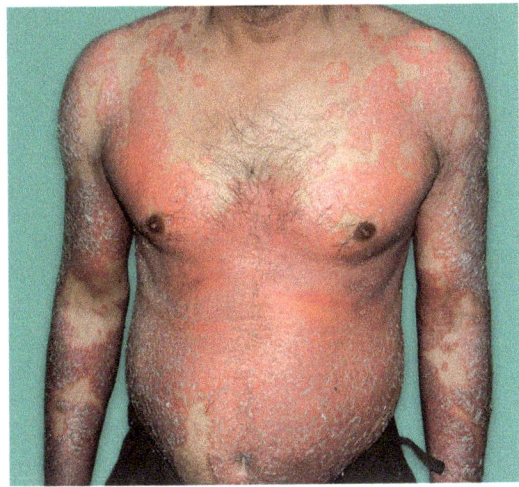

a. Potent topical steroid cream all over the body.
b. Coconut oil or plain vaseline
c. Calcipotriol ointment
d. Dithranol ointment

50. A middle age female complains of flushing on taking spicy food along with following facial lesions. What is the clinical diagnosis?

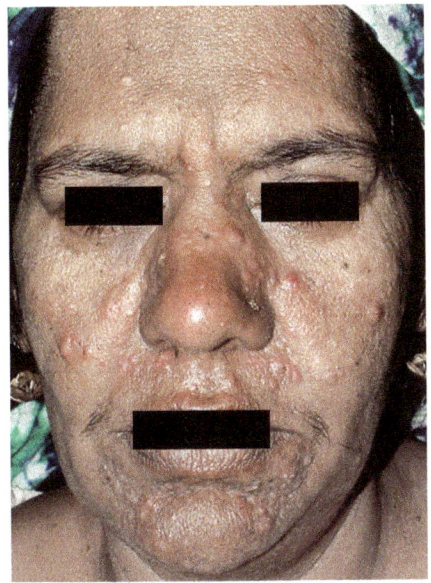

a. Acne vulgaris
b. Acne rosacea
c. Acute urticaria
d. Drug induced acne

51. This patient presented with hyperkeratosis and scaling that involved both soles. What is the closest clinical diagnosis?

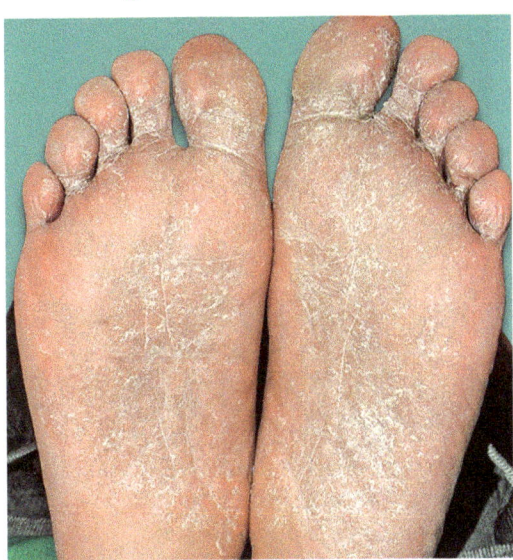

a. Diffuse keratoderma of soles
b. Squamous hyperkeratotic type tinea pedis
c. Candidiasis soles
d. Eczema soles

52. This patient gives a history of painless swelling, rupture and formation of ulcer. Ulcer has thin bluish and undermined margins with watery discharge. Which of the following statements is not true?

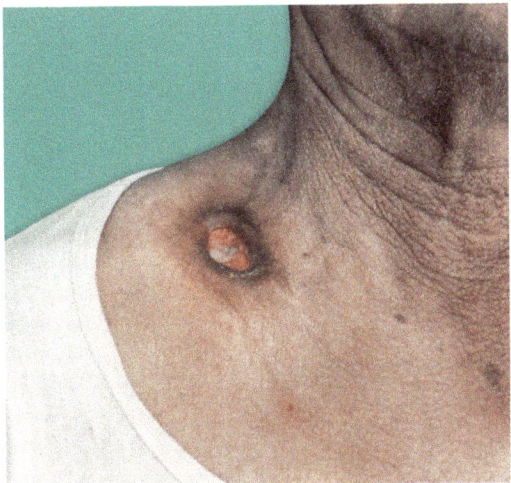

a. It is a cutaneous tuberculosis called scrofuloderma
b. It is exogenous tuberculosis with high degree of immunity.
c. It heals with peculiar puckered scarring.
d. It is endogenous tuberculosis with poor immunity.

53. What is the diagnosis of this patient?

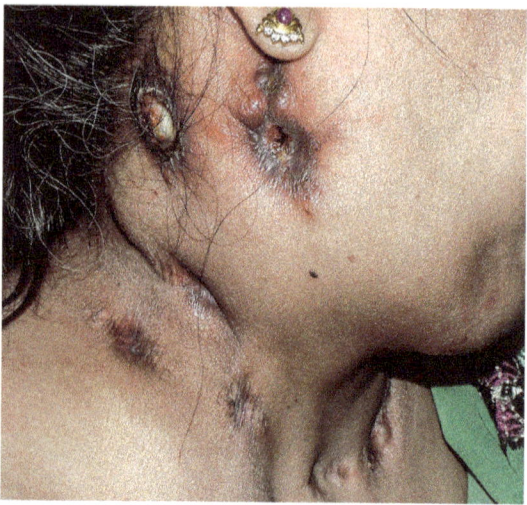

a. Untreated scrofuloderma involving multiple cervical lymph nodes.
b. Hidradenitis suppurativa
c. Multiple bacterial sinuses
d. Osteomyelitis

54. Which one of the following drugs used by this leprosy patient is causing brownish black pigmentation of skin and skin lesions?

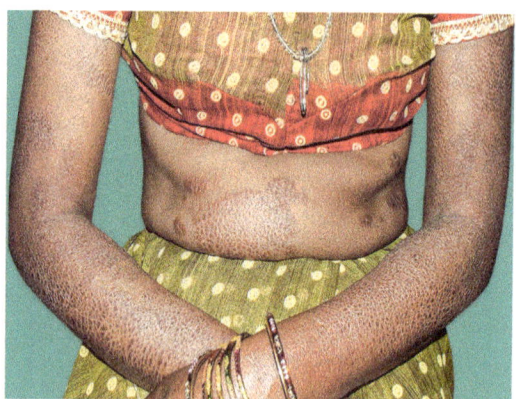

a. Rifampicin
b. Dapsone
c. Clofazimine
d. Thalidomide

55. This patient presented with recurrent herpes zoster. Which one of the following interpretations is correct?

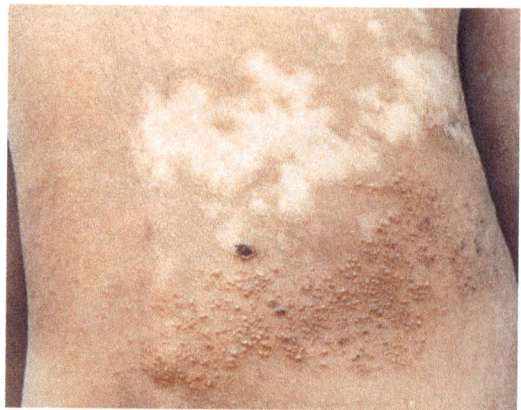

a. Nothing alarming, rarely it can occur
b. It can occur in a diabetic patient
c. It is alarming and underlying HIV infection should be ruled out
d. It can occur in a patient receiving systemic steroids

56. A pediatrician gave ceftriaxone for acute suppurative otitis media to a one month old baby. Next day the child developed blisters on trunk and extremities with no mucosal involvement. Dermatologist's opinion was sought. Which one of the following statements is true?

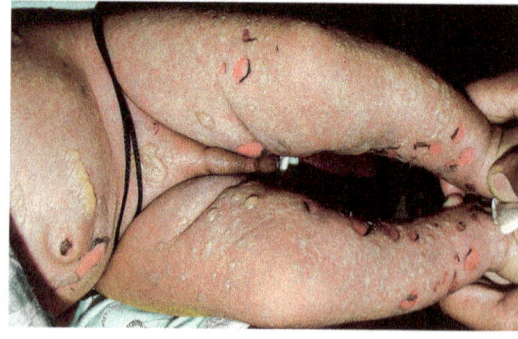

a. It is a drug induced pemphigus in a child
b. It is staphylococcal scalded skin syndrome (SSSS)
c. Stevens-Johnson syndrome (SJS)
d. Toxic epidermolysis necrolysis (TEN)

57. A child presented with gradually progressive plaque on buttock that had crusting, induration at the periphery and scarring in the centre. What is the clinical diagnosis?

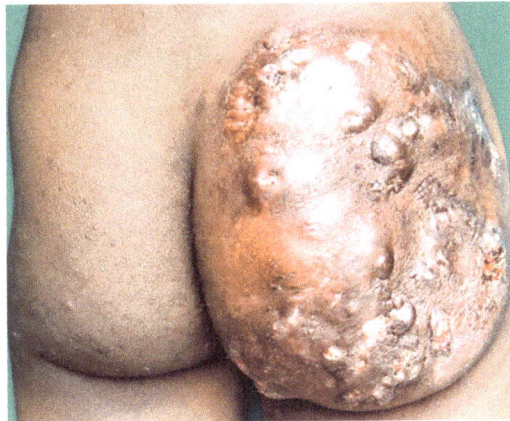

a. Mycetoma
b. Cutaneous leishmaniasis
c. Lupus vulgaris
d. Untreated injection abscess

58. A 16-year-old female complained of slowly progressive excessive hair fall. Which one of the followings is the closest clinical possibility?

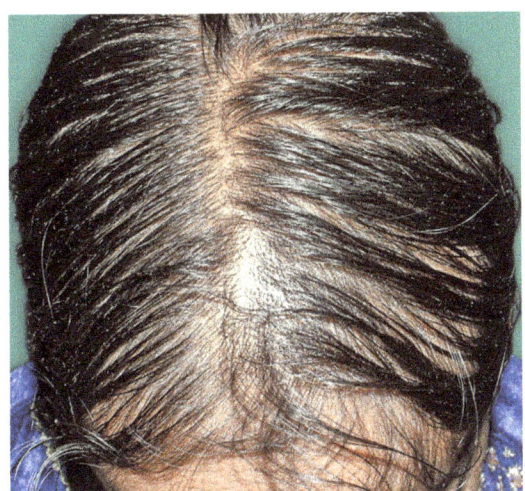

a. Lupus hair due to SLE
b. Alopecia areata
c. Trichotillomania
d. Female pattern androgenic alopecia

59. This infant is having minute papules and pustules involving trunk, scalp and soles *(MCQ 74)*. The child is irritable, cries and unable to sleep at night. Baby's mother is also having generalized pruritus which is more at night. What is the closest clinical diagnosis?

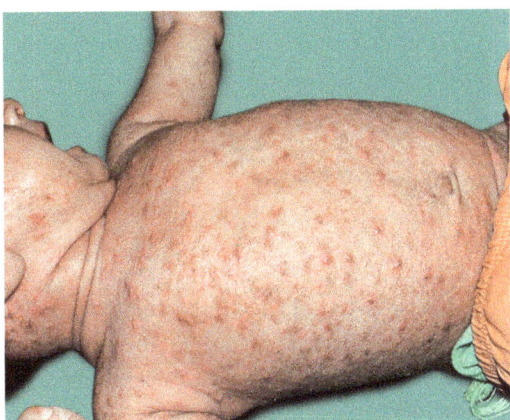

a. Seborrheic dermatitis (SD) with secondary infection
b. Miliaria rubra with secondary infection
c. Infantile scabies
d. Atopic dermatitis (AD) with secondary infection

60. What is the diagnosis of this patient?

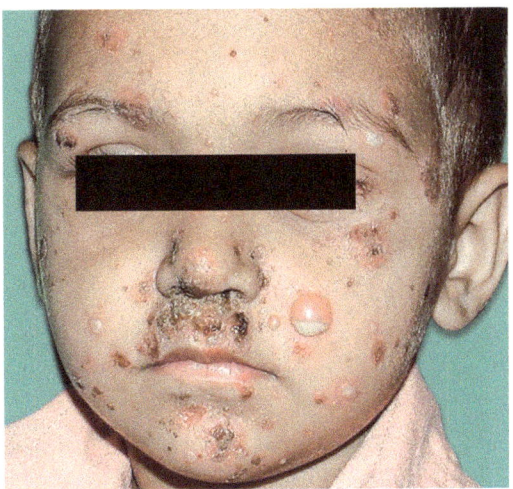

a. Insect bite hypersensitivity (IBH) with secondary infection
b. Chickenpox
c. Pemphigus vulgaris
d. Impetigo contagiosa

61. Which one of the following statements is not true about pediculosis pubis?

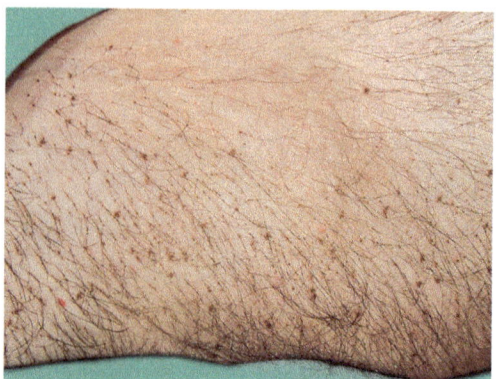

a. It is caused by *Pthirus pubis*
b. Transmitted by sharing clothing and bedding only
c. Many a times diagnosis is made by patient himself
d. Other hairy areas of body may also be infested by *P. pubis*

62. Following patient complained of generalized pruritus more at night. He is also having itchy papules on his genitals. What is the clinical diagnosis?

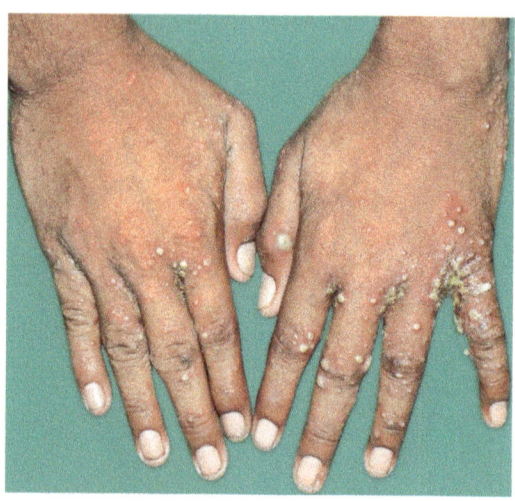

a. Pompholyx with secondary infection.
b. Infected scabies
c. Id eruption
d. Candidiasis

63. Overlying skin of multiple subcutaneous nodules break down to form multiple undermined ulcers and sinuses that are not adherent to underlying tissues. What is the clinical diagnosis?

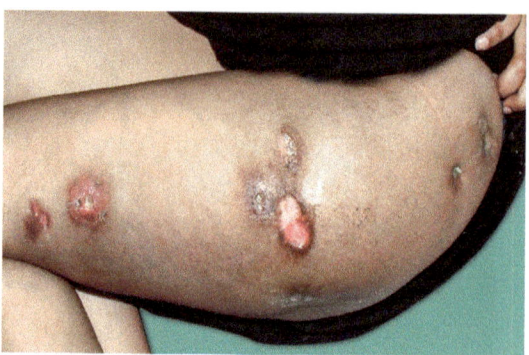

a. Lymphangitic form of sporotrichosis
b. Osteomyelitis
c. Tuberculous gumma on lateral aspect of thigh.
d. Multiple boils

64. This patient presented with hyperkeratotic non itchy lesion on hand since infancy. What can be the closest clinical diagnosis?

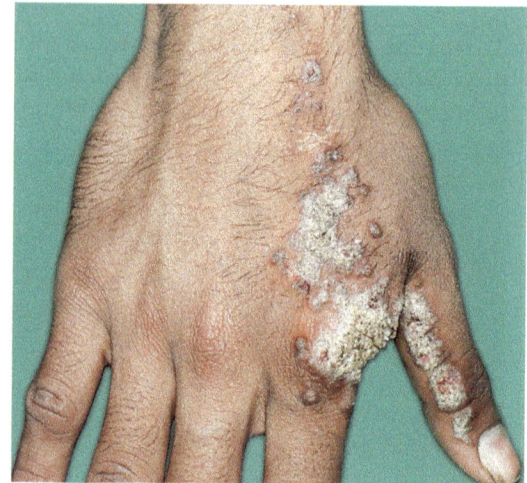

a. Hyperkeratotic eczema
b. Tuberculosis verrucosa cutis (TVC)
c. Hyperkeratotic nevus
d. Lichen planus hypertrophicus (LPH)

65. Which one of following statements is not true for scabies?

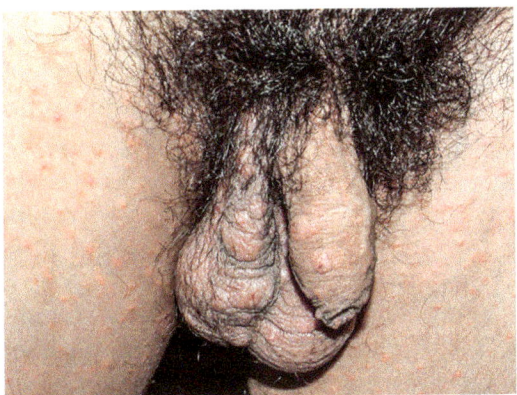

a. Intractable itching which is worse at night
b. Incubation period is 3-4 weeks (average 1 month)
c. Pruritic papules on genitals are pathognomonic of scabies
d. Other family members are also affected

66. Which one of the following statements is not true about this patient?

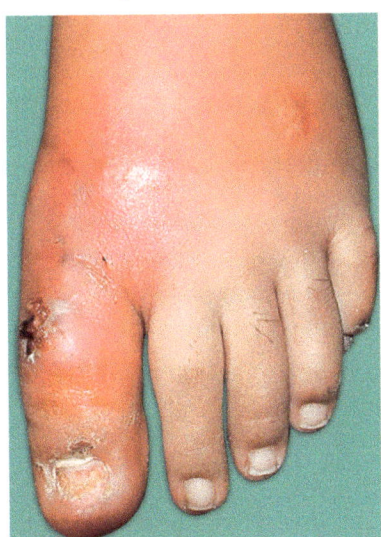

a. It is erysipelas
b. It is cellulitis around a wound showing erythema with indistinct margins
c. It is caused by β-hemolytic streptococci and rarely by *S. aureus*
d. It is an inflammation of subcutaneous tissue

67. A 70-year-old patient complained of mildly pruritic dirty white crusts on elbows, lower abdomen and buttocks *(MCQ 647)*. Few of the family members are suffering from severe pruritus. What is the closest clinical diagnosis?

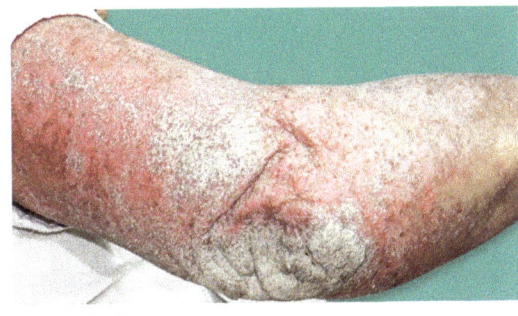

a. Psoriasis
b. Tinea corporis
c. Eczema
d. Crusted or Norwegian scabies

68. Discoid, circumscribed, red and well-defined plaques present on face and V-area of neck. Plaques are covered with adherent scales extending in to orifices of hair follicles. What is the clinical diagnosis?

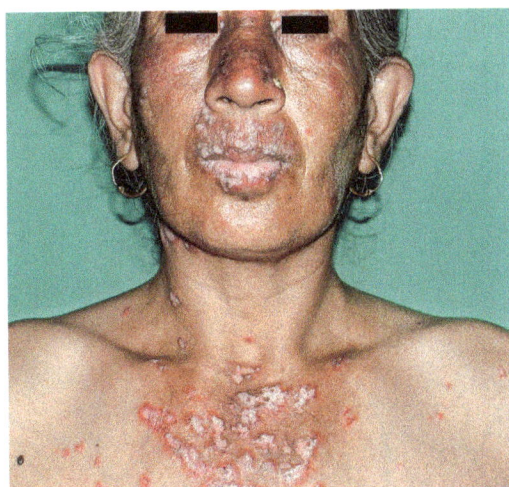

a. Lichen planus
b. Psoriasis
c. Lupus vulgaris
d. Chronic cutaneous lupus erythematosus

69. This patient presented with an asymptomatic, non-hairy, non-scaly, faintly purplish, circumscribed, indurated plaque on back and is attached to underlying tissues with no loss of sensation. What is the clinical diagnosis?

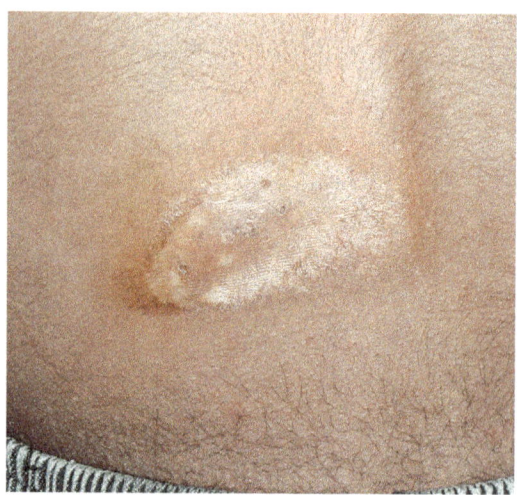

a. Tuberculoid leprosy
b. Keloid or hypertrophic scar
c. Cutaneous nevus
d. Localized morphea

70. Which one of the following options is correct advice to a 58-year-old female who came on 2nd day of herpes zoster rash?

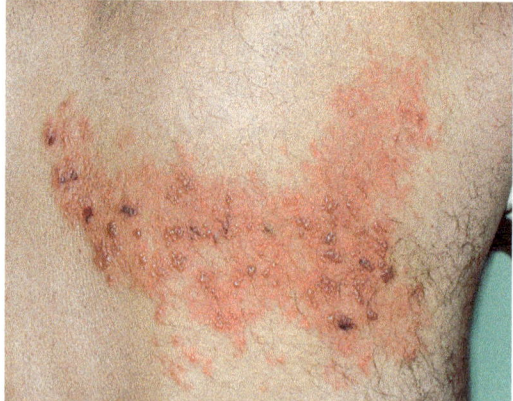

a. Analgesics + systemic antiviral therapy + topical antiviral cream
b. Analgesics + systemic antiviral therapy + calamine lotion
c. Analgesics + calamine lotion
d. Only analgesics because it is a self-limiting disorder

71. Which one of the following statements is not true about this patient?

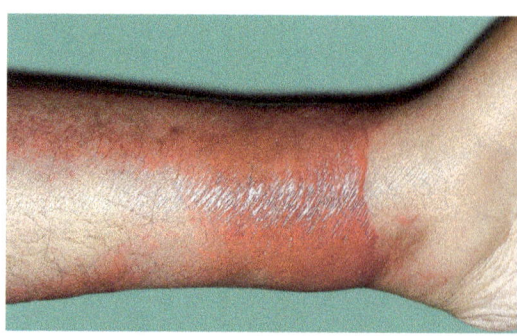

a. It is cellulitis because it is erythematous and edematous
b. It is erysipelas because it has sharp well-defined raised edge to normal tissue
c. It is involving dermis and upper subcutaneous tissue
d. It is a superficial bacterial infection

72. A 2-year-old child presented with chronic and recurrent episodes of symmetrically distributed itchy papules on the exposed extensor surfaces of extremities. Similar papules were also present on face. Genitals were normal. Parents, siblings are not involved. What is the clinical diagnosis?

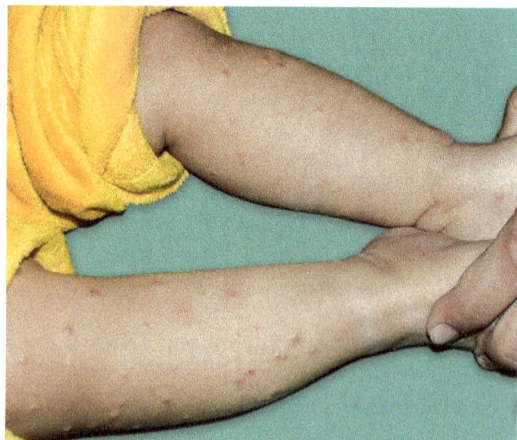

a. Papular urticaria or insect bite hypersensitivity (IBH)
b. Scabies
c. Lichen planus
d. Pityriasis lichenoides chronica (PLC)

73. Which one of the following statements is not true for this patient of pediculosis capitis?

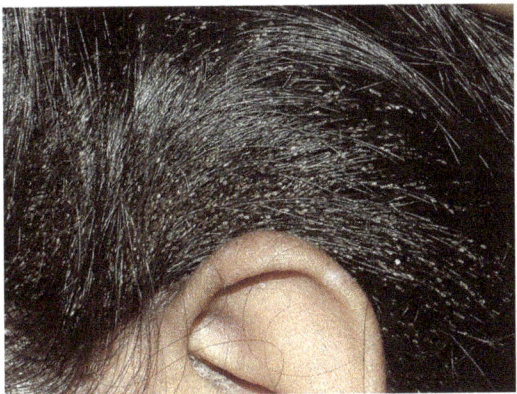

a. Apply 1% permethrin lotion for 12 hours
b. Give two doses of ivermectin separated by an interval of 10 days
c. Parietal and occipital regions are more densely infested. Occipital lymph nodes persist even after treatment
d. Lice survive for only 1–2 days away from host

74. An infant is having papules and pustules on both soles, on trunk *(MCQ 59)* and scalp. The child is irritable, cries and unable to sleep at night. Mother is also having generalized pruritus which is more at night. Which one of following diagnoses is correct?

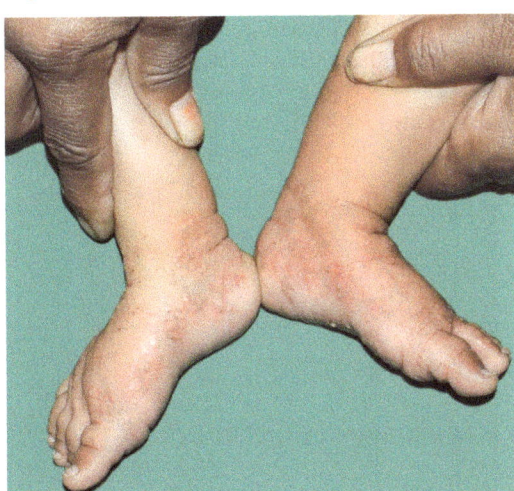

a. Papular urticaria with secondary infection
b. Atopic dermatitis with secondary infection
c. Infantile scabies with secondary infection
d. Pyoderma

75. Which one of the following statements is not true about phthiriasis palpebrarum?

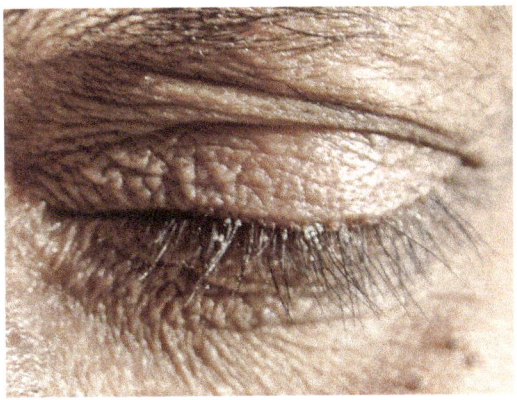

a. Eyebrows and eyelashes may be found involved simultaneously with pubic hair
b. It is caused by pediculosis pubis
c. Lice and eggs can be removed easily mechanically
d. Application of petrolatum, lindane is recommended for eye lashes

76. This patient presented with hair loss on scalp that showed scarring, atrophy, pigmentation and depigmentation. She also had discoid scaly lesions on sun exposed parts of face. What is the clinical diagnosis?

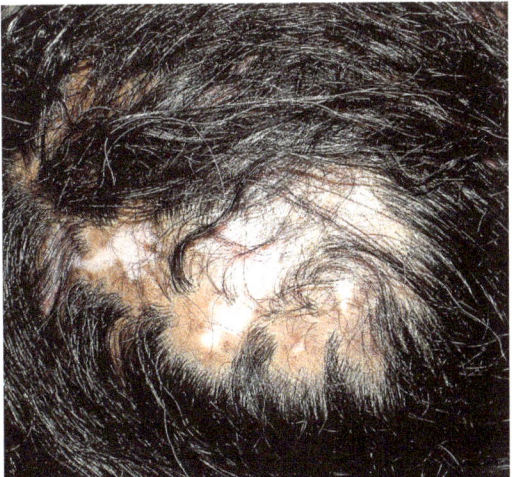

a. Cicatricial alopecia due to lichen planus (LP)
b. Cicatricial alopecia due to chronic cutaneous lupus erythematosus (CCLE)
c. Trichotillomania
d. Alopecia areata

77. What is the antihistamine of choice in this patient of renal dysfunction having uremic pruritus?

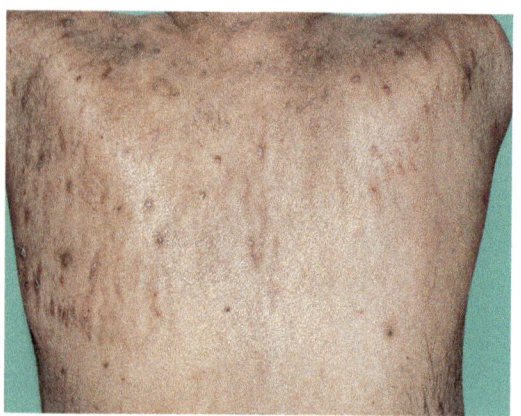

a. Levocetrizine
b. Cetrizine
c. Fexofenadine
d. Loratadine

78. Nail changes in this patient consist of tendency to form pterygium, thinning of nail plate, exaggeration of longitudinal lines and brittleness. In which of the following diseases are these changes characteristically seen?

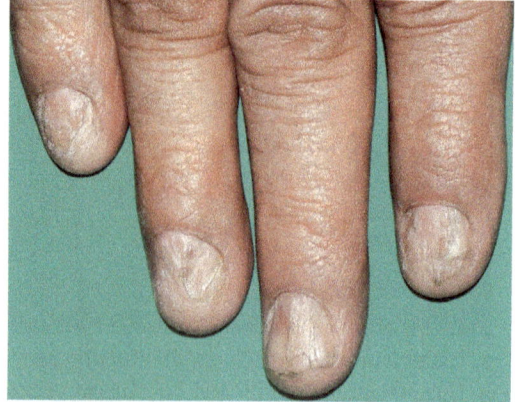

a. Tinea unguium
b. Psoriasis
c. Lichen planus
d. Alopecia areata
e. Darier'disease

79. A 2-year-old child presented with easy blistering of skin in response to minor trauma of upper and lower extremities. There is a no involvement of mucosa, nails, eyes, bones or other internal organs. Which one of the following diseases is he suffering from?

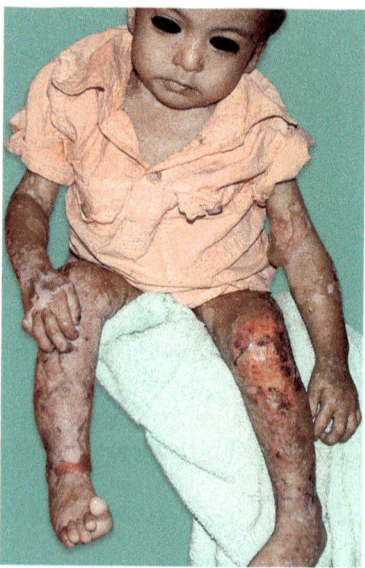

a. Congenital syphilis
b. Pemphigus vulgaris
c. Porphyria cutanea tarda
d. Epidermolysis bullosa simplex

80. This patient presented with eroded plaques with fissured appearance and moist malodorous vegetation in both groins. Other members in family are also suffering from similar disease with remission and relapses. Histopathology shows widespread partial acantholysis. What is the diagnosis?

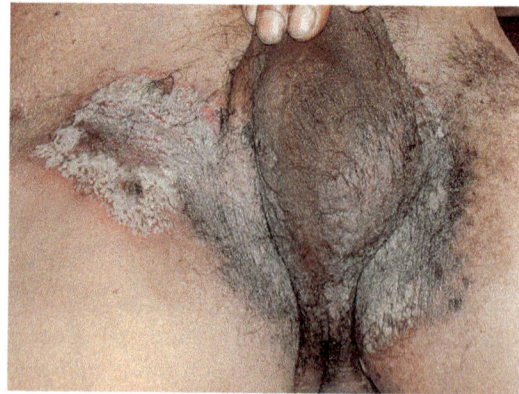

a. Tinea cruris with secondary infection.
b. Hailey-Hailey disease
c. Candidal intertrigo
d. Pemphigus vulgaris (PV)

81. This child came with acute involvement of oral mucosa and conjunctiva. He also had widespread eruption of target shaped lesions (showing partial coalescence) on trunk *(MCQ 304)* involving less than 10% of body surface area. What is the clinical diagnosis?

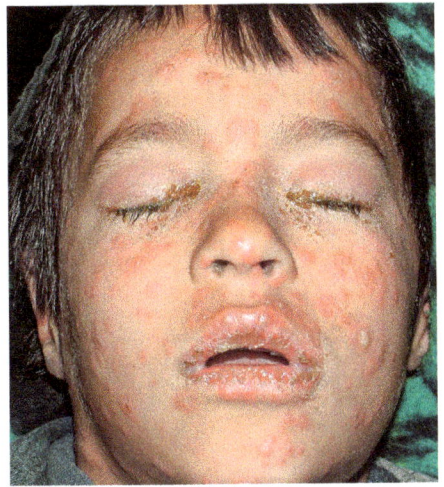

a. Erythema multiforme major
b. Stevens-Johnson syndrome (SJS)
c. Fixed drug eruption (FDE)
d. Measles

82. A 52-year-old patient having renal dysfunction with creatinine clearance 35 mL/min. presented on 3rd day of herpes zoster eruption. Which one of the followings is correct option for him?

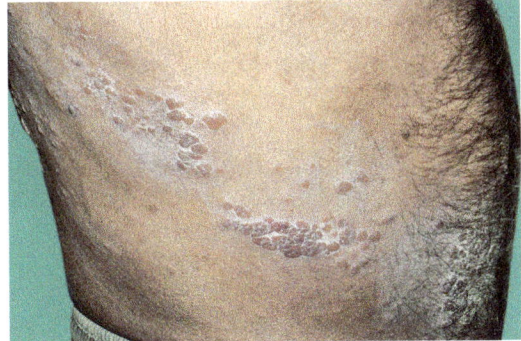

a. Valacyclovir 1 g TDS × 7d
b. Valacyclovir 1 g BD × 7d
c. Valacyclovir 1 g OD × 7d
d. Valacyclovir cannot be given

83. This patient presented with sudden eruption of crop of target or iris shaped lesions accompanied by involvement of oral mucosa only. It is preceded by herpes labialis infection a week before. What is the clinical diagnosis?

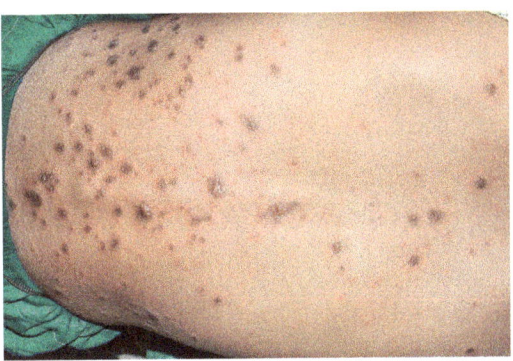

a. Chickenpox
b. Erythema multiforme major
c. Stevens-Johnson syndrome (SJS)
d. Toxic epidermal necrolysis (TEN)

84. This patient presented with involvement of both groins having pink color, white scaling and well defined margins with little itching. Discrete well defined scaly plaques four to five in number are also seen on the scalp. What is the clinical diagnosis?

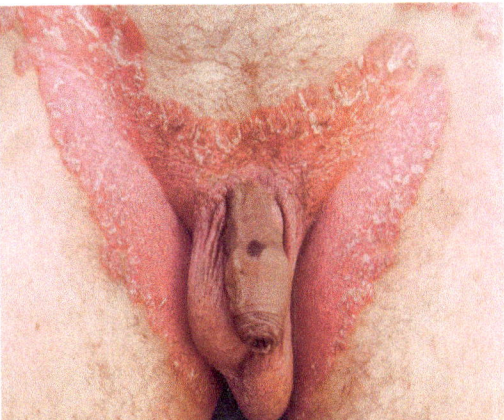

a. Tinea cruris
b. Hailey-Hailey disease
c. Candidal intertrigo
d. Flexural psoriasis

85. A 10-year-old child presented with hypopigmented macule on cheek with powdery white scales. What is possible diagnosis among the following options?

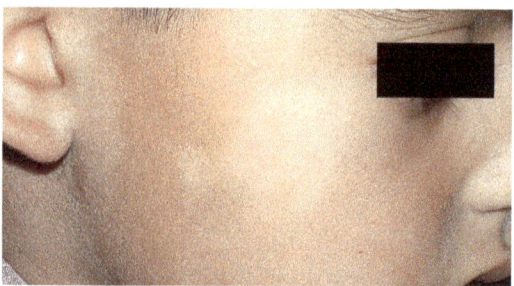

a. Vitiligo
b. Pityriasis alba
c. Nutritional deficiency
d. Manifestation of worm infestation

86. This farmer presented with intractable itching, redness, thickening, pigmentation and lichenification of facial skin. What is the clinical diagnosis?

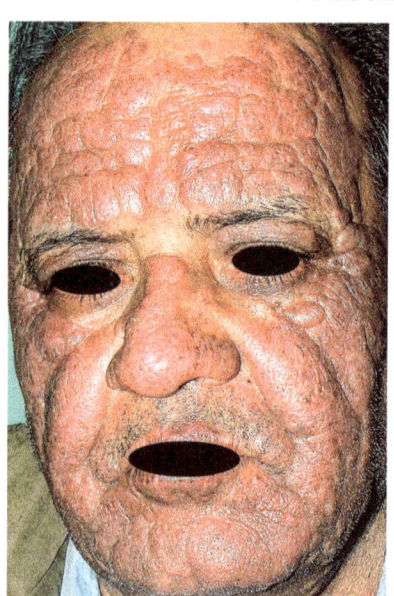

a. Senile eczema
b. It is air-borne contact dermatitis due to *Parthenium hysterophorus*
c. Excessive oil application
d. Lupus pernio
e. Chronic actinic dermatitis (CAD)

87. A 22-year-old man presented with large dry micaceous scales which get separated from the scalp but remain entangled in hairs binding their proximal portions. What is the clinical diagnosis?

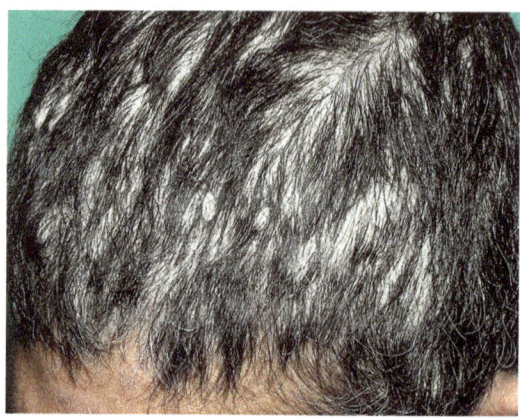

a. Psoriasis
b. Tinea capitis
c. Chronic cutaneous lupus erythematosus (CCLE)
d. Pityriasis amiantacea

88. All the nails show yellow discoloration, subungual hyperkeratosis and onycholysis. These changes are typically seen in which one of the following diseases?

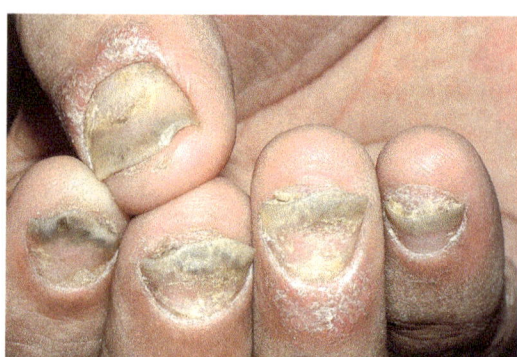

a. Psoriasis
b. Tinea unguium
c. Lichen planus
d. Alopecia areata

89. This young female is having malar rash and non-cicatricial hair loss with broken off hair giving unruly appearance. What is the clinical diagnosis?

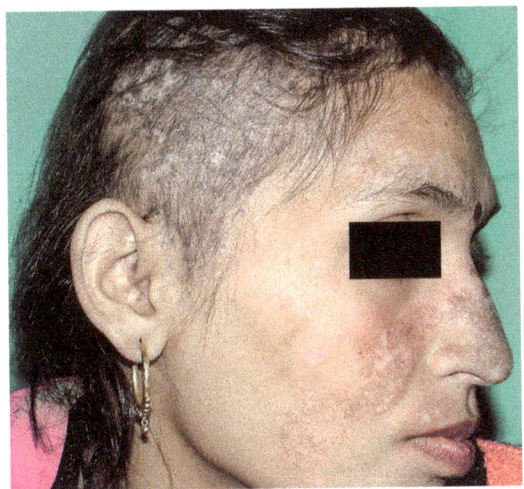

a. Melasma with androgenic alopecia
b. Lichen planus
c. Systemic lupus erythematosus
d. Melasma with alopecia areata

90. Which one of the following antileprotic drugs is causing ichthyotic changes in a leprosy patient?

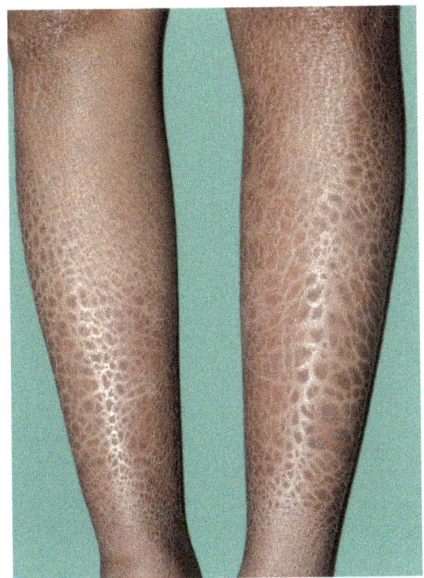

a. Dapsone
b. Clofazimine
c. Rifampicin
d. Thalidomide given in lepra II reaction

91. This man presented with 1-4 mm sized bright red vascular papules on scrotal skin. He complains soreness, itching and bleeding. What is the diagnosis?

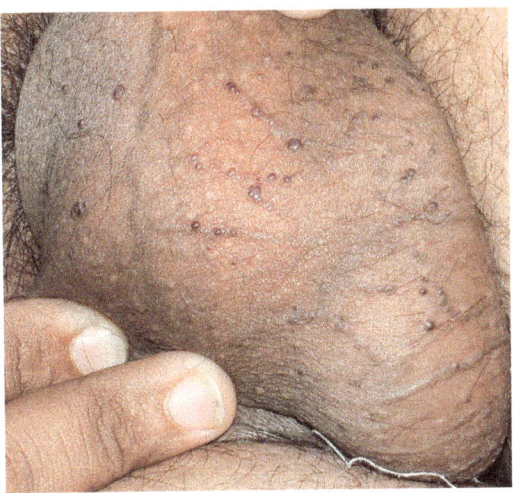

a. Angiokeratoma of scrotum
b. Pediculosis pubis
c. Palpable purpura (PP)
d. Nodular scabies

92. An adult presented with multiple asymptomatic yellow colored, various sized, smooth and elastic swellings on scrotum for the last many years. What is the clinical diagnosis?

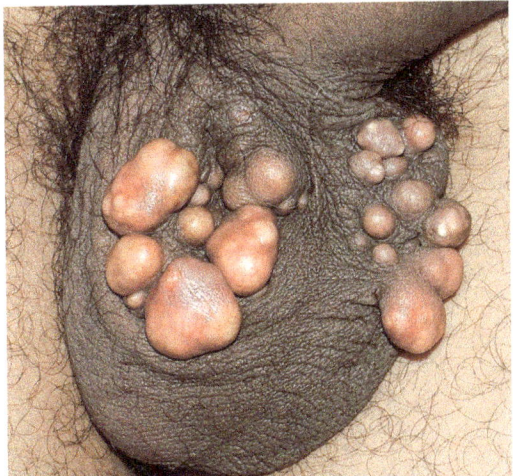

a. Sebaceous cysts
b. Nodular scabies
c. Steatocystoma multiplex on scrotum
d. Strawberry hemangioma

93. A 13-year-old boy presented with moist fissured eczema involving the perioral region adjoining the vermillion border. Which one of the followings is the possible cause?

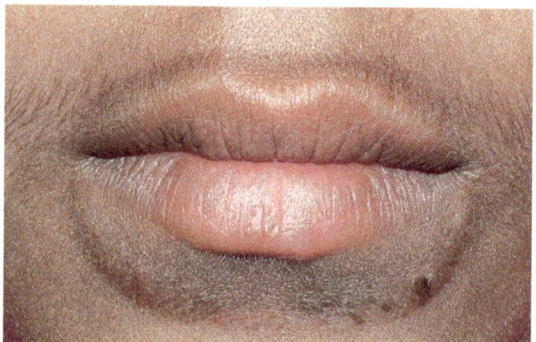

   a. Allergic dermatitis due to tooth paste
   b. Iron or vitamin B_2-Riboflavin deficiency
   c. Dermatitis artefacta
   d. Lip-lick cheilitis

94. An 80-year-old man presented with dry scaly skin of legs with prominent and deep skin markings studded with fine reticulate superficial fissures. What is the clinical diagnosis?

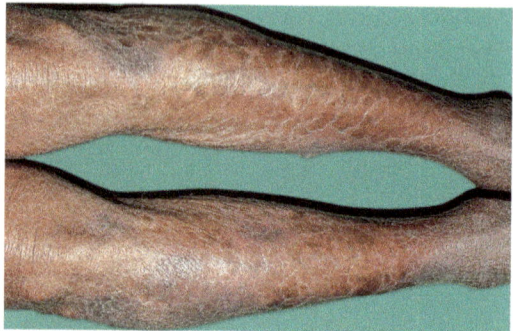

   a. Ichthyosis
   b. Poor hygiene
   c. Asteatotic or senile eczema
   d. Excessive heat exposure

95. Glans shows red discrete plaques with little scaling. There is no history of diabetes or extramarital sexual exposure. In addition, there are few pinkish cutaneous plaques with silvery white scales on other parts of body. What is the clinical diagnosis?

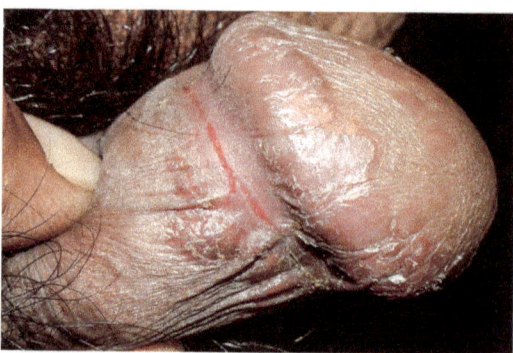

   a. Psoriasis on glans
   b. Lichen planus
   c. Candidal balanoposthitis
   d. Fixed drug eruption (FDE)

96. After intake of co-trimoxazole, this patient had involvement of oral mucosa with eruption of target or iris lesion on back and extremities. Other mucosae were normal. What is the clinical diagnosis?

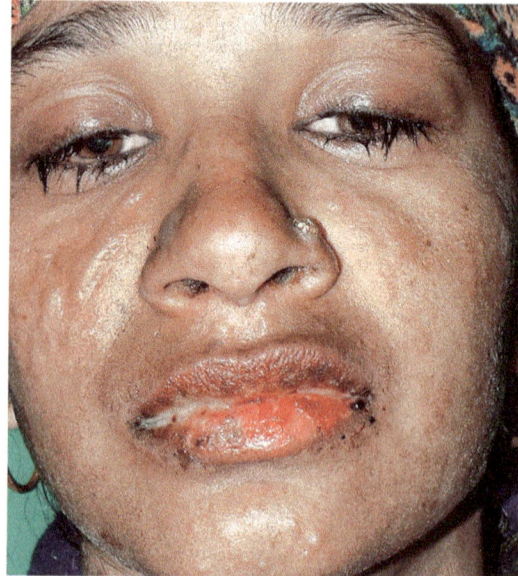

   a. Stevens-Johnson syndrome (SJS)
   b. Erythema multiforme major (EM major)
   c. Fixed drug eruption (FDE)
   d. Toxic epidermal necrolysis (TEN)

97. This patient presented with long standing severe itching on scrotum with a localized lichenified plaque having accentuated skin markings. What is the clinical diagnosis?

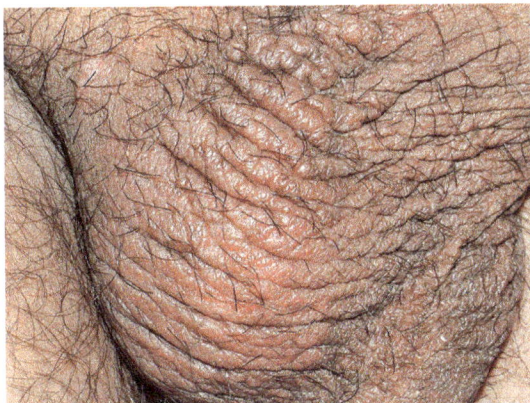

a. Poor hygiene
b. Excessive application of steroid creams
c. Circumscribed neurodermatitis (Lichen simplex chronius)
d. Prolonged application of permethrin

98. She presented with unilateral, persistent and deep red patch in the distribution of sensory branches of trigeminal nerve since birth. What is the clinical diagnosis?

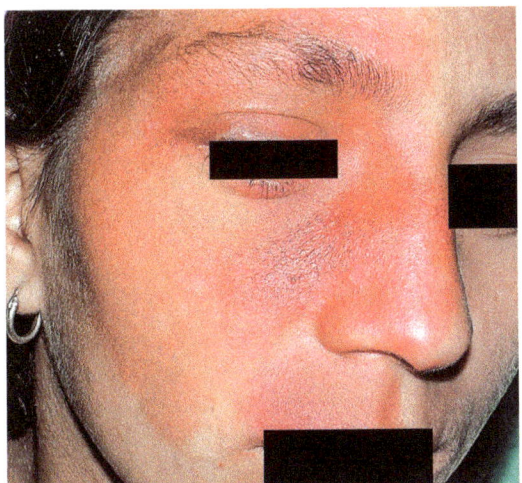

a. Salmon patch
b. Port-wine stain or nevus flammeus
c. Strawberry hemangioma
d. Lymphangioma circumscriptum

99. A child presented with single circumscribed, hairless, slightly raised, waxy, velvety and dark pinkish plaque on the scalp for the last many years. What is the clinical diagnosis?

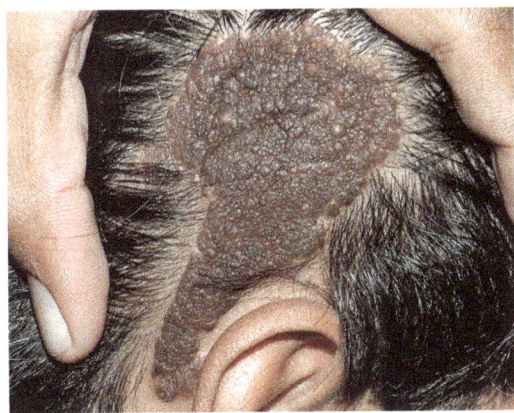

a. Basal cell carcinoma (BCC)
b. Seborrheic dermatitis (SD)
c. Kerion
d. Nevus sebaceous
e. Psoriasis

100. An old man having multiple, discrete, well defined pinkish plaques having slivery white scales. What is the clinical diagnosis?

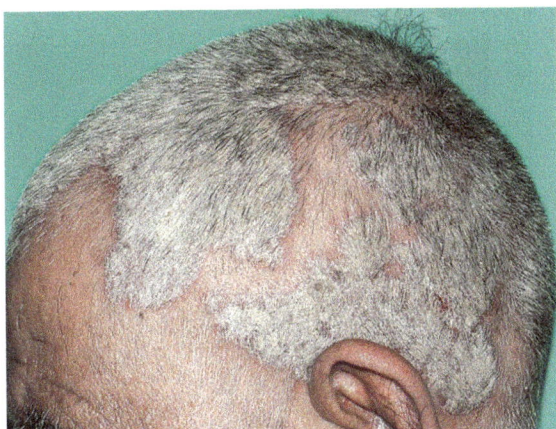

a. Tinea capitis
b. Seborrheic dermatitis (SD)
c. Scalp psoriasis
d. Chronic cutaneous lupus erythematosus (CCLE)

101. She presented with bilateral, asymptomatic, red infiltration of ear lobules with ill defined margins for the last many months. She is also accompanied by numerous scattered maculopapular lesions on trunk. What is the clinical diagnosis?

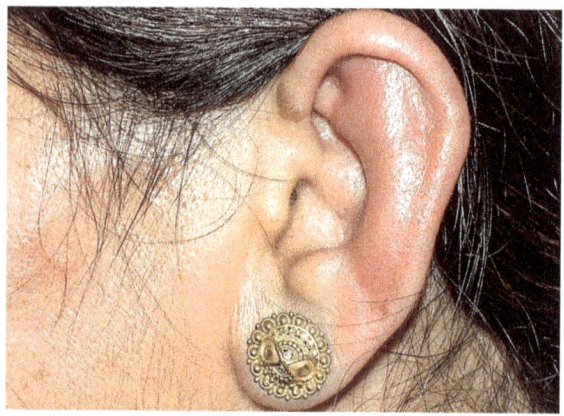

a. Myxedema
b. Chronic urticaria
c. Post-kala-azar dermal leishmaniasis (PKDL)
d. Lepromatous leprosy

102. She presented with painless, single, bright red papule with smooth surface for the last 2 months. She complains of recurrent bleeding from it. What is the clinical diagnosis?

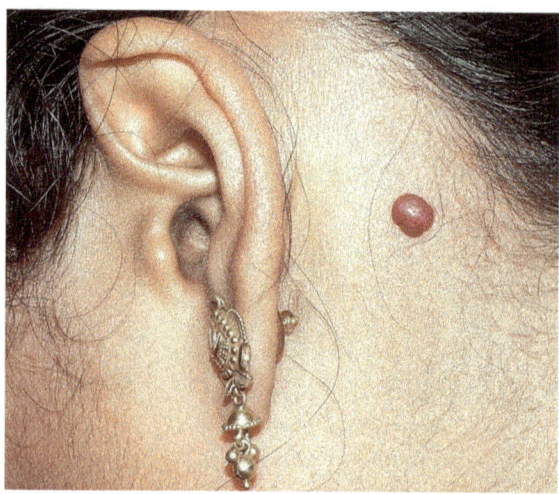

a. Pyogenic granuloma
b. Strawberry hemangioma
c. Cherry angioma
d. Boil

103. A 50-year-old female presented with unilateral, sharply marginated, scaling and crusting of nipple giving an eczematous look. It was accompanied by pain, burning and pruritus also. What is the clinical diagnosis?

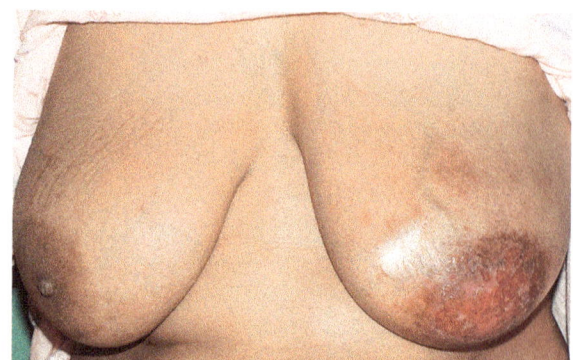

a. Eczema of nipple
b. Psoriasis of nipple
c. Pyoderma of nipple
d. Paget's disease of nipple

104. A 60-year-old man presented with single dark macule about 2 cm sized, showing asymmetry, irregular or notched border and varying color in different areas of lesion. What is probable clinical diagnosis?

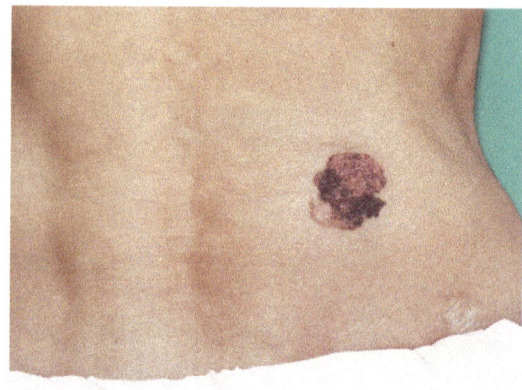

a. Melanocytic nevus
b. Superficial spreading melanoma
c. Cafe-au-lait spot
d. Bowen's disease

Chapter 4 ✦ MCQs of Dermatology, Venereology and Leprology

105. An obese person presented with asymptomatic multiple, 2–5 mm sized, soft, skin, colored round papules on the side neck. What is the clinical diagnosis?

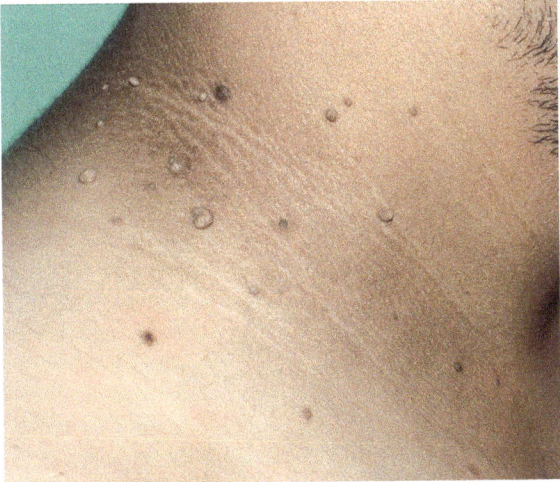

a. Common warts
b. Cutaneous neurofibromas (mollusca fibrosa)
c. Skin tags (soft warts, acrochordon)
d. Dermatosis papulosa nigra (DPN)

106. An adult presented with groups of painless, small vesicles in his right axilla only since childhood. He complains of discharge of watery or blood-stained lymph from vesicles. What is the diagnosis?

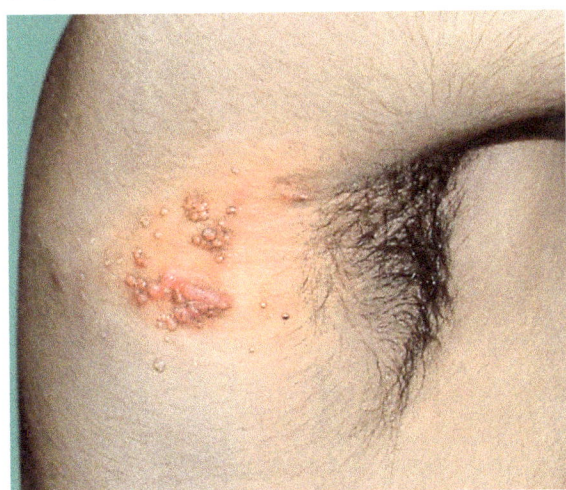

a. Herpes zoster
b. Lymphangioma circumscriptum
c. Recurrent herpes simplex
d. Hailey-Hailey disease

107. This patient presented with claw hand showing flexion deformity of little and ring fingers accompanied by loss of sensation also in the same fingers. What is the diagnosis?

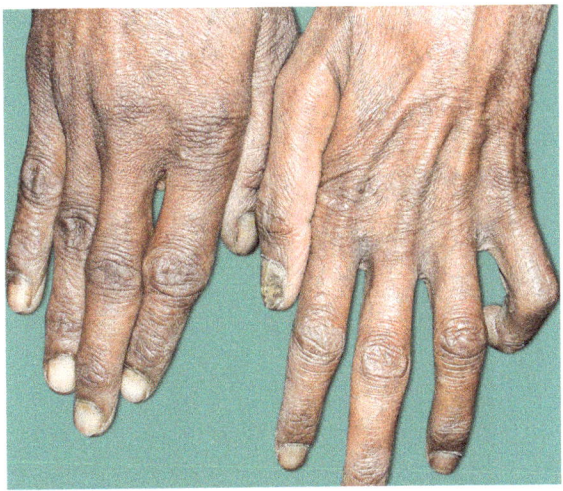

a. Diabetic neuropathy
b. Hansen's disease
c. Carpel tunnel syndrome
d. Amyloid neuropathy

108. A middle-aged female presented with single nodule with central keratotic core on her nose for the last 2 months. What can be the possible diagnosis?

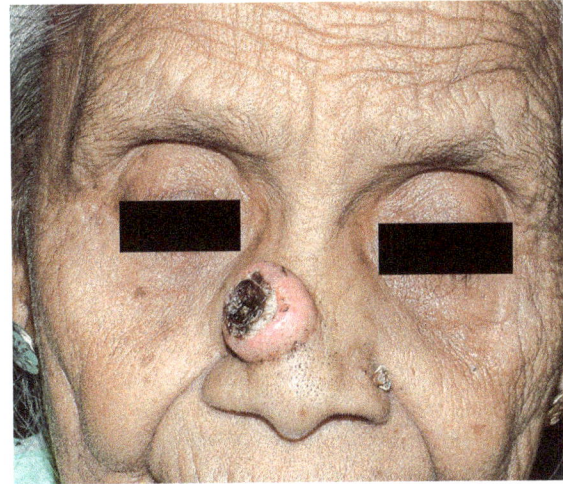

a. Squamous cell carcinoma (SCC)
b. Boil or furuncle
c. Keratoacanthoma (mature stage)
d. Basal cell carcinoma (BCC)

109. A 16-year-old boy presented with closely set asymptomatic hyperkeratosis papules forming plaques since birth in left axilla only along the Blaschko lines.

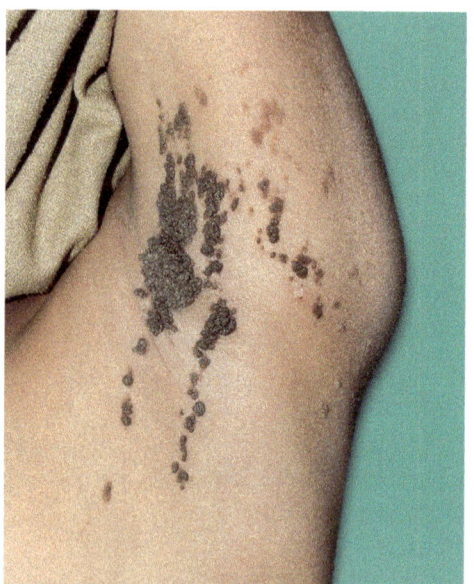

a. Tuberculosis verrucosa cutis (TVC)
b. Common warts
c. Verrucous epidermal nevus
d. Hypertrophic lichen planus

110. This child is having large pigmented hairy hair lesion since birth with increasing in size with age. What is the diagnosis?

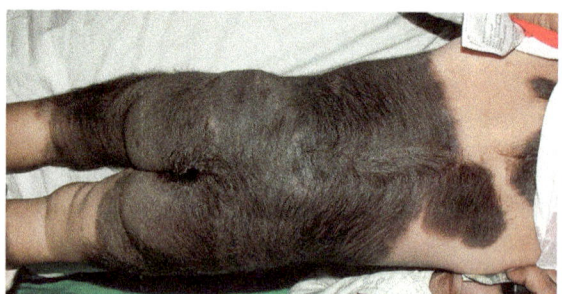

a. Spitz nevus
b. Garment or bathing trunk nevus
c. Halo nevus (Sutton's nevus)
d. Junctional nevus

111. A 35-year-old male presented with recurrent, scattered and widely spaced small abscesses with sinus tracts and scars in both axillae, perianal region *(MCQ 343)* and groins. What is the clinical diagnosis?

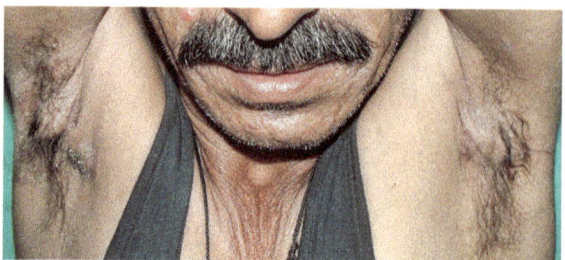

a. Fox-Fordyce disease
b. Hidradenitis suppurativa
c. Tubercular lymphadenitis
d. Multiple boils in a diabetic patient

112. He presented with increased longitudinal striations and fissuring in nail plate with tendency of spontaneous breaking. In which one of the following diseases is it seen typically?

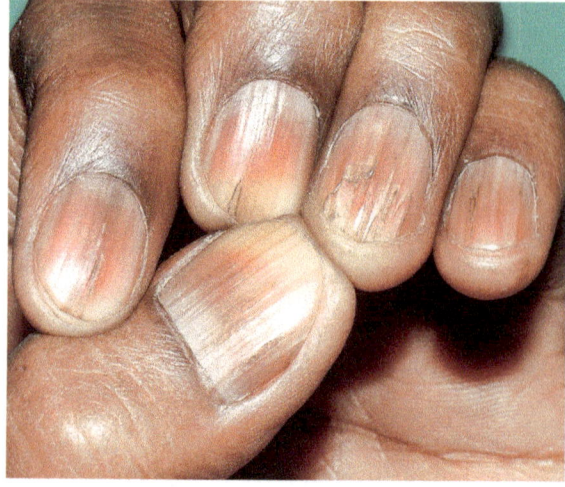

a. Onycholysis seen in psoriasis
b. Onychorrhexis seen in lichen planus
c. Trachyonychia seen in alopecia areata
d. Onychomycosis seen in tinea unguium

113. A 43-year-old farmer presented with a slow growing exophytic tumor having a cauliflower appearance on upper back for last one year. What is the clinical diagnosis?

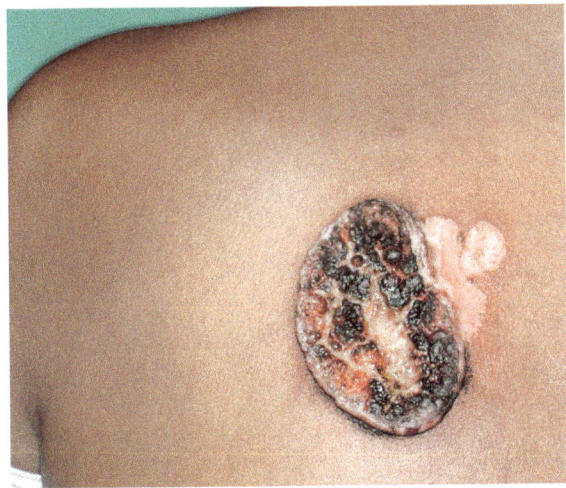

a. Melanocytic melanoma (MM)
b. Basal cell carcinoma (BCC)
c. Lupus vulgaris
d. Verrucous squamous cell carcinoma (VSCC)

114. A 14-year-old child presented with single, soft, red vascular papule on upper lip for the last 2 months with the complain of recurrent bleeding. What the clinical diagnosis?

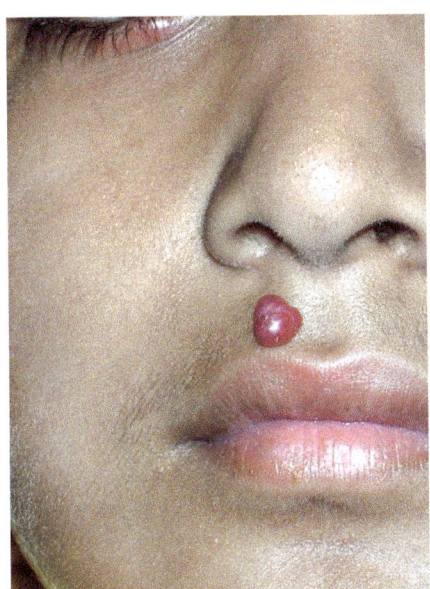

a. Strawberry hemangioma
b. Angiokeratoma
c. Infected sebaceous cyst
d. Pyogenic granuloma
e. Cherry angioma

115. This man presented with superciliary madarosis, nasal collapse, infiltration of ear lobules and broadening of nose. What is the probable diagnosis?

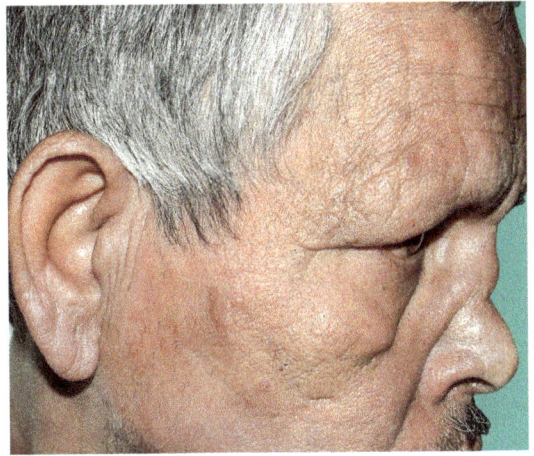

a. Hypothyroidism
b. Late benign syphilis
c. Traumatic nasal collapse
d. Lepromatous leprosy (LL)
e. Wegener granulomatosis (WG)
f. Relapsing polychondritis

116. An old man presented with an elevated plaque on pinna with ulceration, hyperkeratosis, pigmentation and bleeding for the last 3–4 years. What is the clinical diagnosis?

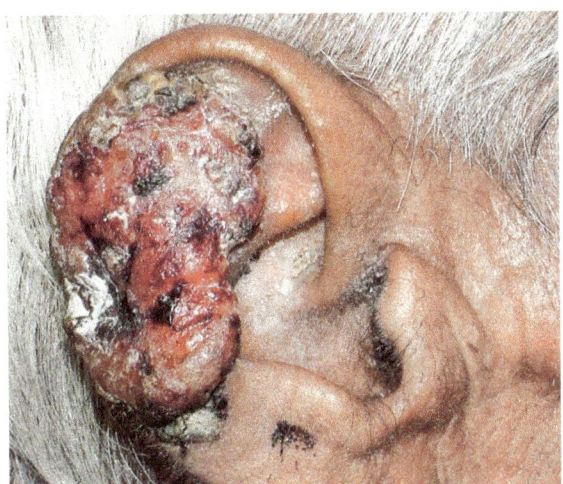

a. Squamous cell carcinoma (SCC) showing pigmentation
b. Granuloma faciale
c. Moist or rural type old world leishmaniasis
d. Lupus vulgaris

117. A 60-year-old male presented with multiple, dark colored well circumscribed, very superficial soft and friable verrucous papules on face for last 2–3 years. Such lesions are present on trunk as well. What is the diagnosis?

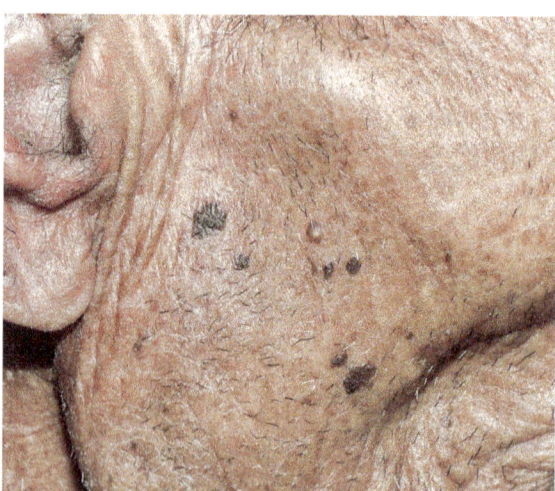

a. The sign of Leser-Trelat
b. Skin tags or acrochordon
c. Actinic keratosis
d. Seborrheic keratosis (SK)

118. In summer, this man presented with unbearable pinpricking and burning sensation or discomfort. It manifested with uniform rash on back consisting of minute red papules. What is the probable diagnosis?

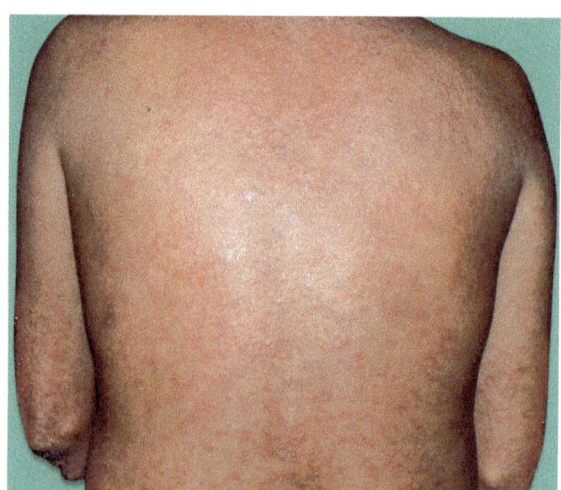

a. Morbilliform rash due to some drug
b. Acute urticaria
c. Miliaria rubra
d. Erythroderma

119. This patient presented with coarse pitting or thumbling of nail plates. What is probable diagnosis?

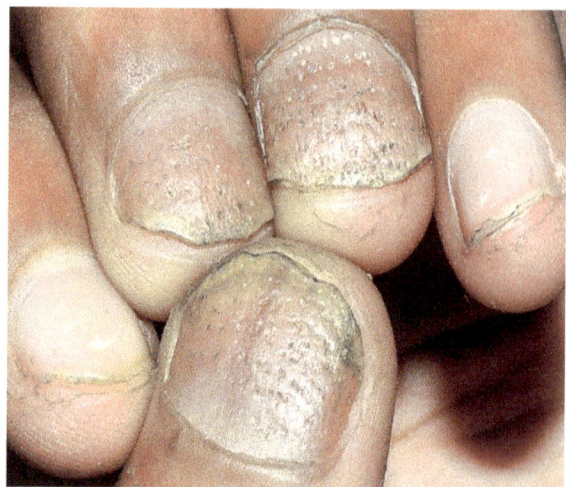

a. Lichen planus (LP)
b. Psoriasis
c. Alopecia areata
d. Darier's disease

120. What is the diagnosis of this patient?

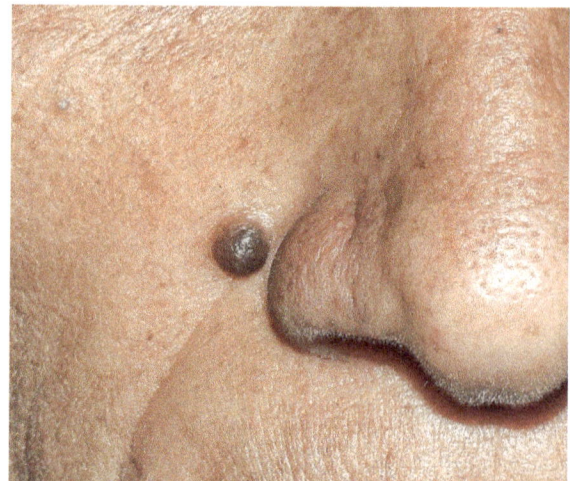

a. Freckles
b. Lentiginosis
c. Compound nevus
d. Intradermal nevus

121. A 70-year-old male is having a brownish black irregular macule on left cheek which is exhibiting slow prolonged radial growth. What is the diagnosis?

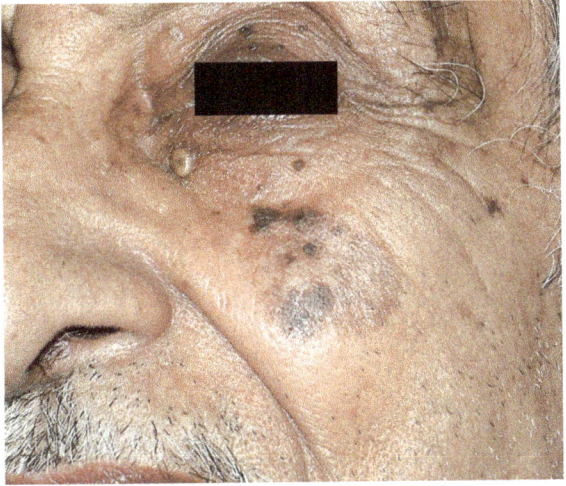

a. Actinic keratosis
b. Lentigo maligna melanoma (LMM)
c. Basal cell carcinoma (BCC)
d. Acquired melanocytic nevus

122. This infant started having in first month of life a superficial, sharply circumscribed round to oval smooth scarlet red tumor which has gradually increased in size. What is the diagnosis?

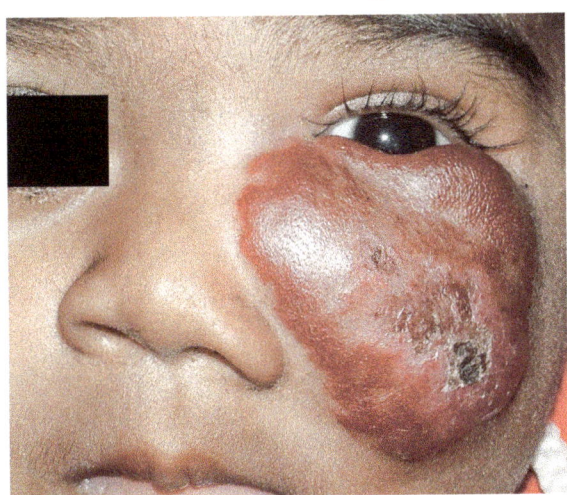

a. Pyogenic granuloma
b. Infantile hemangioma
c. Port-wine stain
d. Salmon patch

123. This old man presented with asymptomatic 1 mm to 10 mm sized dark color macules and papules having rough scaly surface with sharp demarcated edges. Scales are adherent and can be removed with difficulty. What is the diagnosis?

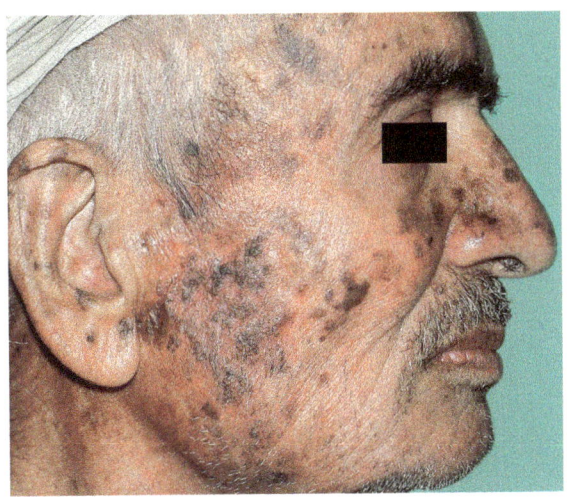

a. Seborrheic keratosis (SK)
b. Plane warts
c. Moles
d. Actinic keratosis

124. Nail plates in this patient show concave shape both in transverse and longitudinal axes. What is it called?

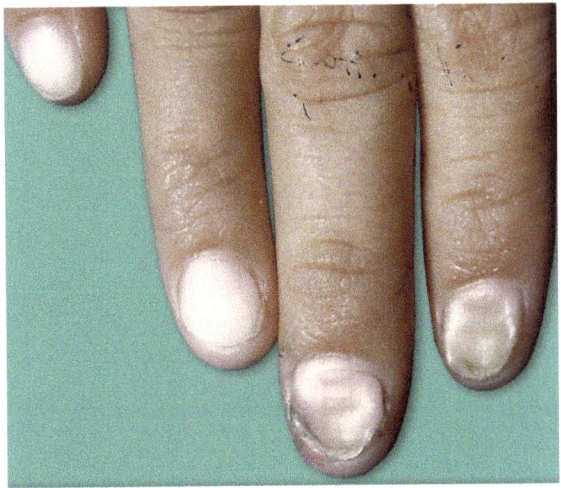

a. Clubbing associated with bronchial carcinoma
b. Beau's line reflecting a systemic disease
c. Koilonychia associated with iron deficiency anemia
d. Yellow nail syndrome associated with respiratory disease

125. This patient has repeated attacks of miliaria rubra. Now presented with 1–3 mm sized, pale and firm papules on limbs and trunk without any discomfort or itching. What is the probable diagnosis?

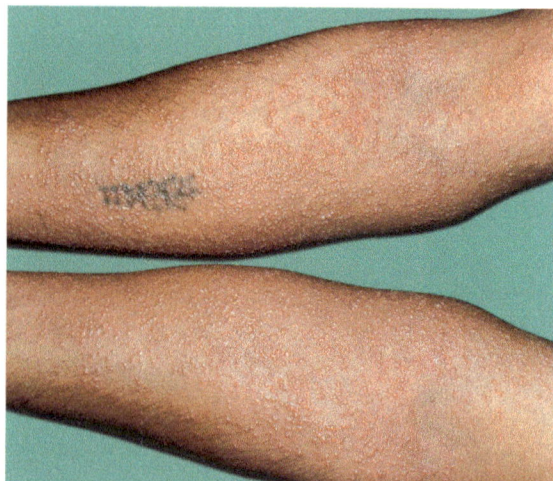

a. Miliaria profunda
b. Miliaria crystallina
c. Miliaria rubra
d. Milia

126. A 60-year-old male presented with a uniformly dark blue or black elevated dome-shaped lesion on trunk for the last 1 year. What is the clinical diagnosis?

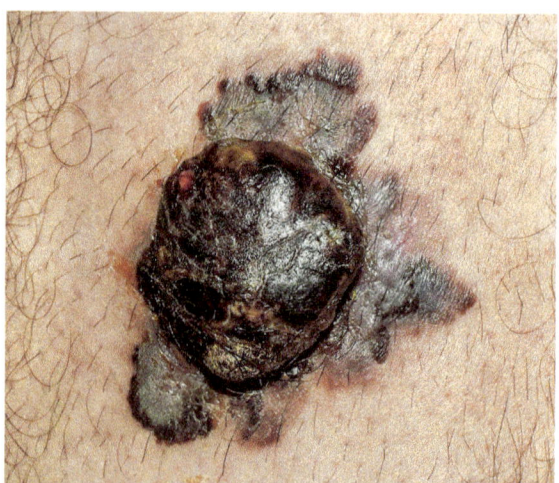

a. Acquired melanocytic nevus
b. Nodular melanoma showing horizontal growth phase
c. Squamous cell carcinoma (SCC)
d. Basal cell carcinoma (BCC)

127. Two weeks after initiation of phenytoin a 50-year-old man developed malaise, fever with sheet like, painful glistening cutaneous erosions involving more than 30% of body surface with positive Nikolsky's sign. It was also accompanied by severe mucosal involvement. What is the diagnosis?

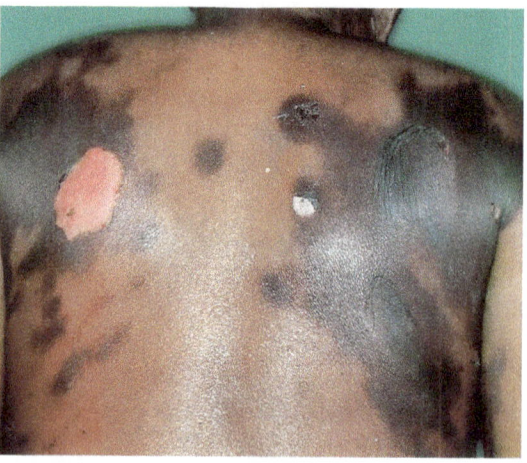

a. Fixed drug eruption (FDE)
b. Erythema multiforme (EM)
c. Toxic epidermal necrolysis (TEN)
d. Steven-Johnson Syndrome (SJS)

128. An 18-year-old female presented with massive loss of scalp hair. On examination by magnifying glass, it revealed firmly anchored partially broken hairs in the bald area, comedo like black spots and empty follicular orifices. What is the possible clinical diagnosis?

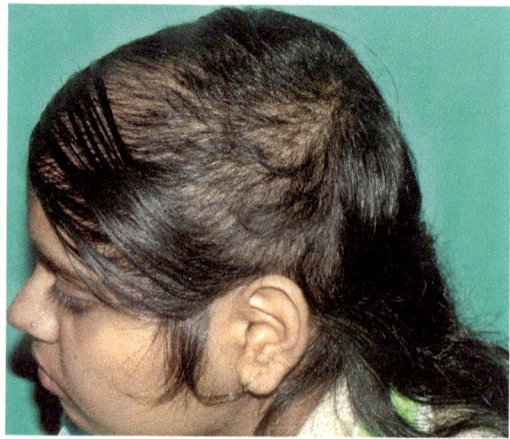

a. Androgenic alopecia
b. Trichotillomania
c. Alopecia due to SLE
d. Alopecia areata (AA)
e. Telogen effluvium

129. This patient presented with fever, joint pain and urticarial rash. Rash is persisting for the last 5–7 days and wheals are slightly painful. What is the clinical diagnosis?

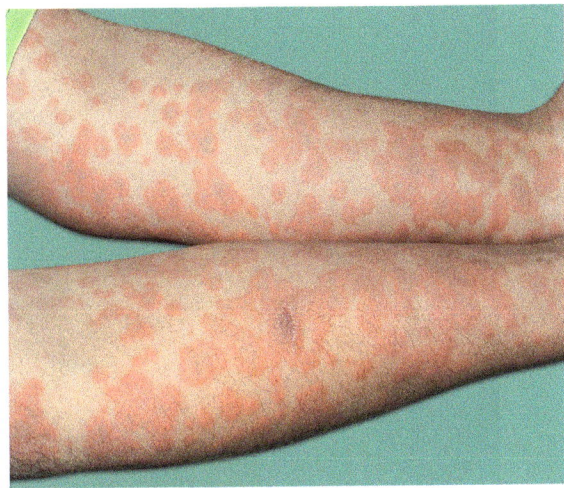

a. Acute urticaria
b. Urticarial vasculitis
c. Morbilliform rash
d. Erythema multiforme (EM)

130. This patient presented with pruritic, purplish, plain toped papules with mild scaling on foot. What is the diagnosis?

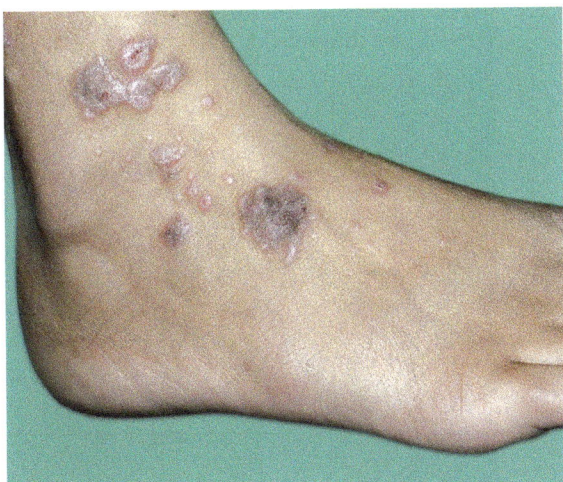

a. Psoriasis
b. Lichen planus
c. Prurigo nodularis
d. Tuberculosis verrucosa cutis (TVC)

131. An 18-year-old female presented with a crop of small vesicles which are surrounded by irregular erythema. It is preceded by fever and malaise. What is the clinical diagnosis?

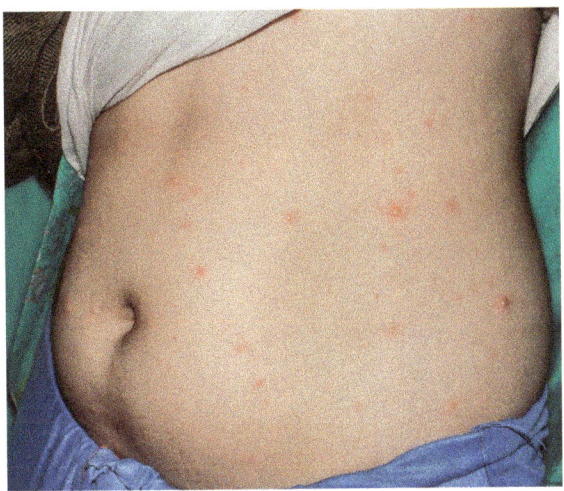

a. Measles
b. Acne vulgaris
c. Acneiform eruption
d. Chickenpox

132. A 50-year-old man having uncontrolled diabetes mellitus presented with painless and non-pruritic bullae on legs with no mucosal involvement. What is the diagnosis?

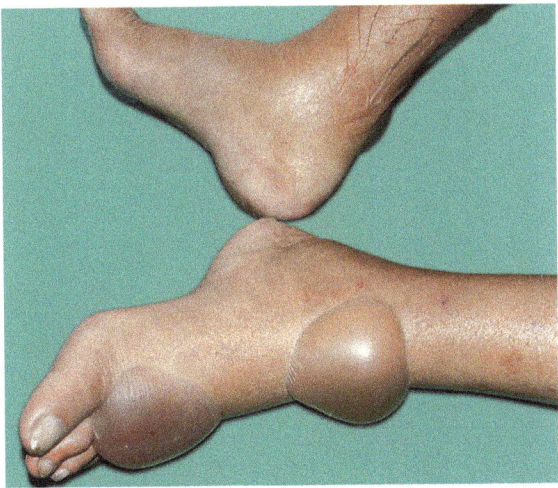

a. Pemphigus vulgaris induced by antidiabetic drugs
b. Erythema multiforme induced by drugs
c. Bullous diabeticorum
d. Bullous pemphigoid

133. This patient presented with bulbous enlargement of terminal phalanx resulting into increased transverse and longitudinal curvatures of nail plate. What is the clinical diagnosis?

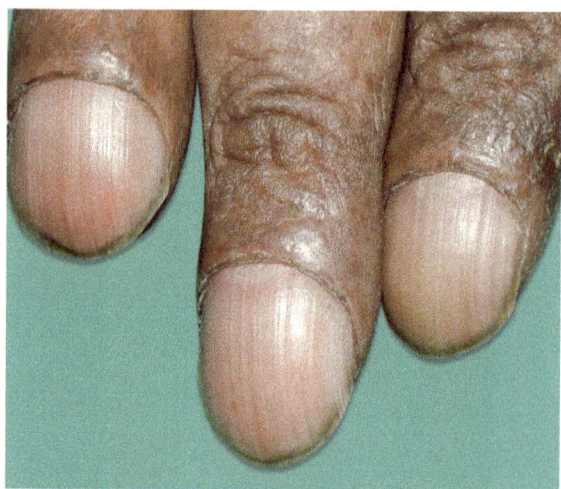

a. Clubbing
b. Koilonychia
c. Subungual hyperkeratosis
d. Onychogryphosis

134. Following herpes simplex, this patient developed profuse number of macules, papules and target lesions on extremities with no mucosal involvement. What is the diagnosis?

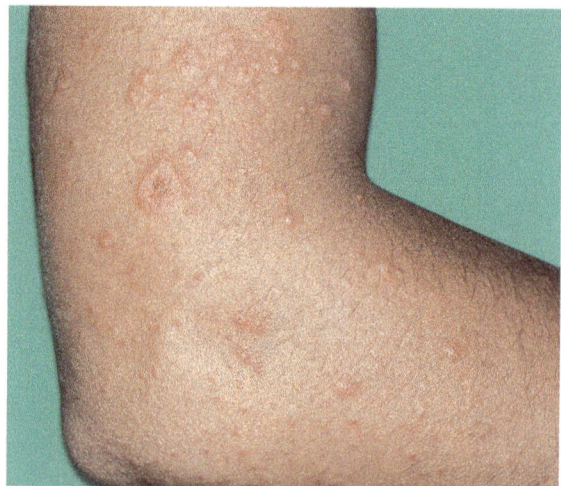

a. Erythema multiforme minor
b. Erythema multiforme major
c. Morbilliform rash
d. Pityriasis rosea

135. This lady presented with discrete pruritic excoriated papules on extensor surfaces of her forearms in late second trimester of pregnancy. What is the diagnosis?

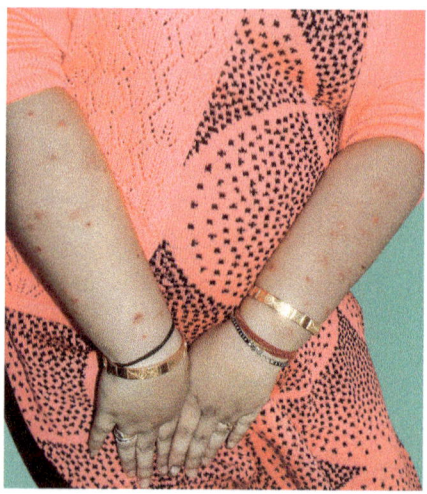

a. Pruritic urticarial papules and plaques of pregnancy (PUPPP)
b. Impetigo herpetiformis
c. Prurigo of pregnancy
d. Pemphigoid gestationis
e. Prurigo gravidarum

136. A 50-year-old man presented with severe itching, darkening and thickening of trunk and extremities. What is the diagnosis?

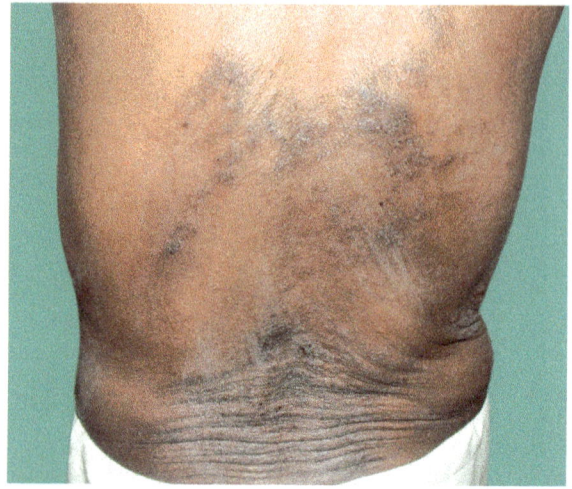

a. Psoriasis
b. Tinea corporis
c. Constitutional eczema with lichenification
d. Generalized lichen planus.

137. An 8-year-old child presented with itching, oozing, crusting and fissuring both soles for the last two years with remissions and relapses. What is the diagnosis?

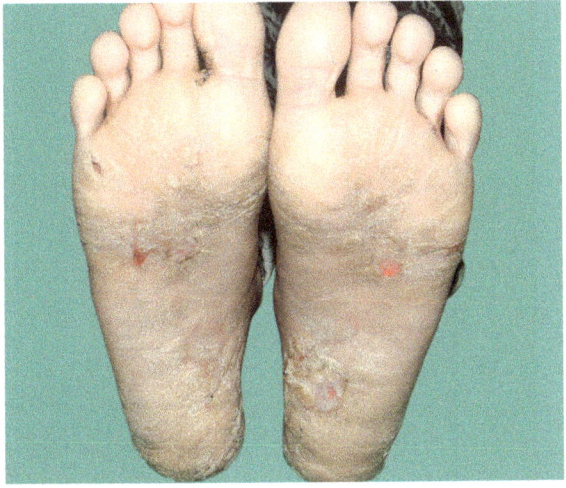

a. Tinea pedis
b. Plantar keratoderma
c. Eczema soles
d. Plantar psoriasis

138. A 2-year-old child presented with a very large patch with fine scaling and well-defined margins. There is little itching with no hair loss. What can be the diagnosis?

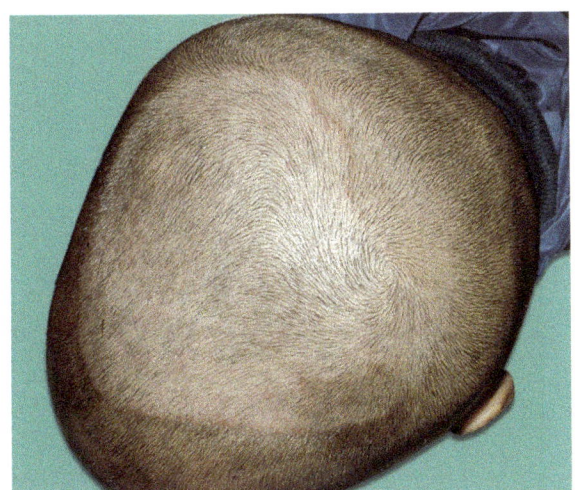

a. Psoriasis
b. Pityriasis capitis
c. Tinea capitis
d. Pityriasis alba

139. She presented with history of Raynaud's phenomenon on exposure to cold. Fingers are swollen with tightly bound skin that is extending proximal to digits. In some of the fingers (index figures) pulp has become atrophied with nails covered on them. Face is expressionless with pinched nose. What is the diagnosis?

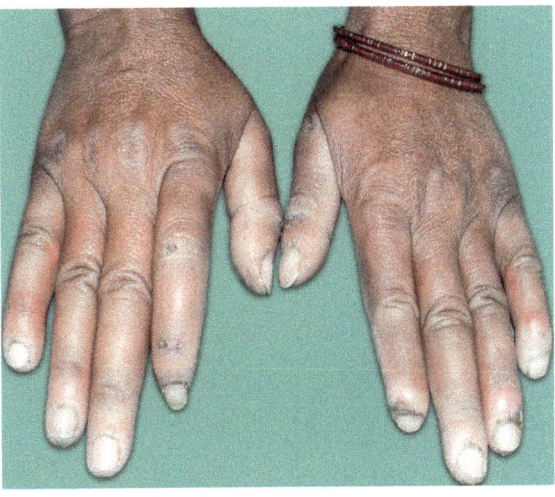

a. Systemic sclerosis
b. Systemic lupus erythematosus (SLE)
c. Generalized morphea
d. Lichen sclerosus et atrophicus

140. With which one of the following conditions match these characteristic target lesions?

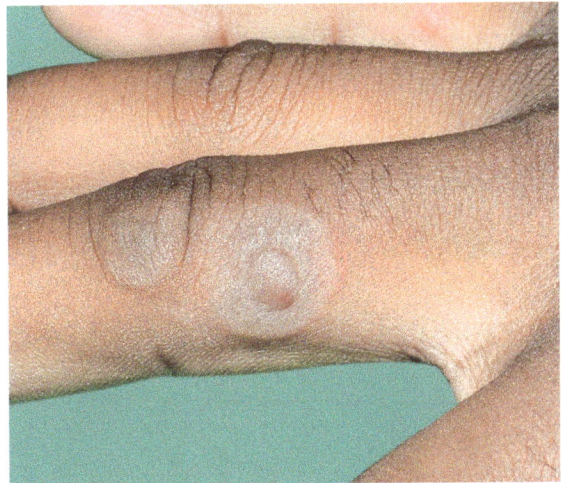

a. Epidermolysis bullosa (EB)
b. Dermatitis herpetiformis (DH)
c. Erythema multiforme (EM)
d. Pemphigus vulgaris (PV)

141. A 14-month-old male child presented with dry, rough skin having diffuse and uniform fish like scaling since the of age of 3 months. Flexures and diaper areas are spared. Extensor surfaces of arms and legs are predominantly involved. What is the clinical diagnosis?

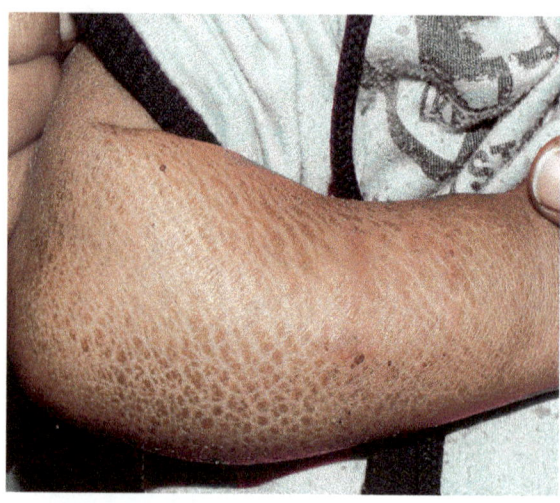

a. X-linked recessive ichthyosis
b. Acquired ichthyosis
c. Ichthyosis vulgaris
d. Malnourishment

142. This patient presented with multiple round erythematous well defined, itchy and dry patches. Borders are active with tendency of central clearing. What is the clinical diagnosis?

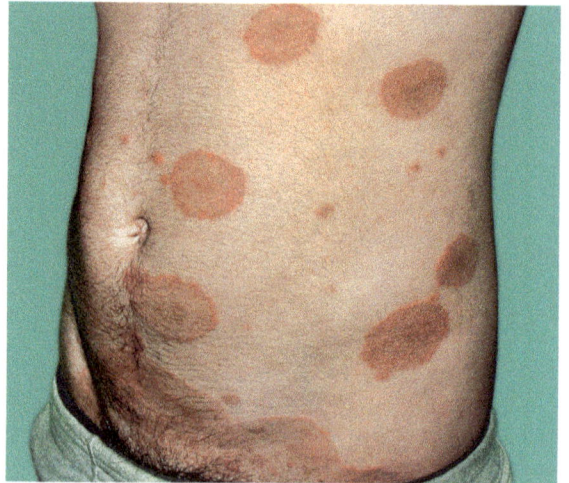

a. Discoid eczema
b. Psoriasis
c. Tinea corporis
d. Fixed drug eruption

143. The thumb of a house wife shows dystrophy of nail plate, loss of cuticle and redness of posterior nail fold. What is the diagnosis and treatment?

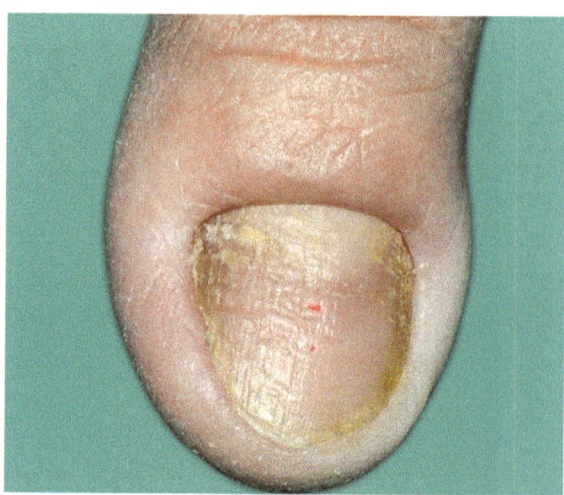

a. Tinea unguium—give systematic antifungal drugs
b. Chronic paronychia—avoid wetting and instill antifungal lotion
c. Traumatic—do nail plate avulsion
d. Koilonychia—give iron capsules only

144. An adult with a history of sexual exposure presented with soft, pink, grouped, pedunculated, filiform, digitate cauliflower like lesions around the preputial orifice. What is the diagnosis?

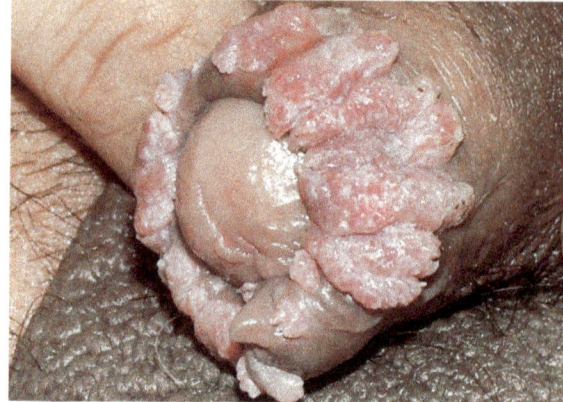

a. Pearly penile papules (PPP)
b. Genital warts
c. Verrucous squamous cell carcinoma (VSCC)
d. Molluscum contagiosum (MC)

145. This man presented with non scarring patchy hair loss in the temporal region. Patches show exclamation mark hair at places. There is loss of hairs in eye brows and moustaches also. What is the clinical diagnosis?

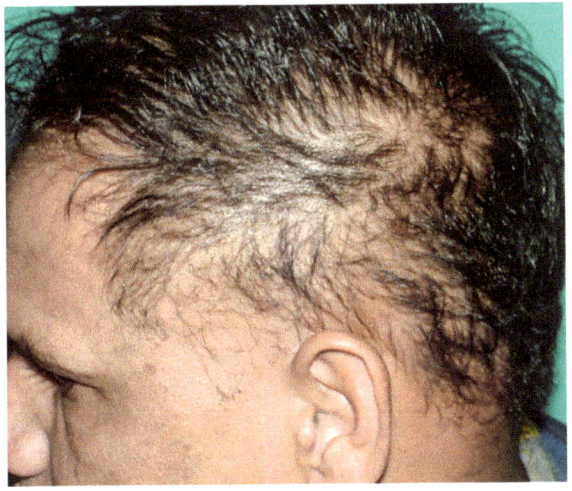

a. Androgenic alopecia
b. Trichotillomania
c. Alopecia areata
d. Telogen Effluvium

146. This man presented with well defined, erythematous raised plaques with silvery white scaling involving back and extensors. What is the diagnosis?

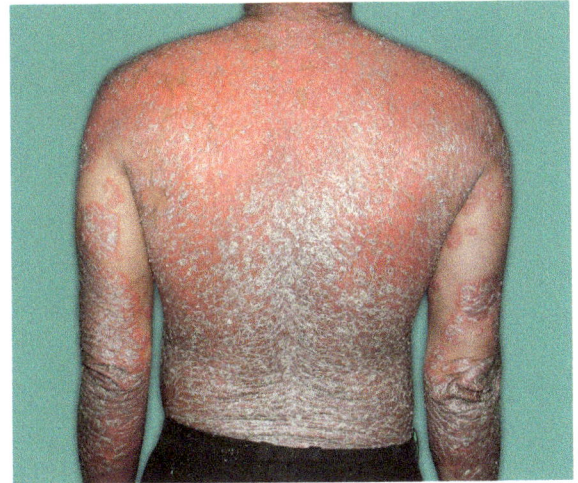

a. Guttate psoriasis
b. Extensive plaque psoriasis progressing to erythroderma
c. Flexural psoriasis
d. Annular psoriasis

147. This patient presented with acute swelling of lower lip with severe unbearable pain with no itching. What is the diagnosis?

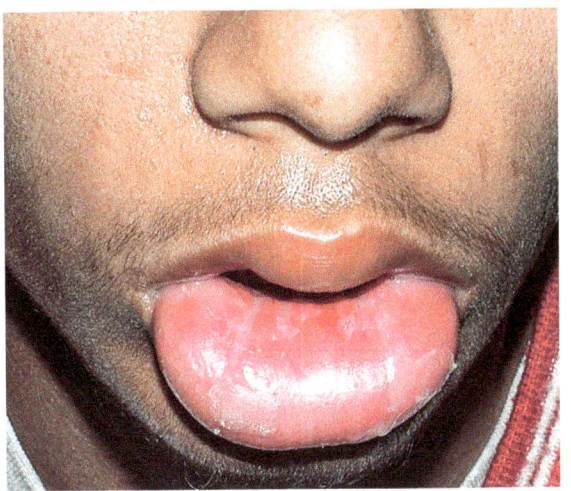

a. Angioedema
b. Boil lower lip
c. Granulomatous cheilitisd
Acute urticaria

148. This old man presented with geometrically-shaped dark purplish patches on arm and forearm. Skin of this patient is dry, scaly, thin with prominent and deep skin markings. What is clinical diagnosis?

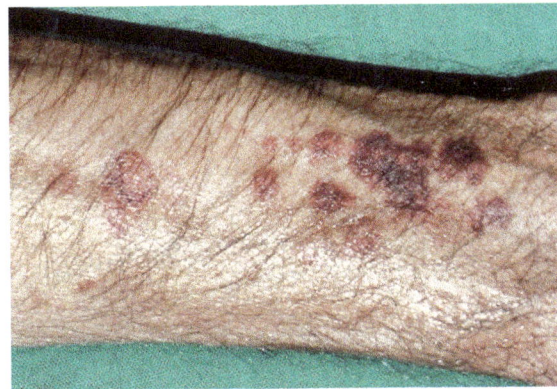

a. Idiopathic thrombocytopenic purpura
b. Henoch-Schonlein purpura
c. Senile purpura
d. Schamberg' disease

149. A compound nevus gets surrounded by a halo of depigmentation. What is the diagnosis?

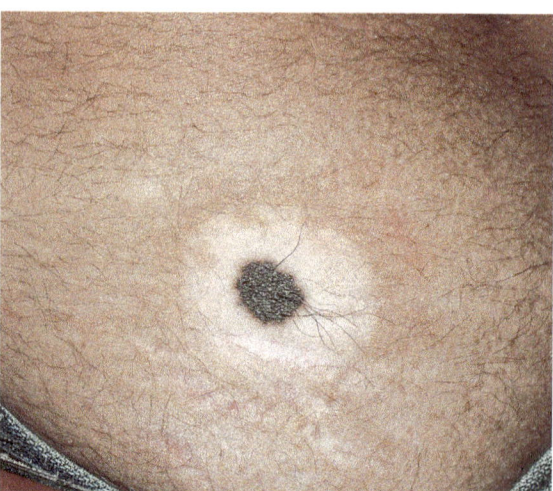

a. Nevus of Ota
b. Intradermal nevus
c. Sutton's nevus
d. Spitz nevus

150. A 50-year-old man presented with itchy ill-defined plaques on both soles. It was accompanied by oozing, crusting, scaling and recurrence for the last 4 years. What is the clinical diagnosis?

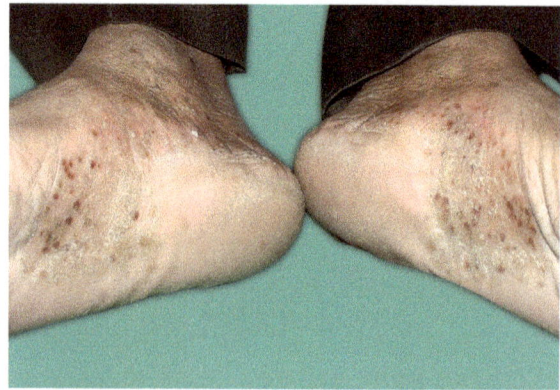

a. Plantar psoriasis
b. Tinea pedis
c. Focal plantar keratoderma
d. Eczema soles

151. A newborn presented with bluish black large patches of hyperpigmentation in the lumbosacral region. Histologically, it showed spindle shaped melanocytes in the deep dermis. What is the clinical diagnosis?

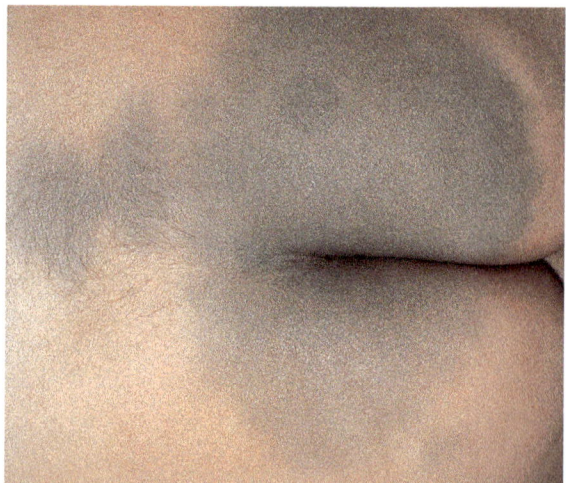

a. Becker's nevus
b. Mongolian spots
c. Congenital melanocytic nevus (CMN)
d. Nevus of Ito

152. Three months after some injection this patient developed depigmentation. Which one of following possibilities could be the reason?

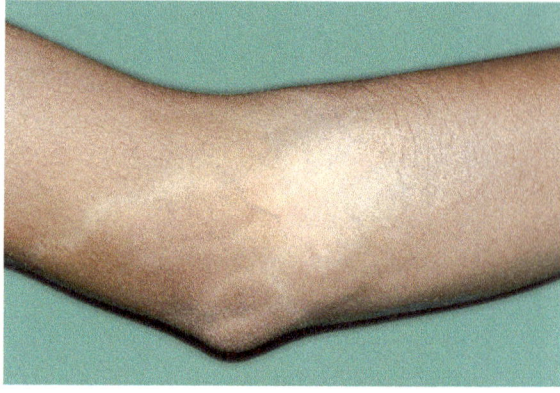

a. It is a vitiligo, injection in just a coincidence
b. It is leukoderma caused by spill over triamcinolone acetonide during intra-articular injection by an orthopedic surgeon
c. It is due to repeated use of analgesic creams
d. Nevus depigmentosus, injection in just a co-incidence

153. A 30-year-old man complained of redness and greasy scales involving whole scalp uniformly and extending beyond frontal hairline. What is the clinical diagnosis?

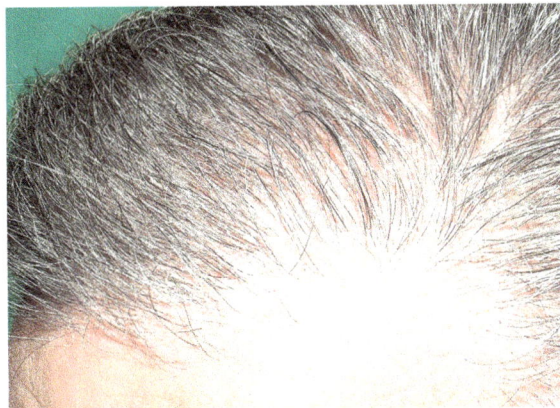

a. Psoriasis scalp
b. Seborrheic dermatitis
c. Tinea capitis
d. Cradle cap

154. This patient has scarring on face after a vesicular rash on face, trunk and extremities. With which one of the following disorders the rash belongs to?

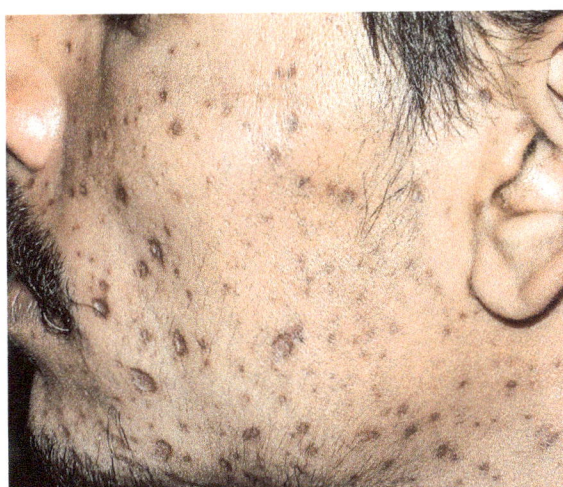

a. Measles
b. Chickenpox
c. Scarlet fever
d. Herpes simplex

155. This patient had uncountable small asymptomatic various sized papular lesions on trunk and extremities for the last few months. He also had infiltration of both pinnae. What can be the diagnosis?

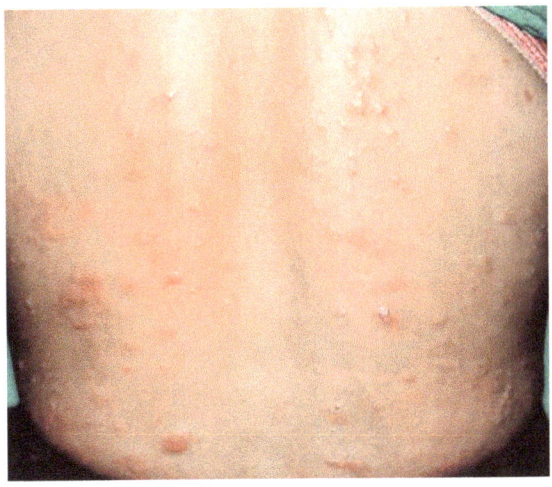

a. Acne vulgaris
b. Lepromatous leprosy
c. Eruptive lichen planus
d. Secondary syphilis
e. Acneiform eruption

156. A 20-year-old boy had multiples variable sized, well defined totally bald patches. The periphery of the lesions showed "exclamation mark hairs". What is the diagnosis?

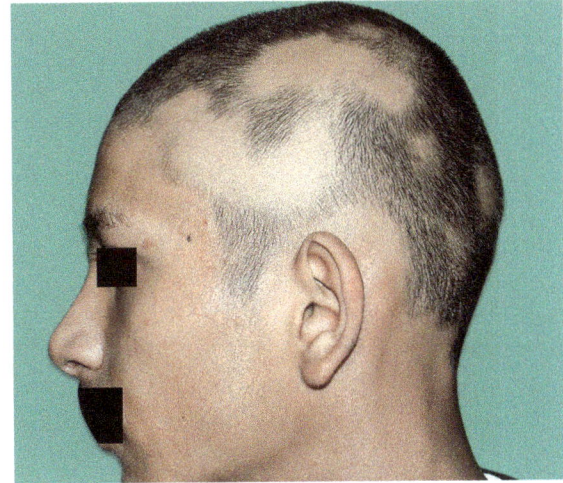

a. Trichotillomania
b. Tinea capitis
c. Alopecia areata
d. Telogen effluvium

157. A 35-year-old patient presented with a single painful dome shaped, reddish hard tender lump on back and has multiple pus discharging follicular openings giving an appearance of a sieve. What is the diagnosis?

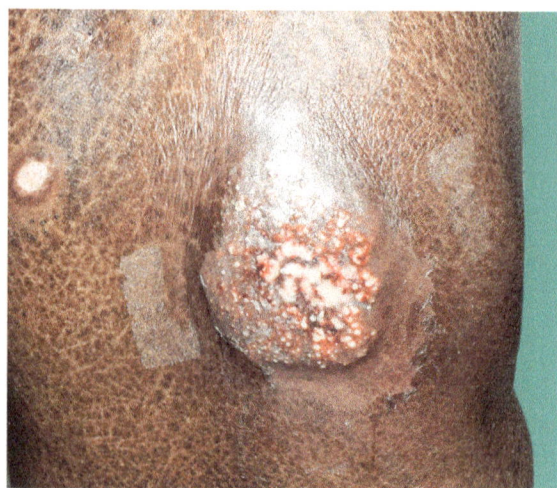

a. Infected sebaceous cyst
b. Furuncle
c. Kerion
d. Carbuncle

158. She complained of bluish gray pigmentation on one side of face in the distribution of first two division of trigeminal nerve since birth. It was accompanied by pigmentation of cornea also. What is the diagnosis?

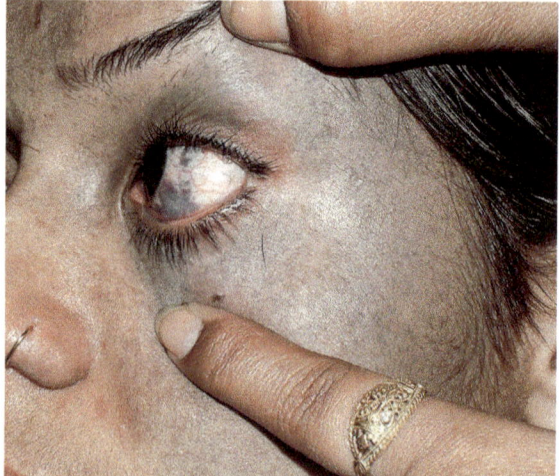

a. Sutton's nevus
b. Nevus of Ota
c. Compound nevus
d. Junctional nevus

159. A 14-year-old child presented with recurrent itching, erythema, oozing in the both popliteal and cubital fossae. What is the clinical diagnosis?

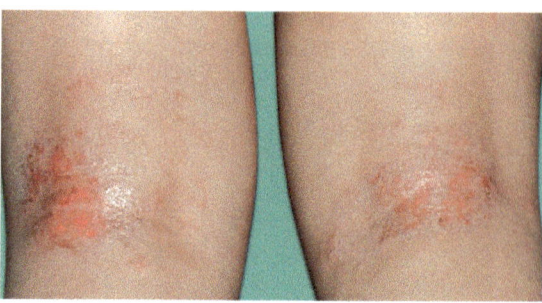

a. Atopic dermatitis (AD)
b. Seborrheic dermatitis (SD)
c. Discoid eczema
d. Flexural psoriasis

160. Few hours after taking some drug, this patient developed itching and burning sensation on glans penis with no accompanying cutaneous lesions. Glans showed dusky discoloration with superficial vesiculation. What is the diagnosis?

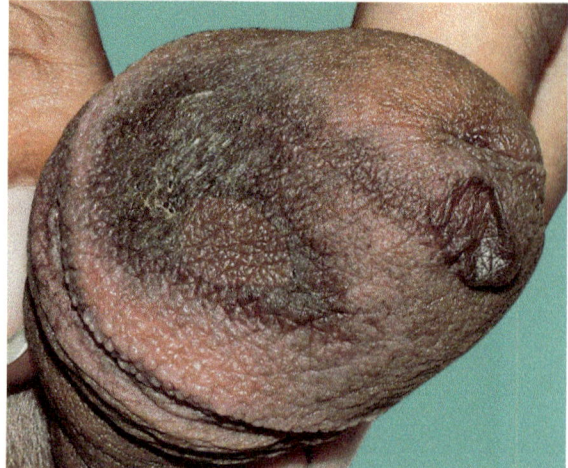

a. Lichen planus
b. Stevens-Johnson syndrome (SJS)
c. Erythema multiforme (EM)
d. Fixed drug eruption (FDE)

161. This patient presented with a crop of asymptomatic small discrete oval macules covered by fine scales. Scales were attached peripherally with free edge towards centre. Lesions were distributed symmetrically on trunk along the ribs. What is the clinical diagnosis?

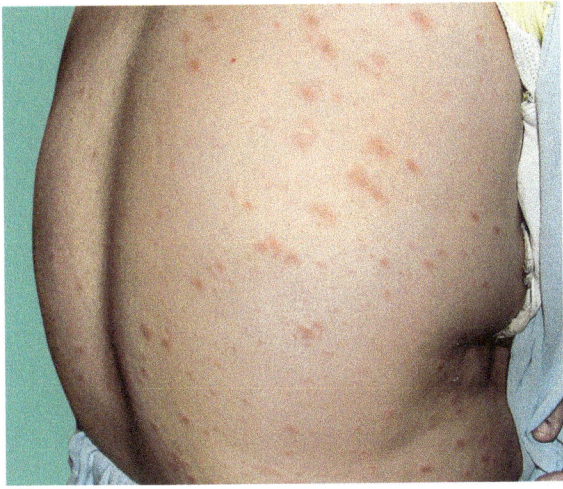

a. Pityriasis rosea
b. Psoriasis
c. Pityriasis lichenoides et varioliformis acuta (PLEVA)
d. Tinea corporis

162. A 9-year-old boy presented with multiple red papules and plaques studded with easily removable silvery white scales. It involved trunk, extremities and scalp. What is the clinical diagnosis?

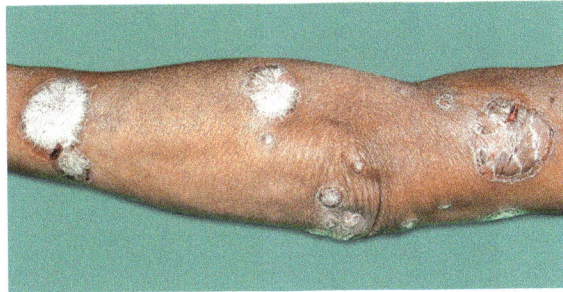

a. Lichen planus (LP)
b. Psoriasis
c. Pityriasis lichenoides chronica (PLC)
d. Parapsoriasis

163. Three months after typhoid fever, she had sudden, diffuse and excessive loss of scalp hair. Which one of the followings in a closest possibility for her?

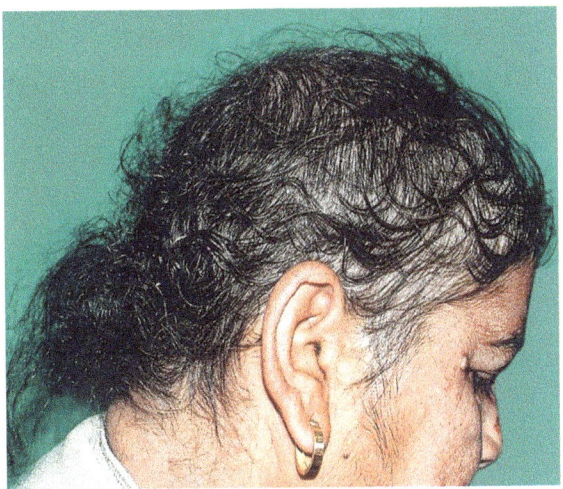

a. Androgenic alopecia
b. Alopecia areata
c. Trichotillomania
d. Telogen effluvium

164. Presence of retroauricular dermatitis favors the diagnosis of which one of the following disorders?

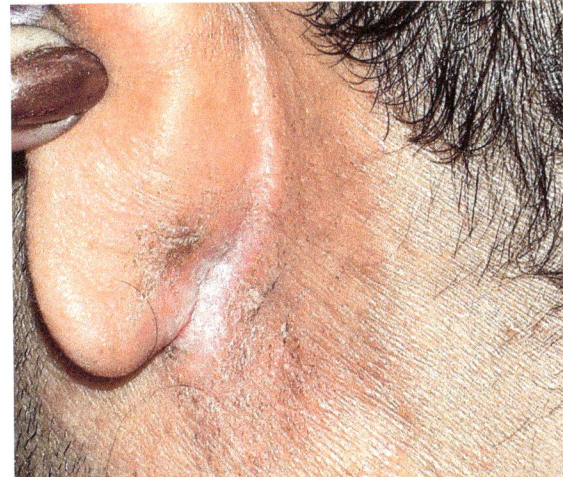

a. Atopic dermatitis (AD)
b. Seborrheic dermatitis
c. Psoriasis
d. Candidal intertrigo due to underlying diabetes

165. A 35-year-old female started having fever and malaise. It was followed by appearance of crop of vesicles on face. It spread down to chest and back. Vesicles are surrounded by irregular rim of erythema. What is the diagnosis?

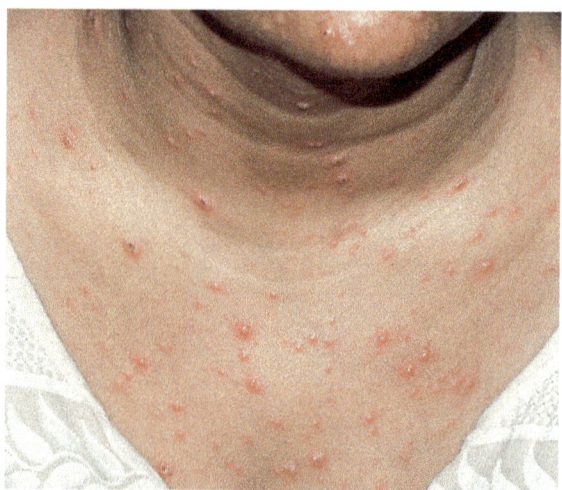

a. Chickenpox
b. Measles
c. Acne vulgaris
d. Erythema multiforme (EM)

166. This obese patient complained of itching, redness and soreness in both groins. What is clinical diagnosis?

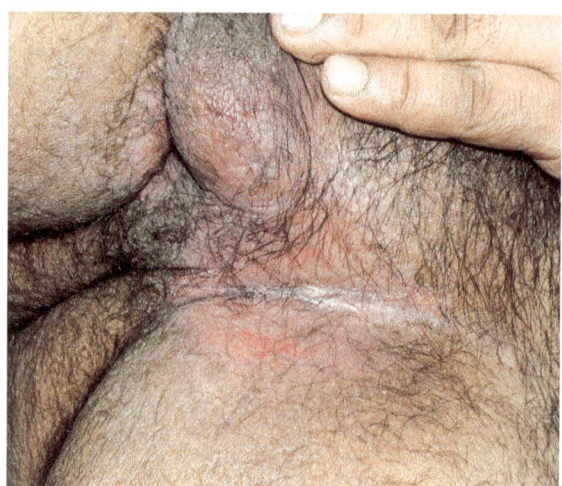

a. Candidal intertrigo
b. Flexural psoriasis
c. Intertrigo
d. Tinea cruris

167. A 14-year-old girl presented with a big patch of hair loss on frontotemporal side of scalp in a span of one year. What is the diagnosis?

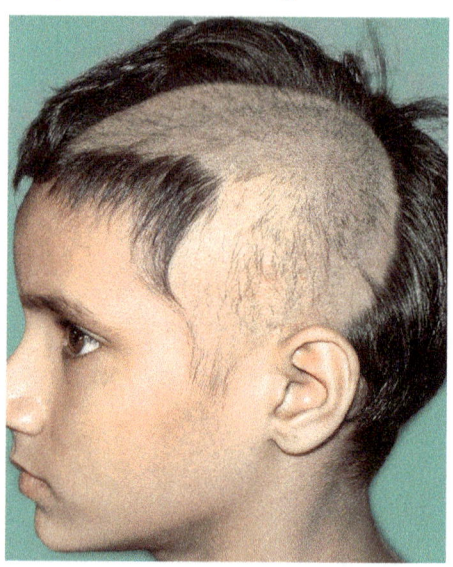

a. Alopecia areata
b. Telogen effluvium
c. Trichotillomania
d. Androgenic hair loss

168. A 2-month-old infant presented with adherent greasy scales on scalp. It is a manifestation of which one of the following disorders?

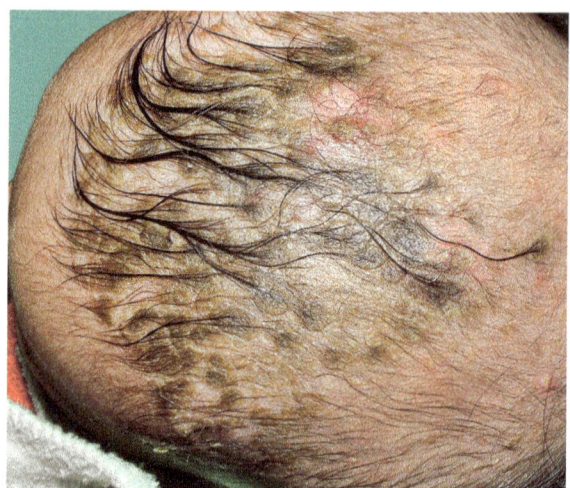

a. Atopic dermatitis (AD)
b. Seborrheic dermatitis (SD)
c. Tinea capitis
d. Psoriasis

169. This patient complained of asymptomatic, discrete, skin-colored papules with hyperkeratotic surface. What is the clinical diagnosis?

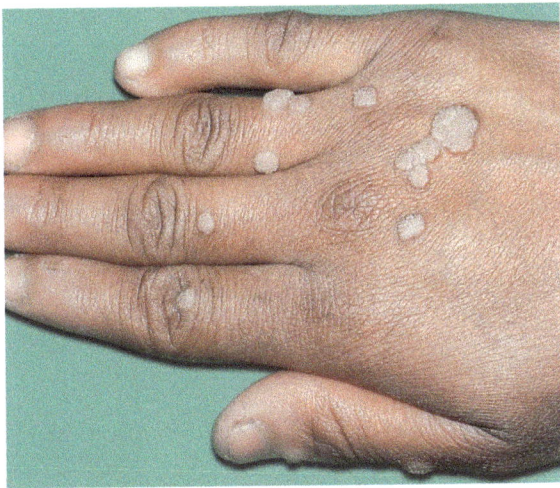

a. Common warts
b. Lichen planus
c. Psoriasis
d. Molluscum contagiosum (MC)

170. This patient presented with extremely itchy, hard papulonodular lesions with raised warty surface on lower extremities for the last 2–3 years.

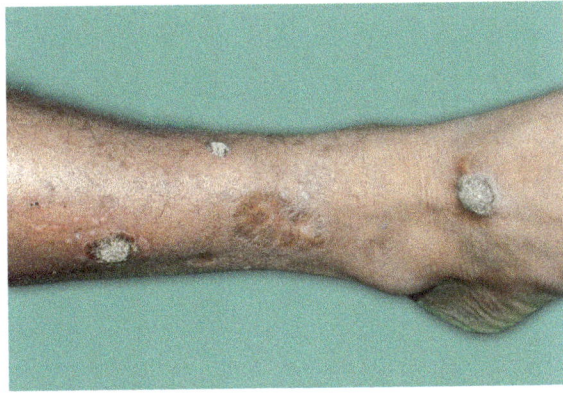

a. Lichen simplex
b. Lichen planus (LP)
c. Prurigo nodularis (PN)
d. Common warts

171. This patient complained of erythema and itching on face along with scaling on eyelashes and nasolabial folds and moustache. What is the clinical diagnosis?

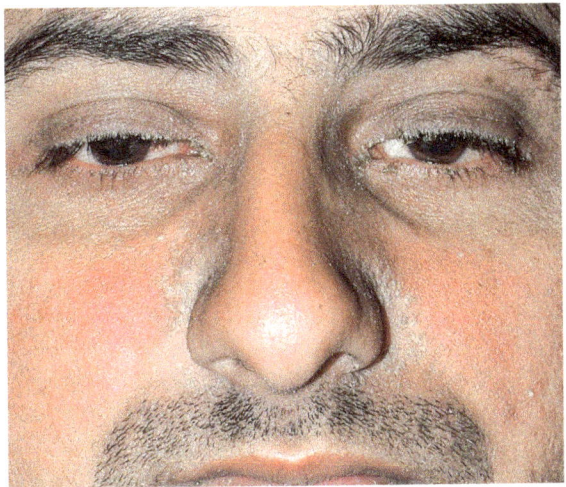

a. Atopic dermatitis
b. Tinea faciei
c. Seborrheic dermatitis (SD)
d. Airborne contact dermatitis (ABCD)

172. A 2-year-old child presented with persistent itchy red papular with central punctum on face and extensor surface of extremities. Other family members are normal. What is the diagnosis?

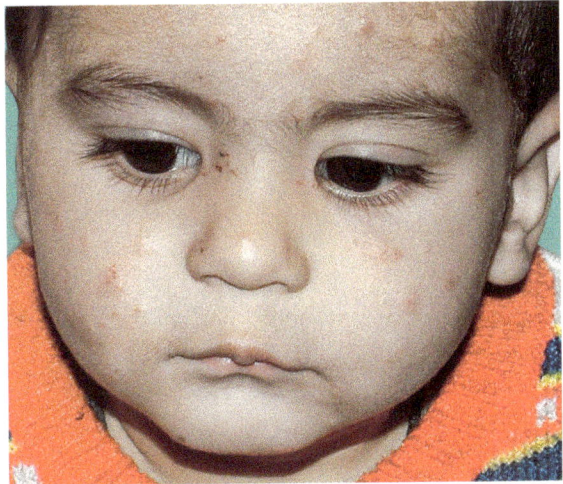

a. Papular urticaria (Insect bite hypersensitivity)
b. Molluscum contagiosum (MC)
c. Scabies
d. Impetigo contagiosa

173. She presented with a crop of vesicles surrounded by erythema on face, trunk and extremities. It was preceded by fever and malaise. What is the diagnosis?

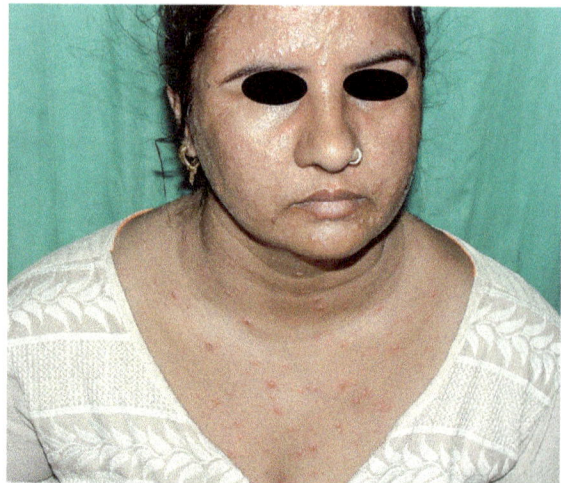

a. Impetigo contagiosa
b. Pemphigus vulgaris
c. Chickenpox
d. Measles

174. A 10-month-old child was having erythema, oozing and crusting on his face for the last few months. He was also having discrete and confluent edematous and exudative plaques on extensor surfaces of limbs. What is the clinical diagnosis?

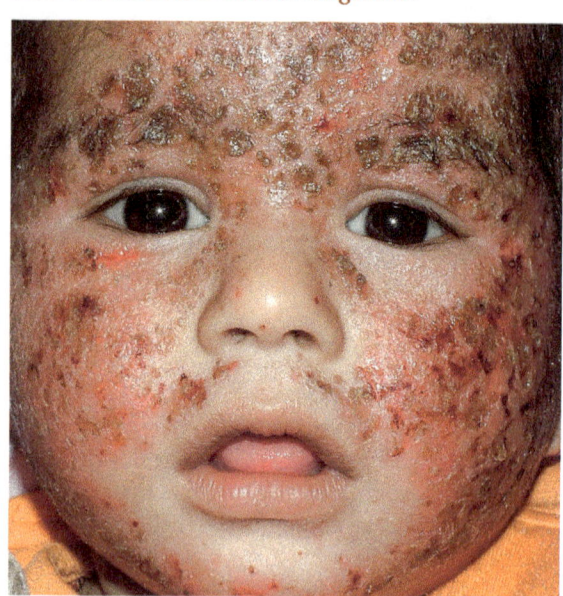

a. Seborrheic dermatitis (SD)
b. Infantile phase of atopic dermatitis (AD)
c. Impetigo contagiosa
d. Measles

175. This patient complained of itching, erythema and greasy white scales in the cervical, presternal and submammary regions. What is the clinical diagnosis?

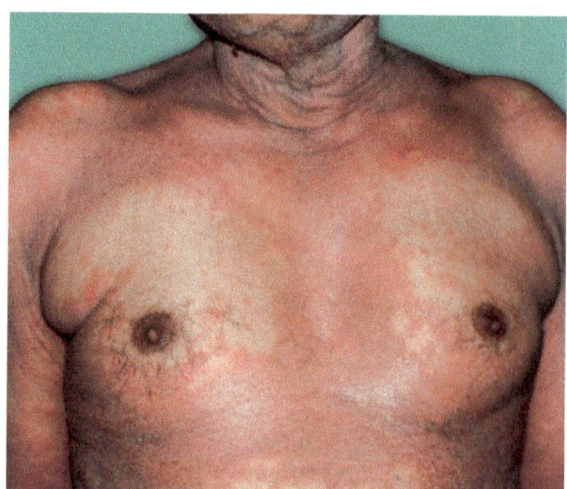

a. Atopic dermatitis (AD)
b. Tinea corporis
c. Seborrheic dermatitis (SD)
d. Flexural psoriasis

176. This patient presented with itchy red papules and nodules on chest. What is the clinical diagnosis?

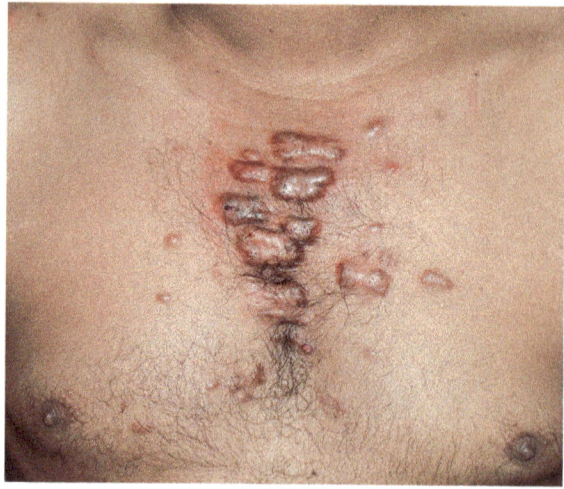

a. Hypertrophic lichen planus
b. Hypertrophic scars
c. Chronic cutaneous lupus erythematosus (CCLE)
d. Keloids on chest

177. This patient presented with a thick, itchy plaque with hyperpigmentation and increased skin markings. What is the clinical diagnosis?

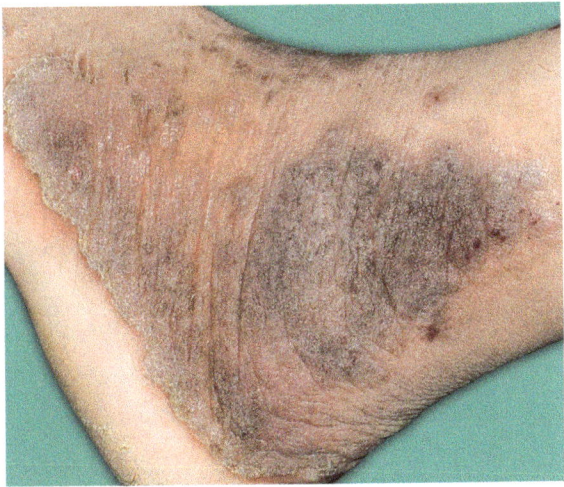

a. Psoriasis
b. Lichenified chronic eczema
c. Lichen planus hypertrophicus (LPH)
d. Tuberculosis verrucosa cutis (TVC)

178. Nails in this patient shows red longitudinal bands which end in V-shaped notch at the free margin of nail. In which of the following conditions are seen these changes?

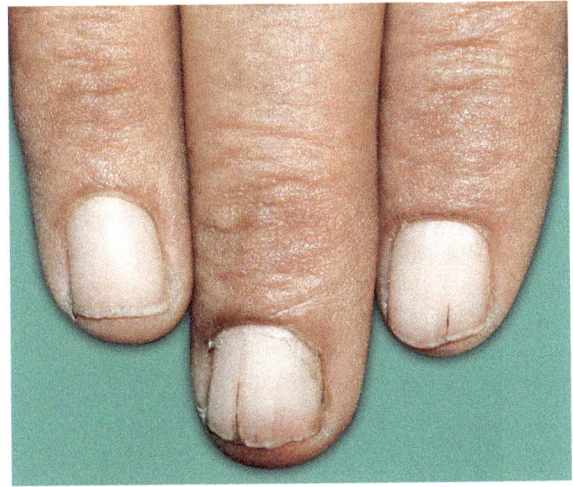

a. Lichen planus
b. Alopecia areata
c. Darier's disease
d. Psoriasis

179. This man presented with red macerations in both groins. Involvement is extending beyond the area of contact and is showing fringed irregular margin with satellite vesicles and pustules at the periphery. What is the clinical diagnosis?

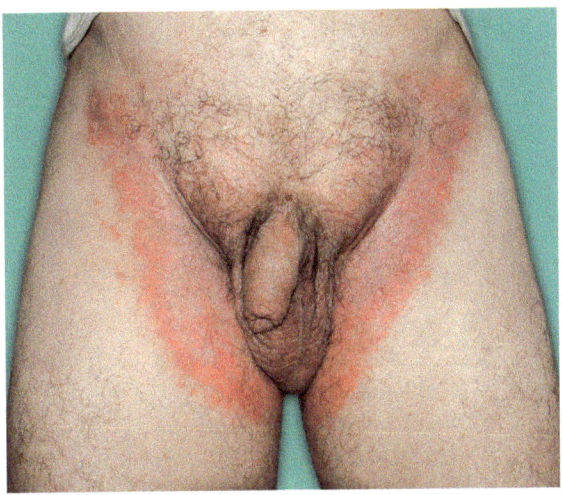

a. Tinea cruris
b. Candidal intertrigo
c. Flexural psoriasis
d. Intertrigo

180. This patient presented with itchy small vesicles on the sides of fingers for the last 2 months. Genitals and buttocks are normal. But he is having infected and inflamed foot injury. What is the clinical diagnosis?

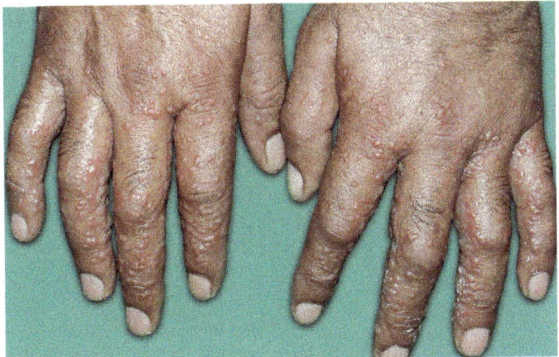

a. Infected scabies
b. Id eruption
c. Contact dermatitis due to cement
d. Pompholyx

181. This girl presented with depigmented macules on left side face for the last one year. What is the clinical diagnosis?

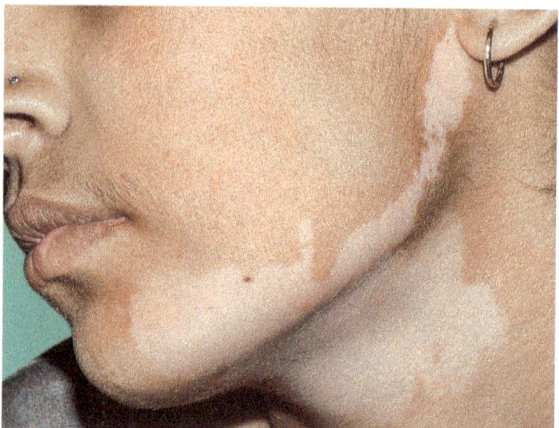

a. Nevus depigmentosus
b. Nevus anemicus
c. Segmental vitiligo
d. Focal vitiligo

182. This male presented with brownish pigmentation on both cheeks for the last 2–3 years. What is the clinical diagnosis?

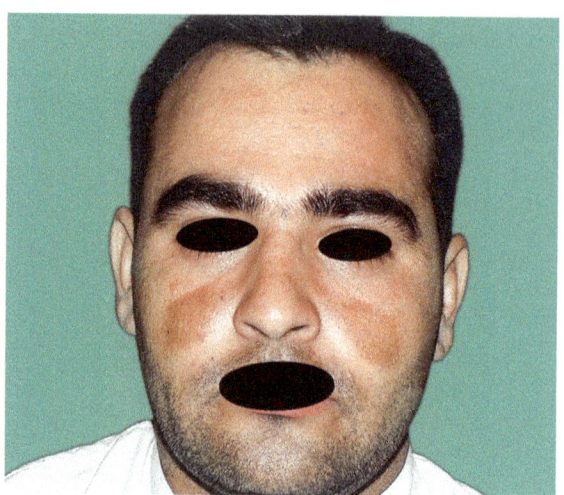

a. Butterfly rash due to SLE
b. Melasma
c. Chloasma
d. Phototoxic reaction

183. This housewife presented with red, macerated finger web spaces accompanied by itching. What is the diagnosis?

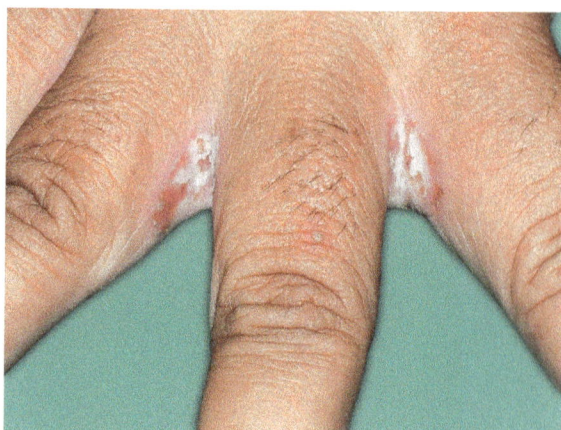

a. Scabies
b. Candidal intertrigo
c. Id eruption
d. Tinea manuum

184. A 40-year-old female presented with oral ulcers and painful hemorrhagic crusting of lips for the last 3 months. She also had large, painful erosions on face and trunk. Nikolsky's sign was positive. What is the clinical diagnosis?

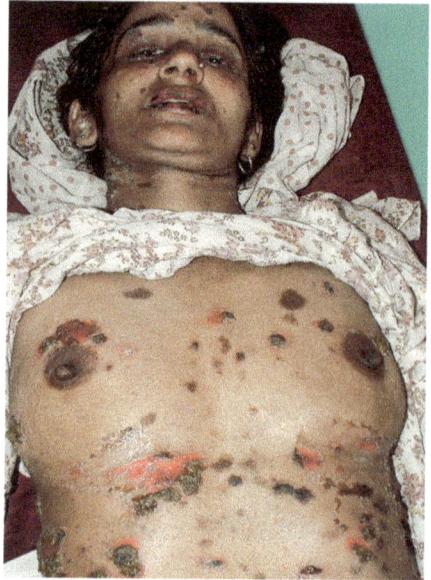

a. Bullous pemphigoid (BP)
b. Linear IgA dermatosis
c. Pemphigus vulgaris
d. Stevens-Johnson syndrome (SJS)

185. A 50-year-old female presented with baldness in central part of scalp with intact frontal hair line. What is the diagnosis?

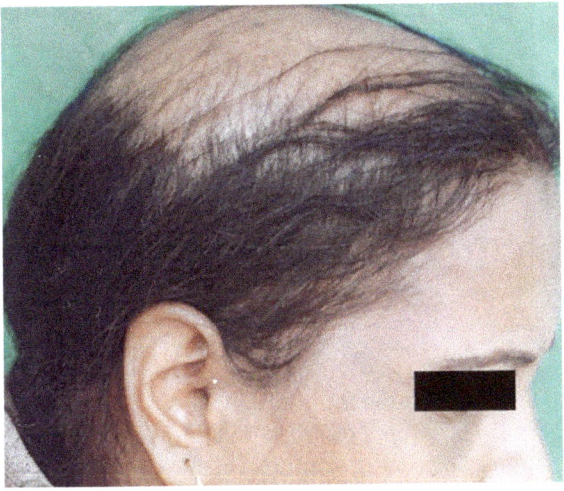

a. Androgenic hair loss
b. Trichotillomania
c. Alopecia areata
d. Telogen effluvium

186. An 18-year-old boy presented with cicatricial type hair loss on scalp. He was also having pruritic purplish colored papules on peripheral parts of body. What is the clinical diagnosis?

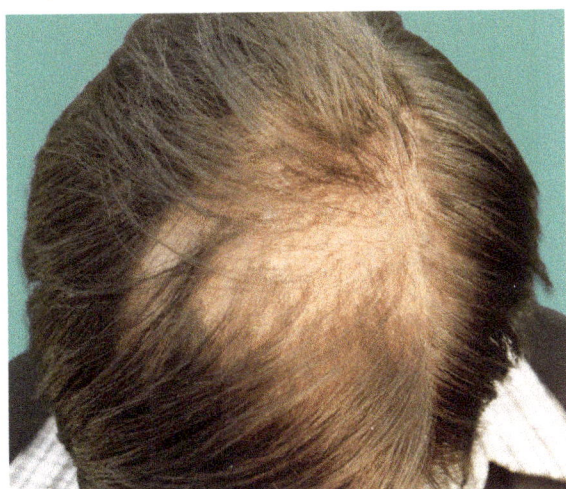

a. Lichen planus
b. Chronic cutaneous lupus erythematosus (CCLE)
c. Trichotillomania
d. Tinea capitis

187. This child presented with sharply circumscribed, round, scarlet red single tumor on the side of nose since the age of 1 month. What is the clinical diagnosis?

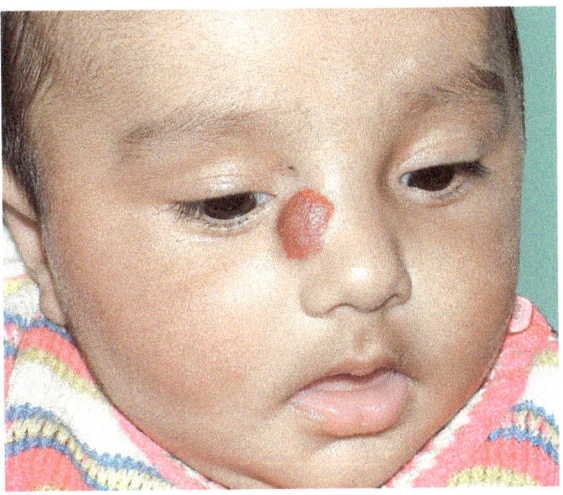

a. Pyogenic granuloma
b. Port-wine stain
c. Cherry angioma
d. Strawberry hemangioma

188. A 22-year-old male presented with dry, rough skin with fish like uniform scaling on various parts of body since his childhood. What is the clinical diagnosis?

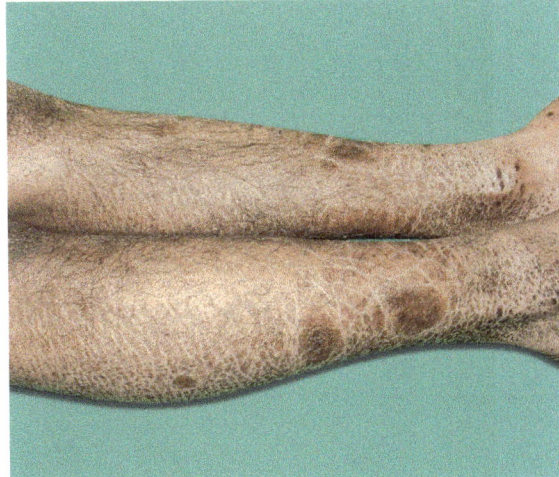

a. Asteatotic eczema
b. Ichthyosis
c. Ichthyosis due to clofazimine
d. Hypothyroidism

189. This patient presented with these linear lesions on left upper and lower extremities. The lesions appeared overnight and patient was unable to give clear history of appearance and evolution of lesions. What is the clinical diagnosis?

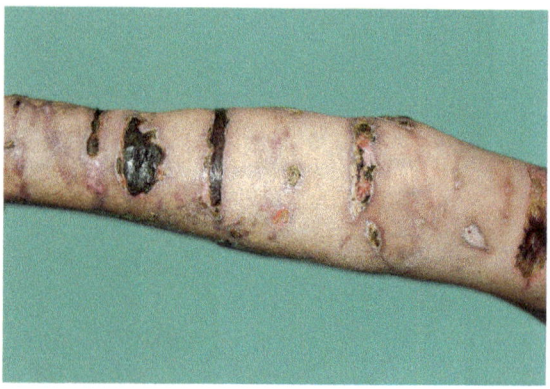

a. Discoid eczema
b. Lupus vulgaris
c. Dermatitis artefacta
d. Psoriasis
e. Ecthyma

190. A 40-year-old female complained of diffuse loss of hair along the midline of scalp in the last couple of years. What is the clinical diagnosis?

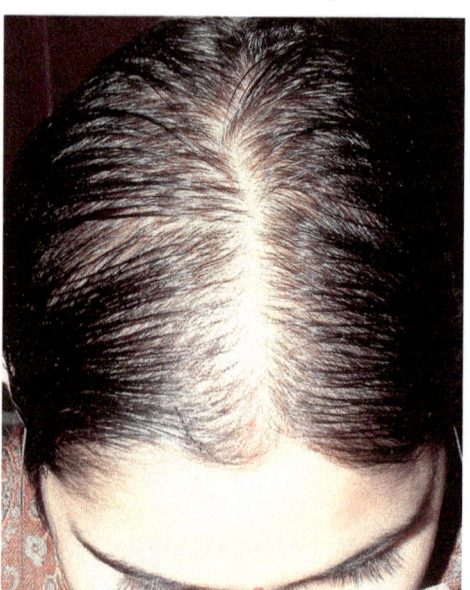

a. Telogen effluvium
b. Alopecia areata
c. Trichotillomania
d. Androgenic alopecia

191. Few hours after intake of cotrimoxazole this patient developed dusky colored large patches surrounded by rim of erythema. There was no mucosal involvement. What is the clinical diagnosis?

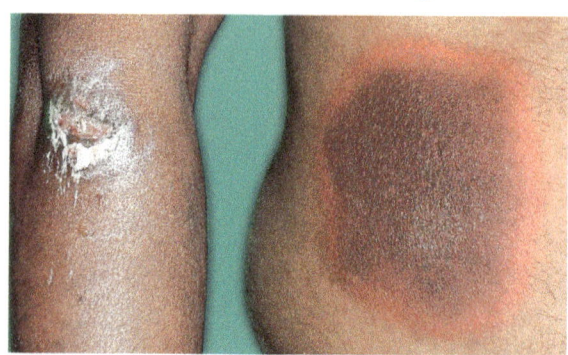

a. Erythema multiforme major (EM major)
b. Erythema multiforme minor (EM minor)
c. Fixed drug eruption (FDE)
d. SJ Syndrome (SJS)

192. This patient presented with asymptomatic yellowish waxy uniform thickening of both soles for the last many years. What is the clinical diagnosis?

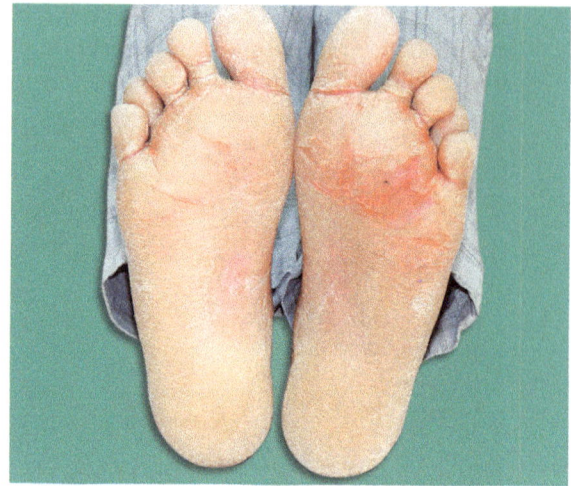

a. Eczema soles
b. Diffuse plantar keratoderma
c. Plantar psoriasis
d. Tinea pedis

193. This old patient presented with a single varied colored patch having raised pigmented irregular and thread like margins. Central part of the lesion is showing atrophy and some scaling. What is the clinical diagnosis?

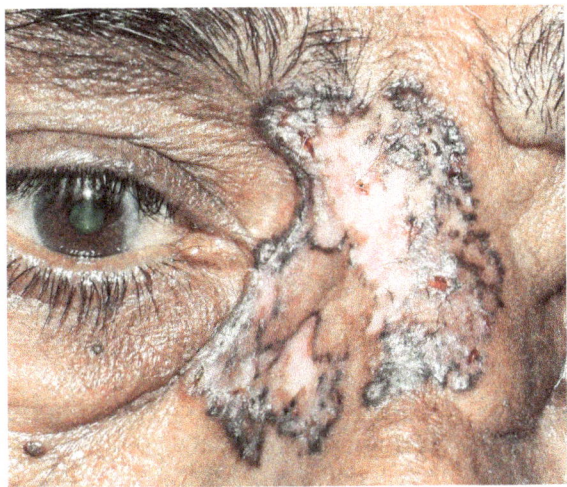

a. Squamous cell carcinoma (SCC)
b. Chronic cutaneous lupus erythematosus (CCLE)
c. Superficial basal cell carcinoma (BCC)
d. Lupus vulgaris (LV)
e. Malignant melanoma (MM)

194. This patient presented with disc-shaped itchy lesions having oozing and crusting. What is the clinical diagnosis?

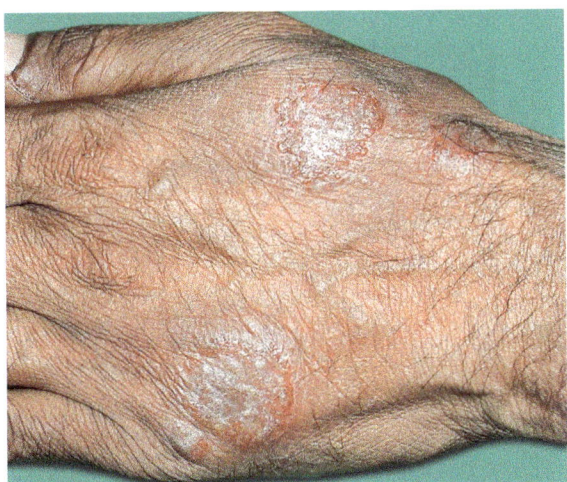

a. Tinea corporis
b. Psoriasis
c. Discoid eczema
d. Lichen planus

195. This patient presented with a single, about 3 cm sized, asymptomatic patch with dark peripheral zone and central wrinkled area. It was followed by appearance of a crop of similar but smaller lesions on trunk along the ribs. What is the clinical diagnosis?

a. Mother patch of pityriasis rosea
b. Guttate psoriasis
c. Pityriasis versicolor
d. Pityriasis lichenoides et varioliformis acuta (PLEVA)

196. A 58-year-old patient presented with symmetrical pinkish red, shiny infiltrative plaques mainly on sun exposed areas of face. It is sparing the area covered by turban and the area below lower eyelids. It is severe in summer. What is the clinical diagnosis?

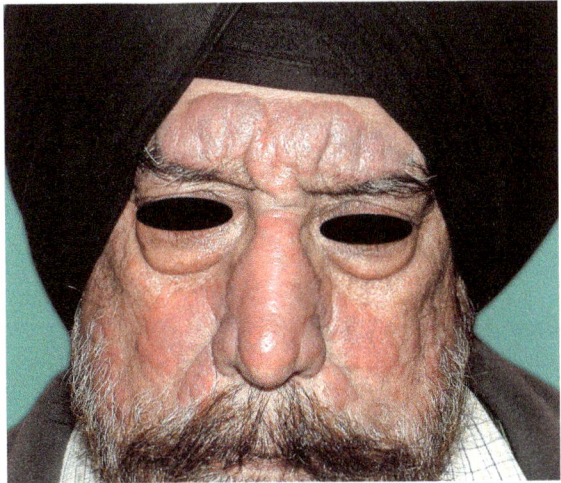

a. Airborne contact dermatitis (ABCD)
b. Chronic actinic dermatitis (CAD)
c. Lupus pernio
d. Polymorphous light eruption (PMLE)

197. She presented with severe itching of vulva for the last 2-3 years along with thickening, dark coloration, increased cutaneous markings and ill defined margin. There was no history of vaginal discharge or diabetes. What is the clinical diagnosis?

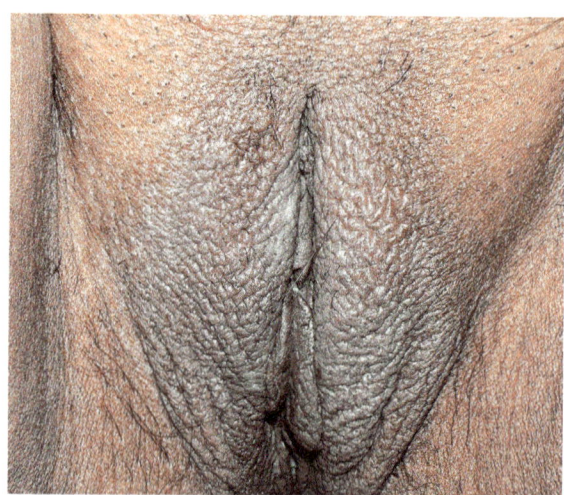

a. Lichen simplex chronicus (LSC)
b. Vulvovaginal candidiasis (VCC)
c. Lichen sclerosus et atrophicus
d. Herpes simplex

198. Within few hours of sun light exposure, this young lady developed erythema, macules and papules on face in a symmetrical manner accompanied by itching. What is the closest clinical diagnosis?

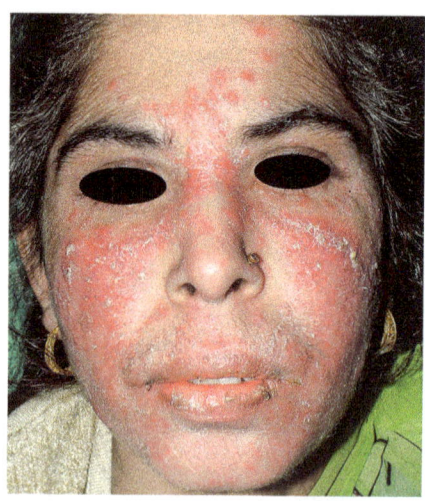

a. Chronic actinic dermatitis (CAD)
b. Polymorphous light eruption (PMLE)
c. Actinic prurigo
d. Hydroa vacciniforme
e. Solar urticaria

199. Within few hours of taking some drug, this patient developed itching and erosions of lips. It was followed by grayish pigmentation of both lips extending to perioral area. What is the clinical diagnosis?

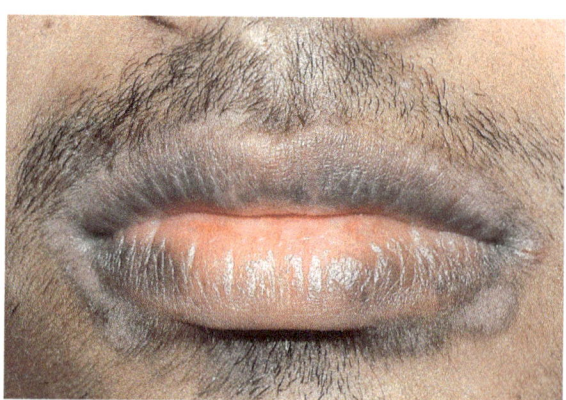

a. Lip-lick cheilitis
b. Fixed drug eruption (FDE) lips
c. Lichen planus lips
d. Tooth paste allergic dermatitis

200. Few hours after taking some drug, this patient developed a large bullous lesion on glans penis with no cutaneous lesions. What is the clinical diagnosis?

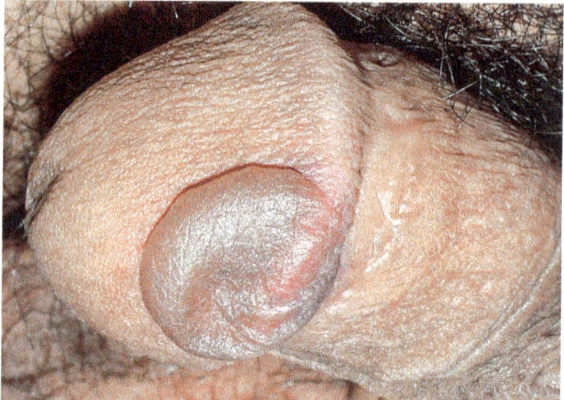

a. Lichen planus (LP)
b. Erythema multiforme (EM)
c. Fixed drug eruption (FDE)
d. Stevens-Johnson syndrome (SJS)

201. This patient shows well-defined thickening, redness, roughness, ulceration and crusting of lower lip. Bridge of the nose is also having red plaque with adherent crust. What is the clinical diagnosis?

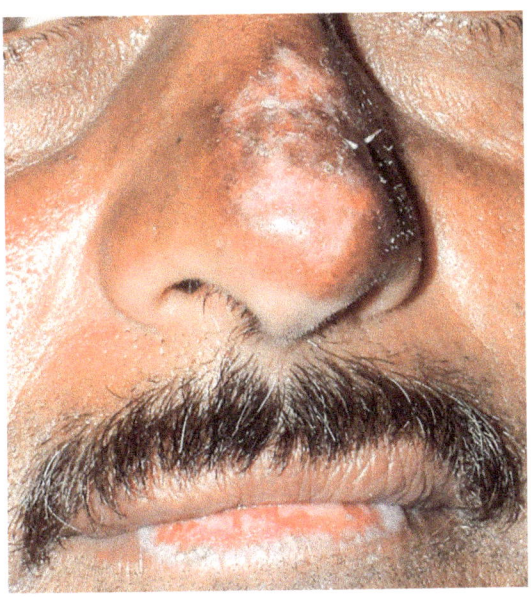

a. Lichen planus
b. Psoriasis
c. Chronic cutaneous lupus erythematosus (CCLE)
d. Lupus vulgaris

202. This patient complains of redness and itching both feet. What is the clinical diagnosis?

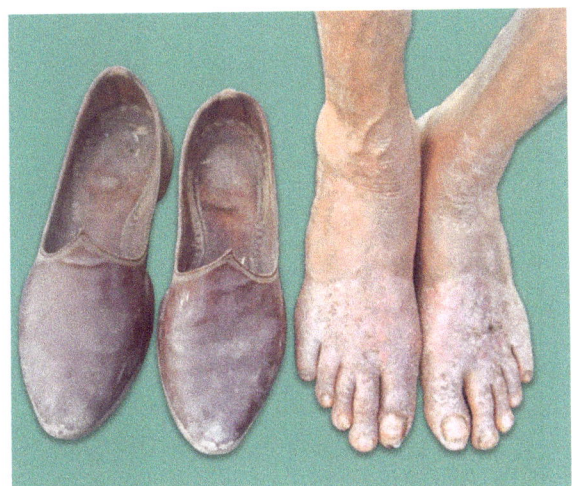

a. Candidiasis feet
b. Tinea pedis
c. Allergic contact dermatitis (ACD) due to shoes
d. Psoriasis of feet

203. This patient developed excessive hair loss on scalp, axillae, suprapubic region and extremities during chemotherapy for breast cancer. What is the clinical diagnosis?

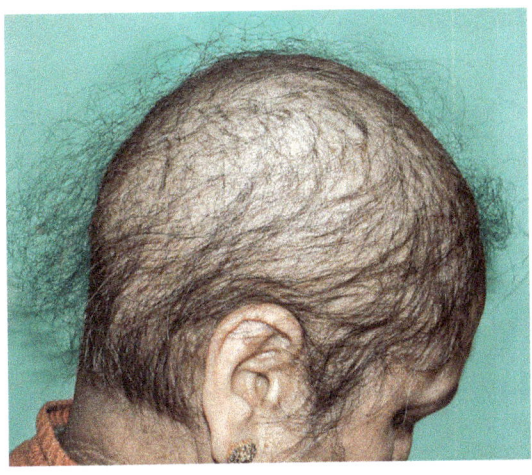

a. Alopecia universalis
b. Telogen effluvium
c. Anagen effluvium
d. Trichotillomania

204. A 1-year-old child presented with a large, red and well-defined plaque on scalp studded with white scaling. This child had red scaly plaques on other parts to body also. It is a manifestation of which one of the following disorders?

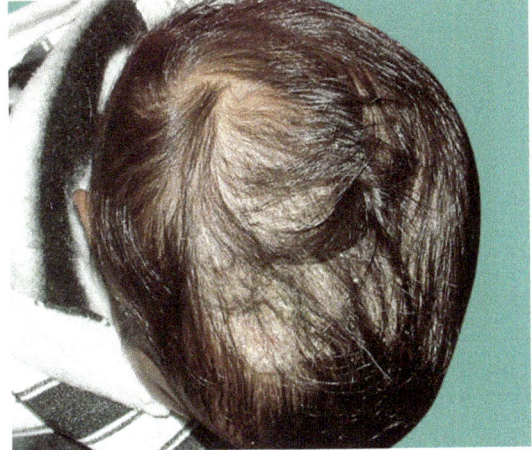

a. Psoriasis scalp
b. Seborrheic dermatitis (cradle cap)
c. Tinea capitis
d. Atopic dermatitis

205. Few weeks after surgery, this patient developed asymptomatic thickening of scar which is confined to the surgical incision. Which one of the following diagnoses it deserves?

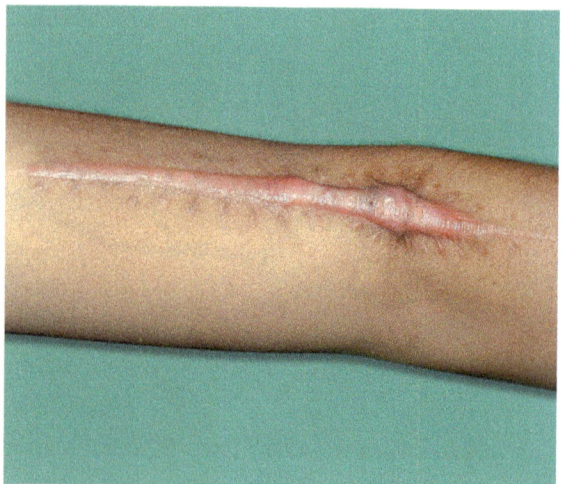

a. Keloid
b. Hypertrophic scar
c. Scar sarcoidosis

206. This patient is getting itchy, well demarcated erythematous pale swellings of skin for the last few days. Swellings last for few hours to reappear again at other site. What is the diagnosis?

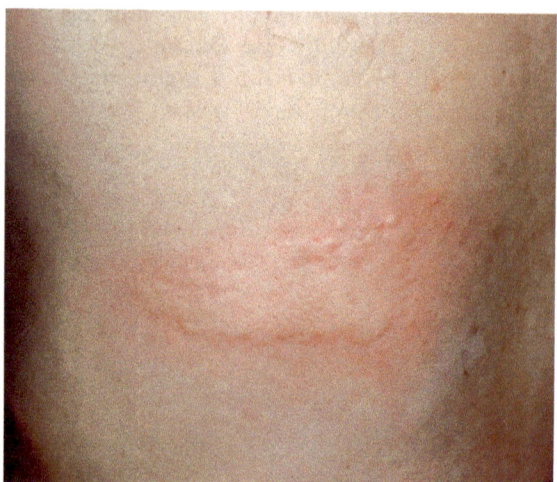

a. Symptomatic dermatographism
b. Acute urticaria
c. Chronic urticaria
d. Angioedema

207. A 15-year-old patient presented with itching, erythema and scaling with ill-defined margins in both cubital fossae for the last one year. What is the diagnosis?

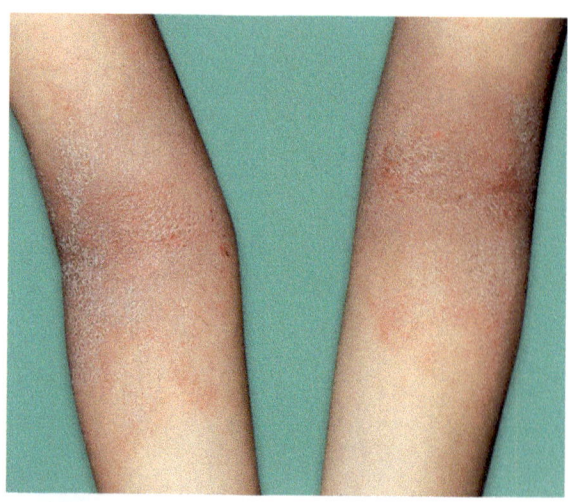

a. Tinea corporis
b. Atopic dermatitis (AD)
c. Seborrheic dermatitis (SD)
d. Flexural psoriasis

208. A 50-year-old patient presented with itchy violaceous papules and plaques five month after antitubercular treatment (ATT). What is the most appropriate diagnosis for this patient?

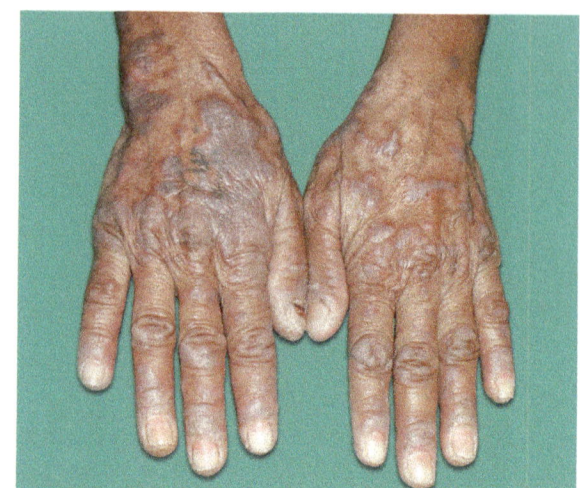

a. Psoriasis
b. Lichenoid eruptions
c. Common warts

209. This young patient presented with multiple, shiny, pearly white dome shaped and umbilicated papules in the suprapubic region for the last three months. What is the clinical diagnosis?

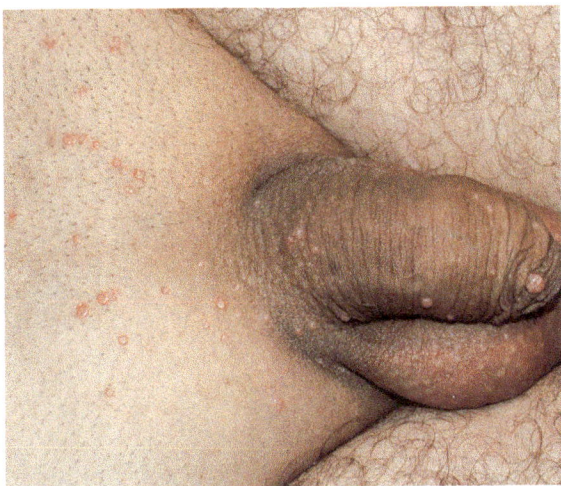

a. Lichen planus (LP)
b. Common warts
c. Molluscum contagiosum (MC)
d. Bacterial folliculitis

210. This patient complained of redness maceration, Itching and soreness of both soles for the last many months. What can be the clinical diagnosis?

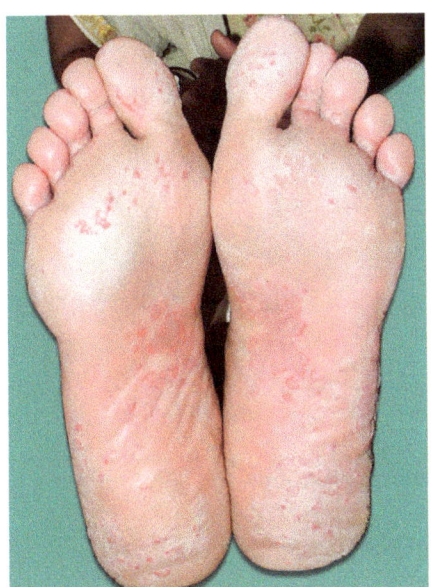

a. Tined pedis
b. Eczema soles
c. Candidiasis soles
d. Pitted keratolysis

211. This patient presented with 4–5 erythematous, scaly, well defined lesions with central clearing giving annular appearance. Sensations are impaired in the center. What is the clinical diagnosis?

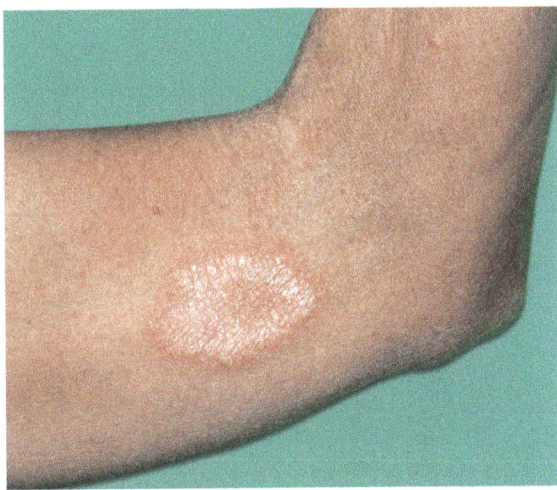

a. Tuberculoid leprosy
b. Mid-borderline leprosy
c. Indeterminate leprosy
d. Lepromatous leprosy

212. She presented with multiple mildly itchy reddish small patches with greasy scales in the interscapular area. There are no vesicles or crusting. Greasy scales were present in eye brows, eyelashes, nasolabial folds and flexures. What is the clinical diagnosis?

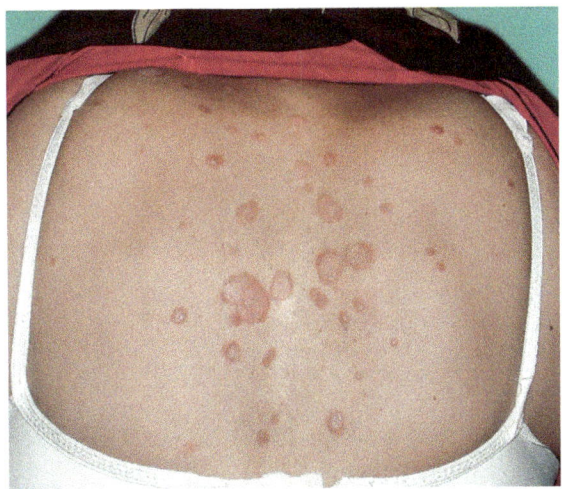

a. Pemphigus foliaceous (PF)
b. Tinea corporis
c. Pityriasis rosea (PR)
d. Pityriasis versicolor
e. Seborrheic dermatitis (SD)

213. This patient presented with itching, oozing thickening of dorsa of both feet with no well-defined margins. What is the clinical diagnosis?

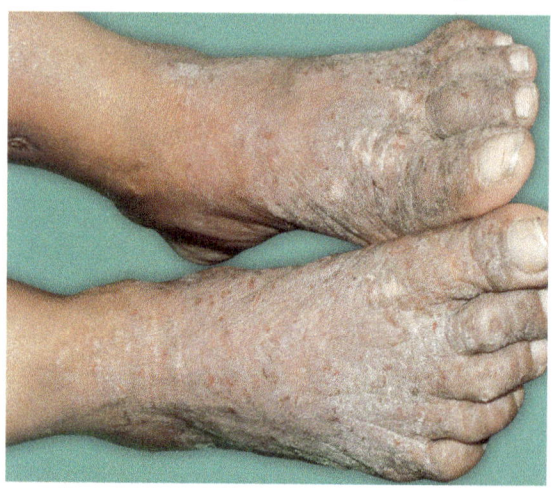

a. Tinea pedis
b. Eczema both feet
c. Contact dermatitis shoes
d. Psoriasis of feet

214. A 30-year-old male presented with asymptomatic papular or papulosquamous rash on palms for the last two months. Similar rash was also seen on lower extremities and trunk *(MCQ 293)* also. What is the clinical diagnosis?

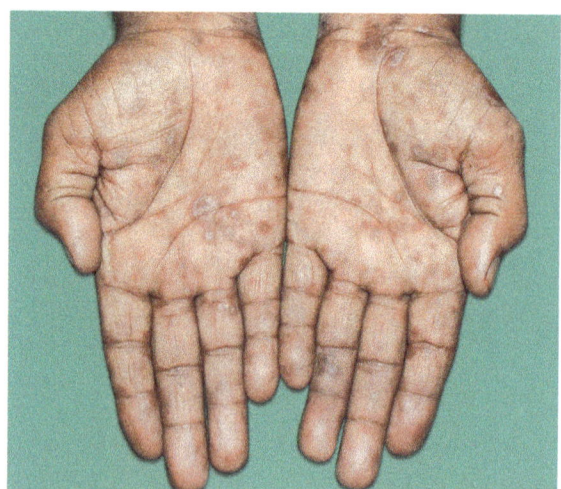

a. Lichen planus
b. Secondary syphilis
c. Erythema multiforme (EM)
d. Psoriasis of palms

215. Gum hypertrophy in this patient is due to which one of the following antiepilepsy drugs?

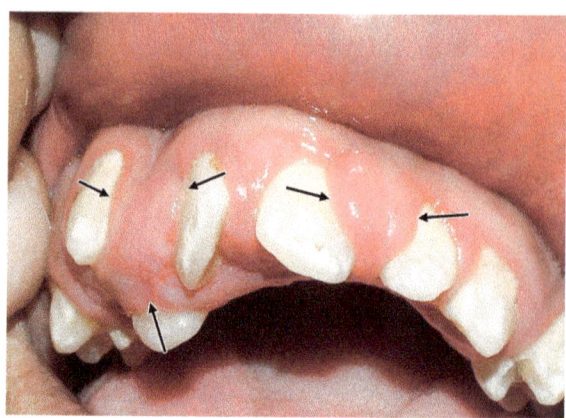

a. Phenobarbitone
b. Carbamazepine
c. Phenytoin
d. Lamotrigine

216. An adult male presented with papules, pustules and comedones on face. What is the clinical diagnosis?

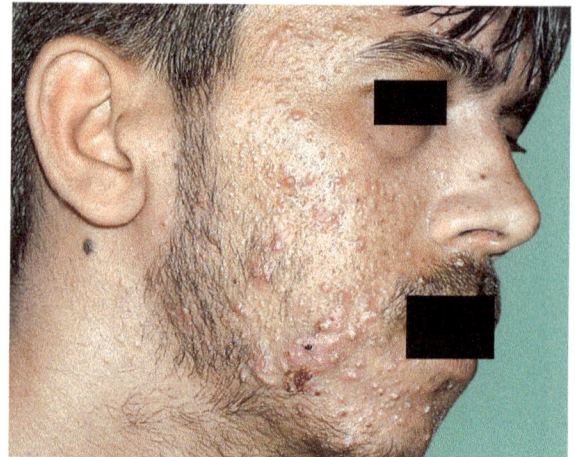

a. Acne rosacea
b. Acneiform eruption
c. Milia
d. Acne vulgaris

217. This patient presented with thickening of lips, puffiness of eyelids and face. She also complained of malaise, lethargy, constipation and hoarseness of voice. What is the clinical diagnosis?

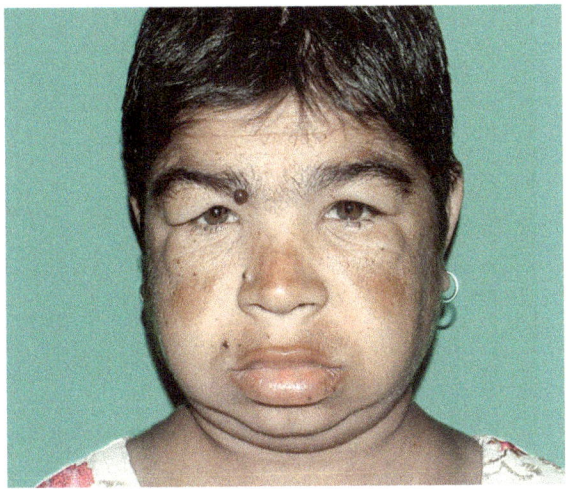

a. Lepromatous leprosy (LL)
b. Nephrotic syndrome
c. Myxedema (hypothyroidism)
d. Hepatic cirrhosis

218. A 10-year-old boy presented with eruption of vesicles on both palms with severe itching. What is the clinical diagnosis?

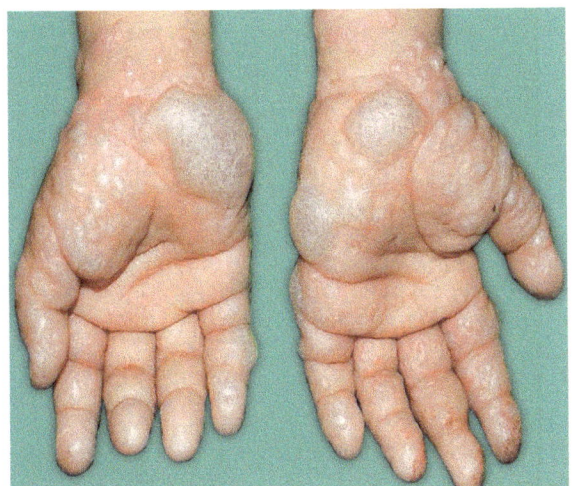

a. Contact dermatitis palms
b. Pompholyx
c. Id-eruption
d. Scabies with secondary infection

219. This patient complained of red colored, large, incomplete rings on the leg for the last many years. There was no itching or loss of sensation. What is the clinical diagnosis?

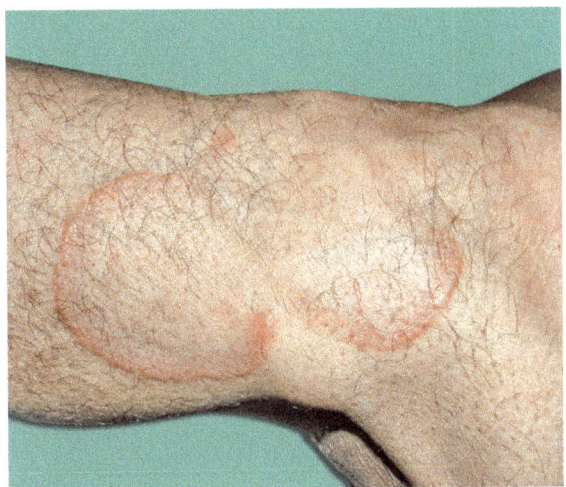

a. Tinea corporis
b. Annular lesions of mid-borderline leprosy
c. Granuloma annulare
d. Annular psoriasis

220. This patient complained of recurrent, oozy and itchy plaques with crusting on the dorsa of both hands. What is the clinical diagnosis?

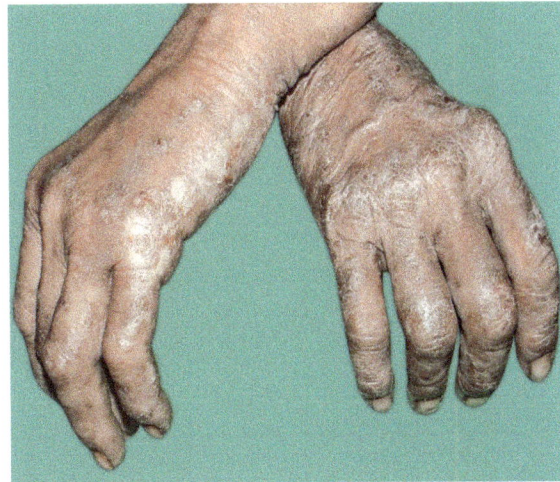

a. Psoriasis of hands
b. Tinea manuum
c. Eczema hands
d. Infected scabies

221. A 70-year-old lady presented with multiple 3–6 mm sized, asymptomatic cherry red colored vascular lesions on abdominal wall. What is the closest clinical diagnosis?

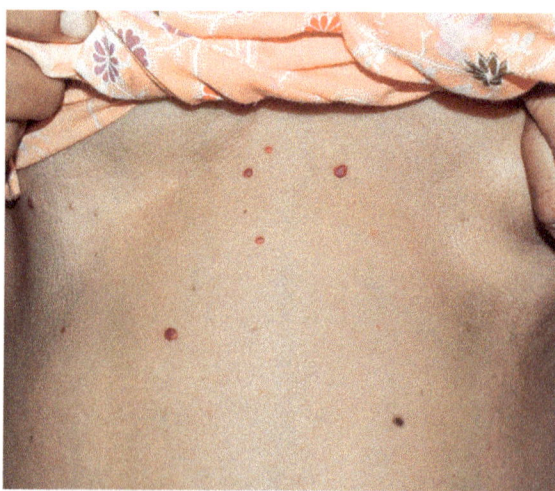

a. Pyogenic granuloma
b. Strawberry hemangioma
c. Cherry angiomas
d. Angiokeratomas

222. This girl presented with itching, oozing and crusting involving both breasts with intact nipples. What is the clinical diagnosis?

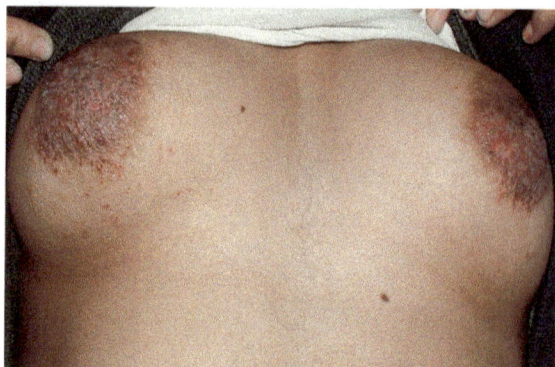

a. Paget's disease
b. Eczema of breasts
c. Pyoderma
d. Psoriasis

223. This patient presented with small papules around nasolabial folds and cheeks with a positive family history. What is the clinical diagnosis?

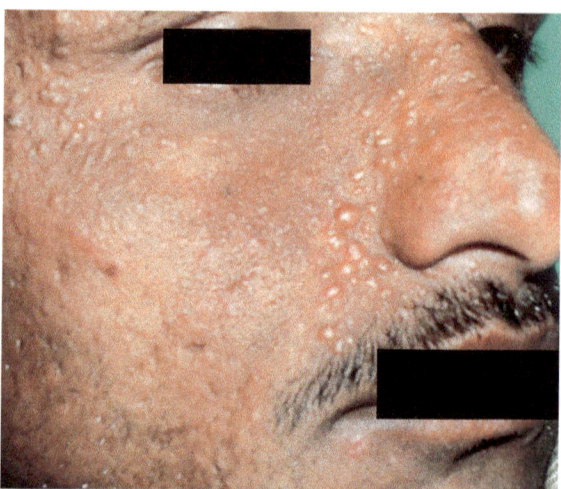

a. Syringoma
b. Trichoepithelioma
c. Acne vulgaris
d. Milia

224. This child presented with small, pearly white, dome shaped and umbilicated papules on face. What is the clinical diagnosis?

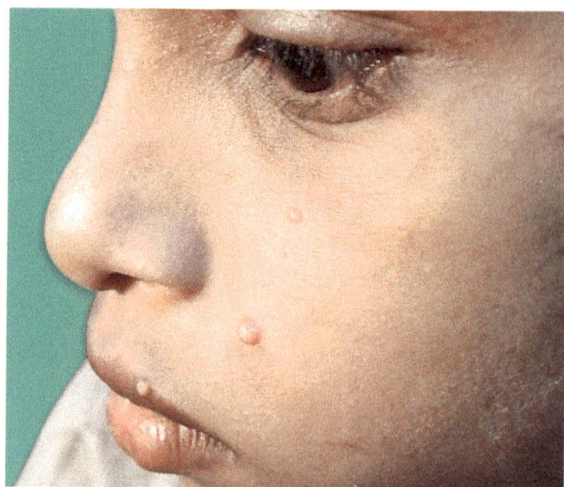

a. Chickenpox
b. Milia
c. Acne vulgaris
d. Molluscum contagiosum (MC)

225. A mason presented with itching, oozing and crusting on dorsa of hands and fingers for the last 3 years. What is the clinical diagnosis?

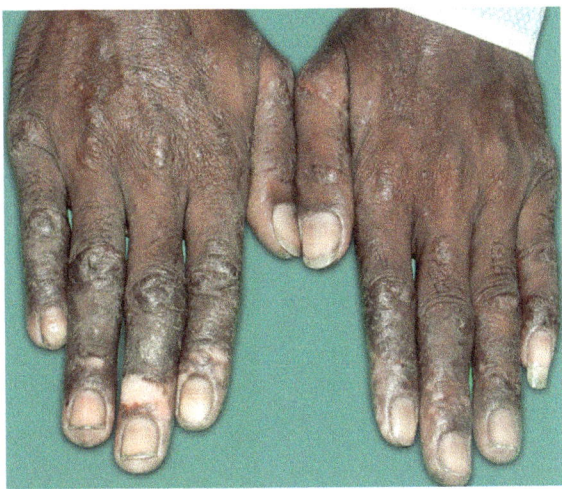

a. Acute irritant contact dermatitis (ICD) due to cement
b. Discoid eczema
c. Allergic contact dermatitis (ACD) due to cement
d. Pompholyx due to cement

226. This elderly patient presented with a single, persistent, red, thin plaque having well defined borders with overlying crust that resembles psoriasis. What can be the closest clinical diagnosis?

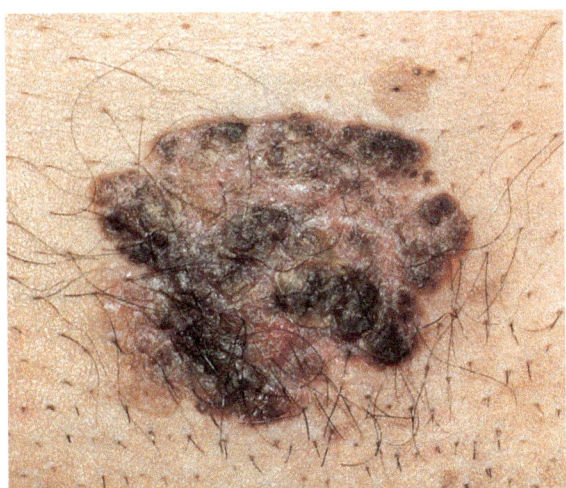

a. Psoriasis
b. Superficial spreading melanoma (SSM)
c. Basal cell carcinoma (BCC)
d. Bowen's disease

227. A 20-year-old boy presented with asymptomatic various sized, 10–12 in number light brown macules on abdominal skin. In addition, there were multiple, skin colored, dome shaped, soft and sessile skin tumors. What is the clinical diagnosis?

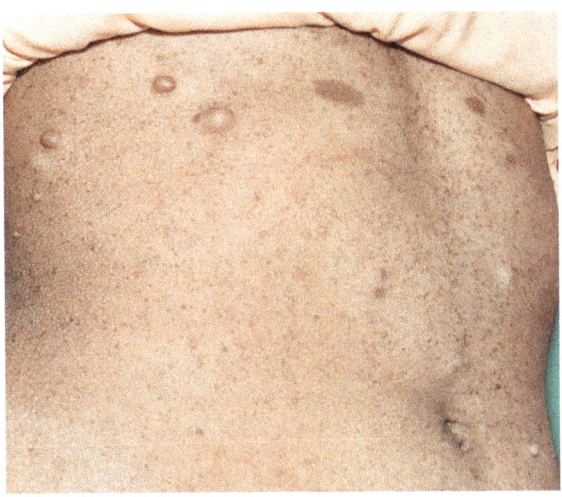

a. Superficial spreading melanoma (SSM)
b. Tuberous sclerosis complex (TSC)
c. Neurofibromatosis type 1
d. Mongolian spots

228. A 50-year-old patient presented with asymptomatic, multiple, small, brown papules on face. What is the clinical diagnosis?

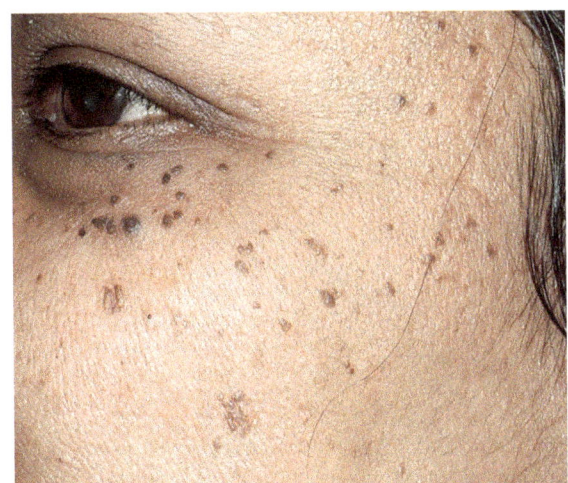

a. Milia
b. Senile comedones
c. Warts
d. Dermatosis papulosa nigra (DPN)
e. Skin tags

229. An 18-year-old boy presented with a crop of red scaly plaques of less than 1 cm size on the back and front of trunk for the last 3 months. It was also accompanied by mild itching. What is the clinical diagnosis?

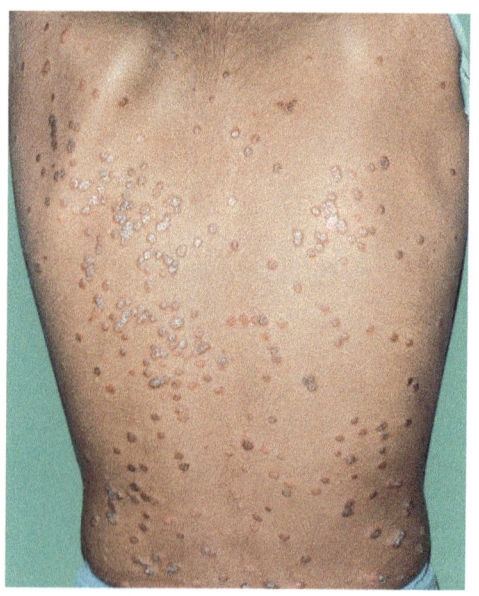

a. Secondary syphilis
b. Pityriasis rosea
c. Guttate psoriasis
d. Discoid eczema

230. A 50-year-old nonsmoker male presented with a painless, persistent, flat, irregular and verrucous white plaque (about 2 cm × 2 cm in size) on the inner side of left cheek. What is the clinical diagnosis?

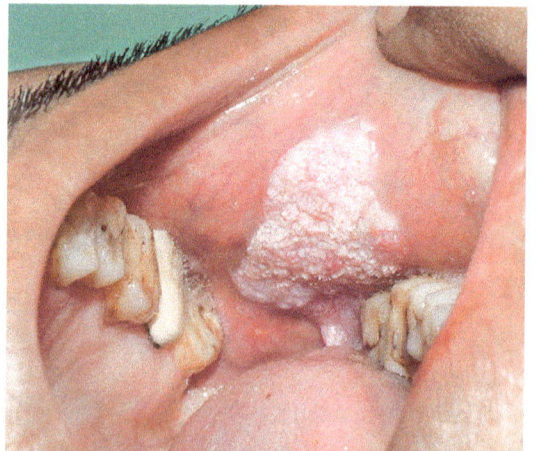

a. Oral leucoplakia (OL)
b. Oral lichen planus (OLP)
c. Oral thrush
d. Smoker's keratosis

231. This patient is presented with multiple, itchy, violaceous papules with little scaling on both palms. What is the clinical diagnosis?

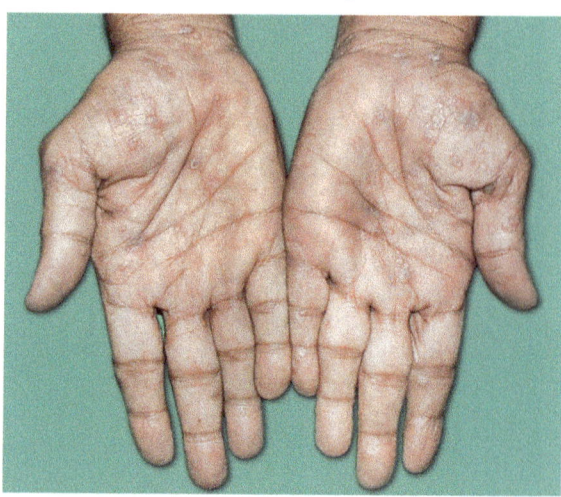

a. CCLE of palms.
b. Psoriasis of palms
c. Lichen planus of palm
d. Tinea manuum

232. She presented with intensely itchy, small, discrete, dome-shaped, pigmented and follicular papules in both axillae. What is the clinical diagnosis?

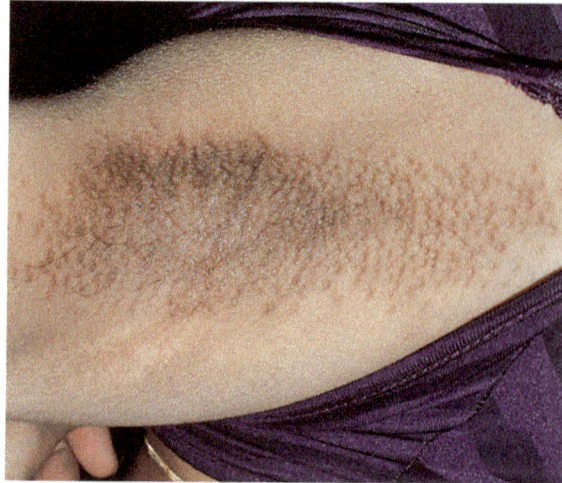

a. Intertrigo
b. Chromhidrosis
c. Bromhidrosis
d. Fox-Fordyce disease

233. This patient presented with mildly itchy erythematous plaques on both palms. Plaques show white scaling and become confluent at places leaving normal skin in between. What is the clinical diagnosis?

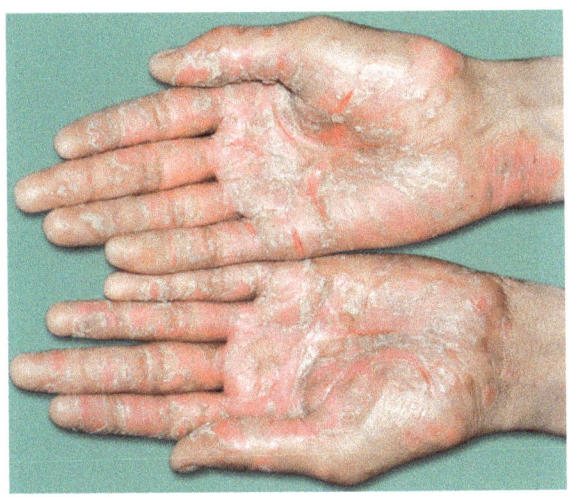

a. Tinea manuum
b. CCLE of palm
c. Psoriasis of palms
d. Eczema of palms

234. This patient presented with asymptomatic multiple skin colored, dome shaped, sessile skin tumors on back. In addition, there were multiple light brown macules also. What is the clinical diagnosis?

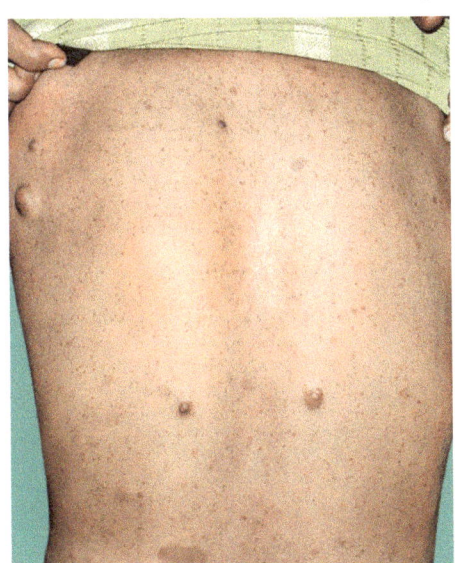

a. Common warts
b. Skin tags
c. Neurofibromatosis type 1
d. Mongolian spots

235. This child presented with pain and swelling upper lip for the last 4–5 days. What is the clinical diagnosis?

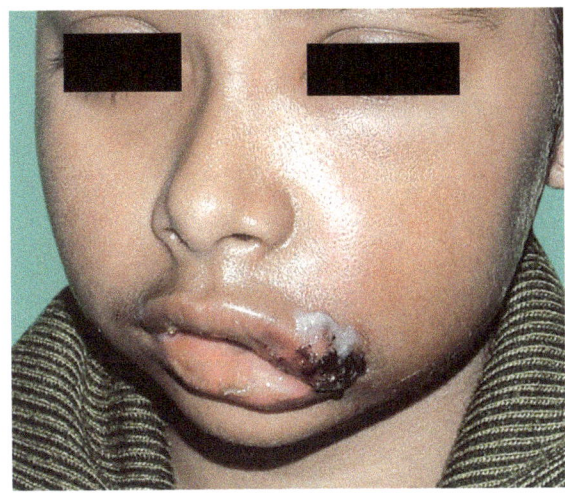

a. Pyogenic granuloma
b. Boil upper lip
c. Angular cheilitis
d. Herpes simplex labialis

236. This patient presented with asymptomatic, 1–3 mm sized, skin-colored papules on eye lids and cheeks with no family history. What is the clinical diagnosis?

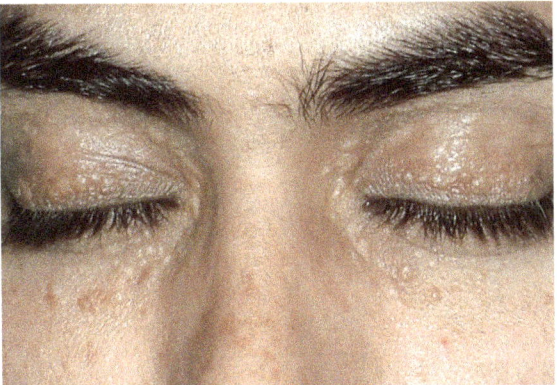

a. Molluscum contagiosum (MC)
b. Milia
c. Trichoepithelioma
d. Syringoma

237. A 63-year-old male presented with reddish brown firm plaque on forehead for the last six months. Histopathology showed diffuse dermal infiltrate of lymphocytes, histiocytes and plasma cells. Numerous red colored pin head sized bodies are identified inside and outside the histiocytes. What is the diagnosis?

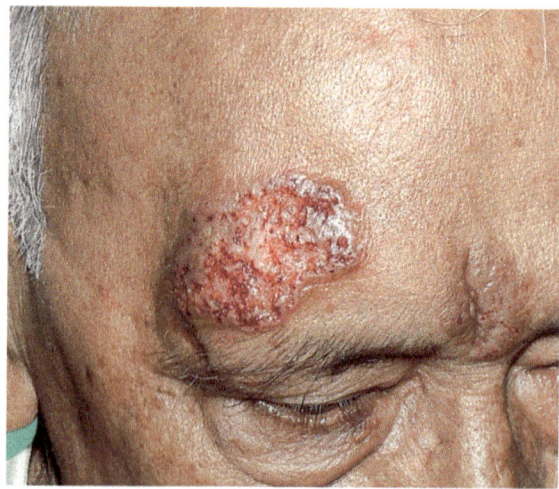

a. Tuberculosis verrucosa cutis (TVC)
b. Moist or rural type old world leishmaniasis
c. Basal cell carcinoma (BCC)
d. Sarcoidosis

238. After taking some drug this patient developed itching and maculopapular rash on trunk and extremities. The rash comprised of 2–10 mm sized red macules that are confluent at places. What is the clinical diagnosis?

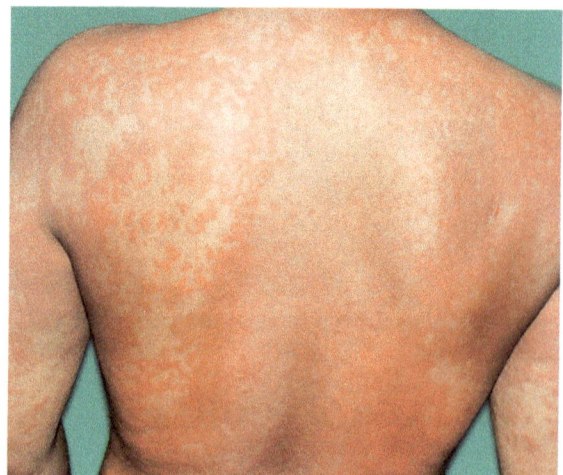

a. Drug-induced morbilliform rash
b. Erythema multiforme (EM)
c. Drug-induced exfoliative dermatitis
d. Drug-induced urticaria

239. This patient presented with red papules and plaques studded with silvery white scaling on extremities, trunk and scalp. What is the clinical diagnosis?

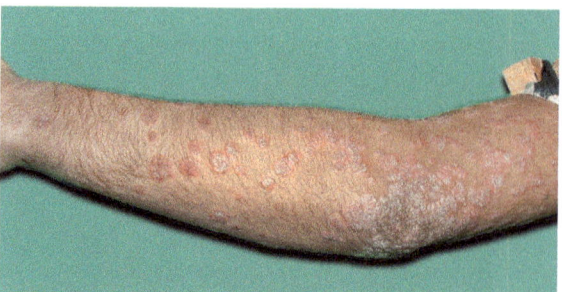

a. Lichen planus hypertrophicus (LPH)
b. Granuloma annulare (GA)
c. Psoriasis
d. Hansen's disease
e. Lupus vulgaris

240. This fair skin girl presented with multiple poorly defined macules about less than 3 mm in size on her face. What is the diagnosis?

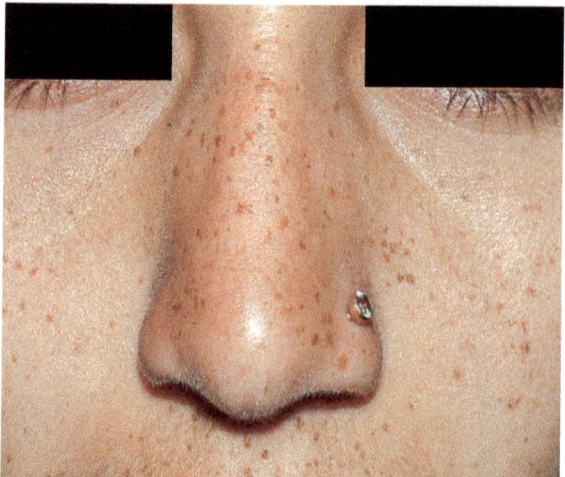

a. Lentiginosis
b. Freckles
c. Cafe-au-lait macules (CALMs)
d. Nevus of Ota

241. This patient complains of a large itchy patch on his face. What is the clinical diagnosis?

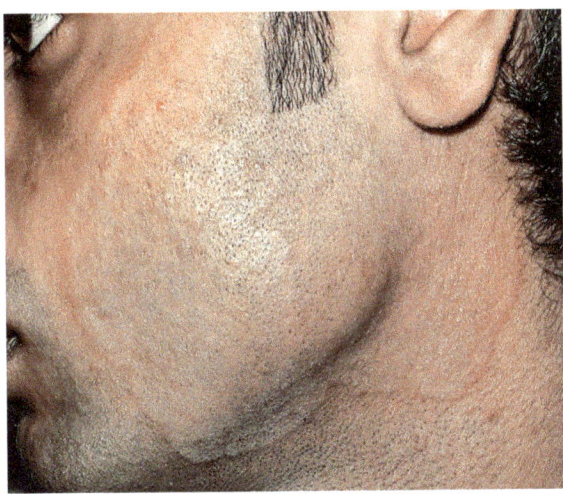

a. Pityriasis versicolor
b. Polymorphous light eruption (PLE)
c. Tinea faciei

242. This patient presented with red, discrete and various sized plaques with adherent scaling on both palms. Lesion showed peripheral hyperpigmentation and central scarring. What is the clinical diagnosis?

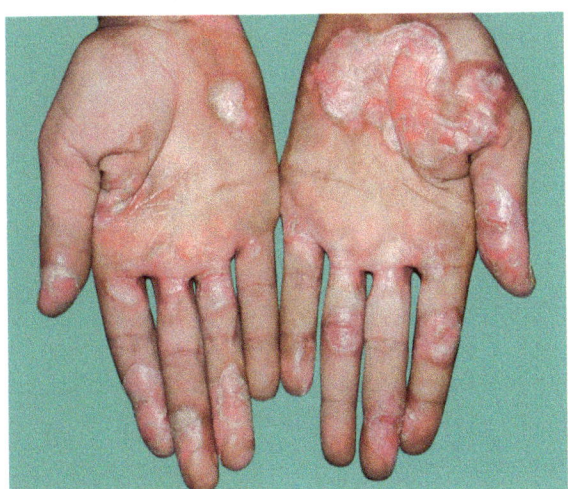

a. Psoriasis of palms
b. Chronic cutaneous lupus erythematosus (CCLE) of palms
c. Tinea manuum
d. Eczema of palms

243. This patient presented with generalized redness and exfoliation of silvery white scales involving almost whole body sparing very little areas in between. What is the clinical diagnosis? There is no fever, lymphadenopathy or internal organ involvement.

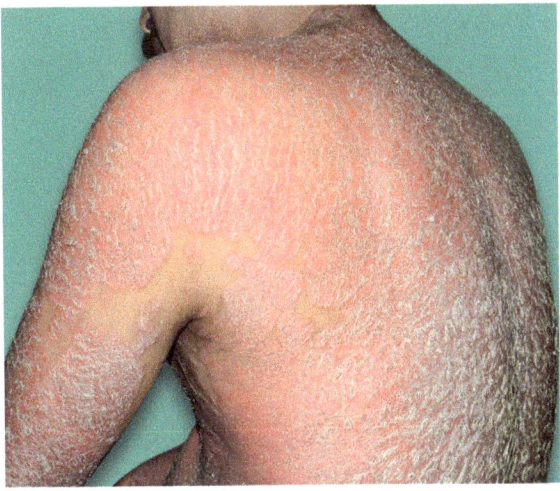

a. Erythroderma due to psoriasis
b. Erythroderma due to seborrheic dermatitis.
c. Drug hypersensitivity syndrome (DHS)
d. Patch or plaque stage mycosis fungoides

244. This patient presented with a raised, dome shaped and nonpigmented nodule on face. What is the closest clinical diagnosis?

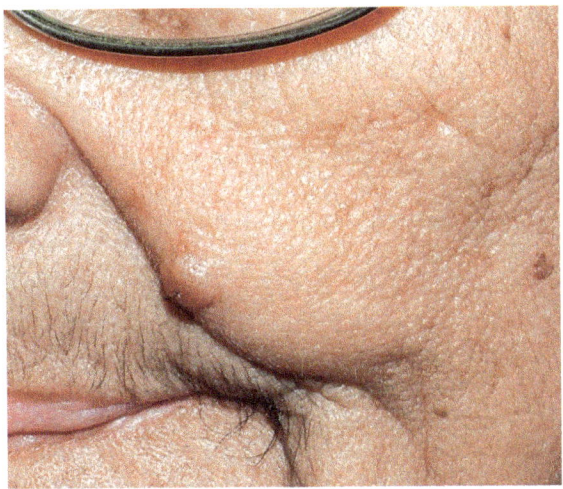

a. Compound nevus
b. Cellular nevus (mole)
c. Intradermal nevus
d. Junctional nevus

245. This lady presented with salmon pink coloration with well-defined margins and white scaling in sub mammary folds and umbilicus. What is the clinical diagnosis?

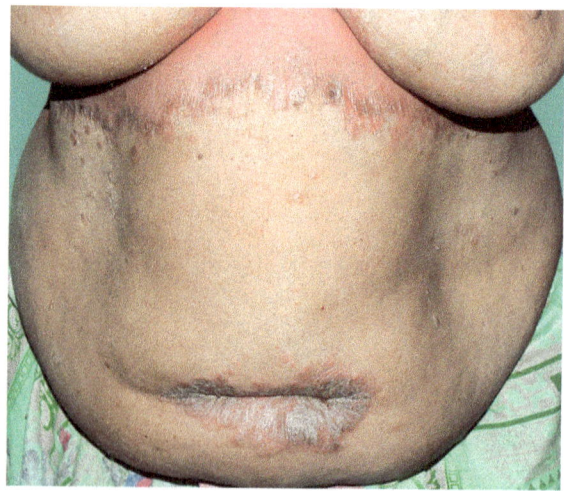

a. Candidal intertrigo
b. Seborrheic dermatitis (SD)
c. Flexural psoriasis
d. Tinea corporis

246. A 10-year-old child presented with a single patch of depigmentation on foot for the last six months. What is the clinical diagnosis?

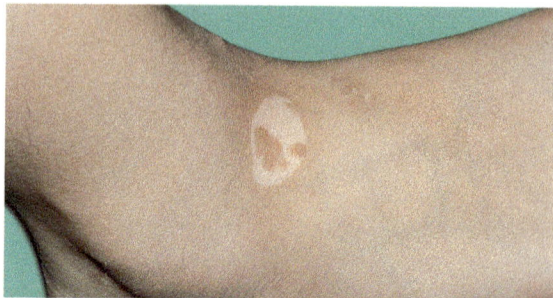

a. Focal vitiligo
b. Segmental vitiligo
c. Nevus depigmentosus
d. Nevus anemicus

247. Nails of this patient show transverse grooves in the nail plate parallel to lunula. What is it called as?

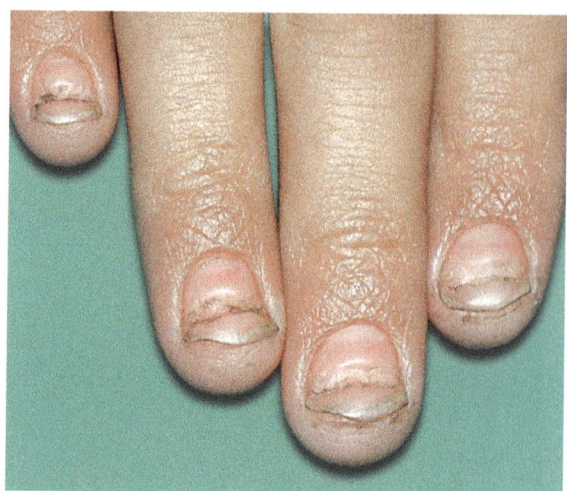

a. Beau's lines
b. Koilonychia
c. Onychogryphosis
d. Clubbing

248. Few hours after taking some drug this man developed multiple gray colored macules on trunk and extremities without involvement of mucosa. What is the possible diagnosis?

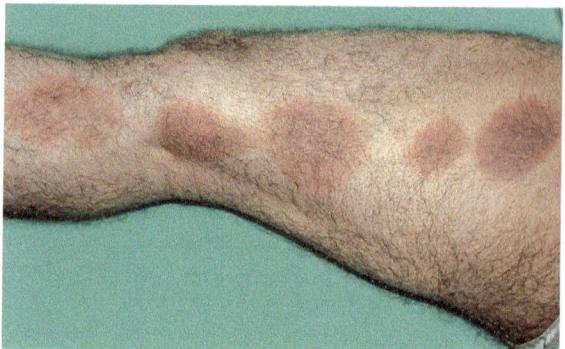

a. Erythema multiforme (EM)
b. Drug induced pemphigus
c. Fixed drug eruptions (FDE)
d. Exanthematous eruptions

249. Two month after the starting of antitubercular therapy, this patient developed generalized erythema, itching, scaling, eosinophilia, fever and lymphadenopathy. What is the clinical diagnosis?

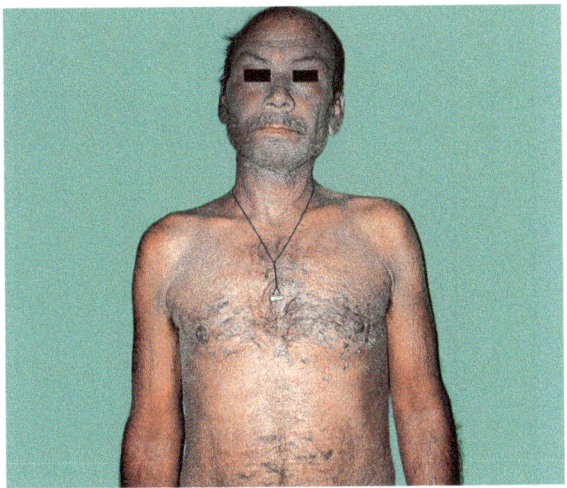

a. Drug-induced morbilliform rash
b. Drug-induced pemphigus foliaceous
c. Drug-induced Ichthyosis
d. Drug hypersensitivity syndrome (DHS)

250. This patient presented with itching, vesicular lesions with oozing and crusting involving both palms. What is the clinical diagnosis?

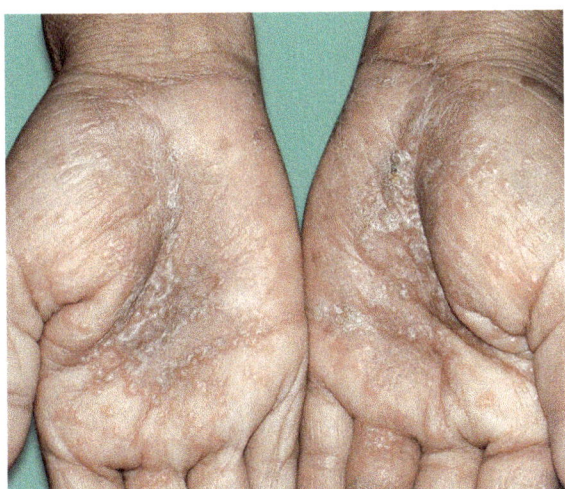

a. Psoriasis of palms
b. Tinea manuum
c. Lichen planus palms
d. Eczema palms

251. A 60-year-old nonsmoker man presented with asymptomatic persistent white patch on lateral side of tongue for the last five years. What is the probable clinical diagnosis?

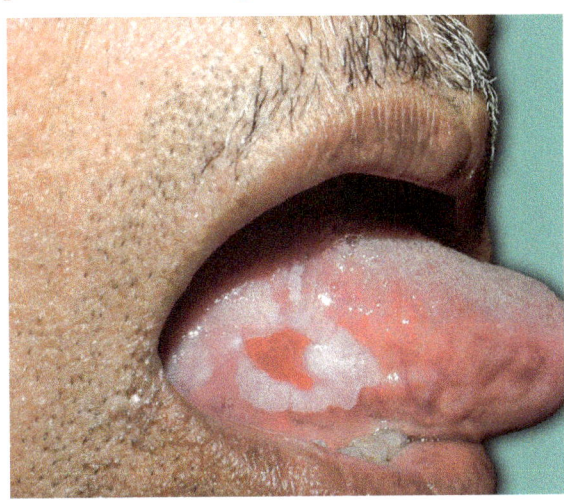

a. Oral lichen planus (OLP)
b. Oral leukoplakia (OL)
c. Hairy leukoplakia
d. Smoker's keratosis

252. This child presented with a circumscribed area of depigmentation on right side of abdomen since birth. What is the possible clinical diagnosis?

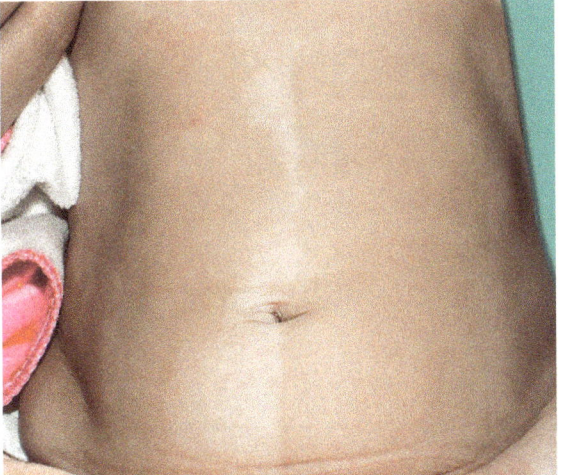

a. Nevus anemicus
b. Focal vitiligo
c. Segmental vitiligo
d. Nevus depigmentosus

253. This lady presented with itchy red macerations under breast extending beyond the area of contact and developed fringed irregular margins with classical satellite vesicles and pustules. What is the clinical diagnosis?

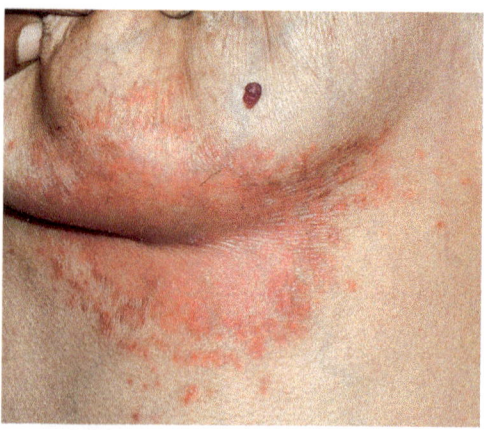

a. Candidal intertrigo (flexural candidiasis)
b. Seborrheic dermatitis (SD)
c. Tinea corporis
d. Flexural psoriasis

254. A male patient presented with multiple deep red patches of various sizes and shapes with little scaling on the front and back of trunk. Patches are asymptomatic and are persisting for last many months. What is the clinical diagnosis?

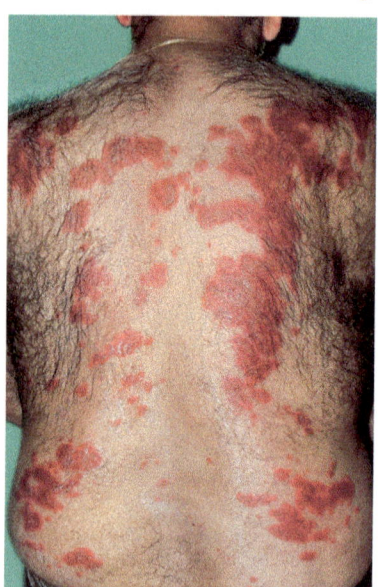

a. Psoriasis
b. Patch stage mycosis fungoides
c. Drug-induced morbilliform rash
d. Urticarial vasculitis

255. This old man presented with single raised, verrucous plaque with central ulceration at the angle of the mouth. What is the closest possible diagnosis?

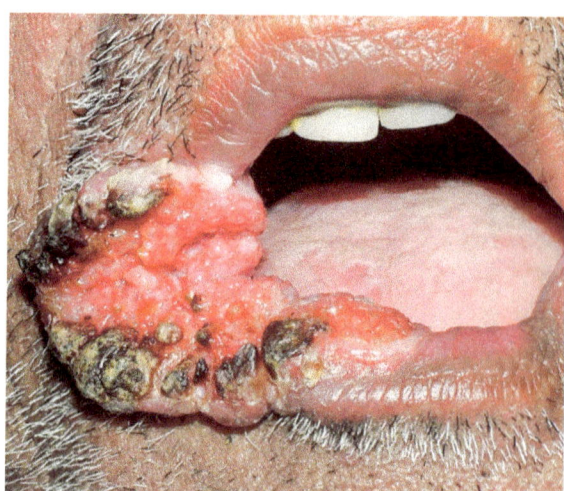

a. Basal cell carcinoma (BCC)
b. Squamous cell carcinoma (SCC)
c. Malignant melanoma
d. Orificial tuberculosis

256. This patient presented with multiple, reddish brown and soft gelatinous plaques on left upper extremity only for the last 1 year. There was no loss of sensations but apple jelly nodules were noticed on diascopy in few lesions. What is the clinical diagnosis?

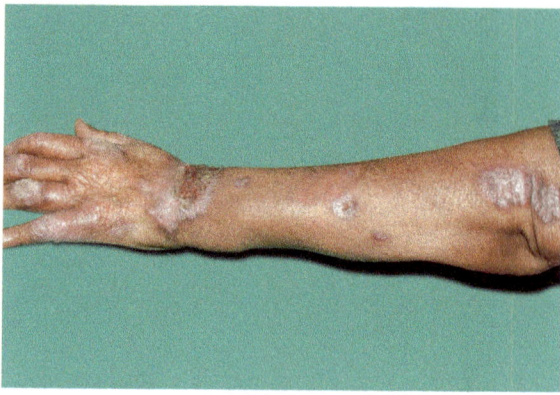

a. Psoriasis
b. Hyperkeratotic eczema
c. Lupus vulgaris
d. Lichen planus hypertrophicus (LPH)
e. Hansen's disease

257. This old man presented with erythema, itching and mild scaling involving the whole body. It developed insidiously in a year all over the body without any history of discrete scaly plaques at the onset of disease process. What is the clinical impression?

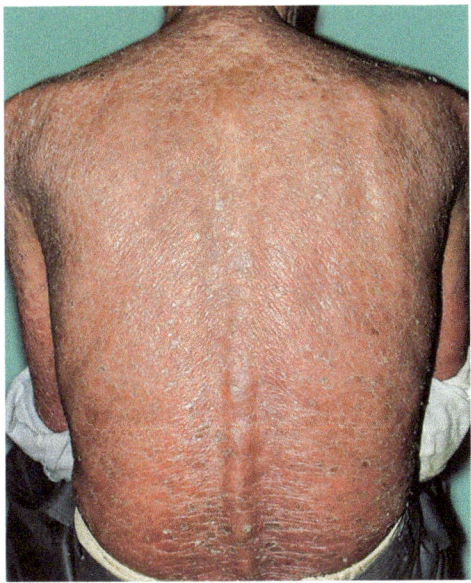

a. Exanthematous eruption
b. Non psoriatic erythroderma
c. Psoriatic erythroderma
d. Exfoliative dermatitis

258. This patient presented with thickening and transverse over curvature of nail plate along its longitudinal axis. To which one of the following nail disorders it belongs to?

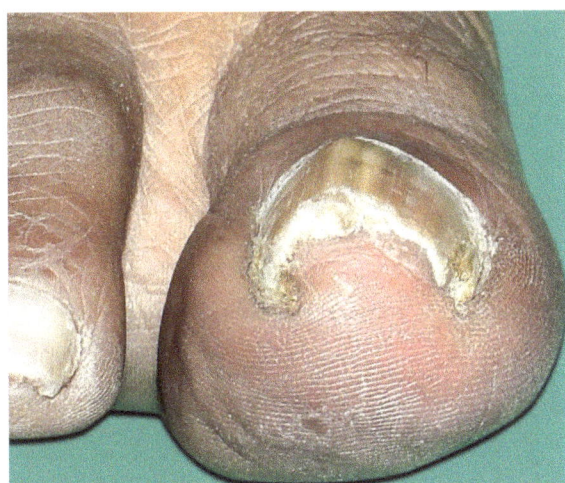

a. Pincer nail dystrophy (PND)
b. Pterygium of nail
c. Subungual hyperkeratosis
d. Onychogryphosis

259. This lady has developed small itchy urticarial papules on abdomen (sparing periumbilical area), upper and lower extremities in 3rd trimester of her first pregnancy. All the lesions are of same morphological type. What is the diagnosis?

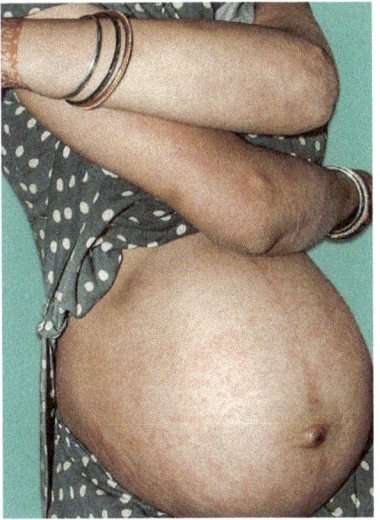

a. Prurigo of pregnancy
b. Toxemic rash of pregnancy
c. Impetigo herpetiformis
d. Pemphigoid gestationis
e. Prurigo gravidarum
f. Chickenpox during pregnancy

260. A patient of generalized psoriasis was taking dexamethasone injections from a village practitioner. She suddenly developed high-grade fever, severe prostration and multiple pinpoint pustules on fiery red skin all over in cervical region, trunk etc. What is the diagnosis?

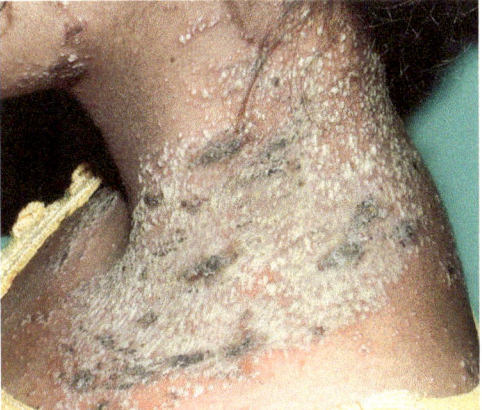

a. Psoriasis with secondary infection
b. Generalized pustular psoriasis (GPP)
c. Psoriatic erythroderma
d. Acropustulosis

261. A 50-year-old male presented with extremely pruritic papules, urticarial wheals and small vesicles on extensors of limbs, buttocks, natal left and shoulders. Lesions have tendency to form groups. Palms, soles and mucous membranes are not involved. What is the clinical diagnosis?

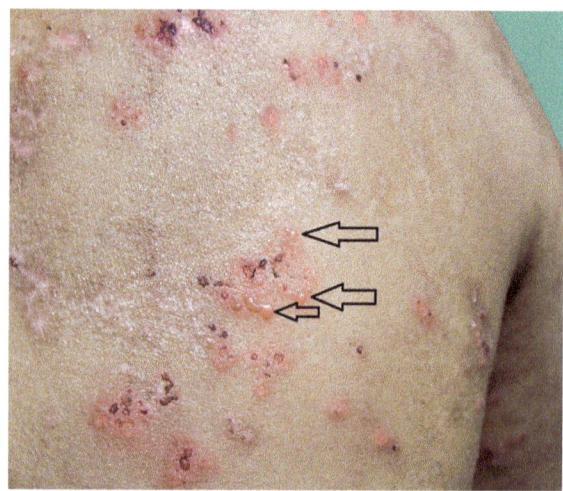

a. Pemphigus foliaceous (PF)
b. Pemphigus vulgaris (PV)
c. Dermatitis herpetiformis (DH)
d. Seborrheic dermatitis (SD)

262. This patient presented with few vesicles and bullae-containing turbid contents. After rupture, dark yellow crust is formed. Nikolsky's sign is negative. Mucosae are not involved. What is the clinical diagnosis?

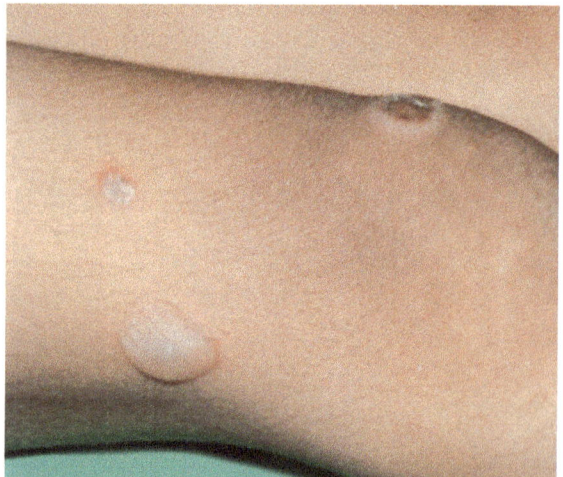

a. Bullous impetigo
b. Bullous pemphigoid (BP)
c. Pemphigus vulgaris (PV)
d. Ecthyma

263. This patient complains of severe itching, thickening, darkening and increased skin markings on the nape of neck only. What is the clinical diagnosis?

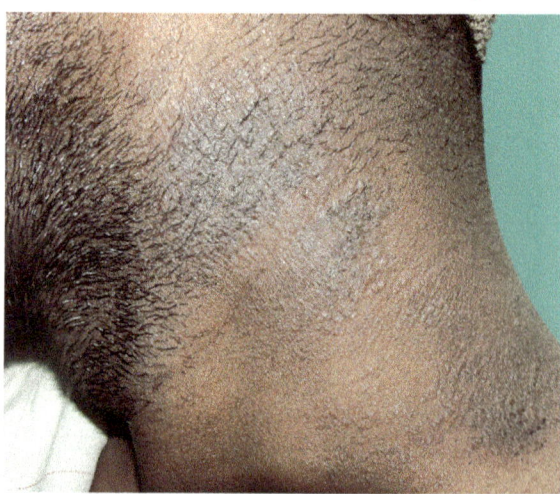

a. Benign acquired acanthosis nigricans (AN)
b. Lichen simplex chronicus (LSC)
c. Chronic actinic dermatitis (CAD)
d. Airborne contact dermatitis (ABCD)

264. She presented with itching soreness, redness and scanty thick curdy white discharge in vulva. It is accompanied by increased frequency of micturition at night. There is no history of extramarital sexual exposure. What is the clinical diagnosis?

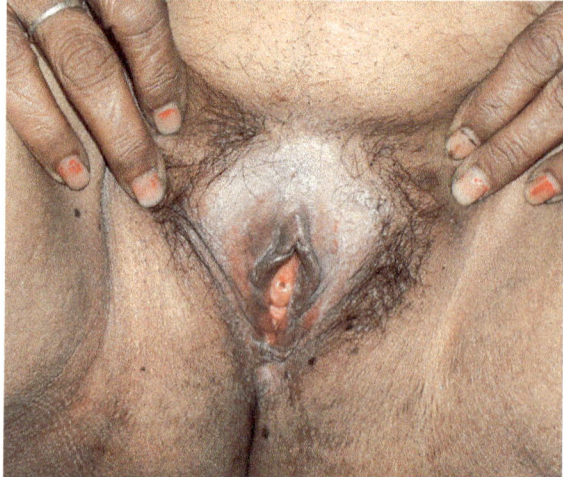

a. Lichen simplex chronicus (LSC)
b. Vulvovaginal candidiasis (VVC)
c. Lichen sclerosus et atrophicus. (LSEA)
d. Gonococcal infection

265. This patient presented with non-itchy, well-defined red plaques studded with silvery scales involving both soles. In addition, he was also having discrete red plaque with white scaling on other parts of body. What is the diagnosis?

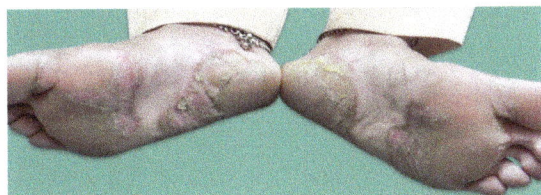

a. Tinea pedis
b. Plantar keratoderma
c. Plantar psoriasis
d. Eczema of soles

266. This child presented with these bullae on erythematous base. Lesions have appeared around the periphery of previous lesion and resulted into "Collarette of blisters". There is a no mucosal involvement. What is the clinical diagnosis?

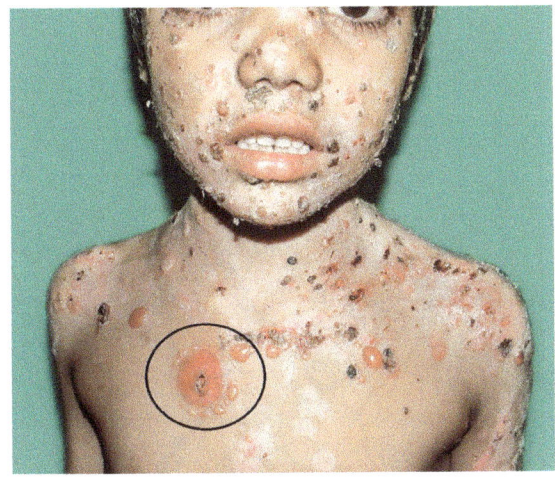

a. Pemphigus vulgaris
b. Bullous pemphigoid
c. Chronic bullous dermatosis of childhood (CBDC)
d. Dermatitis herpetiformis (DH)

267. This patient presented with persistent, multiple, firm gray colored papules (for close picture see) on seborrheic areas of trunk, face and extremities. Nails are showing red longitudinal bands which ends in V-shaped notch at the free margin of nail *(MCQ 178)*. Father is also having similar disease. What is the clinical diagnosis?

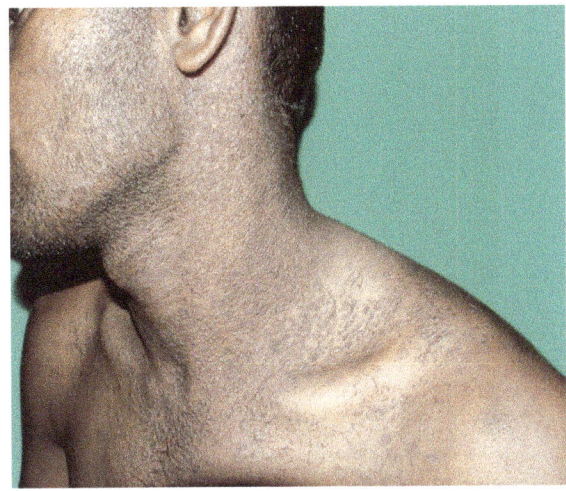

a. Seborrheic dermatitis (SD)
b. Darier's disease
c. Ichthyosis vulgaris
d. Pseudo-acanthosis nigricans (AN)

268. This patient presented with red plaques studded with silvery white scaling on face, scalp, extensors, back and other parts of body. What is the clinical diagnosis?

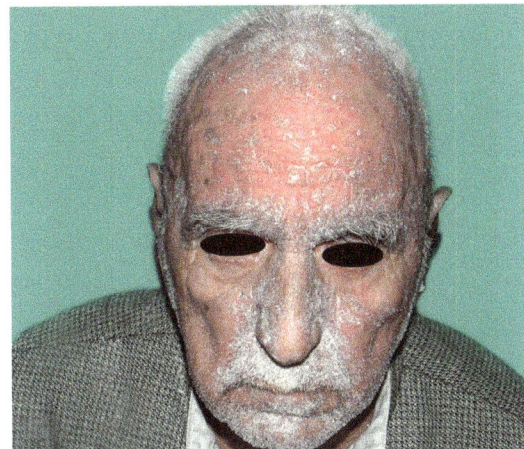

a. Seborrheic dermatitis
b. Widespread psoriasis
c. Generalized discoid lupus erythematosus (Generalized DLE)
d. Tinea faciei
e. Topical steroid damaged face (TSDF)

269. This patient complained of gradual loss of all hairs from his body, namely scalp, eyebrows, eye lashes, moustache, beard, axillae and pubic hairs. What is the clinical diagnosis?

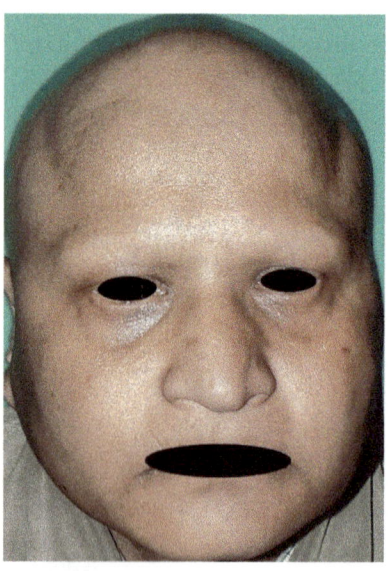

a. Ophiasis
b. Anagen effluvium
c. Alopecia universalis
d. Telogen effluvium

270. This patient presented with small, ivory white, asymptomatic shiny and round macules on trunk around umbilicus. Similar lesions are also seen in the cervical region and other parts of body. There was no history of Raynaud's phenomenon. Foreskin in this patient has become bluish white *(MCQ 320)* and is difficult to retract. What is the clinical diagnosis?

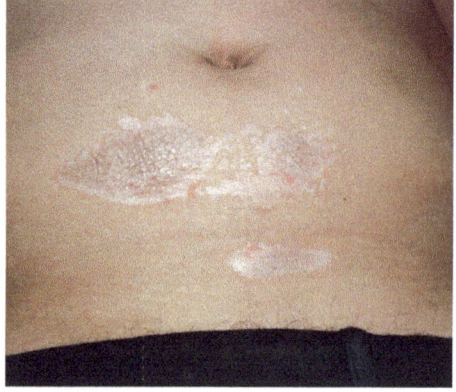

a. Vitiligo
b. Lichen sclerosus et atrophicus
c. Lichen planus
d. Morphea

271. Which one of the following statements is true about a slightly raised, brownish dark, tortuous line about 10 mm in length shown by arrow.

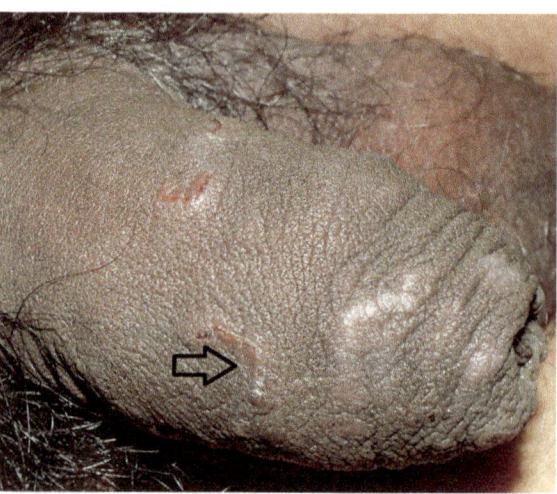

a. It is scabietic burrow
b. It is difficult to detect burrows in good hygienic patients
c. Burrow is pathognomonic of scabies
d. All are true

272. This patient presented with firm, painless swelling of one foot for the last many years. It was studded with multiple sinuses with discharge of granules. What is the clinical diagnosis?

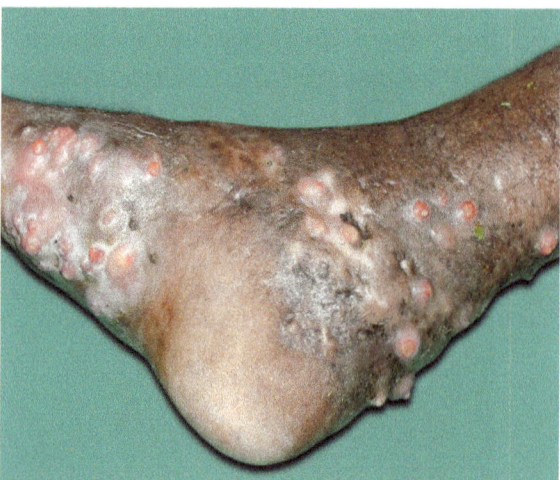

a. Tinea pedis
b. Mycetoma foot
c. Scrofuloderma
d. Osteomyelitis

273. This obese patient presented with pigmentation and cutaneous thickening giving a velvety appearance in the cervical region, axillae and groins. He is having high blood sugar levels but has no itching. What is the clinical diagnosis?

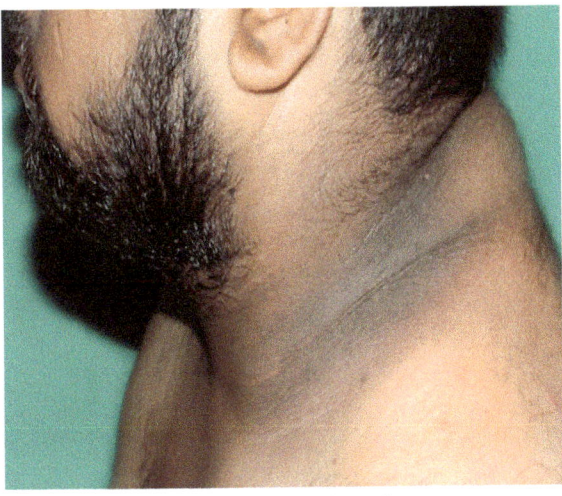

a. Chronic actinic dermatitis (CAD)
b. Benign acquired acanthosis nigricans (AN)
c. Lichen simplex chronicus (LSC)
d. Malignancy associated acanthosis nigricans

274. In 3rd trimester of the pregnancy she developed fever and malaise. It was followed by crop of vesicles that were having surrounding irregular area of erythema. What is the clinical diagnosis?

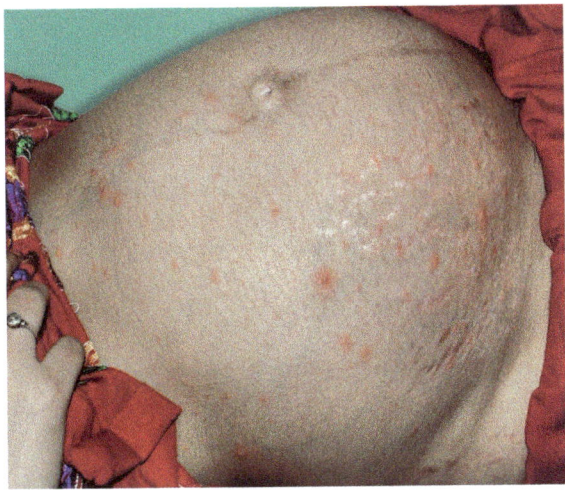

a. Toxemic rash of pregnancy
b. Chickenpox during pregnancy
c. Prurigo of pregnancy
d. Pemphigoid gestationis
e. Prurigo gravidarum

275. On 3rd postpartum day, she developed intensely pruritic tense vesicles and bullae around umbilicus and extremities. There was no mucosal involvement. What is the diagnosis?

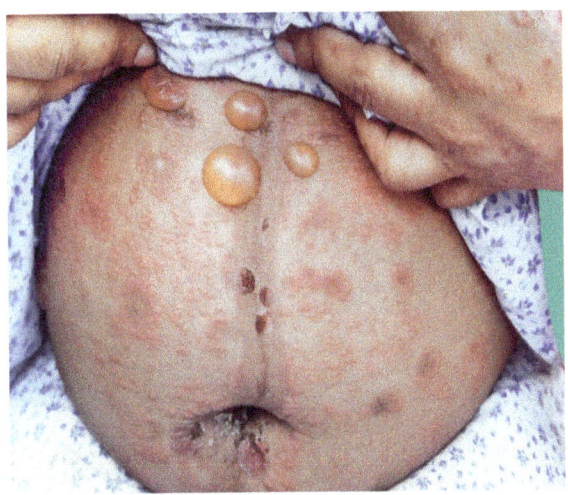

a. Bullous pemphigoid
b. Pemphigus vulgaris (PV)
c. Bullous impetigo
d. Pemphigoid gestationis

276. A 4-month-old baby presented with hair loss in the occipital region. What is the clinical diagnosis?

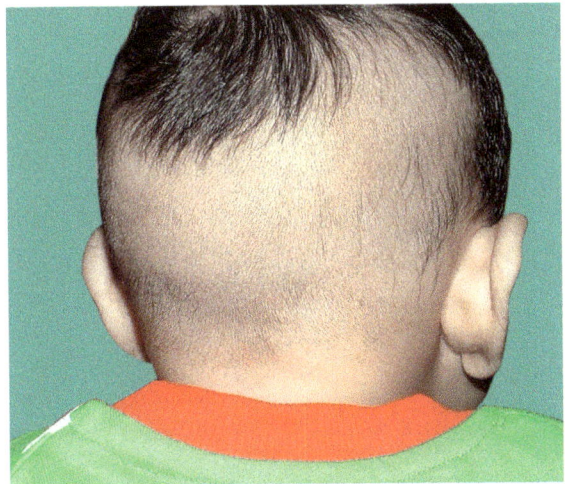

a. Alopecia areata
b. Neonatal occipital alopecia
c. Ophiasis
d. Pseudopelade of Brocq

277. The normal skin in this individual was firmly stroked. It was followed by white line, then a red line, then slight swelling with a red flare in the surrounding skin. It is also accompanied by itching. Which one of the followings is appropriate term for it?

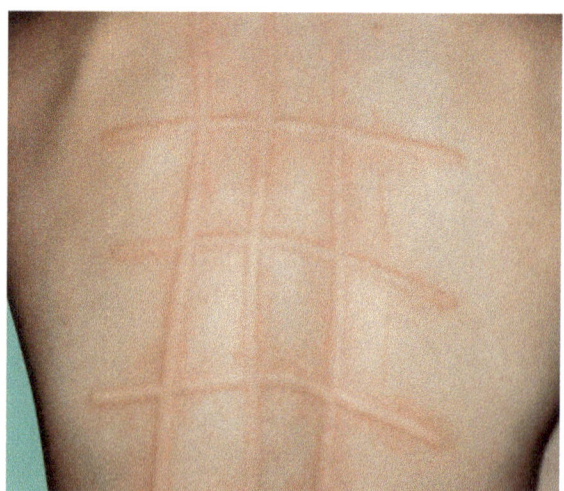

a. Black dermatographism
b. Symptomatic dermatographism
c. White dermatographism
d. Darier's sign

278. An adult presented with 2 cm sized, elastic dome shaped swelling, on mandibular region with central punctum. It is mobile over deeper structures. What is the clinical diagnosis?

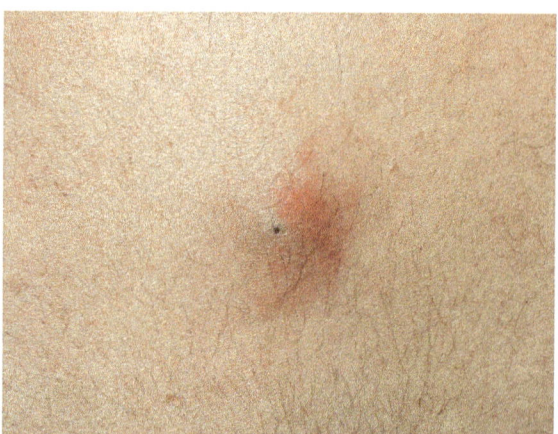

a. Acne cyst
b. Dermoid cyst
c. Sebaceous cyst
d. Boil

279. A 60-year-old man presented with asymptomatic reticular telangiectatic pigmentation of both shins. To which one of the following disorders this patient belongs?

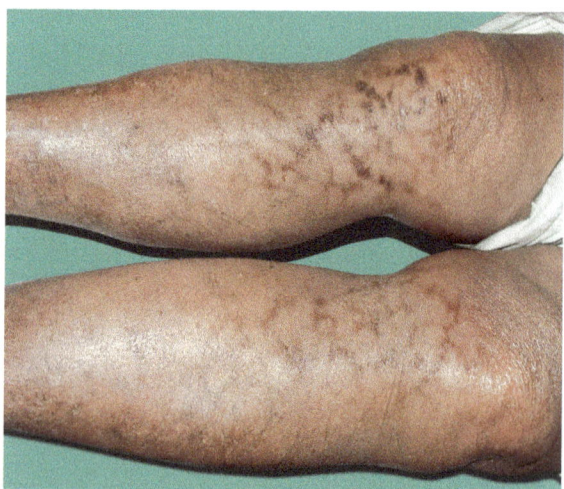

a. Senile purpura
b. Erythema ab igne
c. Asteatotic eczema
d. Ichthyosis

280. A 25-year-old unmarried male presented with asymptomatic off white subpreputial deposits or growth. What is the clinical diagnosis?

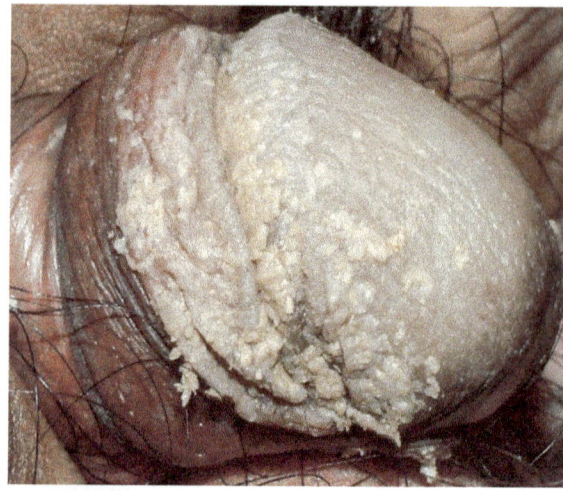

a. Venereal warts
b. Smegma
c. Candidal balanoposthitis
d. Verrucous carcinoma on glans penis

281. Following waxing, this young girl developed multiple Itchy and discrete pustules. What is the diagnosis?

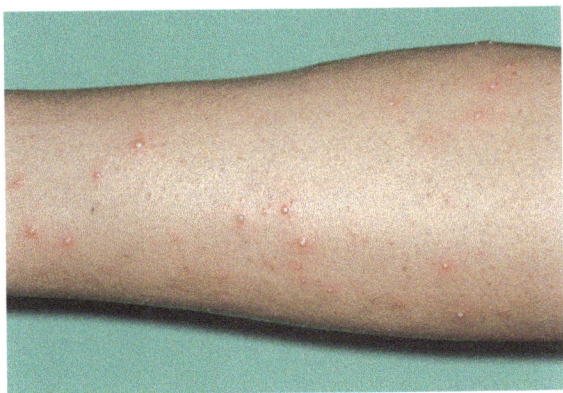

a. Pseudofolliculitis
b. Chronic superficial folliculitis (CSF)
c. Multiple boils
d. Superficial folliculitis

282. This patient complained of plantar hyperhidrosis, malodor and circular-shaped punched out erosions on both soles. What is the clinical diagnosis?

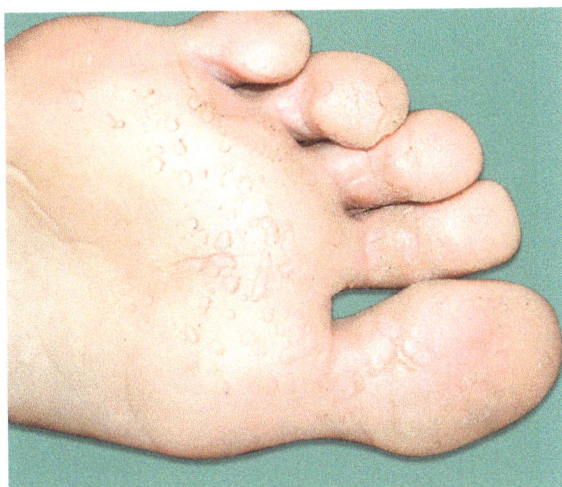

a. Candidiasis soles
b. Tinea pedis
c. Eczema soles
d. Pitted keratolysis

283. A young male presented with soft, pink, grouped, filiform or digitate lesions on coronal sulcus. What is the diagnosis?

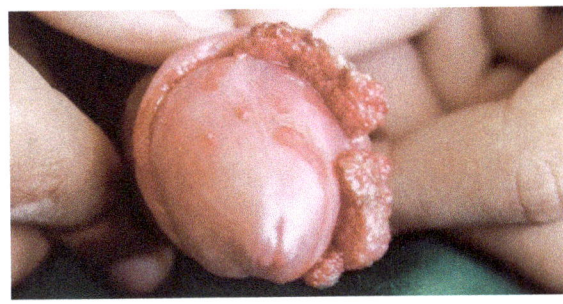

a. Smegma
b. Condylomata acuminata
c. Condylomata lata
d. Pearly penile papules (PPP)

284. She presented with an irregular, smooth, shiny, soft, slightly depressed patch of hair loss on vertex for the last two years. She does not have any cutaneous lesions on other parts of body. What is the clinical diagnosis?

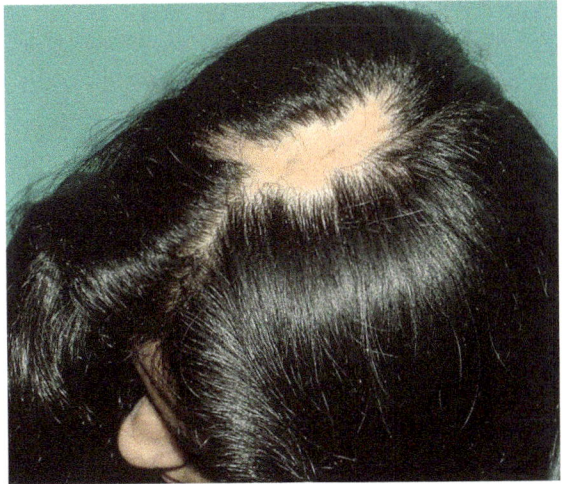

a. Trichotillomania
b. Alopecia areata
c. Folliculitis decalvans
d. Pseudopelade of Brocq

285. A 60-year-old female presented with multiple tense vesicles and bullae on erythematous skin with no mucosal involvement. Nikolsky's sign was negative. What is the clinical diagnosis?

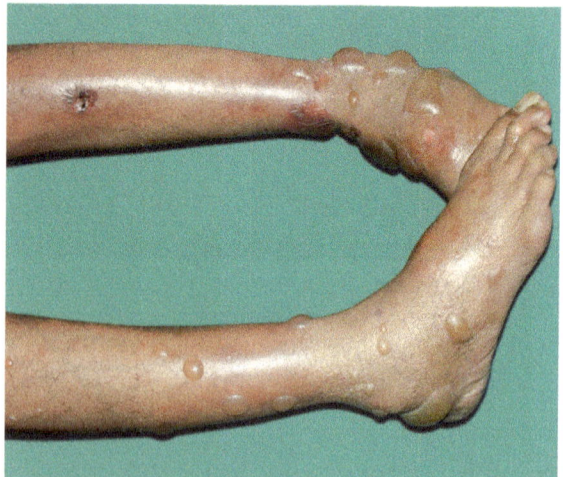

a. Bullous pemphigoid (BP)
b. *Pemphigus vulgaris* (PV)
c. *Pemphigus foliaceus* (PF)
d. Erythema multiforme (EM)
e. Dermatitis herpetiformis (DH)

286. This patient complained of chronic and profuse eruption of follicular pustules on lower extremities. What is the clinical diagnosis?

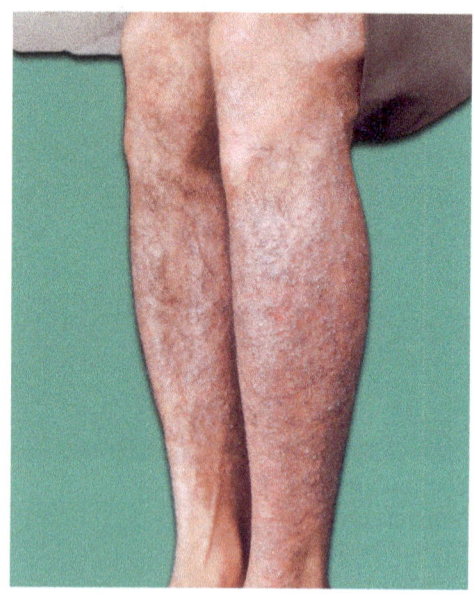

a. Pseudofolliculitis
b. Multiple boils
c. Impetigo contagiosa
d. Chronic superficial folliculitis (CSF)

287. A Young adult presented with multiple, flesh colored flat topped sessile papules in groins, anal region. Additionally, there was asymptomatic maculopapular eruption on trunk, palms and soles. There is a history of unprotected sex with a commercial sex worker (CSW) three months back. What is the clinical diagnosis?

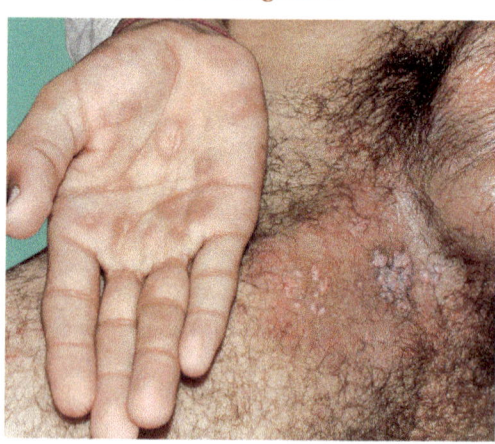

a. Condylomata acuminata
b. Condylomata lata
c. Bacterial intertrigo
d. Tinea cruris

288. This young lady has developed tense vesicles on erythematous base, in clusters on various parts of body for the last one month. Mucosa is not involved. What is the clinical diagnosis?

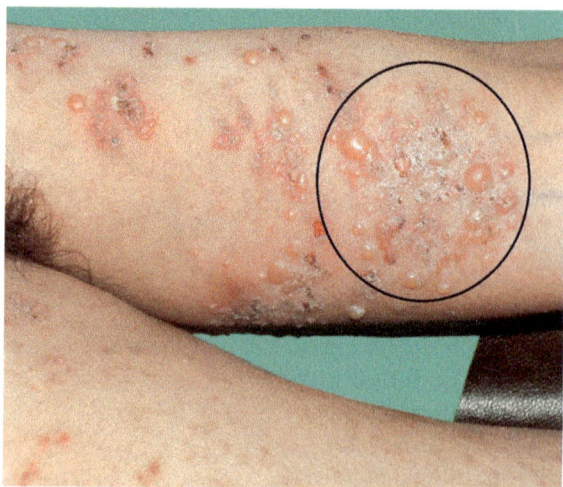

a. *Paederus dermatitis*
b. *Pemphigus foliaceus* (PF)
c. Linear IgA dermatosis in adult
d. Bullous pemphigoid (BP)

289. A 50-year-old man presented with a slow growing exophytic tumor with cauliflower appearance on glans for the last 3 years. It was accompanied by enlargement of inguinal lymph nodes. What is the clinical diagnosis?

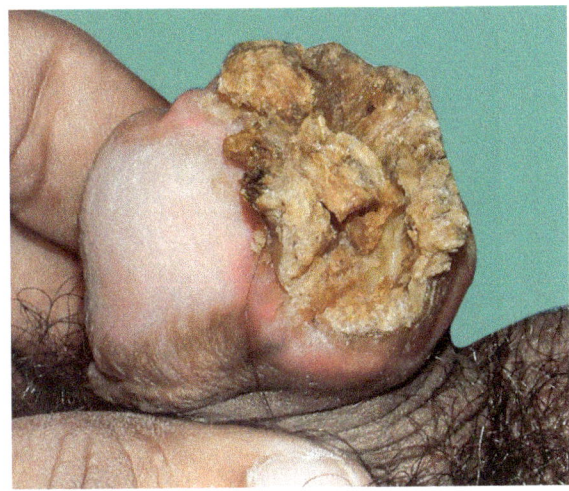

a. Condylomata acuminata
b. Smegma
c. Verrucous squamous cell carcinoma on glans (verrucous SCC)
d. Lichen planus glans

290. A young patient presented with asymptomatic 1–3 mm sized flesh-colored papules at the coronal margin of glans for the last one year. There is a no h/o sexual exposure. What is the diagnosis?

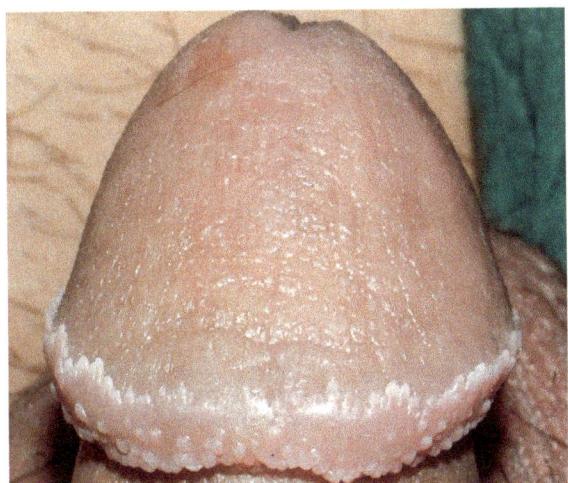

a. Genital warts (condylomata acuminata)
b. Pearly penile papules (PPP)
c. Condylomata lata
d. Lichen planus

291. This male patient having curly hairs complained of tiny red papules and pustules on the shaved beard region accompanied by itching. What is the clinical diagnosis?

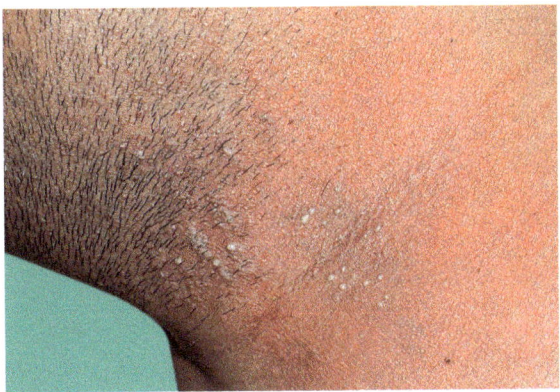

a. Chronic superficial folliculitis (CSF)
b. Pseudofolliculitis barbae
c. Acne vulgaris
d. Multiple boils

292. This patent presented with discrete, well defined red plaques with white scales on the medial side of foot. Similar lesions were also seen on other parts of body. Nails showed subungual hyperkeratosis and coarse pitting. What is the clinical diagnosis?

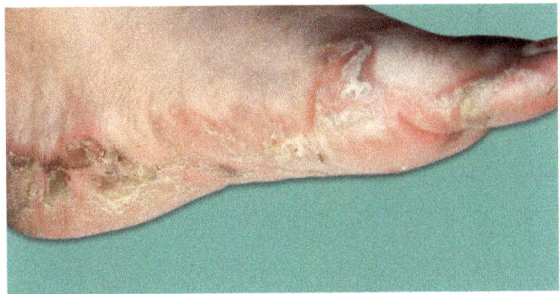

a. Psoriasis
b. Eczema feet
c. Lichen planus
d. Lepromatous leprosy (LL)

293. A 32-year-old patient presented with asymptomatic papular and papulosquamous rash on the front and back of trunk. Similar lesions were also seen on palms and soles. What is the clinical diagnosis?

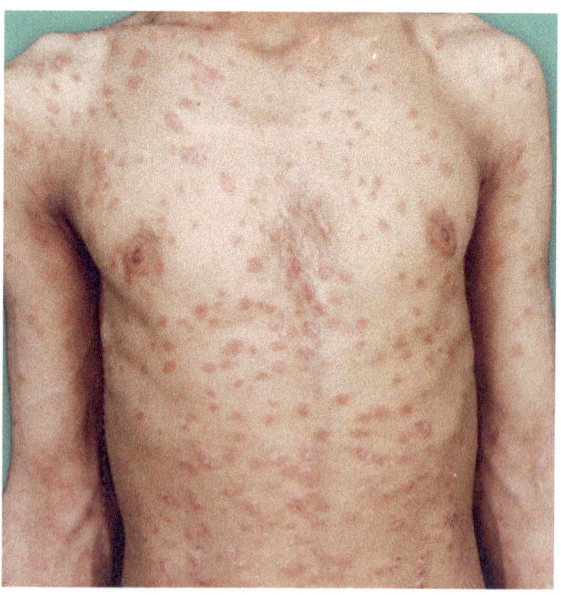

a. Guttate psoriasis
b. Secondary syphilis
c. Lichen planus (LP)
d. Pityriasis rosea

294. This patient presented with multiple large erythematous plaques with silvery white scaling. Lesions show central clearing but no loss of sensation. What is the clinical diagnosis?

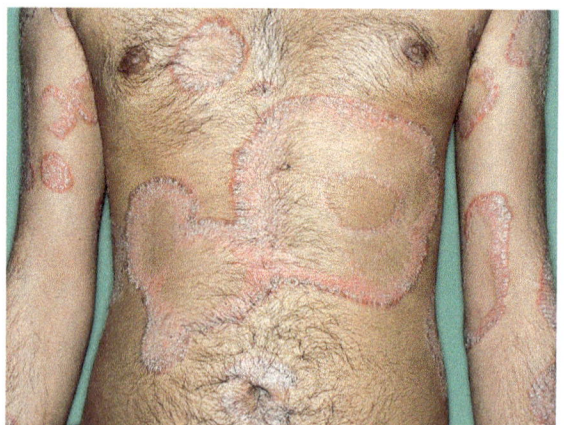

a. Granuloma annulare (GA)
b. Mid-borderline leprosy
c. Annular psoriasis
d. Tinea circinata

295. This patient presented with small and superficial pits on the nail plates of all the fingers. He was also having multiple bald patches on the scalp. What is the closest clinical diagnosis?

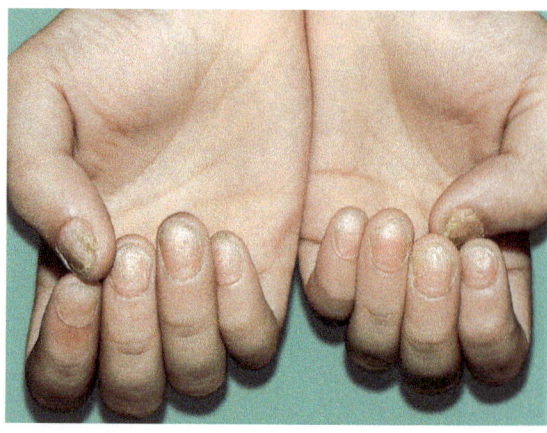

a. Psoriasis
b. Tinea unguium
c. Darier's disease (DD)
d. Alopecia areata (AA)

296. A 10-year-old child presented with huge swelling of lips and eye lids for the last 4–5 days. He was also having itchy wheals over trunk and extremities. What is the clinical diagnosis? It was not accompanied by any GIT or urinary symptoms.

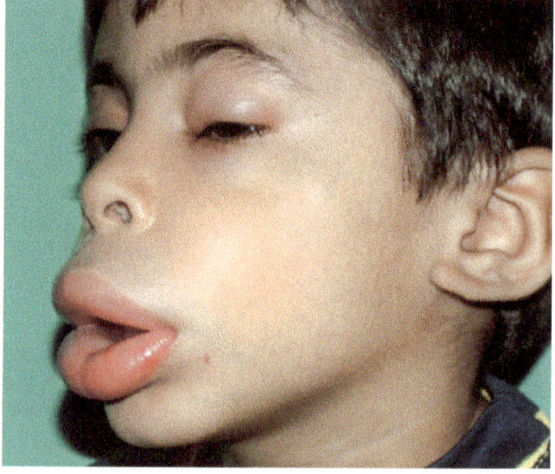

a. Acute urticaria
b. Myxedema
c. Ordinary angioedema
d. Hereditary angioedema

297. This patient presented with loss of hairs in a band like pattern at the periphery of the scalp margin. Which name is given to this condition out of the followings?

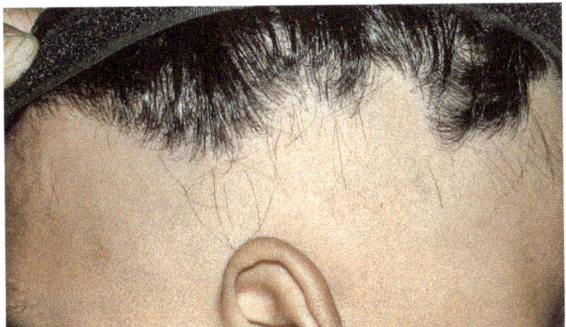

a. Trichotillomania
b. Ophiasis
c. Pseudopelade of Brocq
d. Anagen effluvium

299. This patient presented with multiple lesions having thick adherent crusts that can be removed with difficulty. There is a surrounding erythema with indurated base. What is the clinical diagnosis?

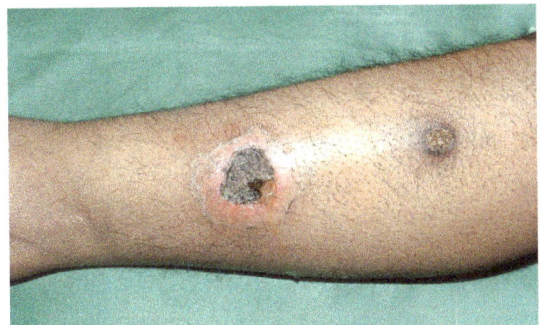

a. Infected discoid eczema
b. Ecthyma
c. Tuberculous gumma
d. Pyoderma gangrenosum

298. This patient complained of itching, thickening and pigmentation of sun exposed areas of skin showing clear margin from covered areas. It is sparing the depth of skin creases and areas behind the ears. Symptoms are severe in summer. What is the clinical diagnosis?

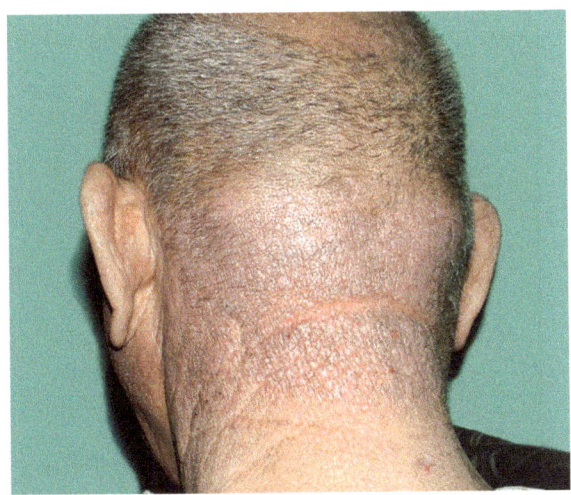

a. Benign acquired acanthosis nigricans (AN)
b. Lichen simplex chronicus (LSC)
c. Chronic actinic dermatitis (CAD)
d. Air-borne contact dermatitis (ABCD)

300. This patient presented with scattered, painful, extensive lesions with scaling, crusting and surrounding erythema at seborrheic sites, e.g., at chest, upper back, axillae, etc. Oral mucosa is not involved. What is the clinical diagnosis?

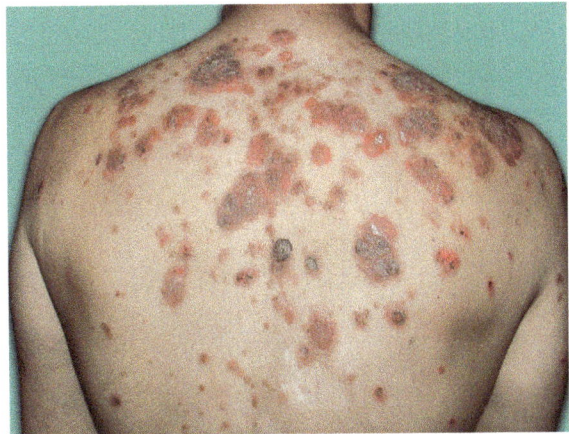

a. Pemphigus vulgaris (PV)
b. Pemphigus foliaceous (PF)
c. Bullous pemphigoid
d. Linear IgA dermatosis of adult

301. This patient presented with numerous asymptomatic skin-colored papules on the back for the last many years. Other siblings are also having similar lesions. What is the clinical diagnosis?

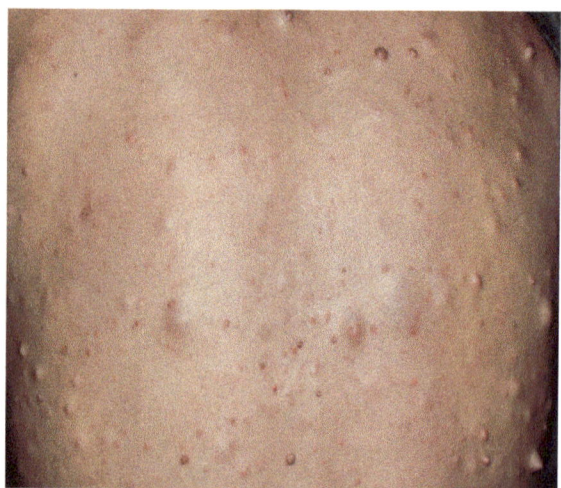

a. Neurofibromatosis type 2
b. Neurofibromatosis type 1
c. Tuberous sclerosis complex (TSC)
d. Darier's disease

302. This obese person is presented with velvety thickening and darkening of cervical skin. Which one of the following options is the closest clinical diagnosis?

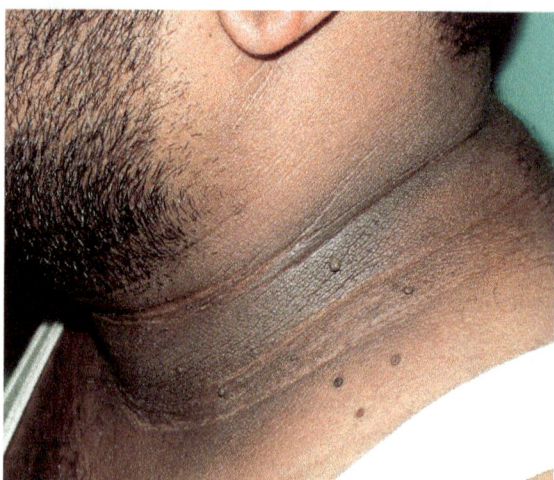

a. Pseudoacanthosis nigricans
b. Darier's disease
c. Polycystic ovarian syndrome (PCOS)
d. Seborrheic dermatitis

303. A 60-year-old female presented with clitoromegaly and sudden onset of facial hirsutism *(MCQ 321)*. What is the closest clinical diagnosis?

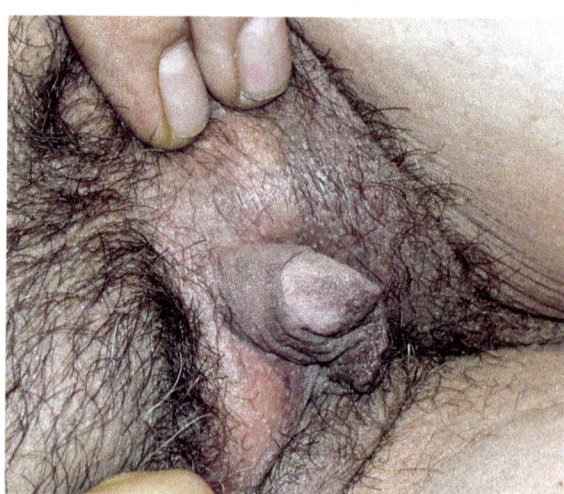

a. Polycystic ovarian syndrome (PCOS)
b. Androgen secreting tumor
c. Cushing syndrome
d. Physiological change in menopause

304. This child developed sudden widespread eruption of erythema multiforme like lesions on trunk and face *(MCQ 81)*. Trunk lesions showed partial coalescence. It was accompanied by involvement of oral mucosa and conjunctivitis. What is the diagnosis?

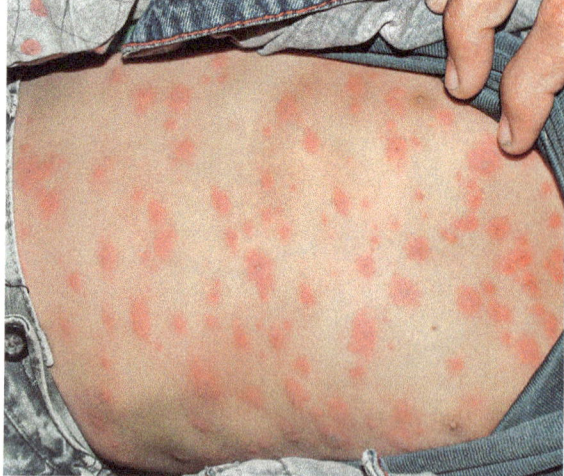

a. Stevens-Johnson syndrome (SJS)
b. Erythema multiforme major
c. Fixed drug eruption (FDE)
d. Toxic epidermal necrolysis

305. This patient developed redness edema and small vesicles on excessive application of anti-inflammatory cream on his forearm. What is the clinical diagnosis?

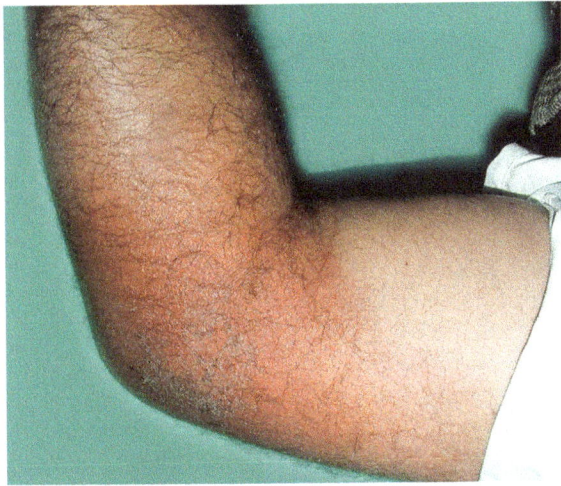

a. Allergic contact dermatitis (ACD)
b. Fixed drug eruption (FDE)
c. Acute irritant contact dermatitis (ICD)
d. Pompholyx

306. This girl presented with epilepsy, low intelligence and multiple red-brown discrete and firm papules on her face. What is the clinical diagnosis?

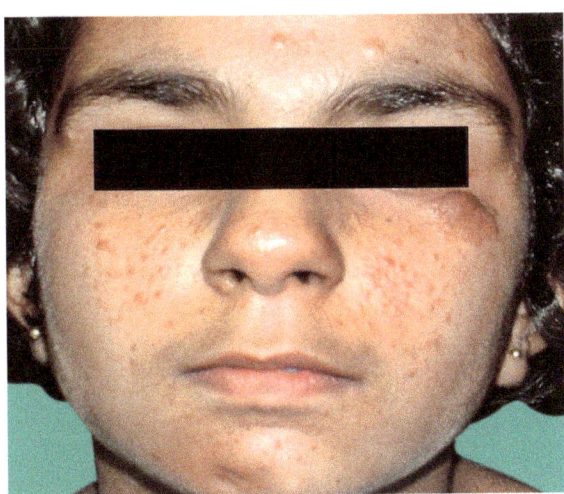

a. Tuberous sclerosis complex (TSC)
b. Neurofibromatosis type 1
c. Plane warts face
d. Acne vulgaris

307. This patient presented with moon shaped face, hair growth on forehead and striae on abdomen and thigh. What is the clinical diagnosis?

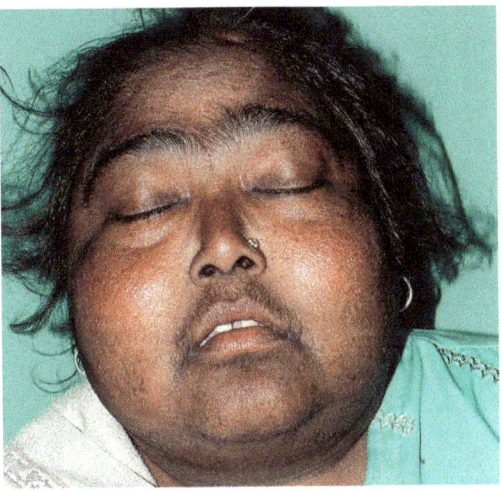

a. Polycystic ovarian syndrome (PCOS)
b. Cushing syndrome due to systemic steroids
c. Androgen secreting tumor
d. Hypothyroidism

308. This patient of psoriasis developed linear psoriatic lesions two weeks after at the site of linear trauma on his back. Which one of the following options is shown in the picture?

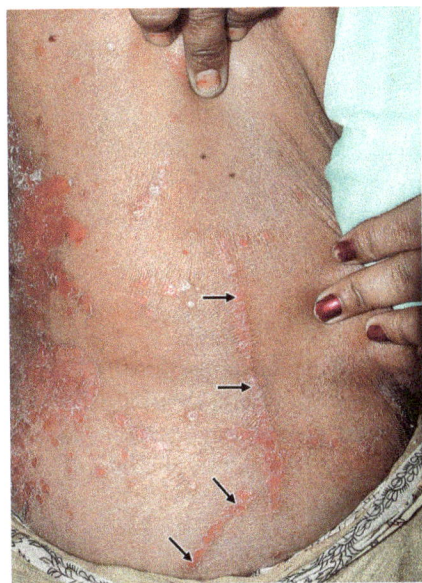

a. Rebound phenomenon
b. Koebner phenomenon
c. Auspitz's sign
d. Grattage test

309. This patient presented with multiple plaques on face and scalp. Plaques on scalp are accompanied by hair loss also. Which one of the followings is closest possibility for this patient?

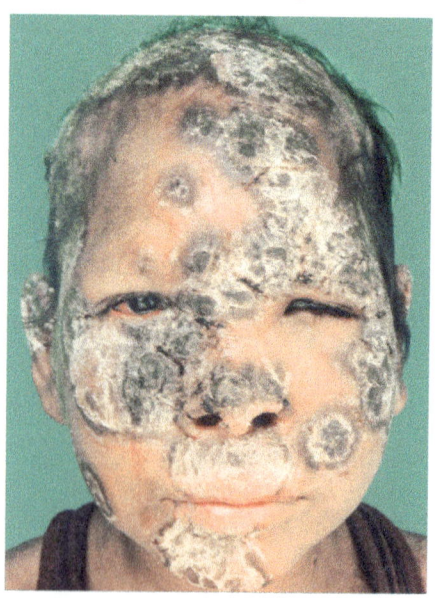

a. Psoriasis
b. Tinea favosa
c. Systemic lupus erythematosus (SLE)
d. Pityriasis amiantacea

310. Which one of the followings is the typical finding in this patient of psoriatic arthritis?

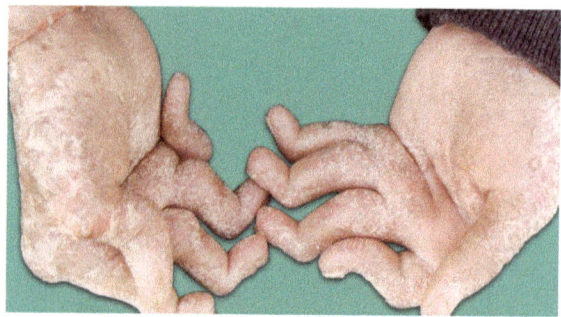

a. Involvement of metacarpophalangeal joint
b. Involvement of carpometacarpal joint
c. Involvement of proximal interphalangeal joint
d. Involvement of distal interphalangeal joint

311. This patient presented with sparse scalp hair, loss of eyebrows, eyelashes and beard hair. He was also having reduced sweating with heat intolerance. He also had hypodontia *(MCQ 323)*. What is the clinical diagnosis?

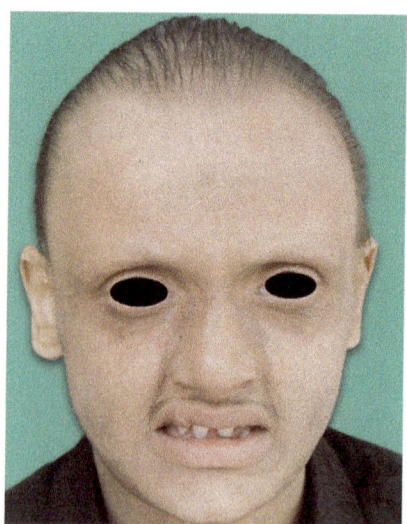

a. Hypothyroidism
b. Anhidrotic ectodermal dysplasia
c. Androgenic alopecia
d. Alopecia universalis

312. This patient presented with 12–15 dark colored asymptomatic macules on front of abdomen for the last many years. Which one of the followings is closest clinical diagnosis?

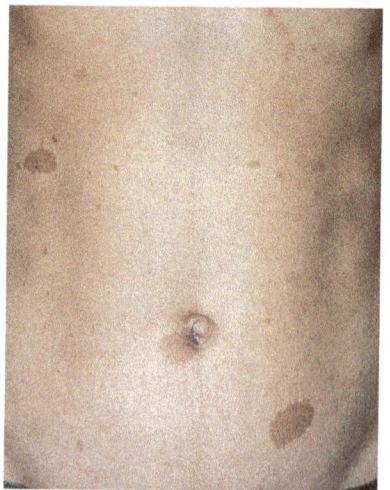

a. Mongolian spots
b. Tuberous sclerosis complex (TCS)
c. Neurofibromatosis type 1
d. Café-au-lait spots (CALMs) in a normal person

313. This typical presentation is seen in which of the following diseases?

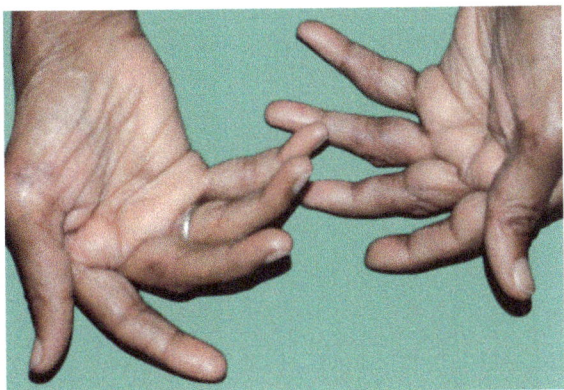

a. Rheumatoid arthritis
b. Psoriatic arthritis
c. Gout
d. Osteoarthritis

314. A 15-year-old boy presented with multiple small plaques (studded with white scales) on scalp. Elbows also showed red plaques with white scales. What is the clinical diagnosis?

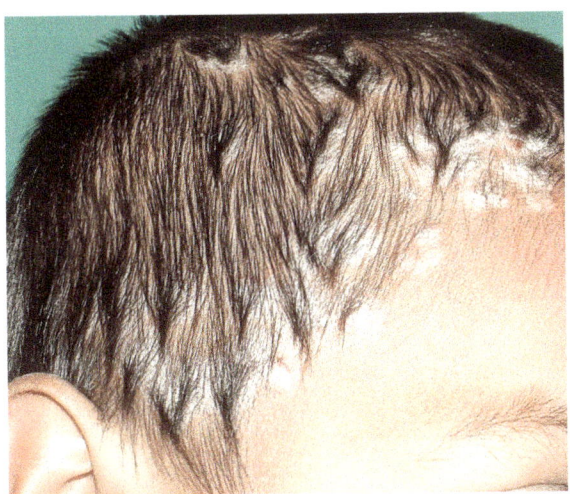

a. Tinea capitis
b. Scalp psoriasis
c. Pityriasis amiantacea
d. Seborrheic capitis

315. A 27-year-old obese lady presented with oligomenorrhea, hirsutism and acanthosis nigricans in the cervical region. What is the clinical diagnosis?

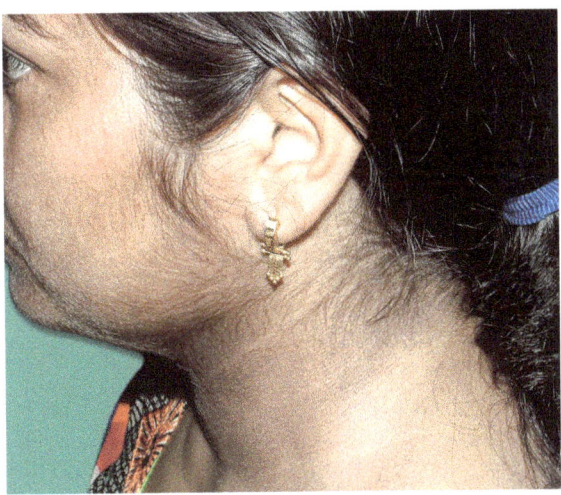

a. Idiopathic hirsutism
b. Androgen secreting tumor
c. Polycystic ovarian syndrome (PCOS)
d. Cushing syndrome

316. This patient of psoriasis received many steroid injections from an unqualified practitioner. It was followed by appearance of profuse number of psoriatic lesions. Which one of the following options it matches?

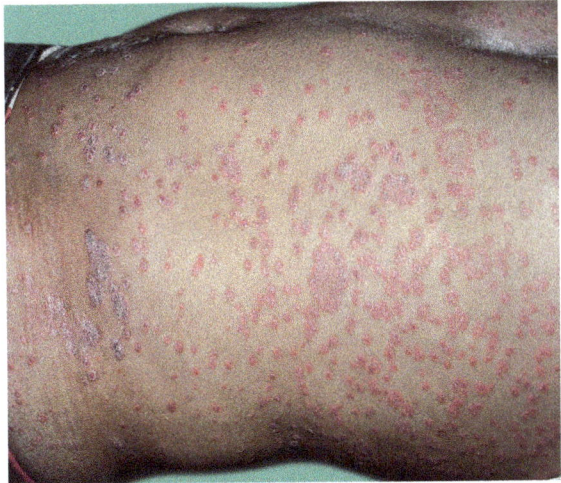

a. Koebner phenomenon
b. Isomorphic phenomenon
c. Auspitz sign
d. Rebound phenomenon

317. This patient developed a smooth, firm and reddish excrescence on the nail fold on her toe after puberty. She was also having epilepsy, low intelligence and adenoma sebaceum on her face. What is the clinical diagnosis?

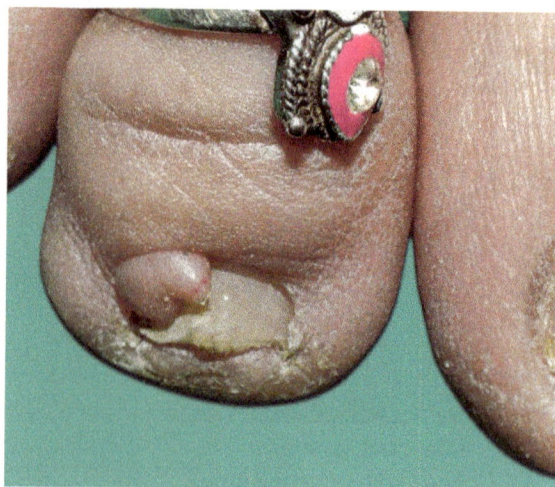

a. Periungual wart
b. Skin tag
c. Periungual fibroma in tuberous sclerosis complex
d. Cutaneous horn

318. Following is the close picture of a patient presented with persistent, multiple, firm, rough, skin or gray-colored papules on seborrheic areas of trunk, extremities, groins and axillae. Nails showed characteristic red longitudinal band which ended in V-shaped notch at margin *(MCQ 178)*. What is the closest diagnosis?

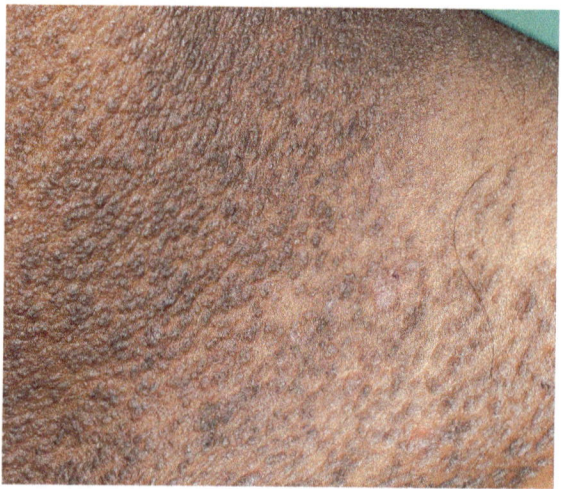

a. Pseudoacanthosis nigricans
b. Seborrheic dermatitis
c. Darier's disease
d. Ichthyosis vulgaris

319. She presented with short squat nose, slanting palpebral fissures, fine and hypopigmented hair. Iris is light colored and shows lighter areas arranged in a ring in outer third (Brushfield's spots). She is also having mental retardation. What is diagnosis?

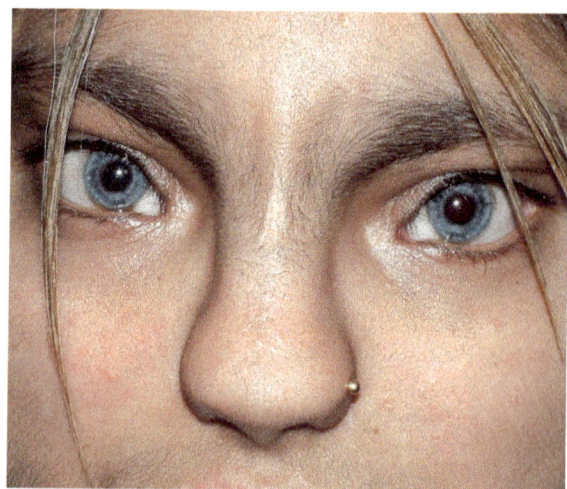

a. Teratogenicity of isotretinoin
b. Down syndrome
c. Teratogenicity of thalidomide
d. Teratogenicity of systemic steroids

320. This patient complained of bluish white foreskin, soreness and difficulty in retracting the prepuce. He is also having few ivory white asymptomatic macules around umbilicus *(MCQ 270)*. What is the possible clinical diagnosis?

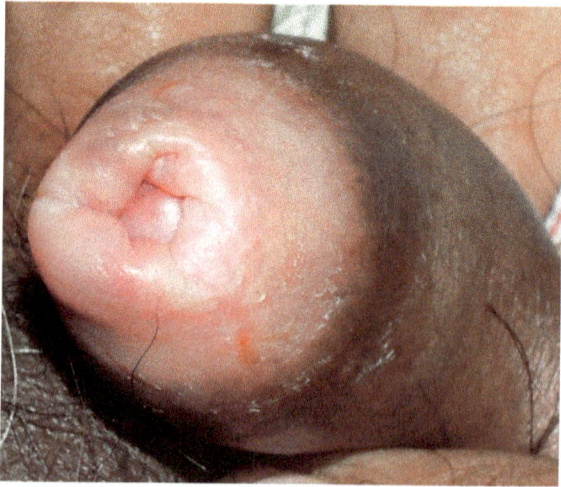

a. Vitiligo
b. Candidal balanoposthitis
c. Balanitis xerotica obliterans (BXO)
d. Smegma

321. A 60-year-old female presented with hirsutism for the last six months accompanied by clitoromegaly *(MCQ 303)*. What is the clinical diagnosis?

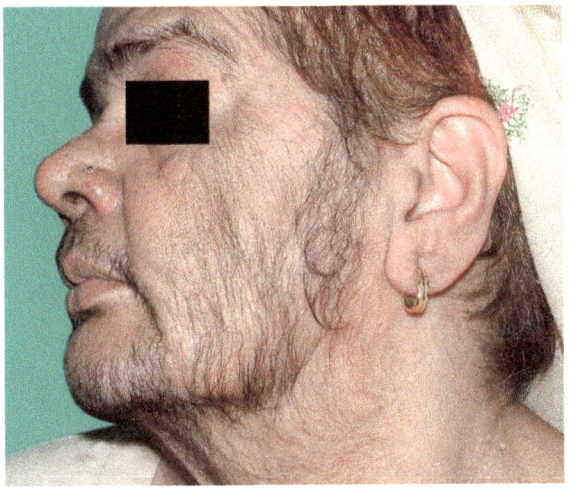

a. Idiopathic hirsutism
b. Polycystic ovarian syndrome (PCOS)
c. Androgen secreting tumor
d. Cushing syndrome

322. The following picture shows the demonstration of easy removal of silvery white scales from a cutaneous lesion with the edge of a glass slide. Which one of the following options is correct for this figure?

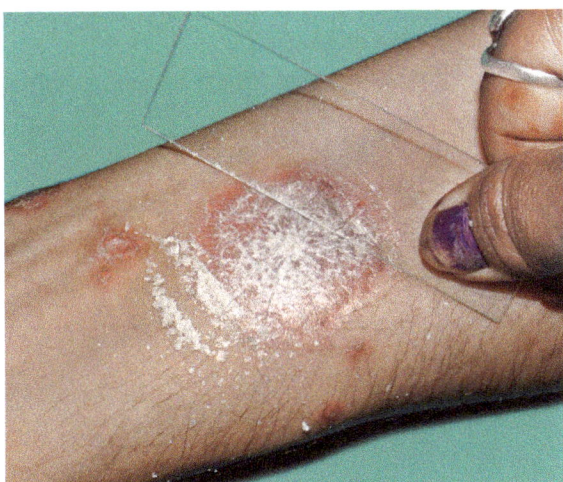

a. Grattage test
b. Koebner phenomenon
c. Auspitz's sign
d. Rebound phenomenon

323. This patient presented with conical and pointed incisors and canines. He was also having sparse hair on scalp, beard and eyelashes *(MCQ 311)*. He also had decreased sweating and heat intolerance. What is the clinical diagnosis?

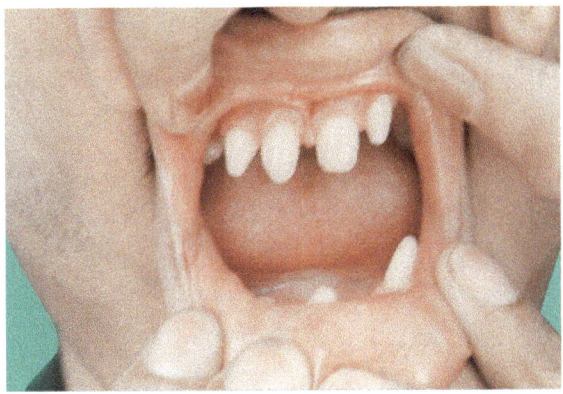

a. Anhidrotic ectodermal dysplasia
b. Hypothyroidism
c. Hutchinson's teeth

324. This child presented with dry rough skin having diffuse and uniform light-colored fish like scales since the age of 6 months. It involved mainly the extensors sparing the diaper area. What is the diagnosis?

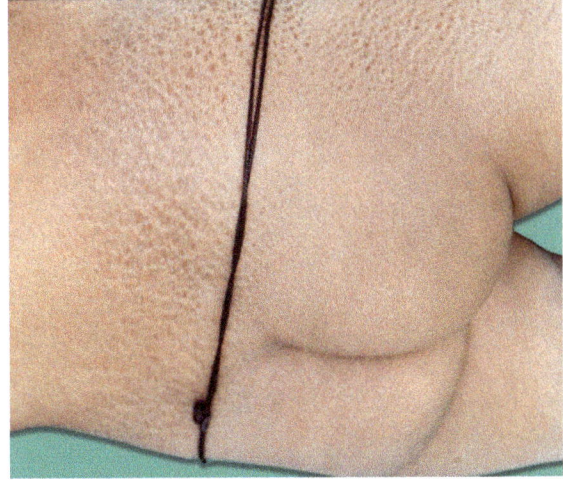

a. X-linked recessive ichthyosis (XLRI)
b. Ichthyosis vulgaris
c. Acquired ichthyosis
d. Atopic dermatitis

325. This patient developed firm rough hyperkeratotic growth on the side of tip of the finger for the last six months. What is the clinical diagnosis?

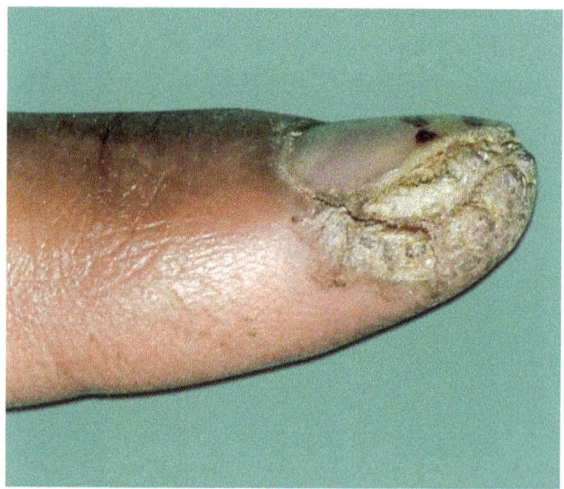

a. Periungual fibroma
b. Periungual wart
c. Cutaneous horn
d. Corn

326. This patient complained of a small perianal papule for the last one year. There is recurrent foul-smelling pus or serosanguinous discharge from it time to time. What is the diagnosis?

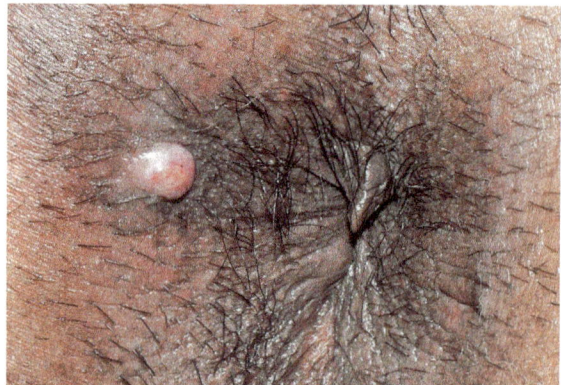

a. Perianal boil
b. Perianal sinus
c. Perianal skin tag
d. Perianal hidradenitis suppurativa

327. A 20-year-old patient presented with a single painful ulcer inside lower lip. He had similar ulcer two three times during the past one year. What is the clinical diagnosis?

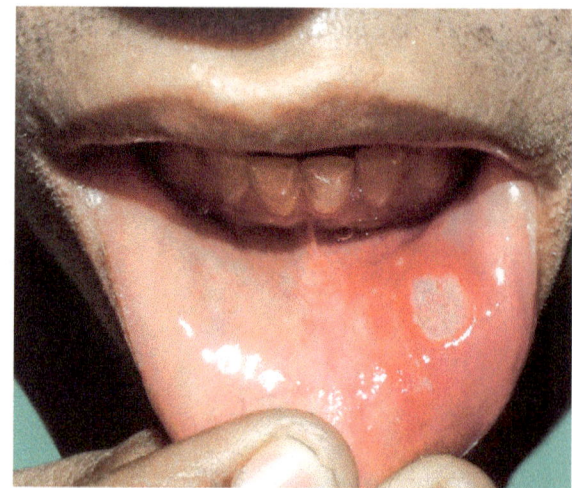

a. Aphthous ulcer
b. Behcet's disease
c. Secondary syphilis ulcer
d. Pemphigus vulgaris

328. A 25-year-old female presented with gradual increased growth of facial hair. She was having no menstrual irregularity or hormonal imbalance. Both ovaries were of normal size (<10 CC). What is the clinical diagnosis?

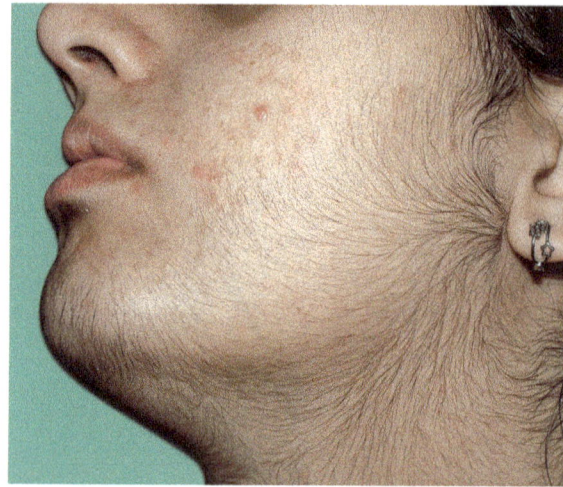

a. Polycystic ovarian syndrome (PCOS)
b. Idiopathic hirsutism
c. Hypertrichosis
d. Steroid induced hirsutism

329. The following picture depicts that after initial removal of silvery white scales from a cutaneous lesion, on further scrapping pin point bleeding spots are visible. Which one of the following options is correct for this figure?

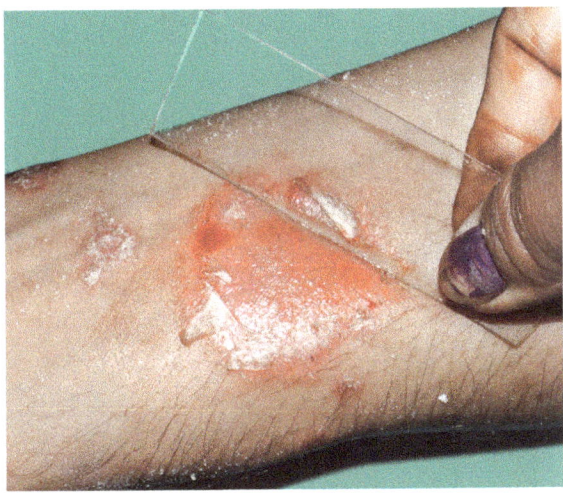

a. Grattage test
b. Auspitz's sign
c. Koebner phenomenon
d. Rebound phenomenon

330. This patient is presented with ocular hypertelorism, short and squat nose, small and deformed ears. He was having mental retardation also. What is the possible diagnosis?

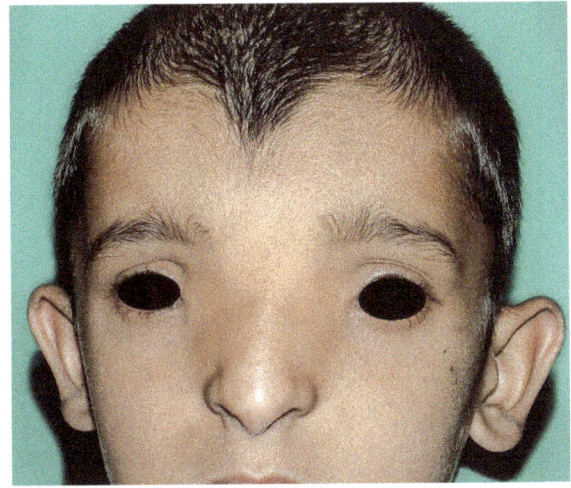

a. Teratogenicity of systemic steroid
b. Teratogenicity of isotretinoin
c. Down syndrome
d. Teratogenicity of thalidomide

331. This patient complained of asymptomatic pedunculated soft growth in medial aspect of upper part of thigh for the last 3–4 years. What is the closest clinical possibility?

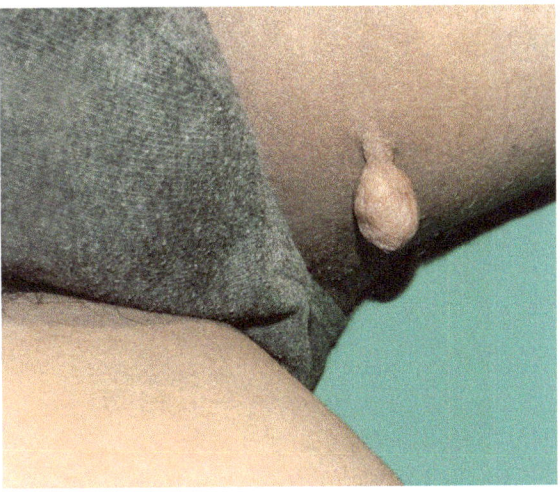

a. Cutaneous horn
b. Molluscum contagiosum
c. Venereal wart
d. Large skin tag

332. This boy presented with widespread purpuric lesions on legs and lower abdomen for the last one week. It was accompanied by mild arthritis. What is the clinical diagnosis?

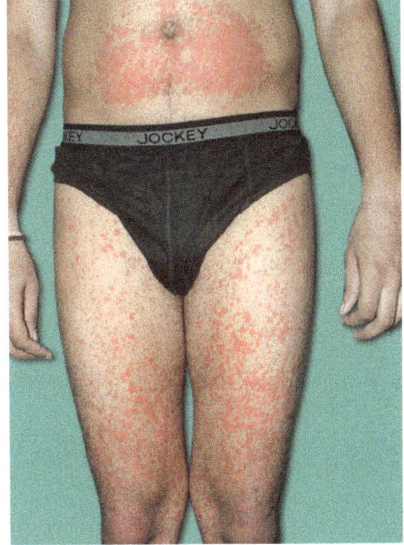

a. Chronic myelocytic leukemia (CML)
b. Henoch-Schonlein purpura (HS purpura)
c. Idiopathic thrombocytopenic purpura (ITP)
d. Senile purpura

333. The patient complaint of the deposition of off white colored cheesy material having foul smell under the foreskin. What is the clinical diagnosis?

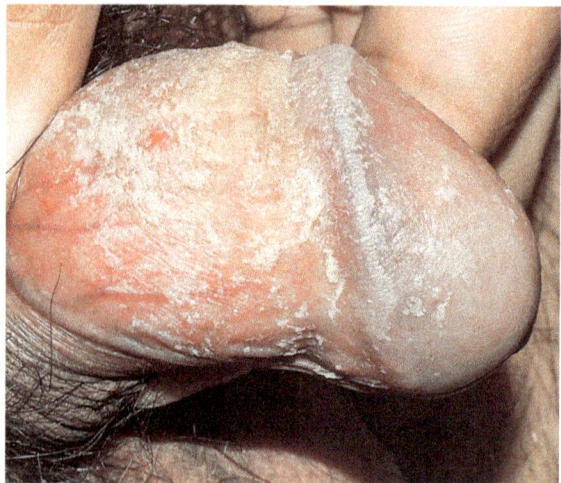

a. Lichen planus
b. Balanitis xerotica obliterans
c. Candidal balanoposthitis
d. Smegma

334. This patient presented with a tuft of coarse terminal hairs in the lumbosacral region for the last many years. What is the clinical diagnosis?

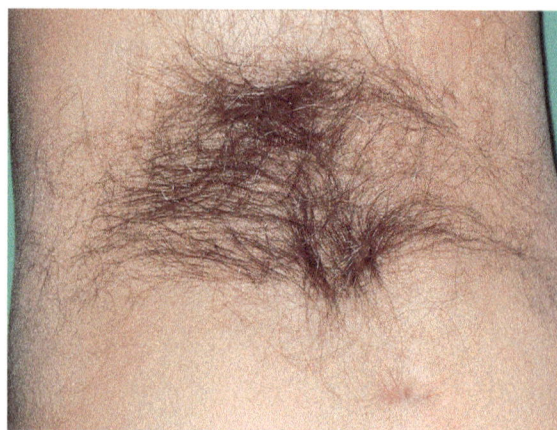

a. Idiopathic hirsutism
b. Androgenic secreting tumor
c. Steroid-induced hypertrichosis
d. Hypertrichosis

335. A 15-year-old boy presented with dark-colored polygonal-shaped scales all over body since first week of his life. Antecubital folds and popliteal folds are spared. What is the possible clinical diagnosis?

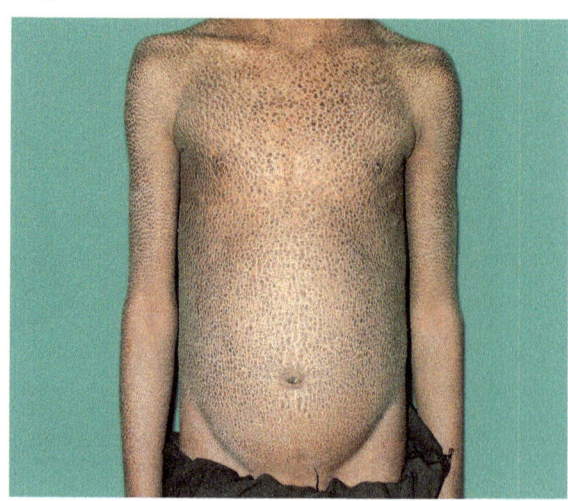

a. X-linked recessive ichthyosis (XLRI)
b. Ichthyosis vulgaris
c. Acquired ichthyosis
d. Atopic dermatitis

336. This patient after taking ciprofloxacin developed itching and maculopapular rash on trunk *(MCQ 236)* and extremities. Rash is comprised of 2–10 mm sized red macules that are confluent at places. What is the diagnosis?

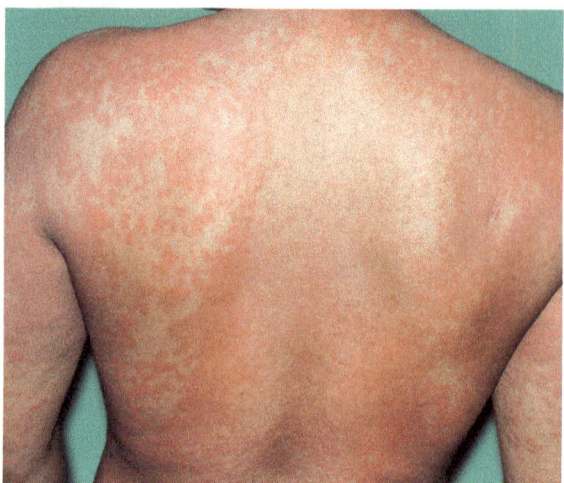

a. Drug-induced urticaria
b. Drug-induced erythroderma
c. Drug-induced morbilliform rash
d. Erythema multiforme (EM)

337. This patient complained of massive thickening of plantar skin at places with difficulty in walking. There is no itching. What is the clinical diagnosis?

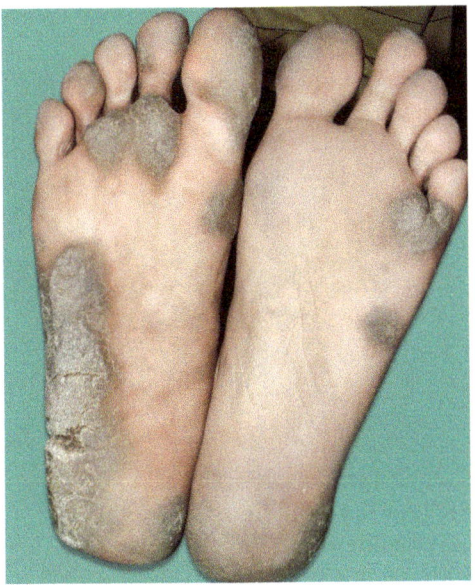

a. Tinea pedis
b. Plantar psoriasis
c. Focal plantar keratoderma
d. Eczema of soles

338. This patient complained of hyperpigmentation studded with coarse terminal hairs in the scapular region since the age of 16 years. What is the clinical diagnosis?

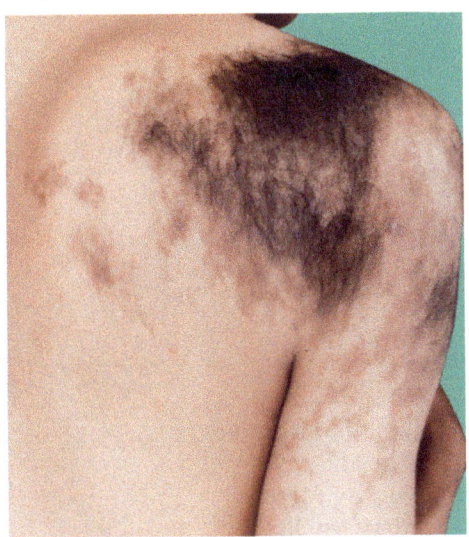

a. Nevus of Ota
b. Nevus of Ito
c. Becker's nevus
d. Congenital melanocytic nevus (CMN)

339. This patient complained of itchy, violaceous, uncountable number of papules on back and extremities. He had mucosal lesions also. What is the closest clinical diagnosis?

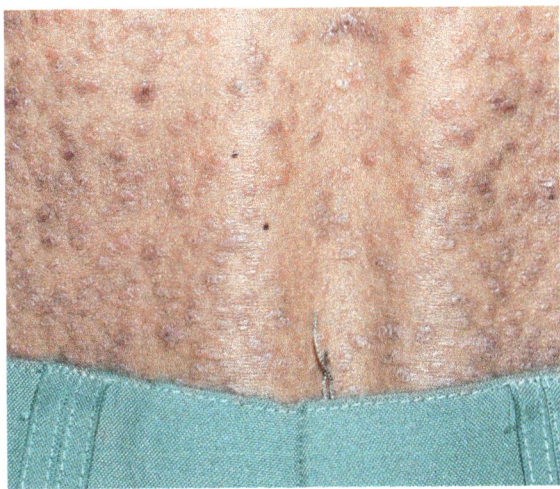

a. Secondary syphilis
b. Lepromatous leprosy (LL)
c. Acne back
d. Lichen planus
e. Acneiform eruption

340. This patient complained of extensive hair loss at vertex with recession of frontal hairline. What is the clinical diagnosis?

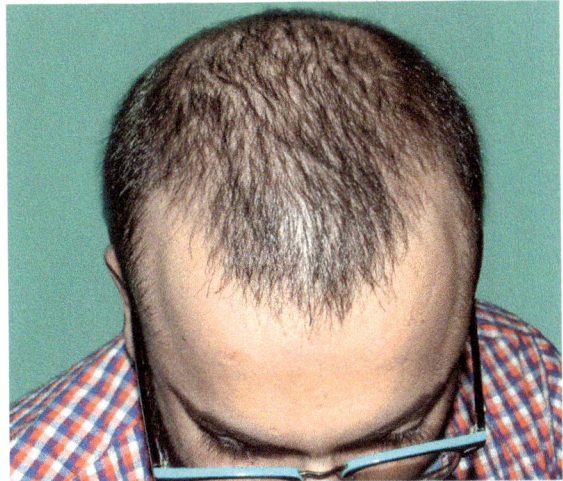

a. Trichotillomania
b. Telogen effluvium
c. Alopecia areata
d. Male androgenic alopecia

341. This patient complained of a big patch of hyper-pigmentation with coarse terminal hairs on forearm since birth. It is gradually enlarging as the body size increases. What is the clinical diagnosis?

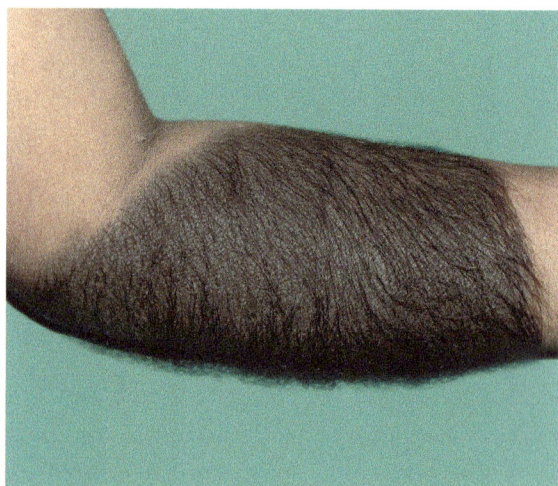

a. Congenital melanocytic nevus (CMN)
b. Becker's nevus
c. Nevus of Ota

342. She noticed red spots in her eye, inside her lower lip, on abdomen and extremities *(MCQ 354)* for the last one week. What is the clinical diagnosis?

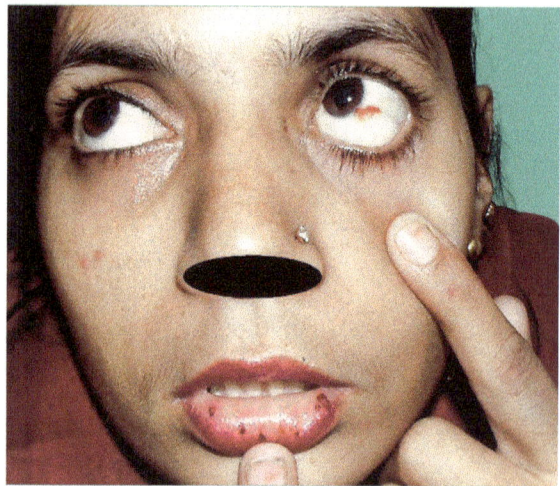

a. Henoch-Schonlein purpura (HS purpura)
b. Chronic myeloblastic leukemia (CML)
c. Senile purpura
d. Idiopathic thrombocytopenic purpura (ITP)

343. A 30-year-old patient complained of multiple recurrent, widely spaced, small abscesses, sinus tracts and scars in the perianal region. He had similar lesions in both axillae also *(MCQ 111)*. What is the possible diagnosis?

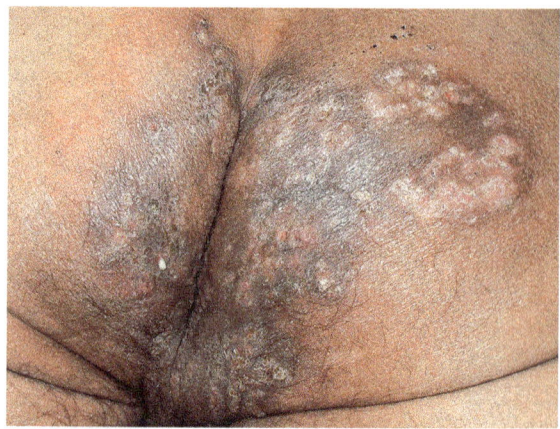

a. Perianal bacterial sinus
b. Scrofuloderma
c. Hidradenitis suppurativa
d. Multiple boils in a diabetic patient

344. She started having oral ulceration about 6 months back. Four months later, she developed multiple flaccid blisters on chest and abdomen which ruptured easily and followed by painful erosions *(MCQ 184)*. What is the clinical diagnosis?

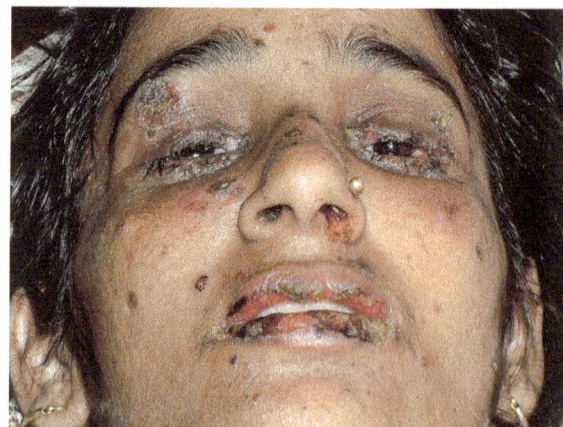

a. Dermatitis herpetiformis (DH)
b. Pemphigoid
c. Pemphigus vulgaris
d. Secondary syphilis

345. This patient presented with a hard yellowish-brown horn like growth on the side of fingertip. What is it?

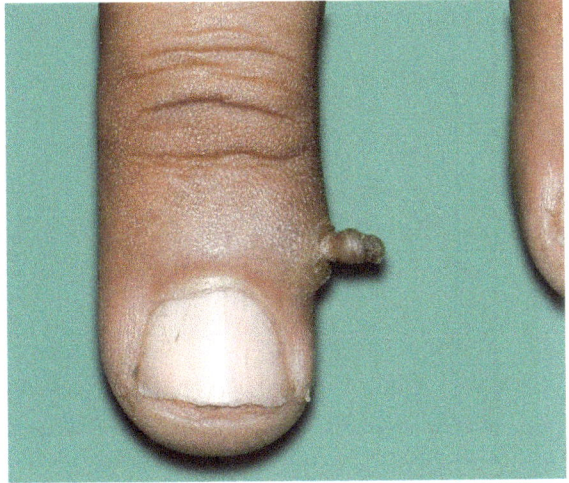

a. Periungual wart
b. Periungual fibroma
c. Cutaneous horn
d. Skin tag

346. Few of the violaceous, itchy papules are forming a linear pattern. Which one of the following phenomena is depicted by the picture?

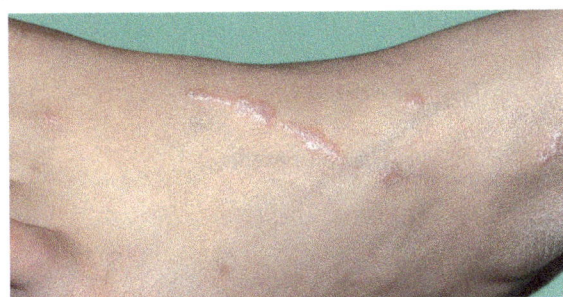

a. Rebound phenomenon
b. Koebner phenomenon
c. Auspitz's sign
d. Grattage test

347. Which one of the following options belongs to the following microphotograph of a KOH smear under high power magnification?

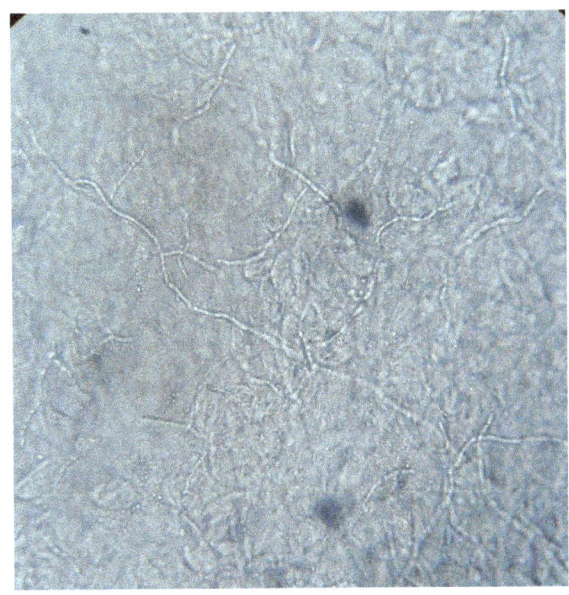

a. Filaments with group of spores in pityriasis versicolor
b. Pseudomycelia of Candida
c. Hyphae of dermatophyte
d. Sclerotic cells of chromoblastomycosis

348. This farmer developed firm irritable but painless papules on both hands. It was followed by formation of dark colored crust on the depressed center of nodules. Which one of the followings is the closest clinical diagnosis?

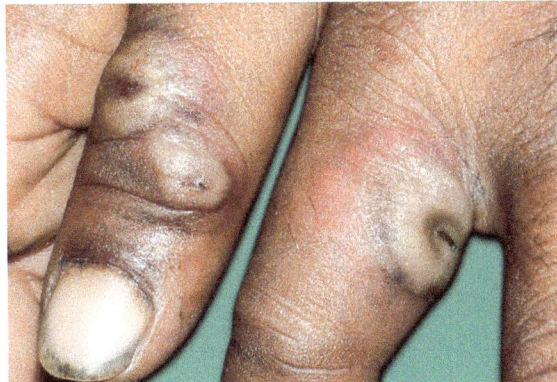

a. Boils
b. Infected molluscum contagiosum
c. Milker's nodule
d. Infected common warts

349. A 6-year-old boy presented with dark-colored scales all over body since the age of one week. It spared axillary folds, cubital folds and popliteal folds. Which one is the closest clinical diagnosis?

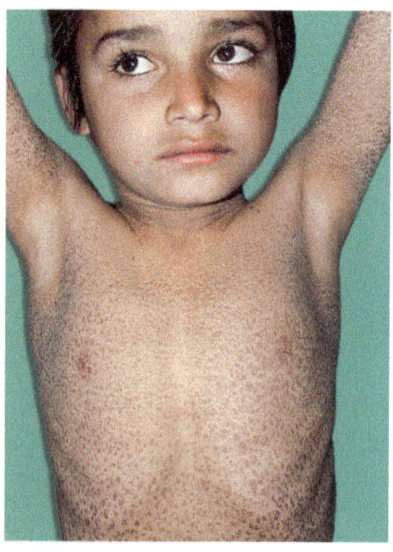

a. Ichthyosis vulgaris
b. Acquired ichthyosis
c. Atopic dermatitis
d. X-linked recessive ichthyosis (XLRI)

350. This patient complained of hard keratotic papule on lateral aspect of fifth toes on both feet. What is the clinical diagnosis?

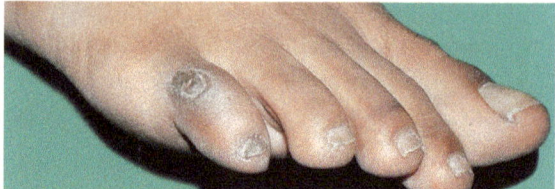

a. Callus
b. Corn
c. Wart
d. Knuckle pads

351. Which one of the following options belongs to the following microphotograph under oil immersion lens?

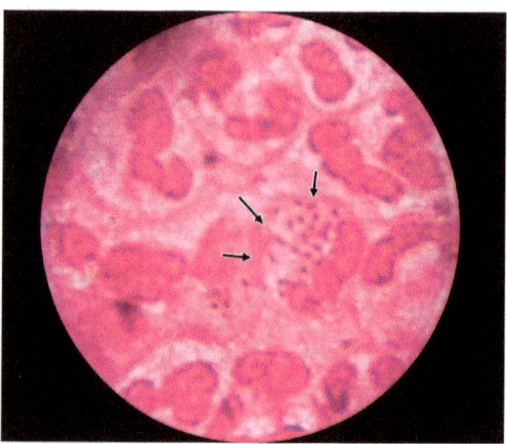

a. Acantholytic cells in Tzanck smear
b. Leishman-Donovan bodies (LD bodies)
c. Gram-negative diplococci inside neutrophils
d. Red stained AFB in slit skin smear

352. Which one of the following statements is not true about this patient showing 15 mm × 15 mm sized induration in tuberculin skin test using PPD as antigen?

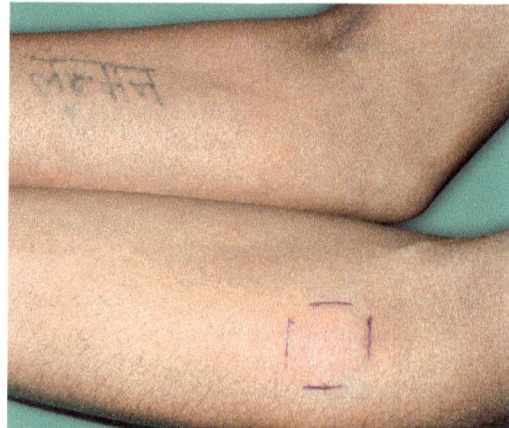

a. It is interpreted as doubtful
b. It suggests a favorable prognosis
c. He is less susceptible to new *M. tuberculosis* infection than PPD negative patient
d. It does not imply immunity to tuberculosis
e. It does not suggest the presence of active disease in vaccinated children or patients above two years of age

353. She complained of recurrence of herpes zoster on the right flank. Previous attack of herpes zoster is evident by the hypopigmentation on left side. Which one of the following statements is correct?

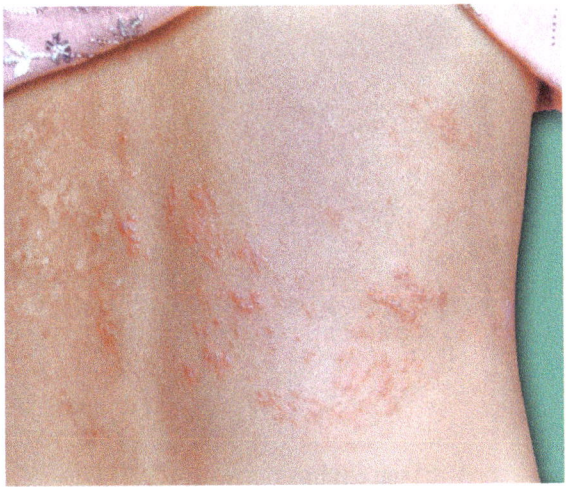

a. It can recur in a patient receiving high dose of systemic steroids
b. It can recur in a diabetic patient
c. It is alarming, HIV infection must be ruled out
d. It is not alarming. Rarely, it can recur

354. She noticed red spots and bluish macules on her extremities and abdomen for the last one week. She also had similar red spots inside her lower lip *(MCQ 342)*. What is the closest clinical diagnosis?

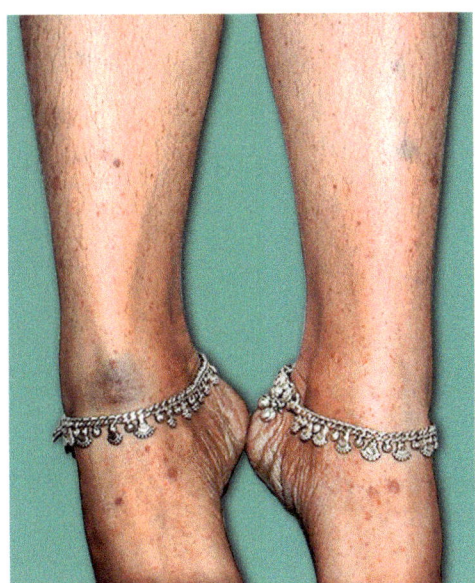

a. Senile purpura
b. Idiopathic thrombocytopenic purpura (ITP)
c. Henoch-Schonlein purpura (HS purpura)
d. Chronic myeloblastic leukemia (CML)

355. This patient presented with circumscribed asymptomatic thickening over the finger joints. What is the clinical diagnosis?

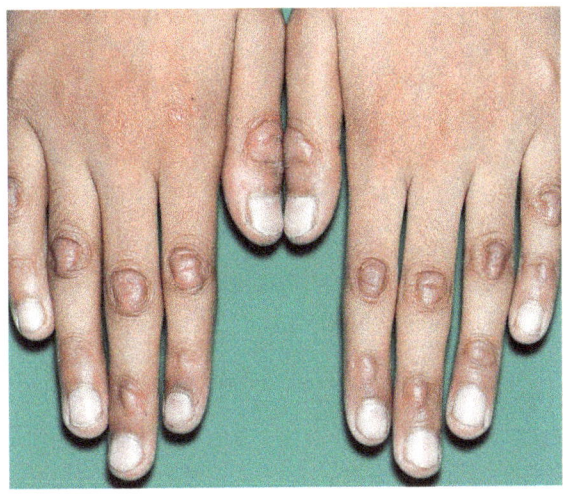

a. Common warts
b. Callus
c. Corns
d. Knuckle pads
e. Gottron papules

356. This patient complained of multiple shiny dome shaped papular lesions on the back. Magnifying glass *(MCQ 375)* revealed central umbilications. What is the clinical diagnosis?

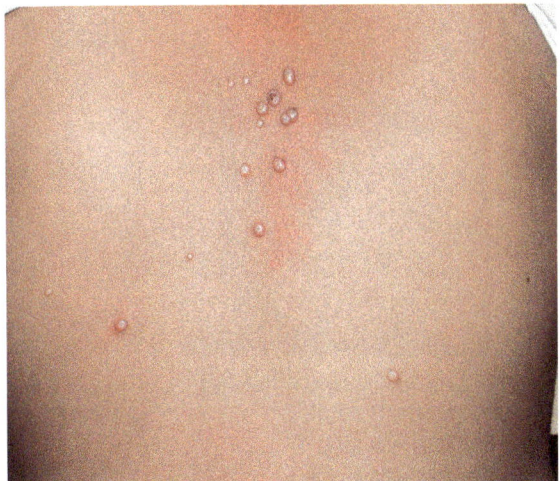

a. Acne vulgaris back
b. Acneiform eruption
c. Acne conglobata
d. Molluscum contagiosum

357. This patient complained of pain, redness and swelling of upper lip for the last six days. What is the clinical diagnosis?

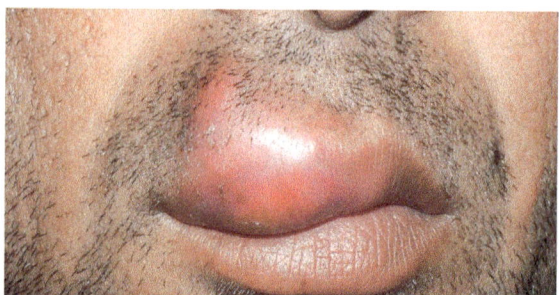

a. Angioedema
b. Boil
c. Granulomatous cheilitis
d. Sycosis barbae

358. She complained of itching and fine white scales on the entire scalp. What is the clinical diagnosis?

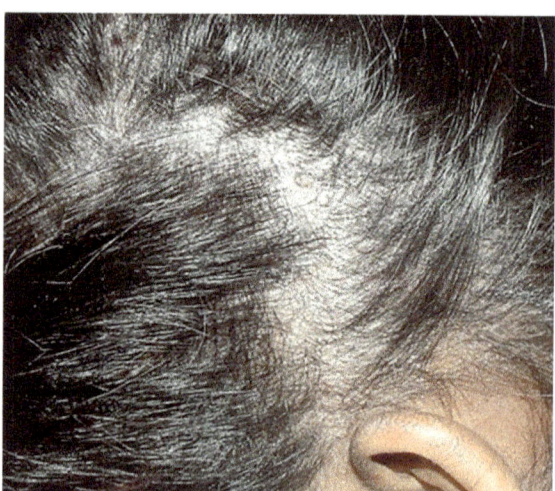

a. Pityriasis versicolor (PV)
b. Pityriasis capitis
c. Pityriasis alba
d. Pityriasis rosea

359. A 60-year-old man presented with itching on face, neck, popliteal fossae and cubital fossae (MCQ 401). What is the closest clinical diagnosis?

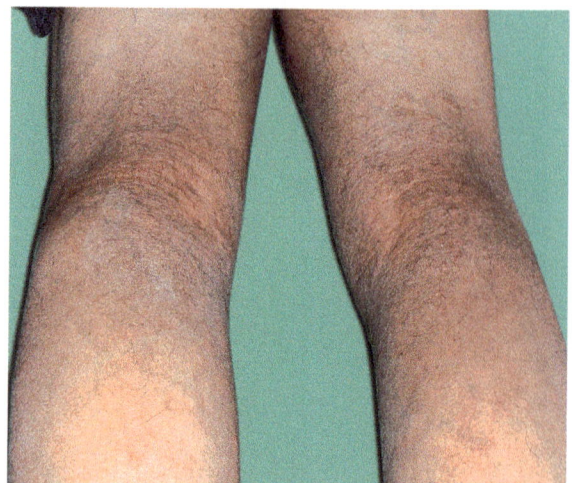

a. Airborne contact dermatitis (ABCD)
b. Adult phase atopic dermatitis
c. Seborrheic dermatitis (SD)
d. Darier's disease (DD)

360. This child complained of itching in the preauricular region. He was also having chronic pus discharge from this ear. What is the clinical diagnosis?

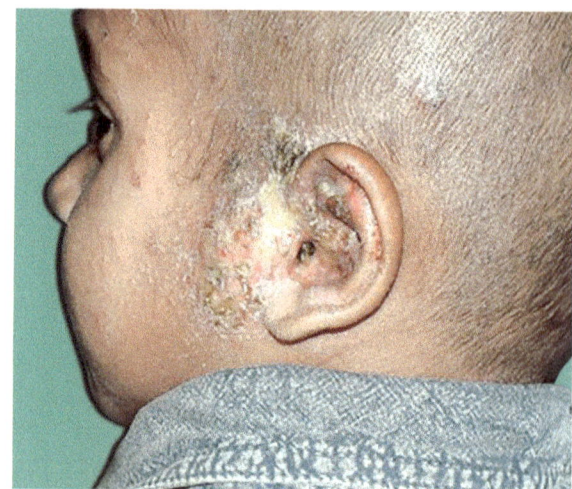

a. Impetigo contagiosa
b. Scrofuloderma
c. Infected dermatitis
d. Ecthyma

361. This patient presented with discrete papules on his face. One year back, he had persistent high undulating fever, hepatosplenomegaly and lymphadenopathy. He also had ashy black pigmentation on face, hands, feet and abdomen. What is the clinical diagnosis?

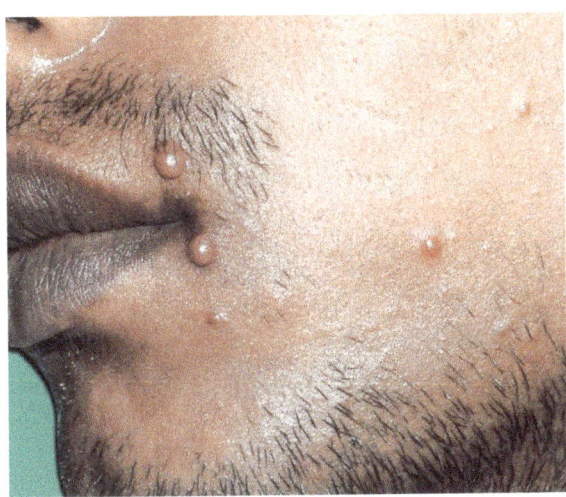

a. Molluscum contagiosum
b. Post kala-azar dermal leishmaniasis (PKDL)
c. Intradermal nevi
d. Trichoepithelioma

362. She complained of redness, itching and fissuring of both lips for the last three months. What is the clinical diagnosis?

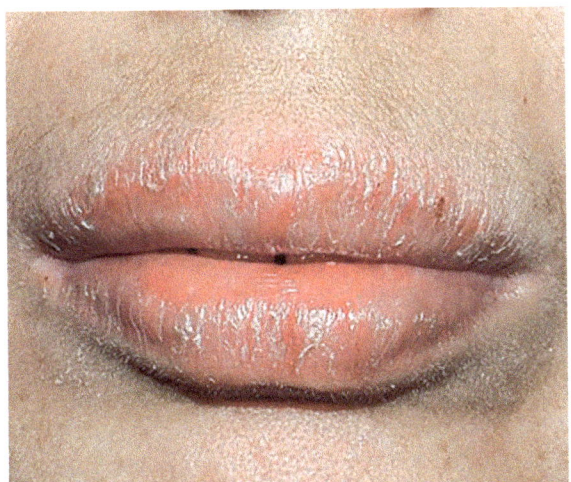

a. Contact irritant dermatitis (CID) due to lipstick
b. Contact allergic dermatitis (CAD) due to lipstick
c. Lip-lick cheilitis
d. Fixed drug eruption (FDE)

363. Which one of the following options belongs to the following microphotograph of KOH smear under high power magnification?

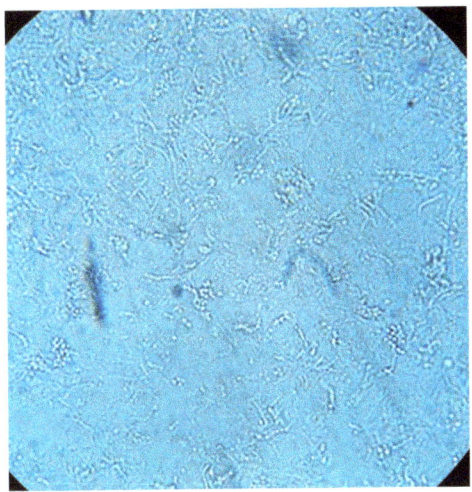

a. Hyphae of dermatophytes
b. Sclerotic cells of chromoblastomycosis
c. Pseudomycelia of Candida
d. Filaments with groups of spores in pityriasis versicolor

364. This patient presented with single thick hyperkeratotic plaque on the medial side of big toe. What is the closest clinical diagnosis?

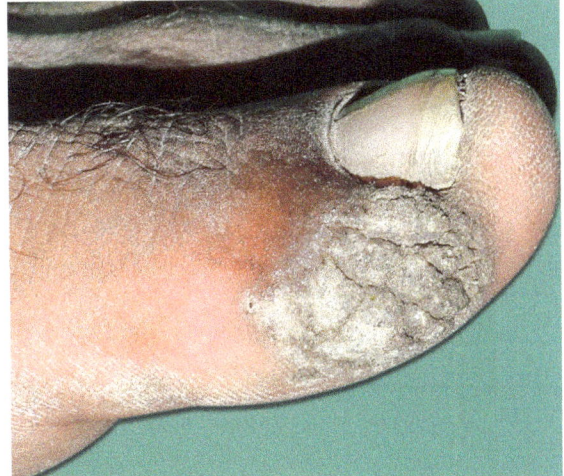

a. Periungual wart
b. Tuberculosis verrucosa cutis (TVC)
c. Periungual fibroma
d. Corn

365. This man very gradually developed pigmentation on his legs in a span of last four years. What is the clinical diagnosis?

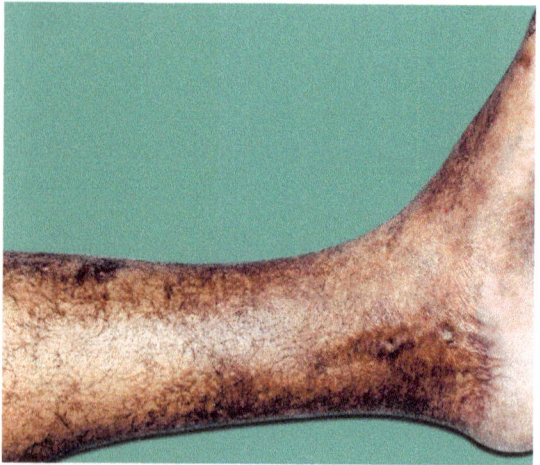

a. Senile purpura
b. Schamberg's disease
c. Lichen planus
d. Chronic myelocytic leukemia (CML)

366. This young patient complained of persistent diffuse painless enlargement of both lips for the last one year. Which one of the following possibilities is the closest diagnosis?

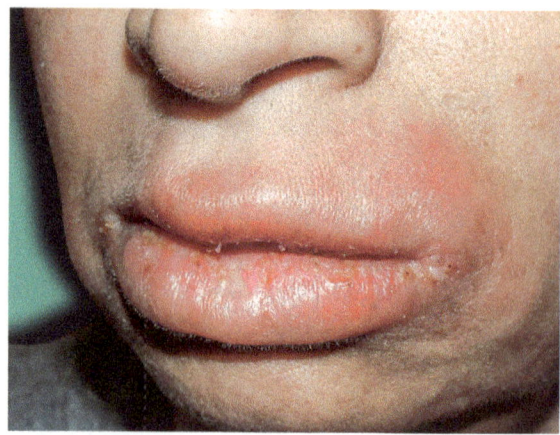

a. Granulomatous cheilitis
b. Angular cheilitis
c. Cheilitis glandularis
d. Actinic cheilitis

367. This patient presented with a painful ulcer which is surrounded by a zone of erythema. Ulcer has violaceous undermined edges and base is covered with pus. What is the closest clinical diagnosis?

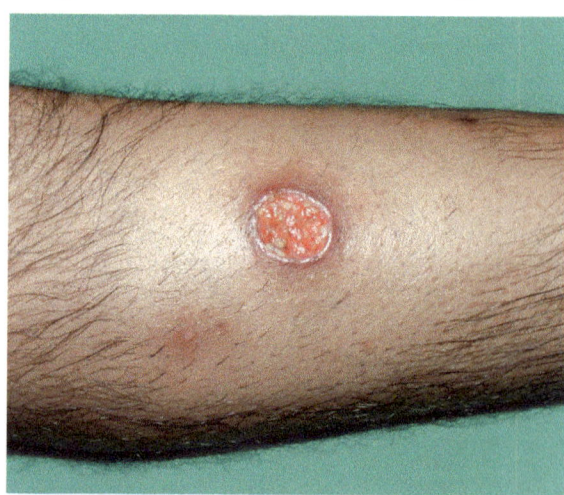

a. Ecthyma
b. Tuberculosis chancre
c. Pyoderma gangrenosum
d. Boil

368. Which one of the following options belongs to this microphotograph under oil immersion lens?

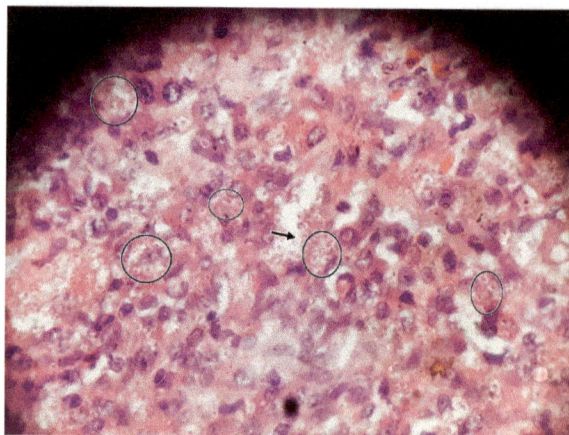

a. Acantholytic cells in Tzanck smear
b. Leishman-Donovan bodies (LD bodies)
c. Gram negative diplococci inside neutrophils
d. Red stained AFB in slit skin smear

369. This patient presented with a painless ill-defined waxy looking yellowish thickened plaque on the sole. What is the clinical diagnosis?

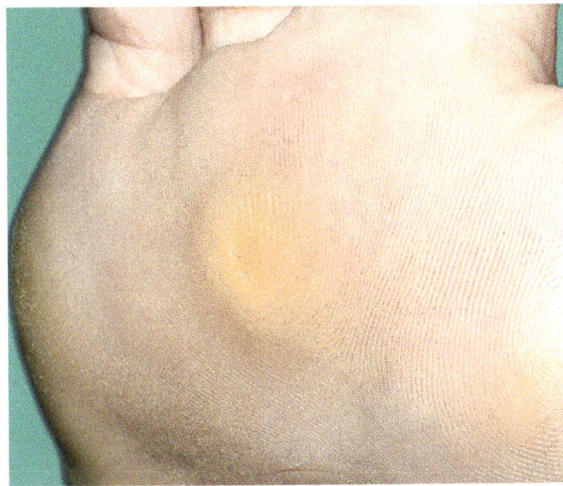

a. Corn
b. Plantar wart
c. Callus
d. Focal keratoderma on sole

370. A 1-month-old female baby was having streaks and whorls of hyperpigmented macules on the trunk and extremities. Whorls on abdomen are studded with vesicles. What is the clinical diagnosis?

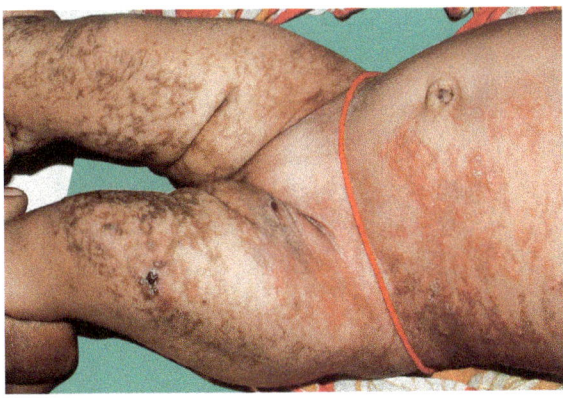

a. Incontinentia pigmenti
b. Dyskeratosis congenita
c. Peutz-Jeghers syndrome
d. Cafe-au-lait macules (CALMs)

371. This patient presented with highly pruritic closely placed papules on the shins. What is the closest diagnosis?

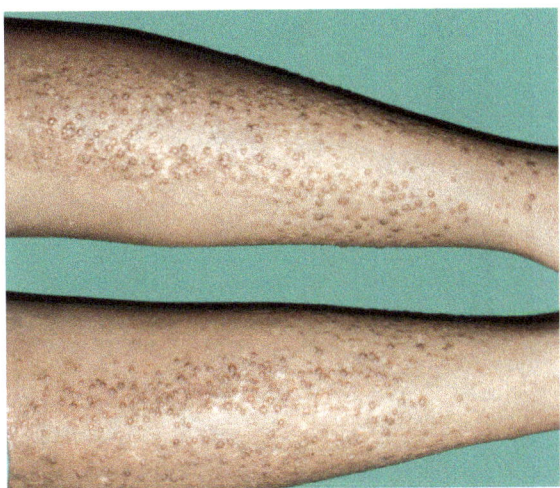

a. Lichen planus
b. Lichen amyloidosis
c. Prurigo nodularis
d. Darier's disease

372. This patient presented with roughness and thickening that involved entire palm of both hands. With magnifying glass, ill-defined superficial rough hyperkeratotic lesions *(MCQ 397)* showing coalescence are well appreciated. What is the clinical diagnosis?

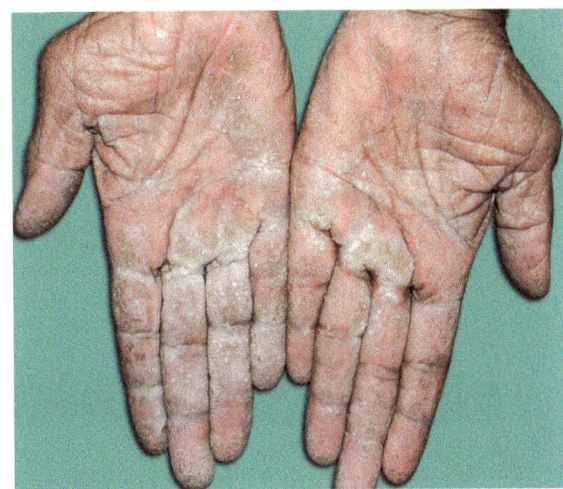

a. Pompholyx
b. Corns
c. Lichen planus
d. Superficial palmoplantar warts (mosaic warts)
e. Deep palmoplantar warts

373. Which one of the following options belongs to the following microphotograph under oil immersion lens?

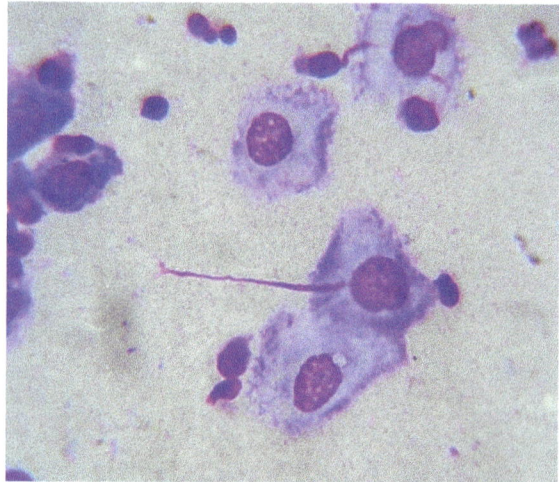

a. Leishman-Donovan bodies (LD bodies)
b. Acantholytic cells
c. Gram negative diplococci inside neutrophils
d. Red stained AFBs in slit skin smear

375. Following picture is a magnified view of multiple papular lesions on back *(MCQ 356)*. What is the clinical diagnosis?

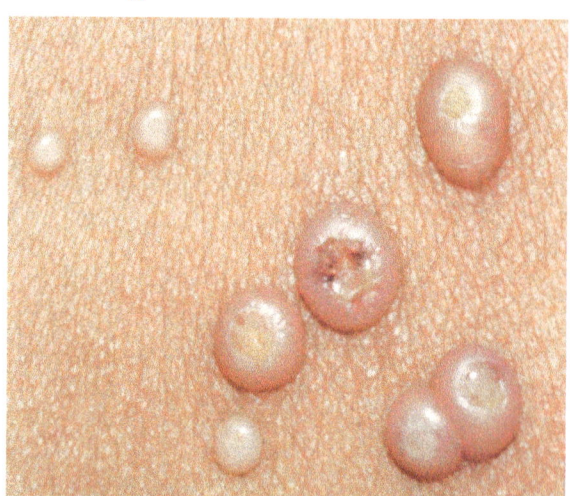

a. Milker's nodule
b. Molluscum contagiosum
c. Common warts
d. Acne conglobata

374. Tuberculin skin test in this patient shows 25 mm × 25 mm sized induration with blister formation. Which one of the following statements is not true?

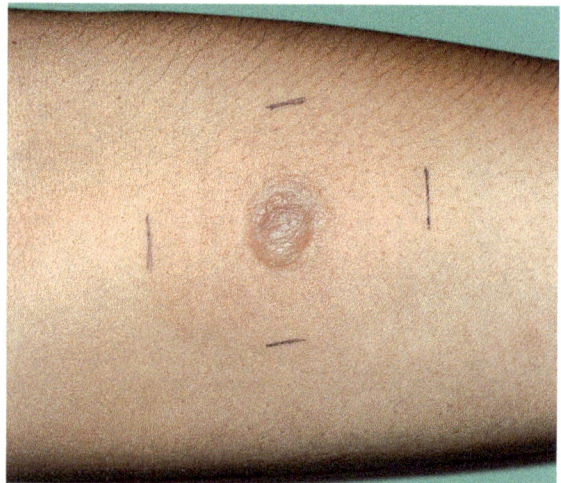

a. He is a strong reactor
b. It suggests susceptibility to tuberculosis infection
c. It suggests presence of active disease
d. It indicates protection from tuberculosis infection

376. This patient complained of bright red scaly patches on the distal parts of the big toe and adjoining toes of both feet. What is the clinical diagnosis?

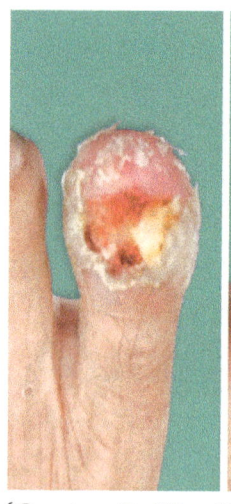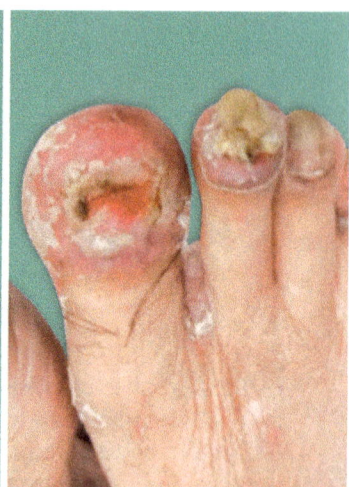

(*Courtesy:* Dr Vijay Singhal)

a. Acropustulosis
b. Keratoderma blennorrhagica
c. Eczema feet
d. Tinea pedis

377. This lady complained of recurrent pruritic, papular lesions on trunk and extremities for the last three years.

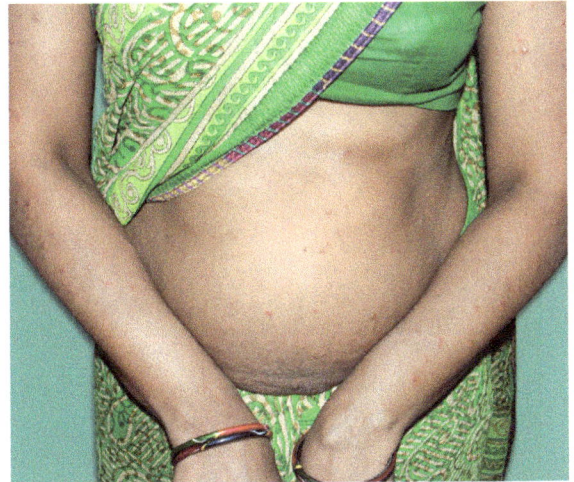

a. Papular urticaria (insect bite hypersensitivity)
b. Cutaneous manifestation of hepatitis B infection
c. Pityriasis rosea
d. Gianotti-Crosti syndrome

378. This patient presented with pinkish brown scar like atrophic macules on pretibial region during his antihypertensive and antidiabetic treatment. What is the clinical diagnosis?

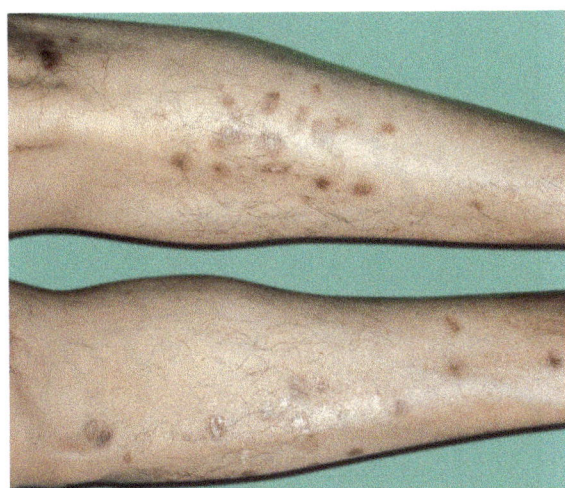

a. Granuloma annulare
b. Lichen amyloidosis
c. Diabetic rubeosis
d. Diabetic dermopathy

379. This patient presented with asymptomatic, indolent, reddish and ill-defined swelling on his forearm for the last three years. Histopathology showed normal epidermis, acellular grenz zone between epidermis and dermis. Dermis showed pan dermal infiltration by lymphocytes. What is the clinical diagnosis?

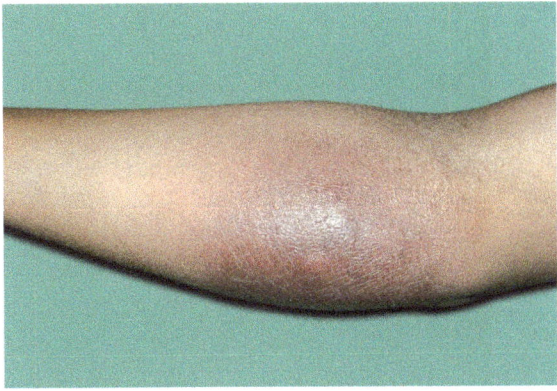

a. Mycetoma
b. Lymphocytoma cutis
c. Mycosis fungoides
d. Actinic reticuloid

380. Seven days after a sexual contact with a commercial sex worker (CSW), he started having burning micturition and pus discharge from urethra. What is the clinical diagnosis?

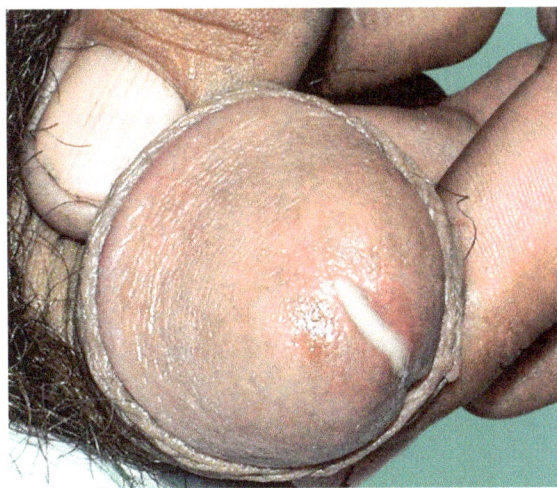

a. Balanoposthitis
b. Reiter's disease
c. Urethral syndrome
d. Smegma

381. This child presented with pruritic, purplish papules on extensors of both legs. What is the clinical diagnosis?

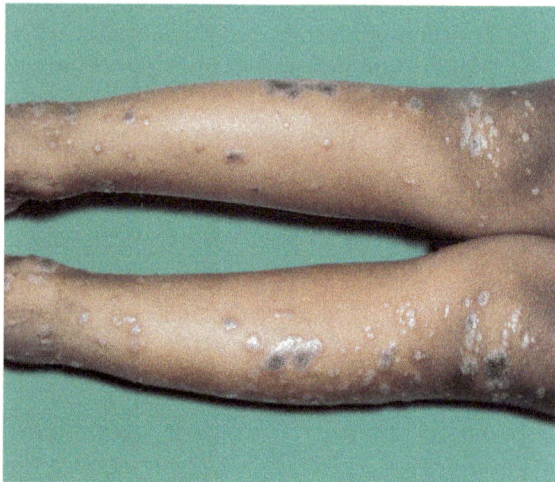

a. Lichen amyloidosis
b. Lichen planus
c. Psoriasis
d. Prurigo nodularis

383. This patient complained of dryness, itching, thickening and fissuring of both palms for the last six months. What is the clinical diagnosis?

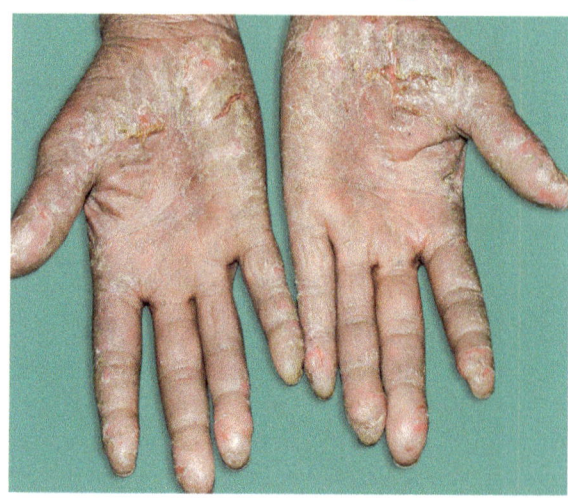

a. Psoriasis palms
b. DLE palm
c. Hyperkeratotic palmar eczema
d. Lichen planus palms
e. Palmar keratoderma

382. This patient presented with single painless ulcer with thin, bluish, undermined margins and watery discharge. What is the closest clinical possibility?

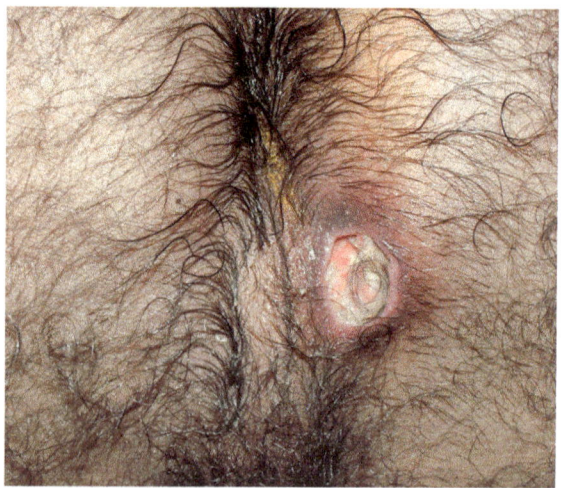

a. Tuberculosis chancre
b. Pyoderma gangrenosum
c. Perianal sinus
d. Carbuncle

384. A 15-year-old child complained of large patch of hair loss in occipital region. What is the closest clinical possibility?

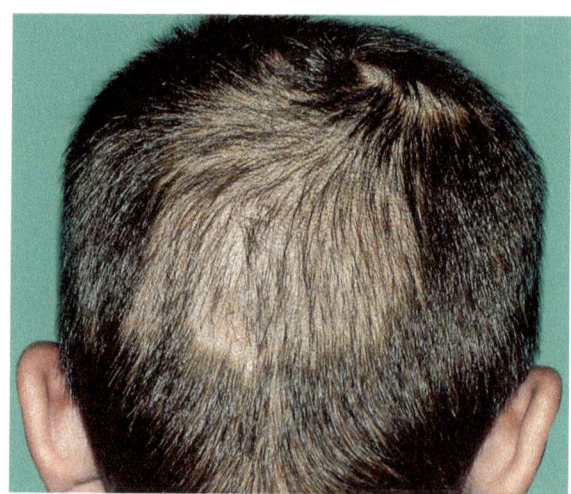

a. Alopecia areata
b. Trichotillomania
c. Pseudopelade of Brocq
d. Tinea capitis

Chapter 4 ✦ MCQs of Dermatology, Venereology and Leprology

385. A caretaker of livestock developed these lesions on face for the last one month. There is no significant itching or pain in these lesions. What is the closest clinical diagnosis?

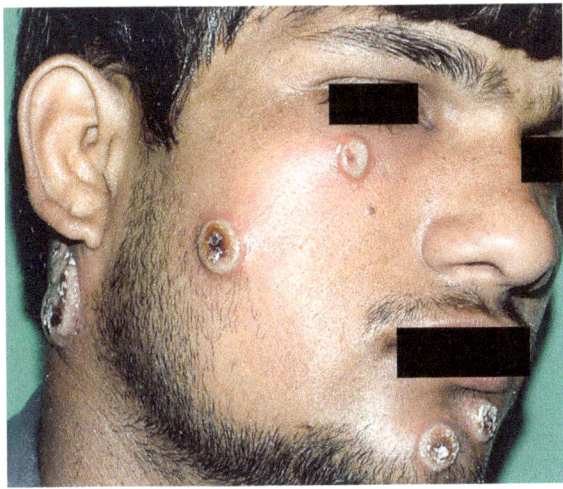

a. Infected molluscum contagiosum
b. Impetigo contagiosa
c. Infected chickenpox
d. Milker's nodule

386. This patient noticed blistering overnight in his one cubital fossa. Blisters are filled with clear fluid. There is no mucosal involvement. What is the closest clinical diagnosis?

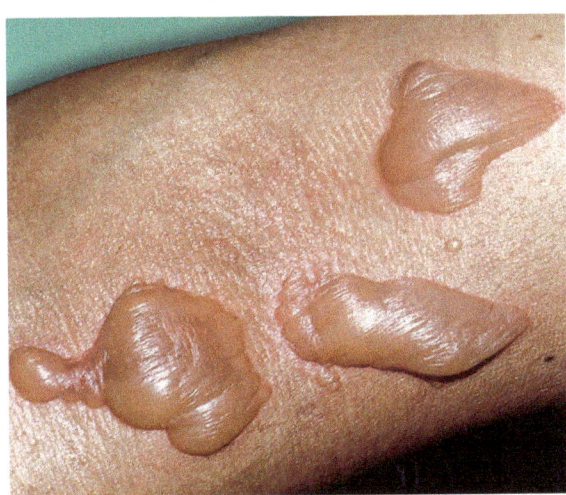

a. Erythema multiforme (EM)
b. Fixed drug eruption (FDE)
c. Bullous impetigo
d. *Paederus dermatitis*

387. This patient complained of red papules and pustules for the last four years in the beard region. What is the clinical diagnosis?

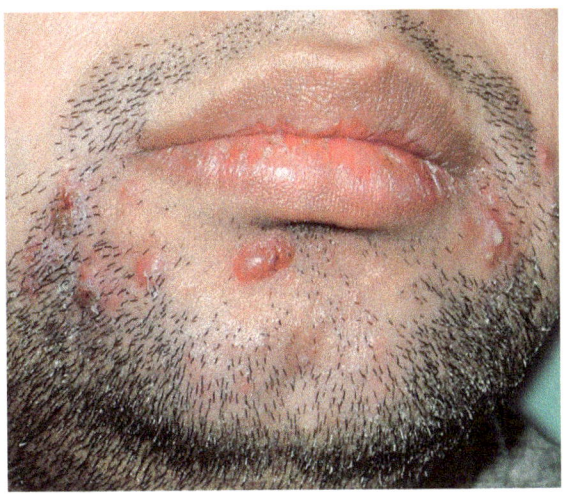

a. Chronic superficial folliculitis (CSF)
b. Sycosis barbae (deep folliculitis)
c. Dermatophytic folliculitis
d. Pseudofolliculitis barbae

388. Which one of the following options belongs to this microphotograph under oil immersion lens?

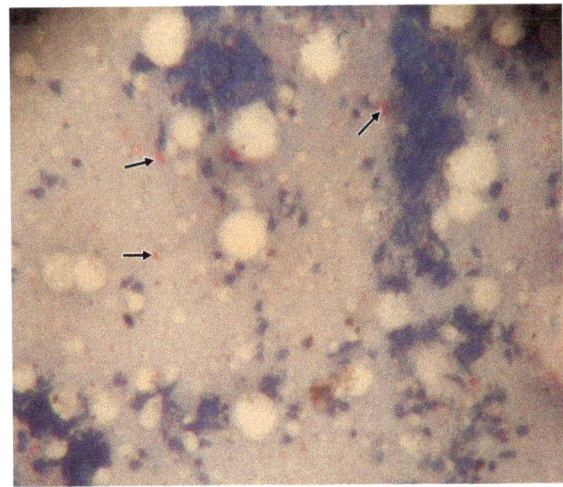

a. Gram-negative diplococci inside neutrophils
b. Acantholytic cells in Tzanck smear
c. Red stained AFB in slit skin smear
d. Leishman-Donovan bodies (LD bodies)

389. She complained of multiple small lesions on face. The appearance of lesions along the line of scratch is showing which one of the following phenomena?

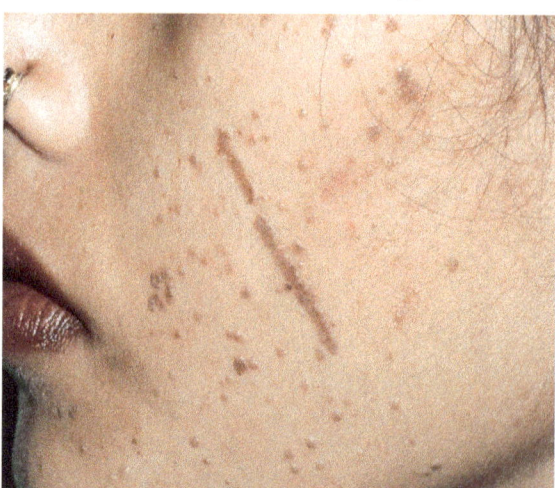

a. Rebound phenomenon
b. Auspitz sign
c. Grattage test
d. Koebner phenomenon

390. A 30-year-old man is developing large ecchymotic patches on various parts of body time to time. What is the clinical diagnosis?

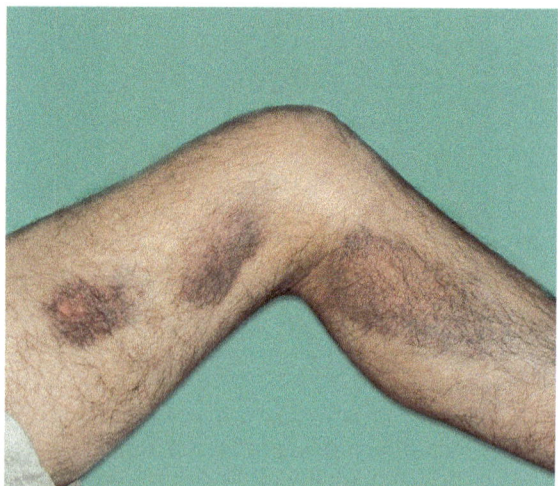

a. Idiopathic thrombocytopenic purpura (ITP)
b. Senile purpura
c. Henoch-Schonlein purpura (HSP)
d. Chronic myelocytic leukemia (CML)

391. A 8-year-old child presented with asymptomatic, symmetric hyperkeratotic and well-defined plaques in the axillae, groins, suprapubic region and around umbilicus since infancy. Hair, nails and mucous membranes are unaffected. Histopathology is nonspecific. Which one of the following options is closest?

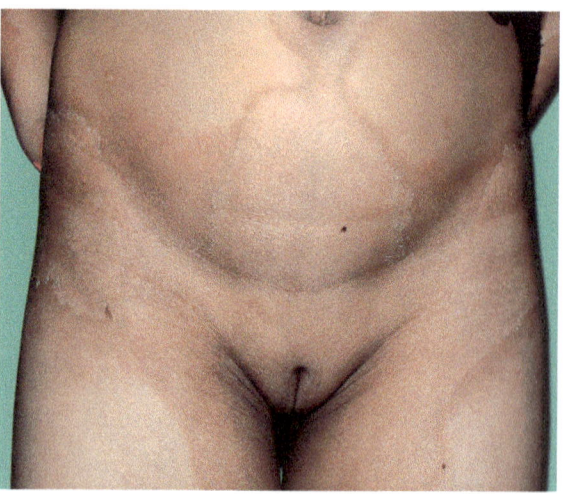

a. Seborrheic dermatitis
b. Tinea incognito
c. Erythrokeratoderma variabilis
d. Flexural psoriasis

392. This child presented with multiple rough asymptomatic lesions on face. What is the clinical diagnosis?

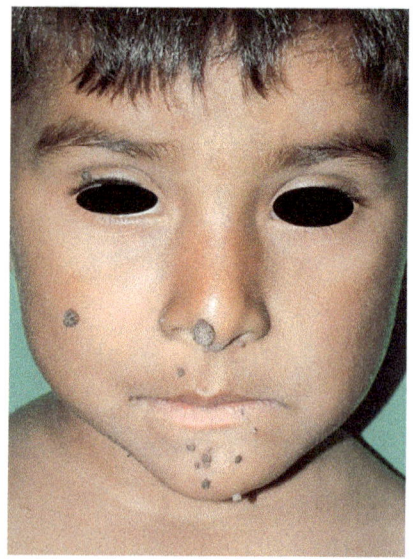

a. Adenoma sebaceum
b. Molluscum contagiosum face
c. Common warts on face
d. Impetigo contagiosa

393. She complained of itching and soreness with superficial tiny erosions between toes in the both feet. What is a clinical diagnosis?

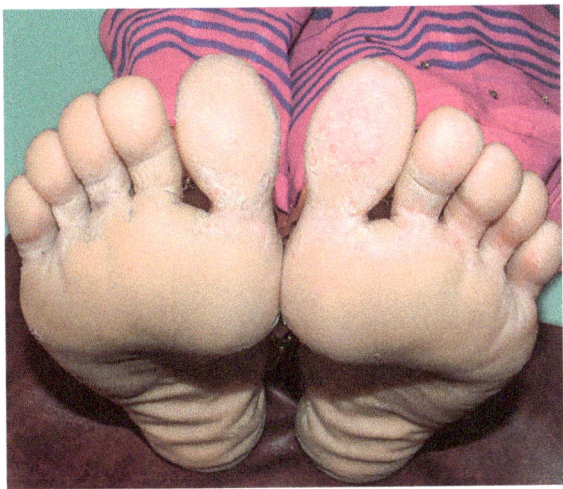

a. Tinea pedis
b. Candidiasis both feet
c. Pitted keratolysis
d. Contact dermatitis to shoes

394. This lady complained of itching, dryness, fissuring and thickening at various places involving the entire palm. What is the clinical diagnosis?

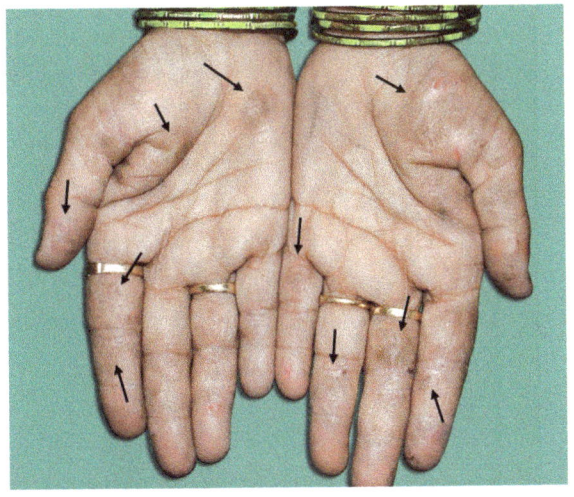

a. Tinea manuum
b. Lichen planus palms
c. Chronic allergic dermatitis due to cement
d. Dry type housewife dermatitis

395. Three days after hair dye, she had swelling over eyelids. There is no history of such problem during last two three applications. What is the clinical diagnosis?

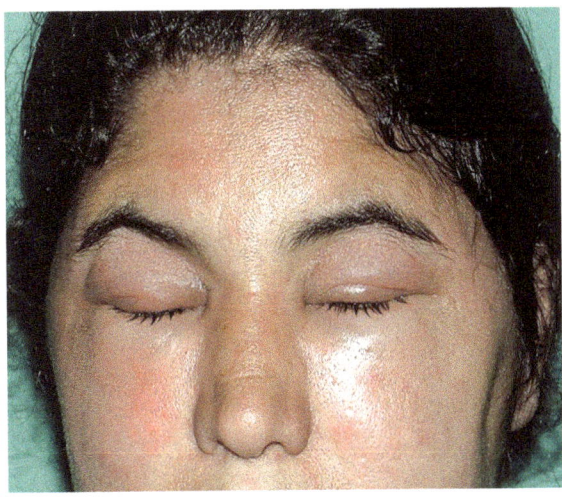

a. Irritant contact dermatitis to hair dye
b. Allergic contact dermatitis to hair dye
c. Angioedema

396. Which one of the following options belongs to this microphotograph of KOH smear under high power magnification?

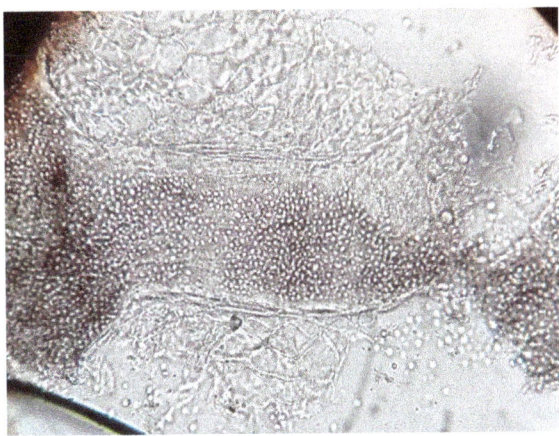

(*Courtesy:* Dr Vijay Singhal)

a. Candidal hyphae
b. Dermatophyte hyphae and spores inside hair follicle
c. Mites, eggs and their fragments of Sarcoptes scabiei
d. Pityriasis versicolor

397. Following is the magnified picture of a patient in which ill-defined superficial rough hyperkeratotic lesions are identified. At places, they show coalescence. He complained roughness and thickening of entire palms on both hands *(MCQ 372)*. What is the clinical diagnosis?

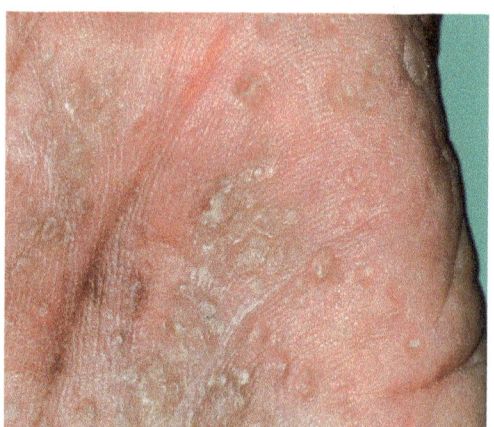

a. Superficial palmoplantar warts (mosaic warts)
b. Lichen planus
c. Pompholyx
d. Corns
e. Deep palmoplantar warts

398. This patient was having multiple dark-colored cauliflower like lesions on the undersurface of prepuce and at coronal sulcus. What is the possible diagnosis?

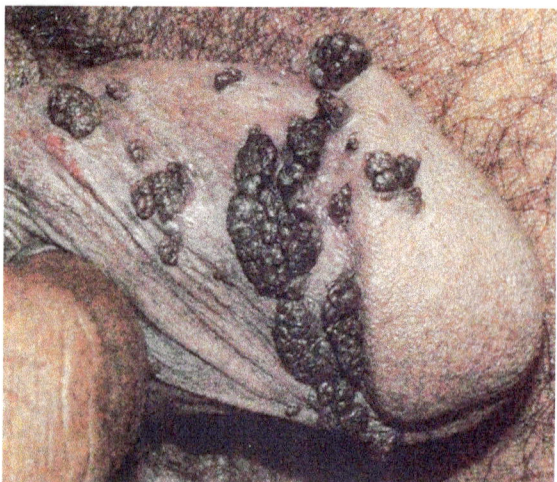

a. Condylomata acuminata
b. SCC penis
c. Seborrheic keratosis
d. Condylomata lata

399. This patient presented with spontaneous development of a single patch of ecchymosis on his shoulder for last seven days only. What is the clinical diagnosis?

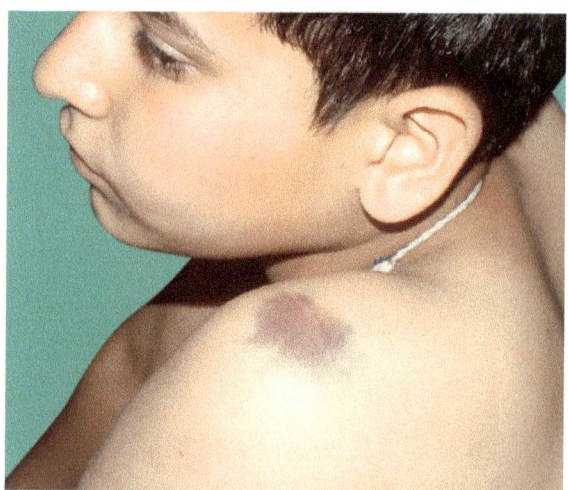

a. Henoch-Schonlein purpura (HSP)
b. Chronic myelocytic leukemia (CML)
c. Actinic purpura
d. Idiopathic thrombocytopenic purpura (ITP)

400. This patient complained of redness, itching and burning on entire face for the last six months. On careful examination, an advancing border was identified *(MCQ 111)*. What is the clinical diagnosis?

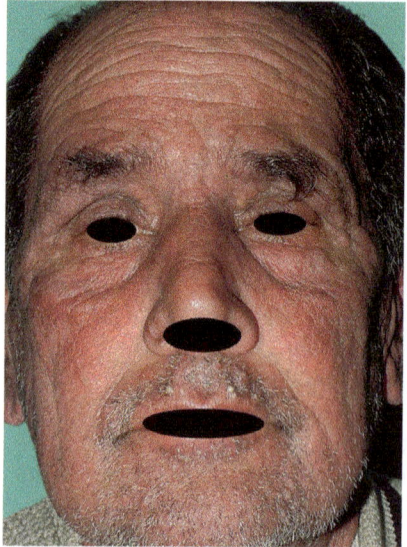

a. Steroid dermatitis
b. Tinea faciei
c. Airborne contact dermatitis (ABCD)
d. Polymorphous light eruption (PLE)

401. A 60-year-old man presented with itching, redness in the cubital fossae, on face, neck and popliteal fossae *(MCQ 359)*. What is the clinical diagnosis?

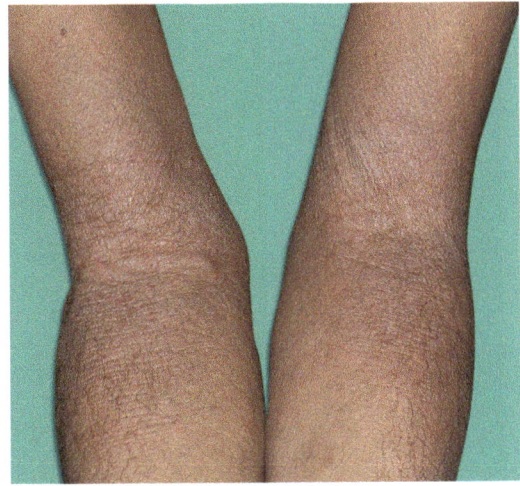

a. Adult phase atopic dermatitis
b. Seborrheic dermatitis (SD)
c. Intertrigo
d. Airborne contact dermatitis (ABCD)

402. Since childhood she is having gradually increasing freckling, dryness, pigmentation on sun exposed areas of body, e.g., face, chest, dorsa of hands. Dark keratotic papules are also present on face in significant number. Her sister is also suffering from the same disease. What is the clinical diagnosis?

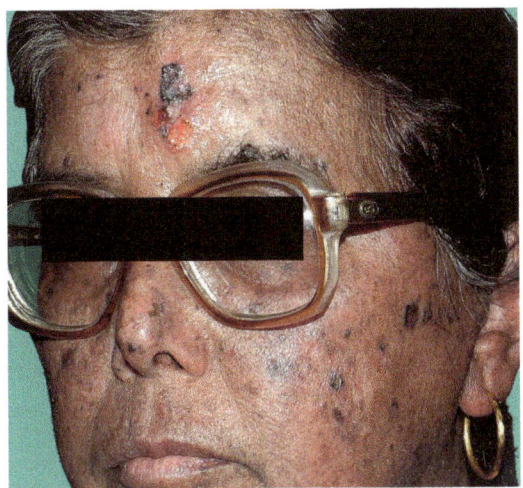

a. Freckles
b. Rothmund Thomson syndrome (RTS)
c. Xeroderma pigmentosum (XP)
d. Actinic keratosis

403. She is presented with eruption of multiple small, flaccid blisters which rupture easily. It was followed by crusting with surrounding erythema. It involved the seborrheic sites. Mucosae were not involved. What is the clinical diagnosis?

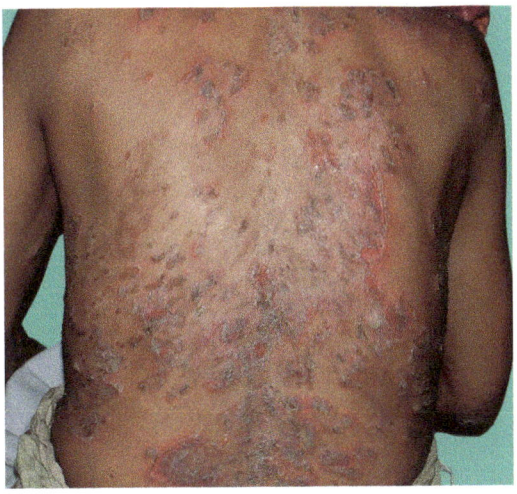

a. Pemphigus vulgaris
b. Pemphigus foliaceus
c. Bullous pemphigoid
d. Linear IgA disease in adult

404. This patient presented with multiple well defined annular or discoid lesions on face. Lesions have deep hyperpigmented center with violaceous thread like edge. What is the clinical diagnosis?

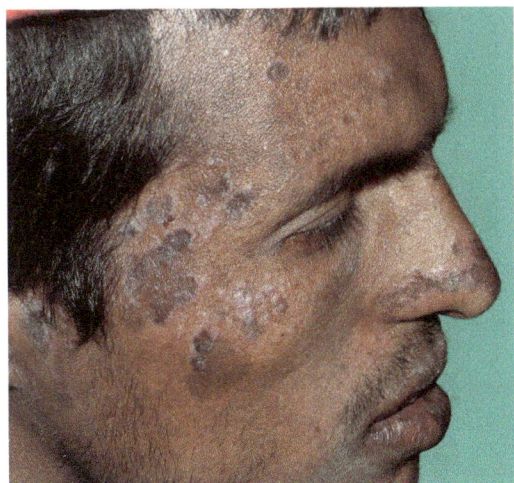

a. Discoid lupus erythematosus (DLE)
b. Actinic keratosis
c. Actinic lichen planus
d. Xeroderma pigmentosum (XP)

405. A 4-month-old baby presented with multiple small lesions on cheeks. What is the clinical diagnosis?

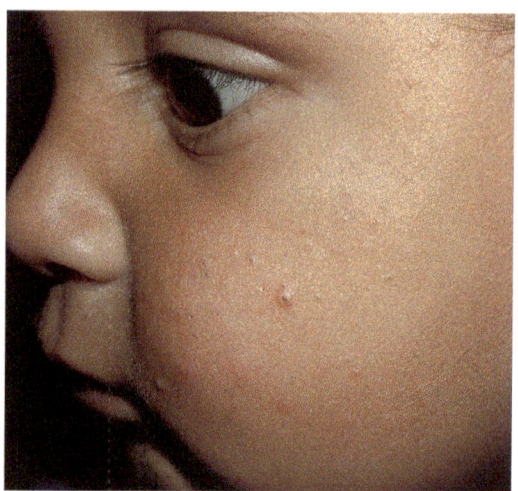

a. Erythema toxicum neonatorum (ETN)
b. Neonatal acne
c. Milia
d. Sebaceous gland hyperplasia

406. This patient presented with small painless, pale white, 1–3 mm sized papules on the penile skin. What is the clinical diagnosis?

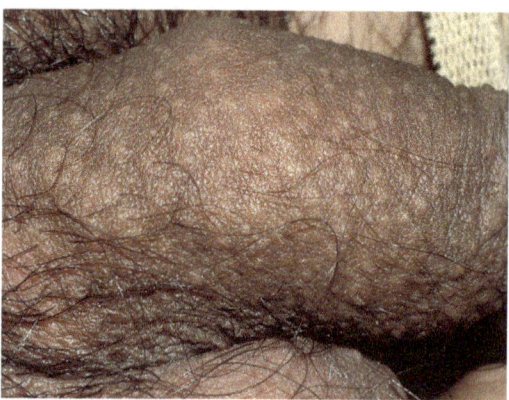

a. Lichen nitidus
b. Fordyce spots
c. Syringoma
d. Molluscum contagiosum

407. She complained of extremely itchy creeping thread like eruption on her abdomen. What is the clinical diagnosis?

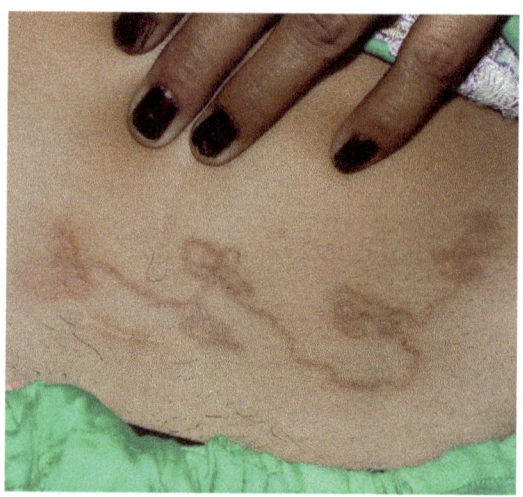

a. Granuloma annulare
b. Larva migrans
c. Tinea corporis

408. A 60-year-old man presented with multiple erythematous plaques and tumors on chest, axillae and abdomen for last 3–4 years. Histopathology showed colonization of lymphocytes along the basal cell layer and clustering of lymphocytes in the epidermis. What is the closest clinical possibility?

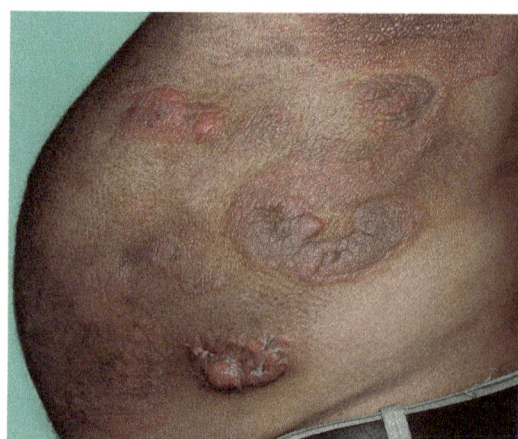

a. Psoriasis
b. Lupus vulgaris
c. Mycosis fungoides tumor stage
d. Squamous cell carcinoma (SCC)

409. This patient complained of diffuse redness of fingers and toes with accompanying itching, burning and pain. There is past history of such symptoms in every winter for the last 3–4 years. What is the clinical diagnosis?

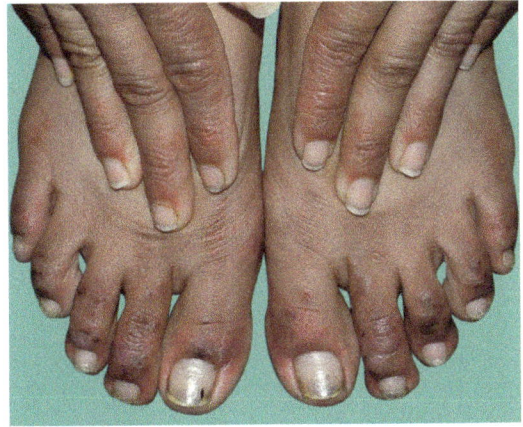

a. Chilblains
b. Raynaud's phenomenon
c. Chronic urticaria
d. Contact dermatitis hands

410. This patient complained of multiple, deep seated and rough hyperkeratotic lesions in his left sole only. What is the clinical diagnosis?

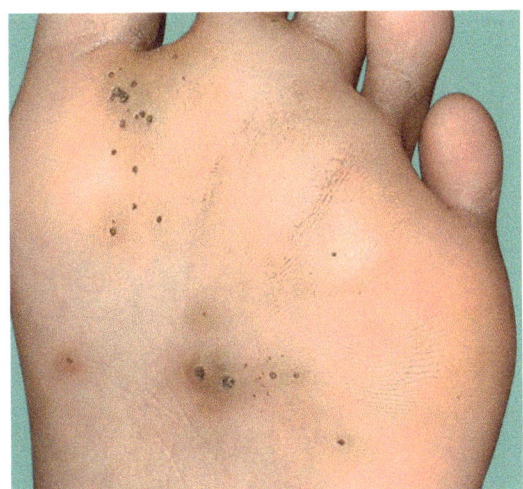

a. Corns
b. Deep palmoplantar warts
c. Pitted keratolysis
d. Superficial palmoplantar warts

411. This patient complained of erythema, itching, and burning sensation on entire face *(MCQ 400)* for last 6 months. What is the clinical diagnosis?

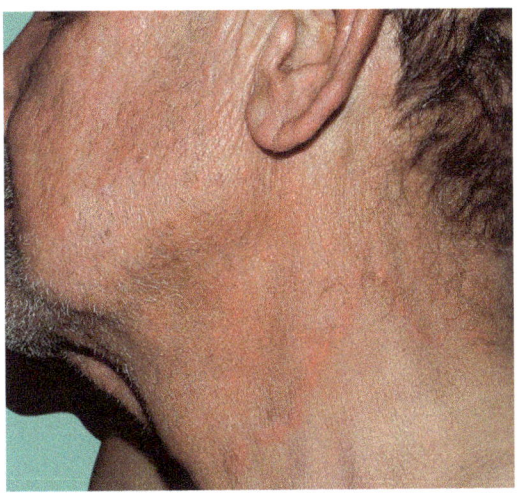

a. Polymorphous light eruption (PLE)
b. Topical steroid damaged face (TSDF)
c. Airborne contact dermatitis (ABCD)
d. Tinea faciei

412. This patient complained of depigmented macule on glans for the last one year. What is the clinical diagnosis?

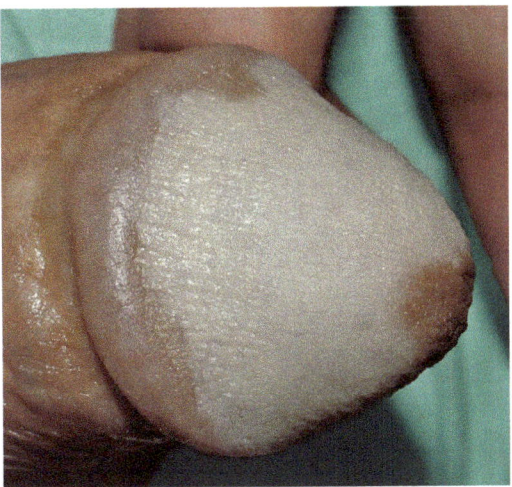

a. Vitiligo glans
b. Lichen planus glans
c. Lichen sclerosus et atrophicus
d. Leucoplakia glans

413. This lady complained of itching, oozing, crusting of both hands for last 3–4 years. What is the clinical diagnosis?

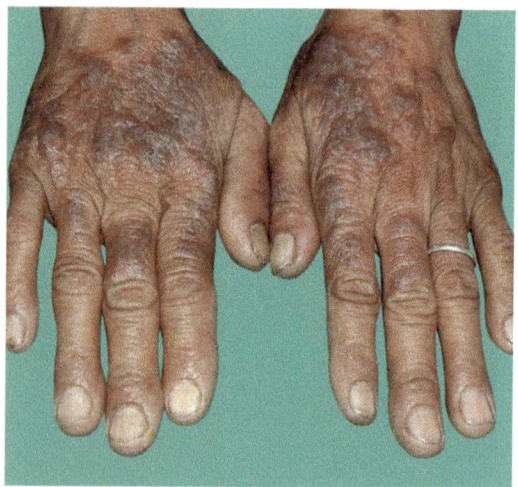

a. Housewife contact dermatitis
b. Discoid eczema
c. Pompholyx
d. Infected dermatitis

414. This infant presented with crop of asymptomatic, tiny and thin-walled vesicles without any surrounding erythema. What is the clinical diagnosis?

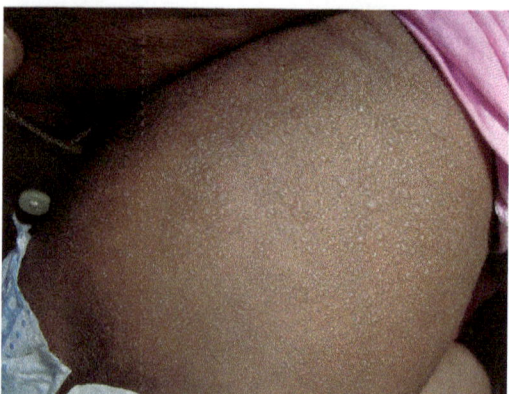

a. Miliaria rubra
b. Miliaria profunda
c. Miliaria crystallina
d. Staphylococcal scalded skin syndrome (SSSS)

415. This patient presented with small tender abscess, scarring and sinuses with seropurulent discharge in both groins. Perianal and axillary regions are also having similar involvement. What is the clinical diagnosis?

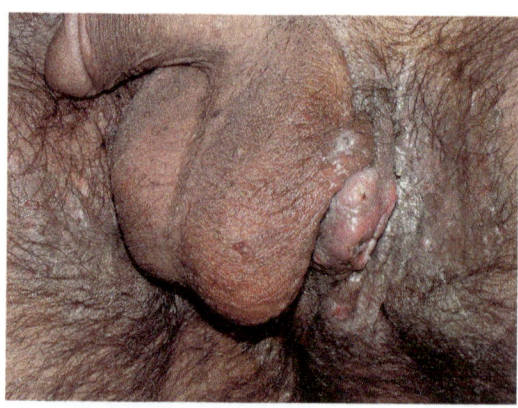

a. Scrofuloderma
b. Hidradenitis suppurativa
c. Fox-Fordyce disease
d. Intertrigo with secondary infection

416. This patient presented with erythema, maceration and whitish deposits at both angles of mouth. What is the clinical diagnosis?

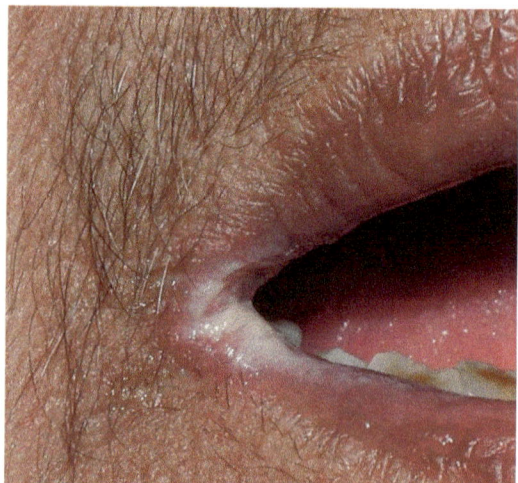

a. Cheilitis glandularis
b. Granulomatous cheilitis
c. Actinic cheilitis
d. Angular cheilitis

417. This patient presented with reddish brown monomorphic papules distributed symmetrically on cheeks, forehead and chin. What is the closest clinical possibility?

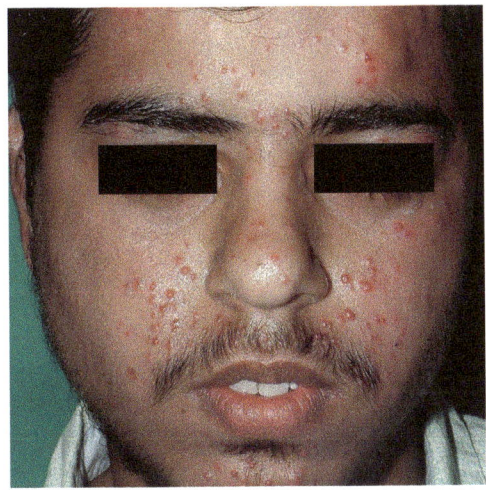

a. Acne vulgaris
b. Acneiform eruption
c. Lupus miliaris disseminatus faciei (LMDF)
d. Perioral dermatitis
e. Acne rosacea

418. For the assessment of superficial erythema, a piece of clear glass or plastic is pressed against the lesion. The observer looks directly at the pressed lesion. Which one of the following options is correct for the name of this test?

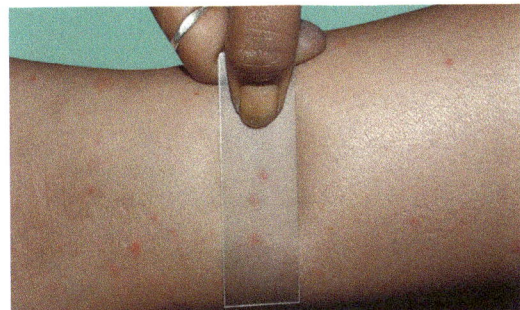

a. Diascopy
b. Dermatoscopy
c. Grattage test

419. At birth, this baby is bright red covered with a translucent membrane. Within hours membrane has dried up to form cracks and fissures on abdomen, extremities and face. The skin over fingers, hands and feet has become taut that has resulted in immobility. Eyelids have turned outwards (ectropion) and lip shows eversion (eclabion). What is the clinical diagnosis of this newborn?

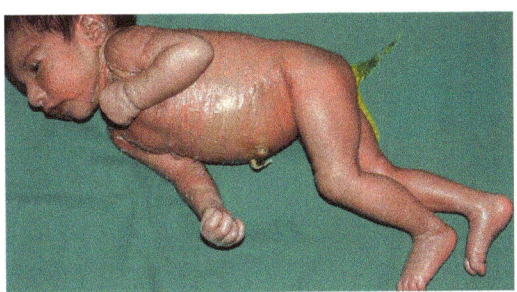

a. Harlequin ichthyosis
b. Collodion baby
c. Restrictive dermopathy

420. This patient complained of multiple projections on eyelid. What is the closest clinical diagnosis?

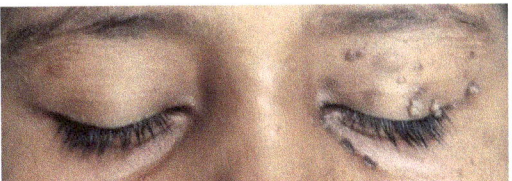

a. Milia
b. Filiform warts
c. Skin tags
d. Molluscum contagiosum

421. This patient presented with asymptomatic discolored macules covered with dust like scales. It involved the trunk and axillae. The lesions tend to become confluent. What is the possible diagnosis?

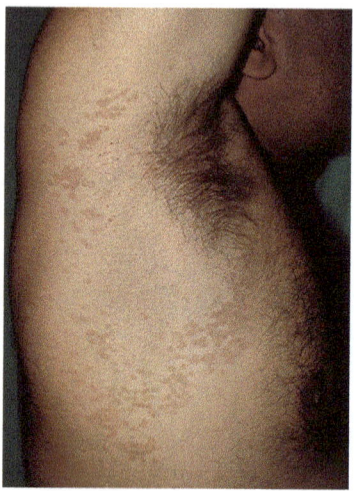

a. Pityriasis alba
b. Pityriasis capitis
c. Pityriasis rosea (PR)
d. Pityriasis versicolor (PV)

422. This young patient complained of gangrenous changes in the tip of his index finger. He is also complaining of pain in legs on walking short distances. He is a smoker for the last 10 years. What is the clinical possibility?

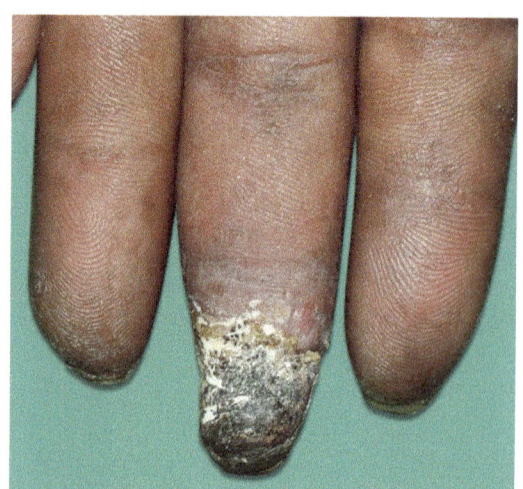

a. Chilblains
b. Raynaud's phenomenon
c. Digital necrosis due to drug
d. Buerger's disease

423. This lady complained of itching and white scaling in her right forefoot. What is the closest clinical diagnosis?

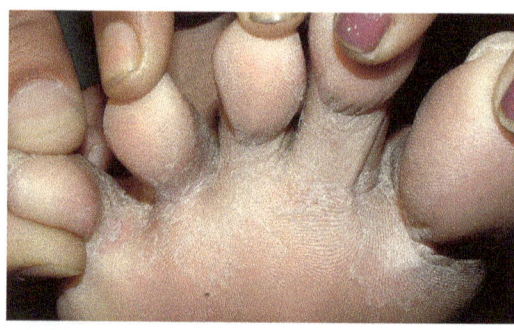

a. Candidiasis foot
b. Tinea pedis
c. Pitted keratolysis
d. Keratolysis exfoliativa

424. This baby was brought with red and tender looking skin in the area covered by diaper. What is the clinical diagnosis?

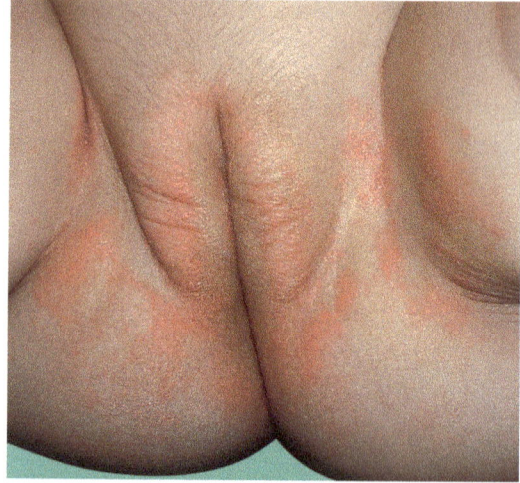

a. Diaper dermatitis
b. Intertrigo
c. Tinea cruris
d. Flexural psoriasis

425. She complained of a small bright red lesion behind her ear for the last six months. What is the possible clinical diagnosis?

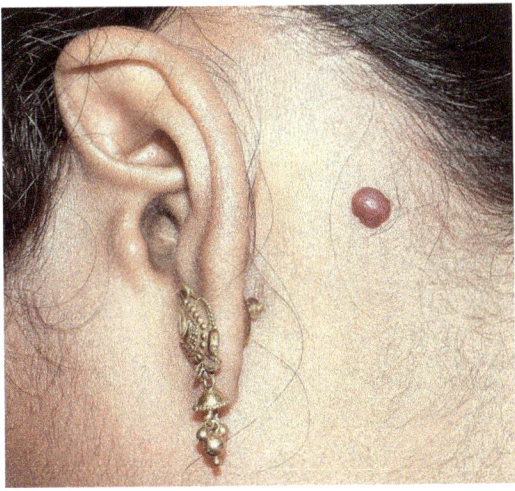

a. Pyogenic granuloma
b. Cherry angioma
c. Strawberry hemangioma
d. Lymphangioma circumscriptum

426. She presented with anterior bulging of eyes and swelling of thyroid gland. What is the clinical diagnosis?

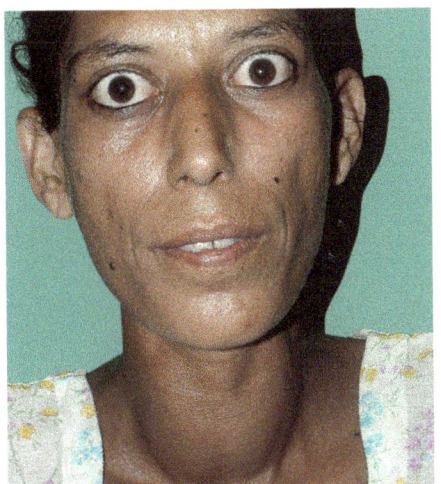

a. Orbital tumor
b. Hyperthyroidism
c. Hypothyroidism
d. Goiter

427. This man presented with hard painful lesions between toes for the last few months. What is the clinical diagnosis?

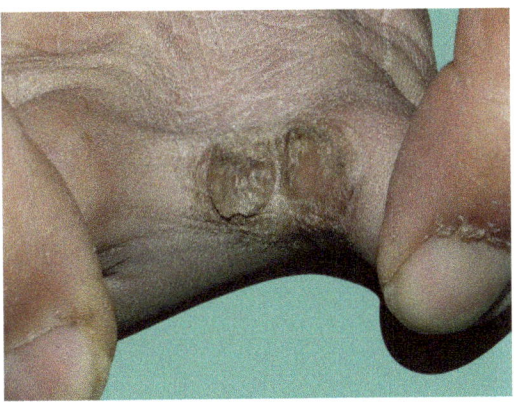

a. Plantar warts
b. Corns
c. Soft corns
d. Callus

428. This child noticed hair loss in the middle of right eyebrow in last six months. What is the clinical diagnosis?

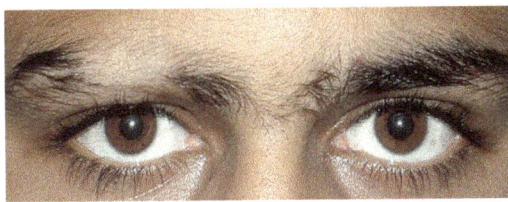

a. Lepromatous leprosy
b. Hypothyroidism
c. Alopecia areata
d. Trichotillomania

429. This patient presented with a large non healing ulcer on his forearm for the last one year. What is the closest clinical diagnosis?

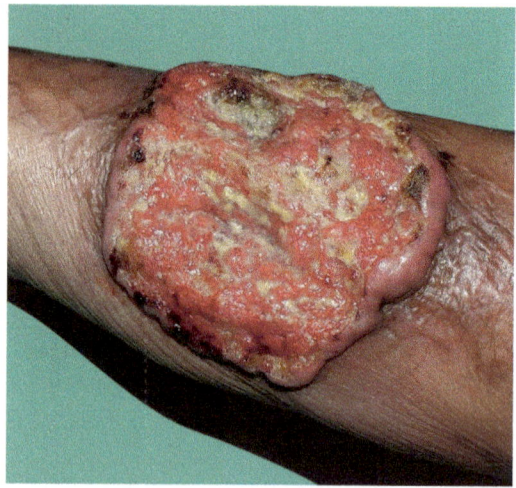

a. Basal cell carcinoma (BCC)
b. Squamous cell carcinoma (SCC)
c. Lupus vulgaris (LV)
d. Malignant melanoma (MM)

430. This patient complained of finger like hyperkeratotic projections in his nostril. What is the clinical diagnosis?

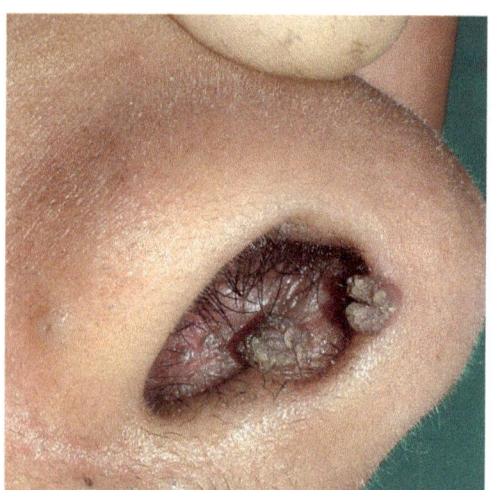

a. Molluscum contagiosum
b. Filiform warts
c. Skin tags
d. Digitate warts

431. This patient complained of chronic infection in his moustache for the last five months. He is not responding to the various types of antibiotics used. What can be the clinical diagnosis?

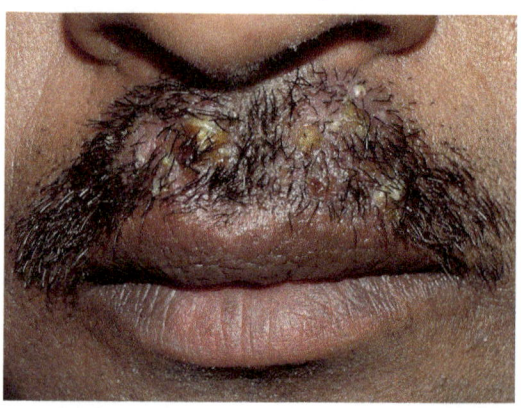

a. Multiple boils
b. Chronic superficial folliculitis (CSF)
c. Tinea barbae
d. Sycosis barbae

432. This full term newborn baby, four days after birth started having blotchy erythematous macules on the face. The macules were having a 1–3 mm sized vesicle or a pustule in the center. What is the clinical diagnosis?

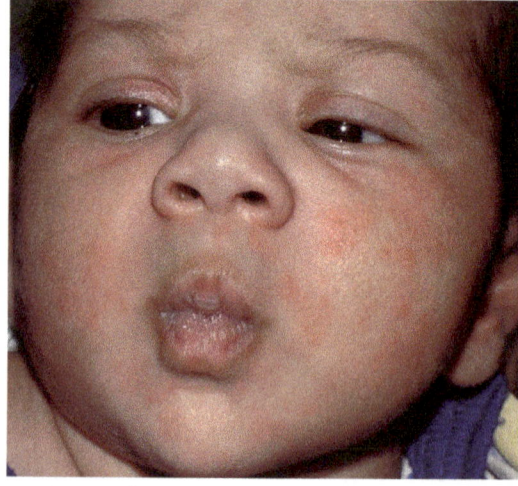

a. Neonatal acne
b. Erythema toxicum neonatorum (ETN)
c. Milia
d. Transient neonatal pustular melanosis (TNPM)

433. This patient complained of loss of sensations in both hands with ulceration at finger tips. On examination, he was having swelling of ear lobules along with hair loss of outer one-third of eyebrows *(MCQ 495)*. What is the diagnosis?

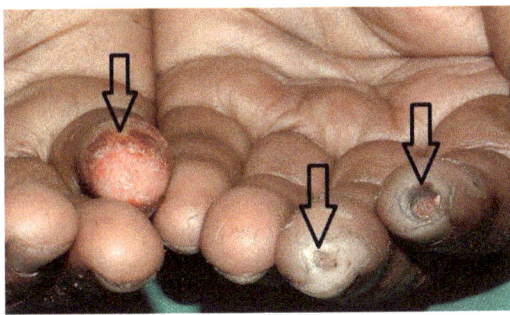

a. Myxedema
b. Lepromatous leprosy (LL)
c. Alopecia areata
d. Systemic sclerosis

434. This patient presented with itchy and crusted lesions on both shins for the last one year. What is the clinical diagnosis?

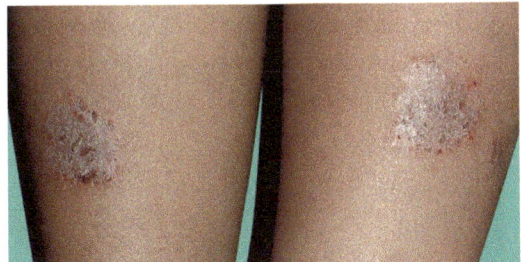

a. Dermatitis artefacta
b. Psoriasis
c. Discoid eczema
d. Tinea corporis

435. This patient complained of pain and small blisters on glans, shaft of penis and scrotum for the last four days. What is the clinical diagnosis?

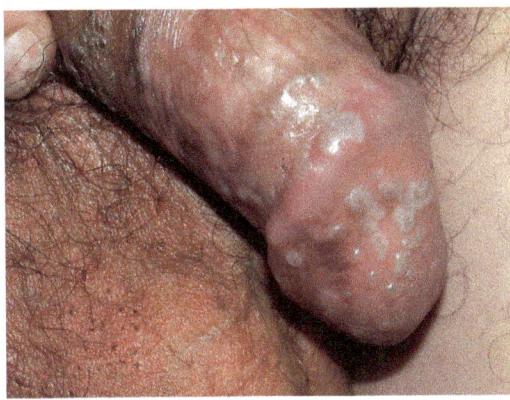

a. *Paederus dermatitis*
b. Scabies
c. Herpes genitalis
d. Herpes zoster

436. This patient complained of soreness in the mouth. On examination, white patches are seen inside the cheeks, on tongue and tonsils. What is the clinical diagnosis?

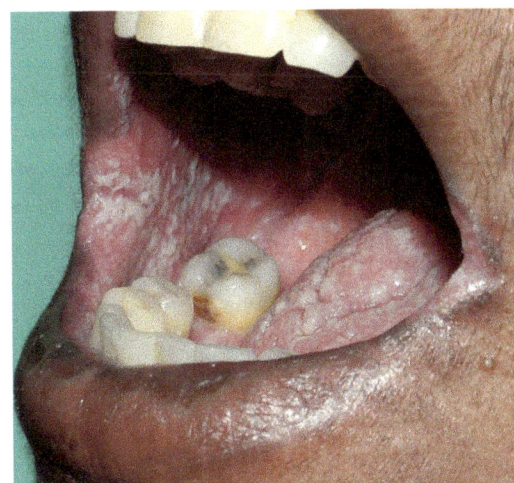

a. Oral leukoplakia
b. Oral lichen planus
c. Oral candidiasis
d. Smoker's keratosis

437. A 10-year-old child presented with violaceous, itchy plaques on both soles extending on to the medial side of both feet. What is the diagnosis?

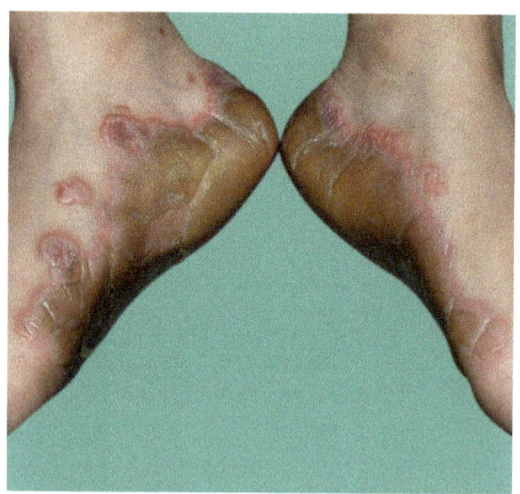

a. Psoriasis soles
b. Lichen planus soles
c. Hyperkeratotic eczema soles
d. Chronic cutaneous lupus erythematosus (CCLE) soles

438. This patient complained of a large sized red plaque on the left side of his face for the last two years. On examination, there were five to six more plaques (1–2 cm sized) on trunk and extremities. Sensations in the plaque were impaired. What is the diagnosis?

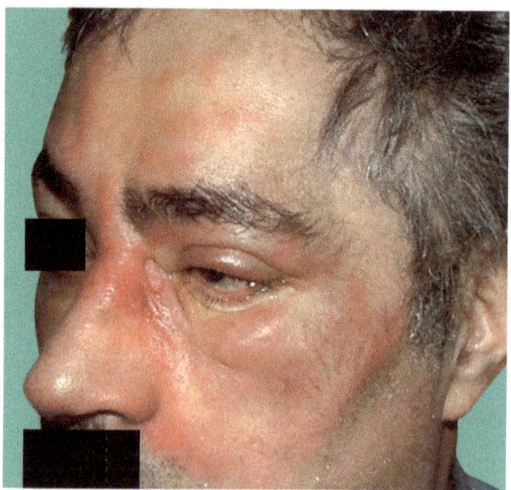

a. Tuberculoid leprosy
b. Mid-borderline leprosy
c. Lepromatous leprosy
d. Indeterminate leprosy

439. This patient complained of itchy umbilicated papules on arms and forearms. He is also having chronic renal failure due to diabetes. What is the closest clinical diagnosis?

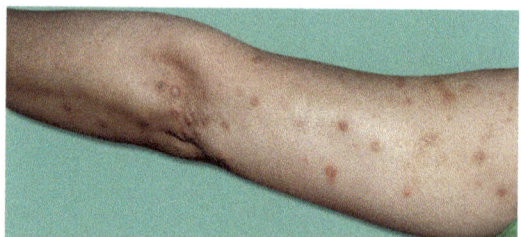

a. Molluscum contagiosum
b. Acquired perforating dermatosis
c. Prurigo nodularis
d. Lichen planus

440. This patient complained of elongated projection at angle of his mouth. What is the clinical diagnosis?

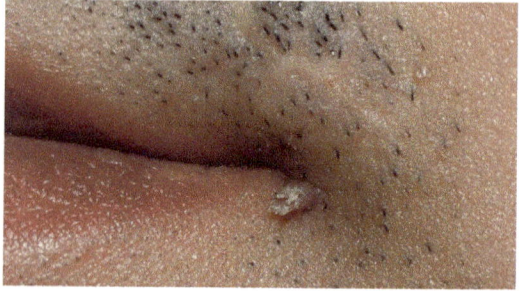

a. Filiform wart
b. Skin tag
c. Plane wart
d. Molluscum contagiosum

441. A 14-year-old child complained of a patch of hair loss in the occipital region. What is the clinical diagnosis?

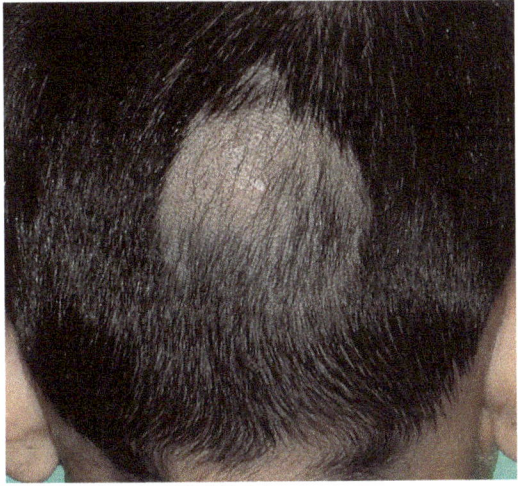

a. Tinea capitis
b. Alopecia areata
c. Trichotillomania
d. Cicatricial alopecia

442. Eight hours after the intake of tinidazole, this patient developed multiple dark brown blisters on chest and arm. There is no involvement of any mucosa. What is the diagnosis?

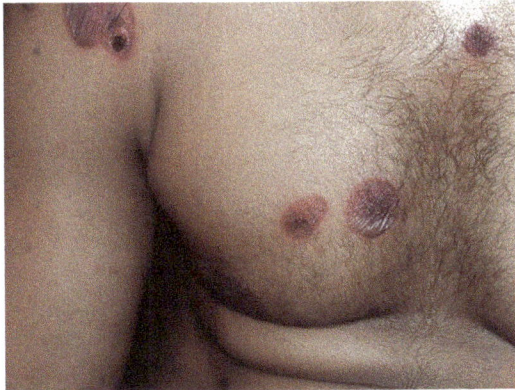

a. Erythema multiforme minor
b. Erythema multiforme major
c. Fixed drug eruption (FDE)
d. Stevens-Johnson syndrome (SJS)

443. A Bihar resident patient complained of multiple nodules of varying sizes along the course of a thick peripheral nerve. There were no skin lesions. What is the closest clinical diagnosis?

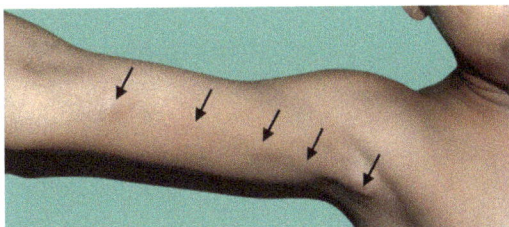

a. Tuberculoid leprosy
b. Segmental necrotizing granulomatous neuritis
c. Amyloid neuropathy

444. This patient developed overnight these lesions on his right thigh accompanied by burning sensation. What is the clinical diagnosis?

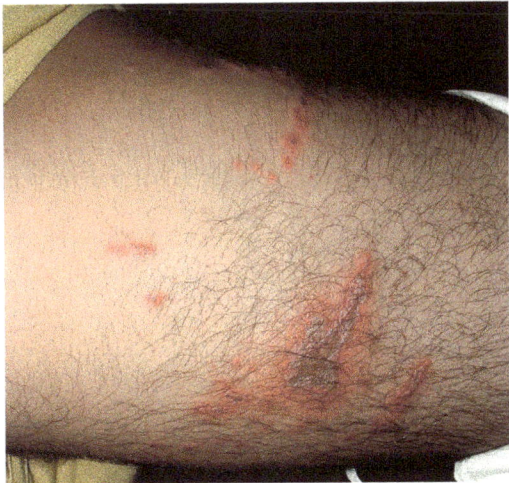

a. Herpes zoster
b. *Paederus dermatitis*
c. Dermatitis artefacta

445. This patient had exposure with a commercial sex worker (CSW). Four days later, he developed on his penile shaft a group of tiny vesicles with surrounding little erythema. What is the clinical diagnosis?

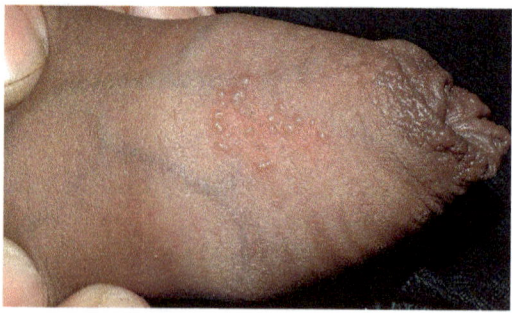

a. Herpes zoster
b. Primary genital herpes
c. Syphilitic chancre
d. Chancroid
e. Lymphogranuloma venereum

446. This patient presented with asymptomatic, soft, pale, velvety plaques on both upper lids for the last two years. What is the clinical diagnosis?

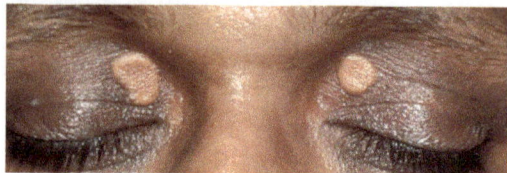

a. Necrobiotic xanthogranuloma
b. Systemic amyloidosis
c. Xanthelasma palpebrarum
d. Palpebral sarcoidosis

447. Skin of the scalp of this patient has become thickened and folded to make furrows like sulci and gyri of brain. He is also having protrusion of lower jaw, i.e., prognathism *(MCQ 473)*. His fingers are also thick *(MCQ 484)*. What is the clinical diagnosis?

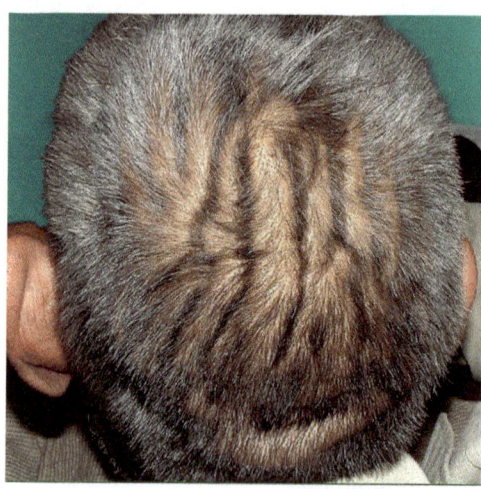

a. Cutis verticis gyrata due to acromegaly
b. Primary hypertrophic osteoarthropathy (PHO)
c. Secondary hypertrophic osteoarthropathy (SHO)

448. Just after weaning, a 6-month-old child started having psoriasiform eczematous lesions symmetrically distributed in perioral and perineal regions, hands and feet. The child had diarrhea and sparse and thin scalp hair. What is the clinical diagnosis?

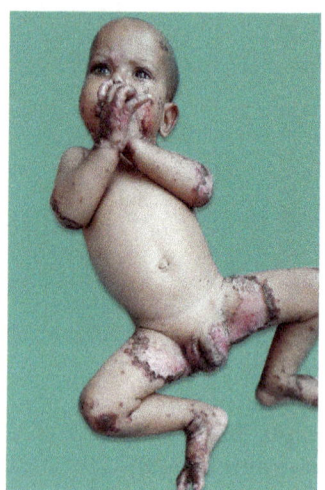

(*Courtesy:* Dr US Pahwa)

a. Vitamin H or B-7 (biotin) deficiency
b. Acrodermatitis enteropathica (ADE)
c. Seborrheic dermatitis
d. Atopic dermatitis

449. This patient complained of burning sensation on use of spicy food stuffs and progressive inability to open mouth. On examination, dark staining of teeth is observed due to habit of betel quid chewing. What is the clinical diagnosis?

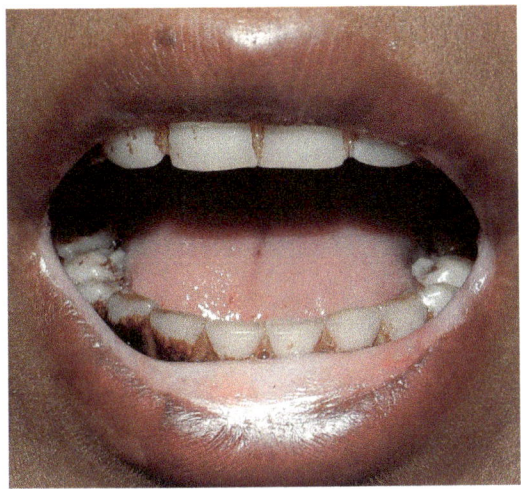

a. Oral submucosal fibrosis
b. Smoker's keratosis
c. Oral presentation of scleroderma

450. This patient complained of multiple rough and thin projections in cervical region. What is the closest diagnosis?

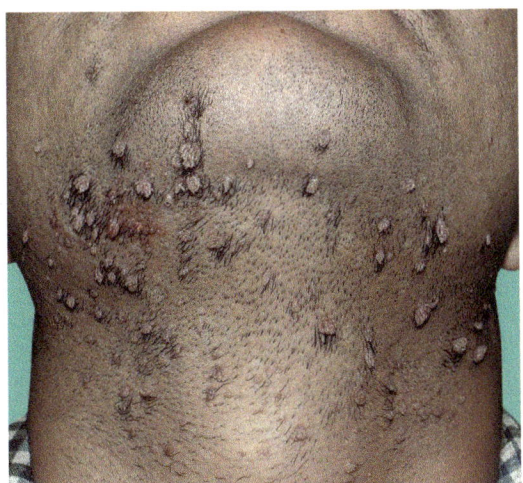

a. Molluscum contagiosum
b. Skin tags
c. Filiform warts
d. Plane warts

451. This patient complained of itchy pustular lesions on the front and back of thighs and lower abdomen. He is not responding to topical and systemic antibiotics and steroids. What can be the possible diagnosis?

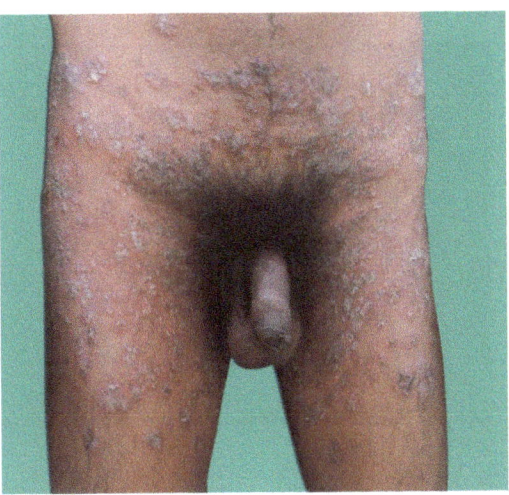

a. Chronic superficial folliculitis (CSF)
b. Tinea corporis
c. Infected scabies
d. Tinea incognito

452. This patient complained of recurrent asymptomatic desquamation of both palms in summer months. What is the closest option for this patient?

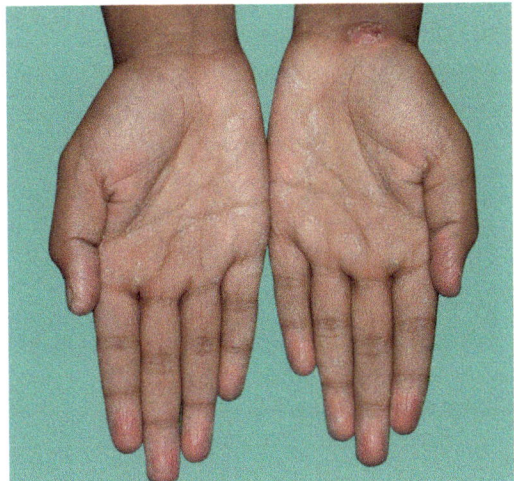

a. Keratolysis exfoliativa
b. Candidiasis palms
c. Eczema palms
d. Tinea manuum

453. This patient had an unprotected sex with a commercial sex worker about 20 days back. Now, he complained of a single painless ulcer on his prepuce. Ulcer is clean, smooth and induration can be easily felt at the base between fingers. What is the clinical diagnosis?

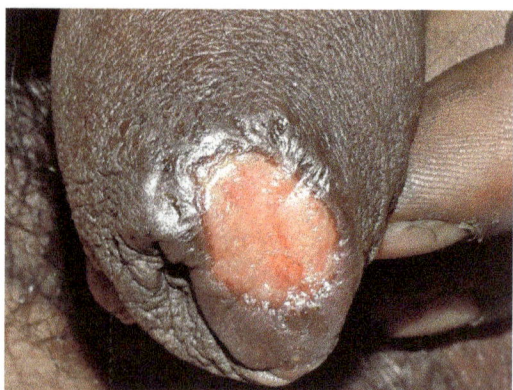

a. Chancroid
b. Syphilitic chancre
c. Lymphogranuloma venereum
d. Granuloma venereum

454. This lady presented with expressionless mask like face. Mouth opening is constricted and has radial furrows with thin lips giving a purse string appearance. She also complained of blue coloration of hands on exposure to cold. What is the clinical diagnosis?

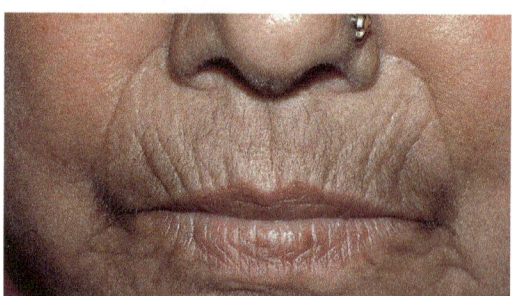

a. Submucosal fibrosis
b. Systemic sclerosis
c. Systemic lupus erythematosus

455. He presented with whiteness of tips of fingers and lips. What is the diagnosis?

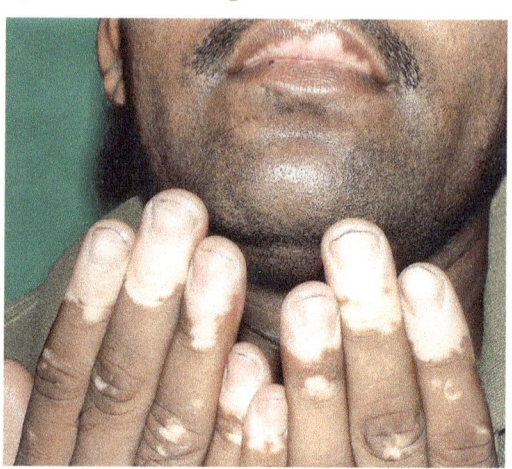

a. Leukoderma
b. Lip and tip vitiligo
c. Generalized vitiligo
d. Universal vitiligo

456. This patient presented with itchy vesicular lesions on the sides of fingers and palms. No distant focus of fungal or bacterial infection was detected. What is the clinical diagnosis?

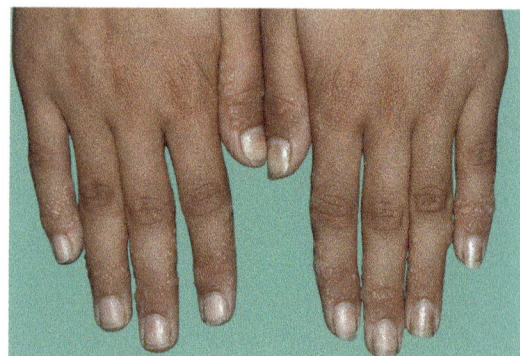

a. Herpetic whitlow
b. Pompholyx
c. Id eruption
d. Infected scabies

457. This lady has a history of multiple extramarital sexual contacts. She presented with multiple, painless, flesh colored, flat topped, sessile papules with oozing and macerations for the last two months. She was also having painless enlargement of axillary and inguinal lymph nodes. What is the clinical diagnosis?

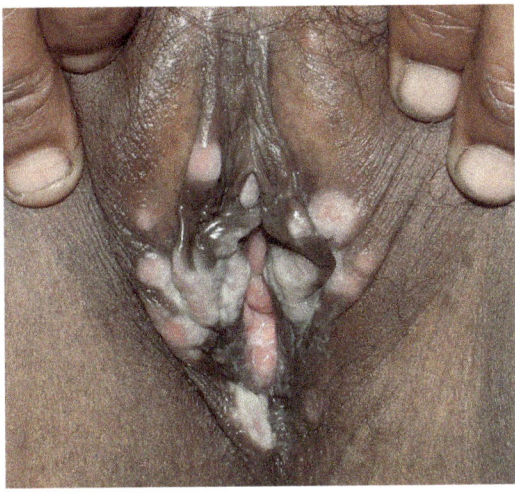

a. Condylomata acuminata
b. Condylomata lata
c. Chancroid
d. Herpes genitalis

458. This patient complained of severe pain in the lateral fold of his finger for the five days. What is the closest clinical diagnosis?

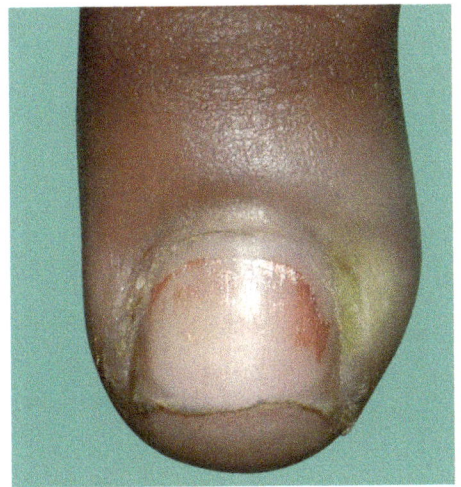

a. Glomus tumor
b. Acute paronychia
c. Chronic paronychia
d. Herpetic whitlow

459. This patient has developed recurrence of herpes zoster lesion on upper back, shoulder and arm. Few years back, he also had herpes zoster in the lumbosacral region which is evident by hypopigmented scarring. Which one of the following statements is most correct for him?

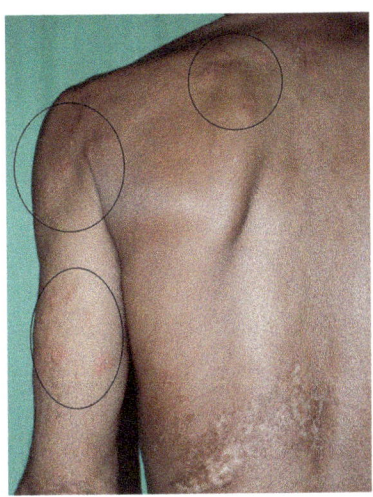

a. Recurrence is due to underlying diabetes
b. Recurrence is due to systemic steroids
c. Recurrence may occur rarely in a normal person
d. Recurrence is always alarming, investigation is must

460. This patient complained of discoloration of nails of left hand. What is the clinical diagnosis?

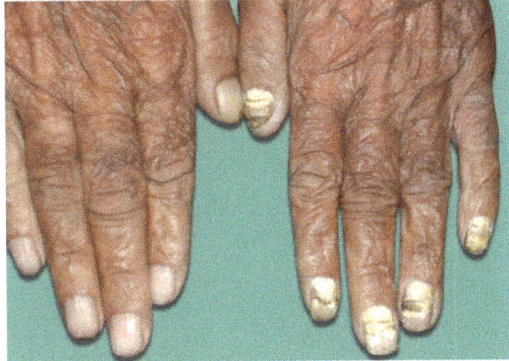

a. Lichen planus
b. Psoriasis
c. Tinea unguium
d. Darier's disease

461. This patient presented on his face a large single well-defined plaque with loss of sensation. Thickened great auricular nerve is easily seen crossing the sternomastoid muscle. What is the clinical diagnosis?

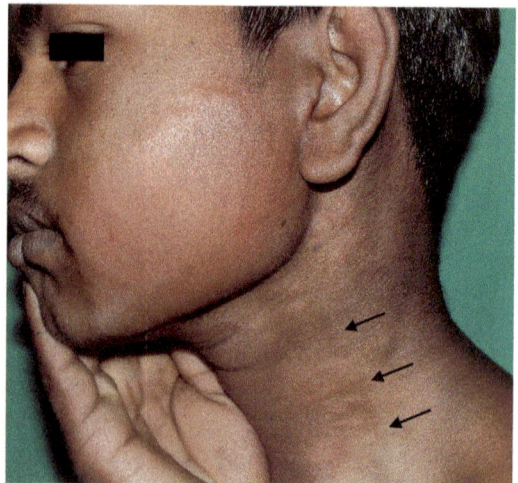

a. Indeterminate leprosy
b. Histoid leprosy
c. Lepromatous leprosy
d. Tuberculoid leprosy

462. This patient complained of painful swelling of lateral nail folds of both big toes for the last one year. What is the clinical diagnosis?

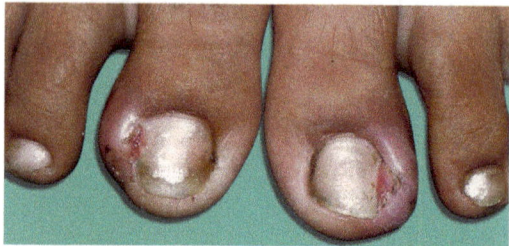

a. Chronic paronychia
b. Tinea unguium
c. Ingrown toenail
d. Acute paronychia

463. This is a magnified view of some small lesions on the face. These are slightly raised lesions with dark-colored keratotic impaction in the center. What are these lesions?

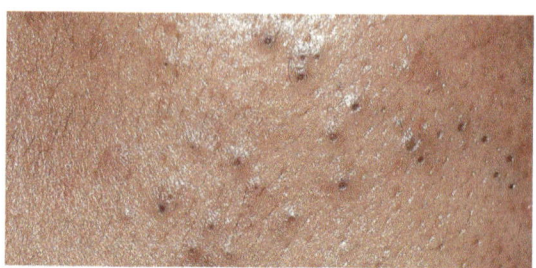

a. White comedones
b. Black comedones
c. Milia
d. Dermatosis papulosa nigra (DPN)

464. A 70-year-old female presented with formation of perivulval plaque. Plaque is 5 × 7 cm sized, asymmetrical, irregular and has notched borders and varied color. It is ulcerated, tender and bleeds. Margins show black pigmentation. The labia minora and majora are no longer visible. What is the closest clinical diagnosis?

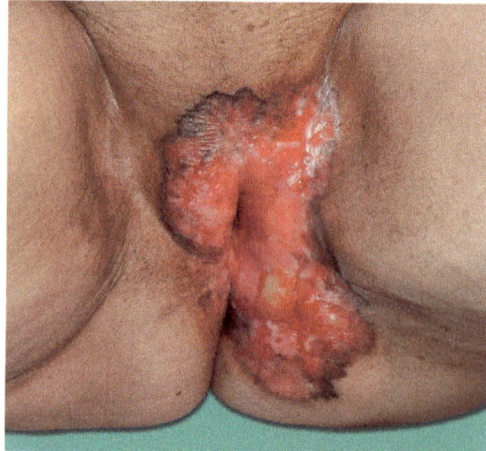

a. Extramammary Paget's disease (EMPD)
b. Superficial spreading melanoma (SSM)
c. Squamous cell carcinoma (SCC)
d. Basal cell carcinoma (BCC)

465. This boy presented with a single non tender nodule on his upper lip for the last six months. Its surface is crusted and complains of recurrent bleeding. What is the clinical diagnosis?

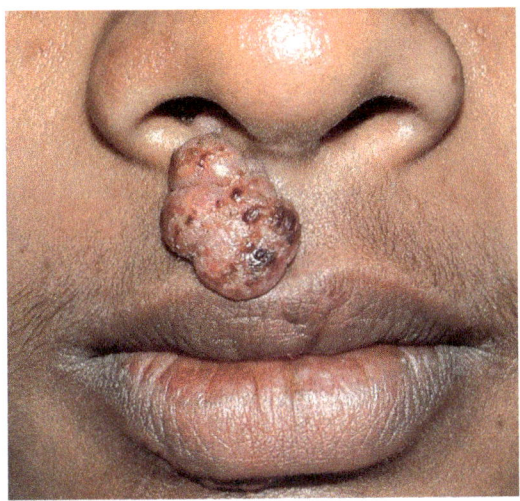

a. Common wart
b. Pyogenic granuloma
c. Strawberry hemangioma
d. Keratoacanthoma

466. A 6-month-old baby was having mild itching with fine white, greasy scales on scalp for the last 4 months. Scalp involvement was extending on the face. What is the clinical diagnosis?

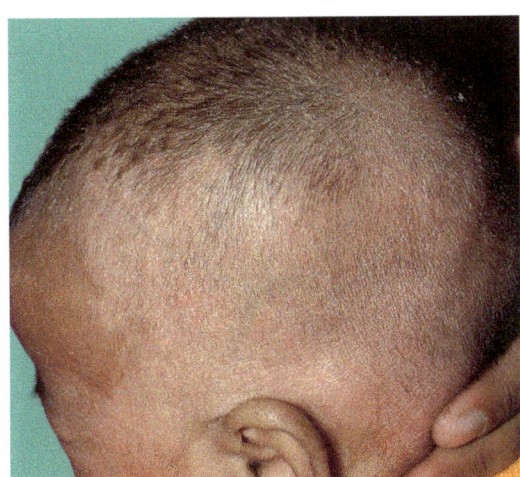

a. Infantile seborrheic dermatitis
b. Atopic dermatitis
c. Tinea capitis
d. Cradle cap

467. She presented with redness on her cheeks and bridge of nose sparing nasolabial folds. She used to have fever of mild and prolonged nature. What is the clinical diagnosis?

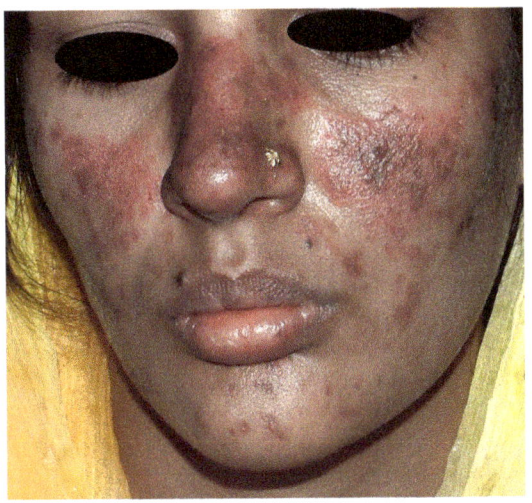

a. Dermatomyositis
b. Malar rash of SLE
c. Polymorphous light eruption
d. Melasma

468. This patient presented with a patch of asymptomatic hair loss on mandibular region for the last one year. What is the diagnosis?

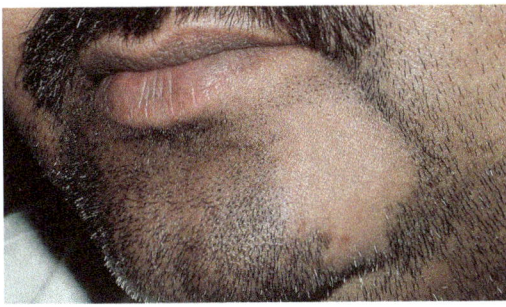

a. Alopecia areata
b. Tinea barbae
c. Alopecia totalis
d. Ophiasis

469. She presented with multiple asymptomatic soft, pink and digitate lesions on her vulva for the last three months. She gives history of multiple sexual exposures. What is the clinical diagnosis?

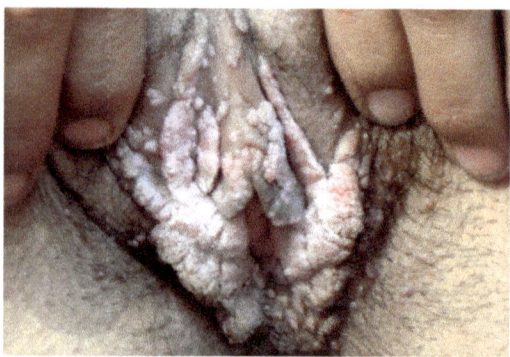

a. Condylomata lata
b. Condylomata acuminata
c. Molluscum contagiosum
d. Angiokeratomas vulva

470. She complained of redness, itching and scaling on her right foot. What is the closest diagnosis?

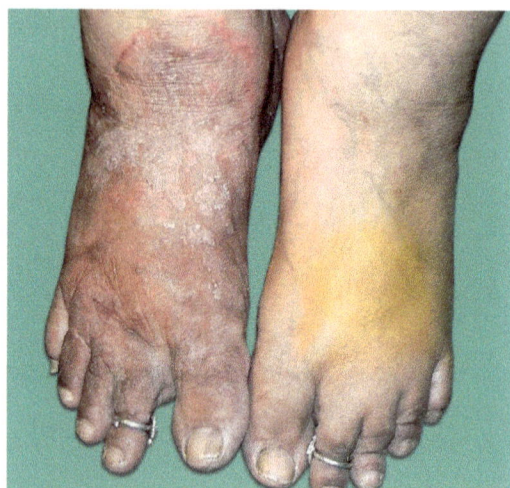

a. Tinea pedis
b. Eczema foot
c. Allergic contact dermatitis (ACD) to shoes
d. Candidiasis feet

471. This patient presented with a group of small superficial erosions on the shaft of penis. There is a history of sexual exposure with the commercial sex worker five days back. What is the clinical diagnosis?

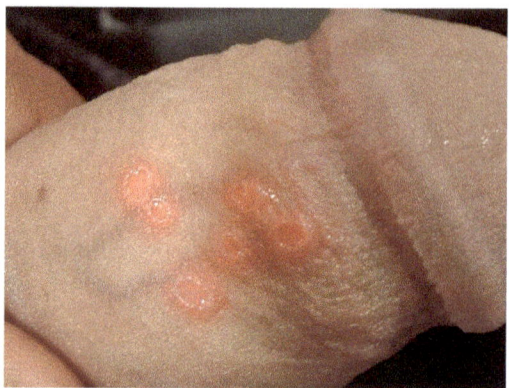

a. Primary genital herpes
b. Herpes zoster
c. Chancroid
d. Syphilitic chancre

472. This patient developed overnight soreness and burning sensation in the popliteal fossa. On examination, two patches of same size and shape with grayish white necrotic slough in the center were seen on the both sides of popliteal crease. What is the clinical diagnosis?

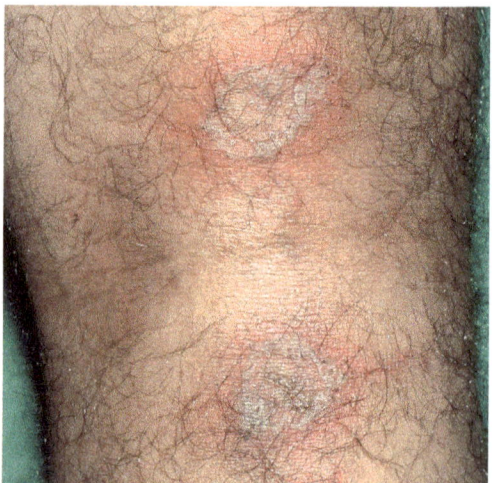

a. Adult phase atopic dermatitis
b. Discoid eczema
c. Kissing lesions of *Paederus dermatitis*

473. This patient complained of protrusion of his lower jaw. His scalp has become thick and folded *(MCQ 447)*. His fingers have also become thick *(MCQ 484)*. What is the clinical diagnosis?

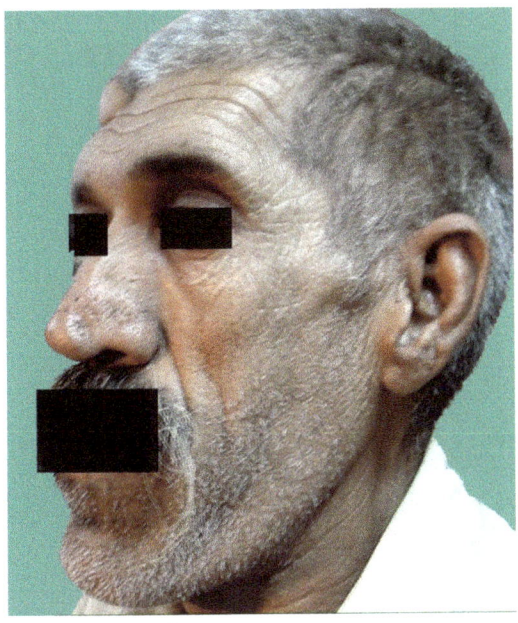

a. Hypothyroidism
b. Acromegaly
c. A normal feature

474. This lady is complaining of loss of pigmentation at the site of bindi application. Which one of the following terms is most appropriate for it?

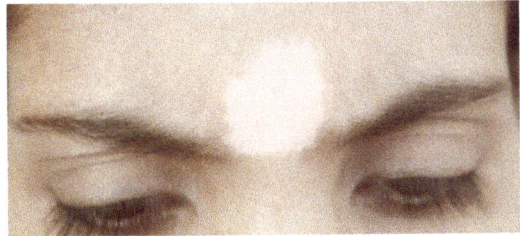

a. Bindi vitiligo
b. Leukoderma due to bindi
c. Focal vitiligo
d. Segmental vitiligo

475. This patient presented with multiple slightly elevated pale papules on cheeks. With stretching of skin, they can be better visualized. Which one of the following terms is used to describe these lesions?

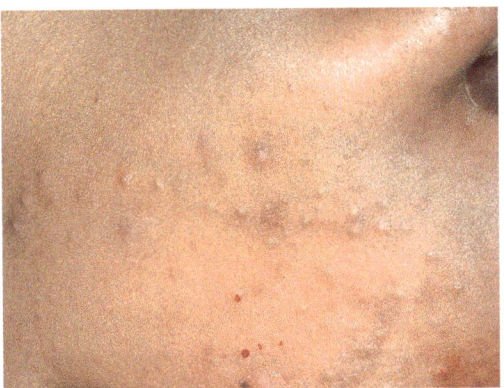

a. Open comedones
b. Closed comedones
c. Miliaria
d. Syringomas

476. She presented with shiny asymptomatic ill-defined plaques on both hands. Similar plaques were also present on her face *(MCQ 505)* and feet *(MCQ 479)*. Involvement tends to be symmetrical. What is the clinical diagnosis?

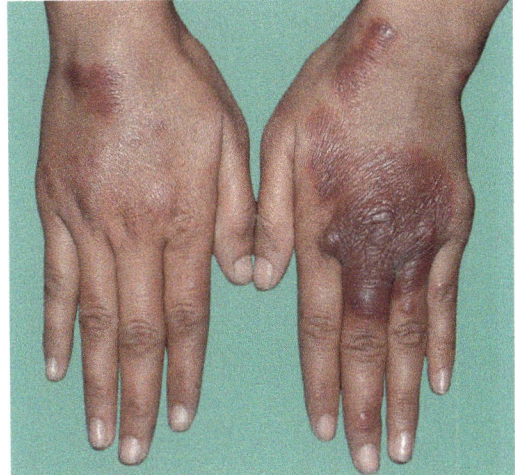

a. Lichen planus
b. Psoriasis
c. Discoid eczema
d. Borderline lepromatous leprosy

477. This baby was uncomfortable with tiny red lesions with erythema on back. What is the clinical diagnosis?

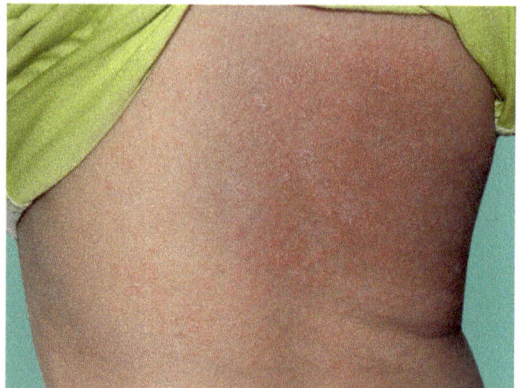

a. Transient neonatal pustular melanosis (TNPM)
b. Erythema toxicum neonatorum (ETN)
c. Miliaria rubra
d. Infantile scabies

479. She presented with multiple shiny erythematous plaques on both feet. She also had similar plaques on face *(MCQ 505)* and hands *(MCQ 476)*. Plaques are multiple but countable and have tendency to be symmetrical. What is the clinical diagnosis?

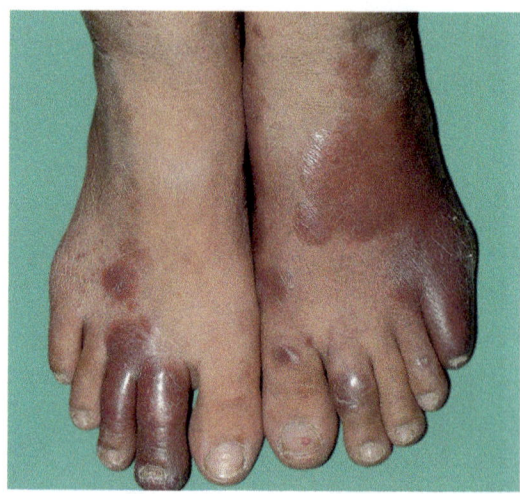

a. Borderline lepromatous leprosy
b. Psoriasis
c. Discoid eczema
d. Lupus vulgaris

478. This young patient complained of pain, dark coloration, ulceration of little toe and heal for the last one year. He is a smoker and has pain in legs on walking short distances. What is the clinical diagnosis?

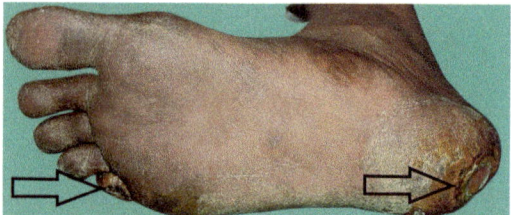

a. Buerger's disease
b. Hypertensive ulcer
c. Venous ulcer
d. Arterial ulcer

480. She complained of discoloration of few nails of left hand and an itchy red patch on right hand. What is the clinical diagnosis?

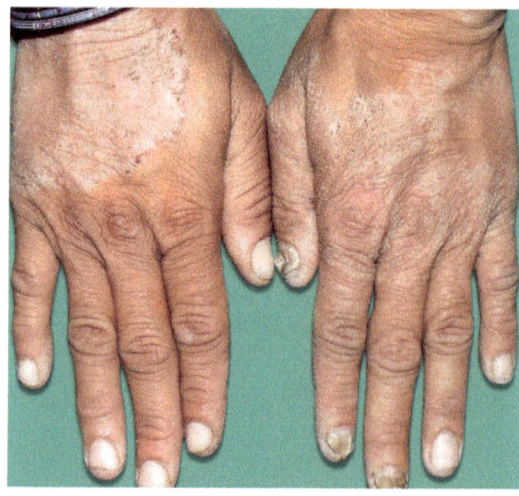

a. Psoriasis involving skin and nails
b. Eczema involving skin and nails
c. Psoriasis of nails and tinea manuum
d. Tinea manuum and tinea unguium

481. This patient complained of dystrophy of nail plates. What is the clinical diagnosis?

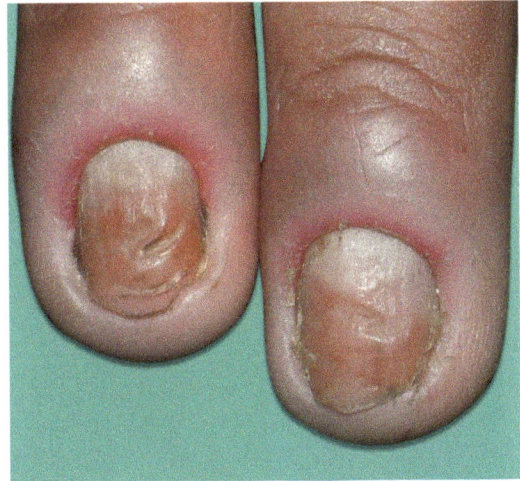

a. Tinea unguium
b. Chronic paronychia
c. Acute paronychia
d. Nail psoriasis

482. This child presented with small red plaques with white scaling on lower extremities with little itching. What is the clinical diagnosis?

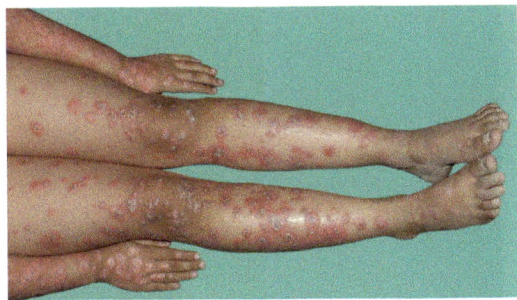

a. Lichen planus
b. Discoid eczema
c. Psoriasis
d. Pityriasis rosea

483. This patient presented with malodorous eroded plaques in the groins and axillae. There is no mucosal involvement. His sister is also suffering from the similar disease. What is the clinical diagnosis?

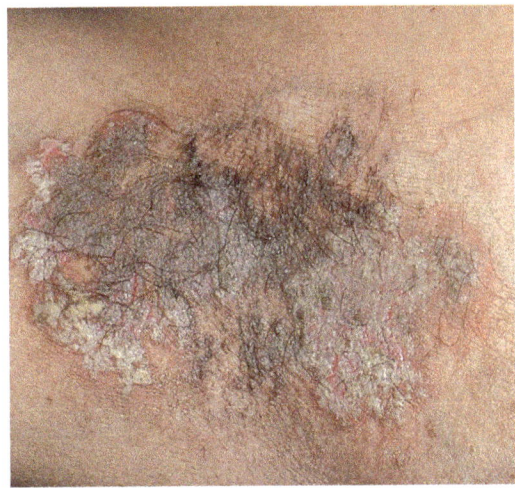

a. Hailey-Hailey disease
b. Intertrigo
c. Candidal intertrigo
d. Flexural psoriasis

484. This patient presented with thickening of fingers of both hands. He was also having protrusion of lower jaw *(MCQ 473)* and scalp skin has become thickened and folded, i.e., cutis verticis gyrata *(MCQ 447)*. What is the clinical diagnosis?

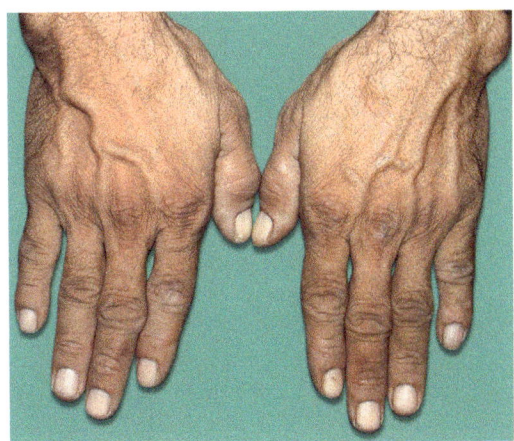

a. Acral hypertrophy in an acromegaly patient
b. Acropachy
c. Insulin resistance

485. A 7-year-old boy complained of itching and scaling on the scalp only. What is the clinical diagnosis?

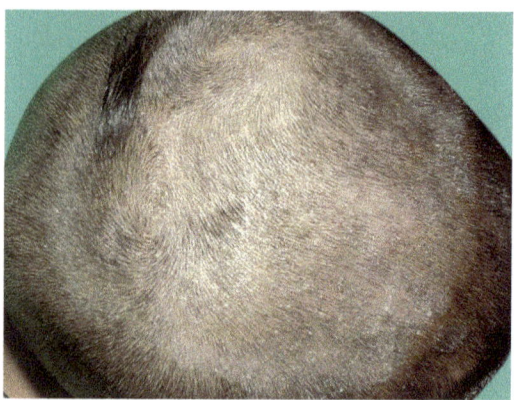

a. Tinea capitis
b. Psoriasis scalp
c. Atopic dermatitis (AD)
d. Seborrheic capitis

486. This patient complained of asymptomatic yellowish uniform thickening of palms and soles since birth. Which one of the followings is the closest diagnosis for this patient?

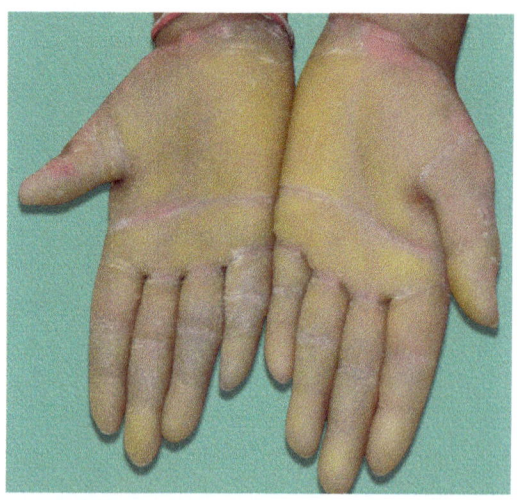

a. Psoriasis of palms and soles
b. Hyperkeratotic eczema palms and soles
c. DLE palms and soles
d. Palmoplantar keratoderma

487. This patient was taking metoprolol as an antihypertensive drug for the last many months. He complained of hardening, pain and black coloration of distal part of his thumb. What is the diagnosis?

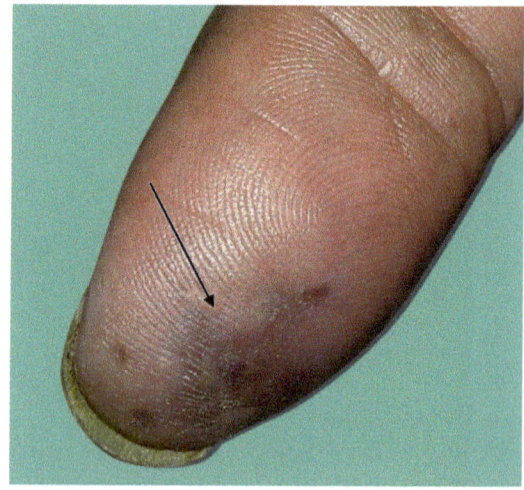

a. FDE due to metoprolol
b. Raynaud's phenomenon
c. Buerger's disease
d. Digital necrosis due to metoprolol

488. This patient presented with a single large plaque on the nape of neck with loss of sensation. What is the clinical diagnosis?

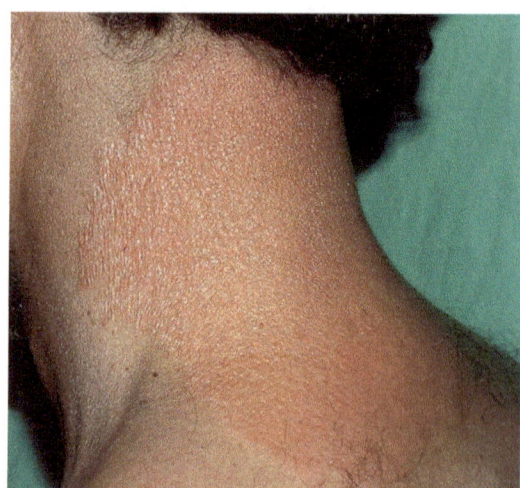

a. Lepromatous leprosy (LL)
b. Indeterminate leprosy
c. Tuberculoid leprosy
d. Mid-borderline leprosy

489. This patient had unprotected sex with a commercial sex worker about seven days back. He is complaining of multiple painful ulcers at the preputial opening. What is the closest clinical diagnosis?

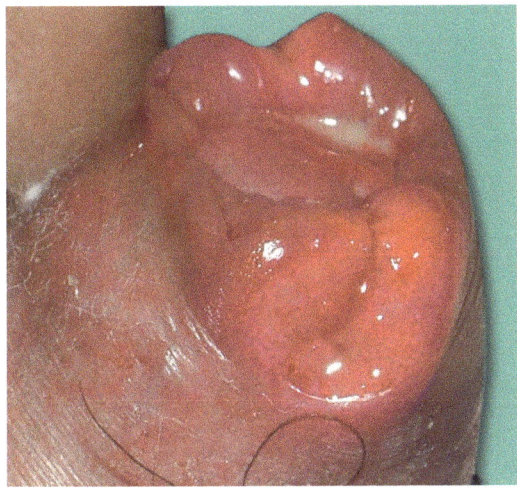

a. Syphilitic chancre
b. Chancroid
c. Lymphogranuloma venereum
d. Granuloma venereum (donovanosis)

490. A housewife complained of maceration of interdigital webs. What is the clinical diagnosis?

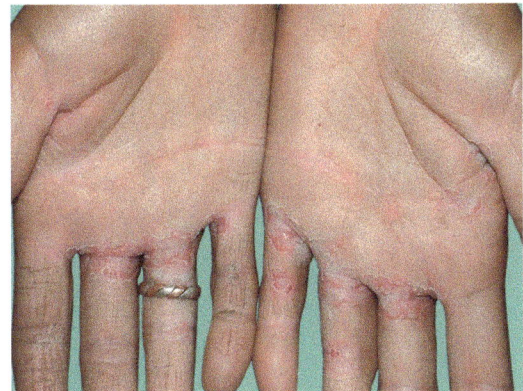

a. Candidiasis
b. Tinea manuum
c. Irritant dermatitis to soaps and detergents
d. Dry type housewife contact dermatitis

491. This patient complained of multiple purplish patches on the tongue. He also had pruritic papular and purplish lesions on the extremities. What is the clinical diagnosis?

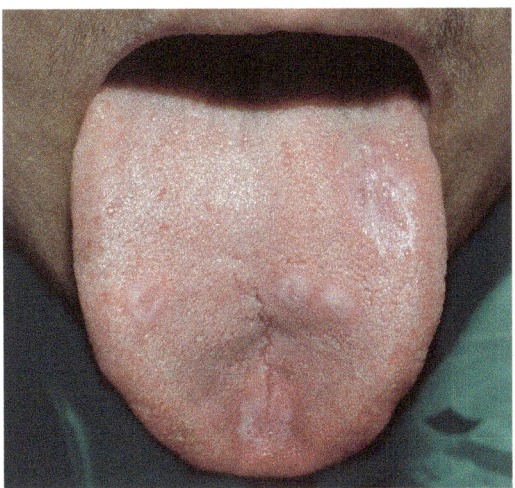

a. Lichen planus tongue
b. Scrotal tongue
c. Geographic tongue
d. Oral leukoplakia

492. This patient presented with swelling and black pigmentation of tip of the finger. There is a history of trauma six months back. What is the clinical diagnosis?

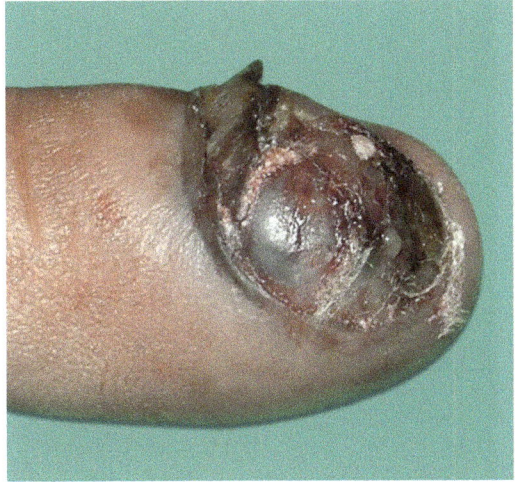

a. Subungual melanoma
b. Subungual hemorrhage
c. Tinea unguium
d. Glomus tumor

493. This patient presented with redness and thickening of lower lip for the last one year. A similar red plaque was also present on his bridge of nose. What is the clinical diagnosis?

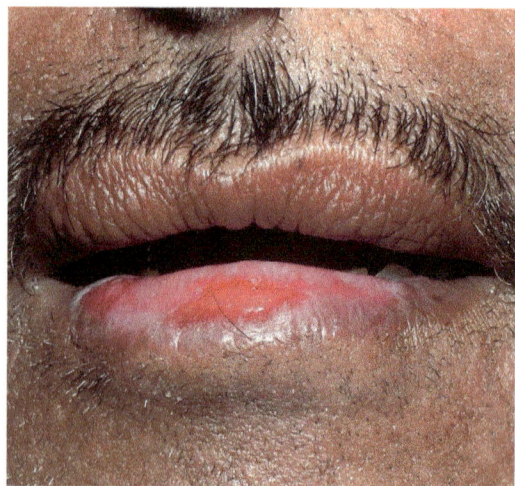

a. Actinic cheilitis
b. Lichen planus lower lip
c. Chronic cutaneous lupus erythematosus
d. Cheilitis simplex

494. A young unmarried girl presented with such lesions on shins and upper extremities for the last few days. What is the clinical diagnosis?

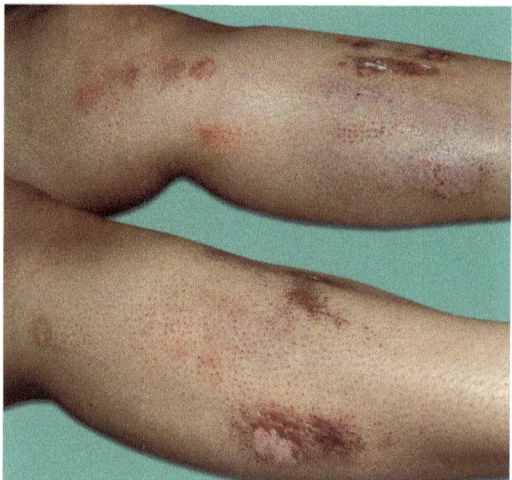

a. Eczema shins
b. Diabetic dermopathy
c. Dermatitis artefacta
d. Pretibial myxedema

495. This patient complained of swelling of both ear lobules. On examination, he was found to have loss of outer one-third of his eyebrows. He was also having loss of sensations in both hands with ulceration of finger tips *(MCQ 433)*. What is the clinical diagnosis?

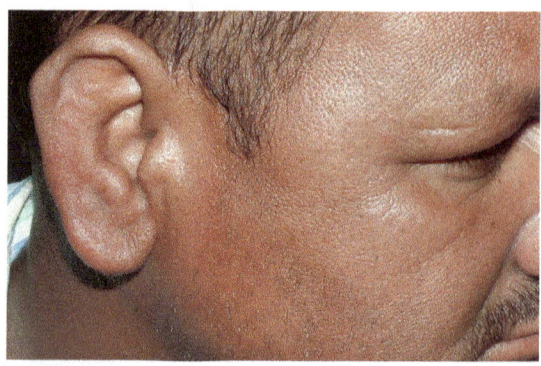

a. Acute urticaria
b. Myxedema
c. Systemic sclerosis
d. Lepromatous leprosy

496. This patient is complaining of episodic digital blanching and blue coloration for the last 5–6 years. She is also having mask life face and her nose is small and pinched *(MCQ 14)*. What is the clinical diagnosis?

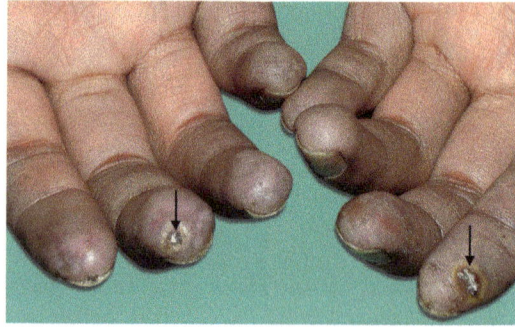

a. Chilblains
b. Raynaud's phenomenon
c. Buerger's disease
d. Deep vein thrombosis (DVT)

497. This newborn presented with multiple 1–2 mm sized papules on cheeks and chin. What is the clinical diagnosis?

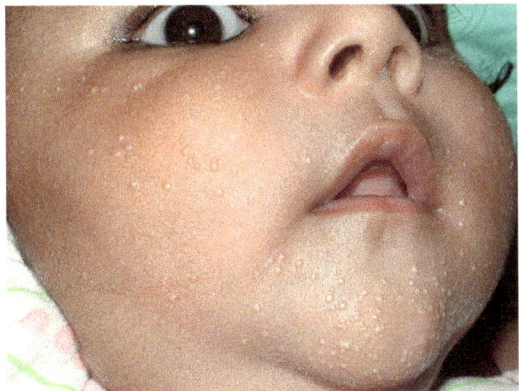

a. Sebaceous gland hyperplasia
b. Milia neonatorum
c. Neonatal acne
d. Transient neonatal pustular melanosis (TNPM)

498. This patient developed itching, vesicles, oozing and crusting around roadside injury on his foot. What is the clinical diagnosis?

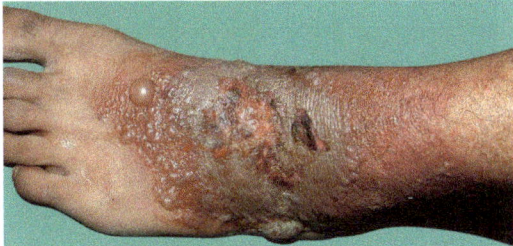

a. Madura foot
b. Infected dermatitis
c. Scrofuloderma
d. Impetigo contagiosa

499. A 12-year-old child presented with itching and little thickening behind both knees. What is the clinical diagnosis?

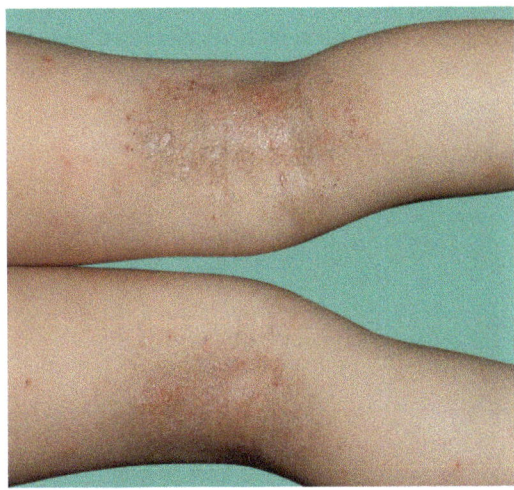

a. Seborrheic dermatitis (SD)
b. Intertrigo
c. Childhood phase atopic dermatitis
d. Tinea corporis

500. This young girl presented with these lesions for the last 3–4 days on her left hand only. What is the clinical diagnosis?

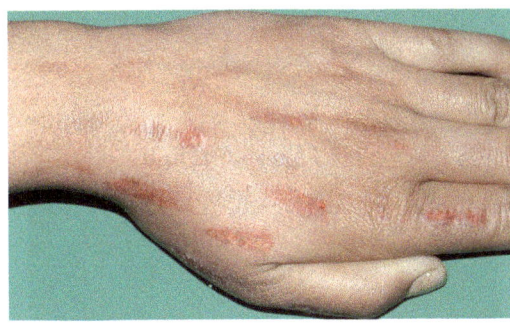

a. Discoid eczema
b. Lichen planus
c. Dermatitis artefacta
d. Housewife's contact dermatitis

501. This lady complained of itching and large red plaques on her trunk. These plaques used to disappear within 24 hours to reappear again at another site. On the back, many plaques have coalesced to form widespread erythema. What is the clinical diagnosis?

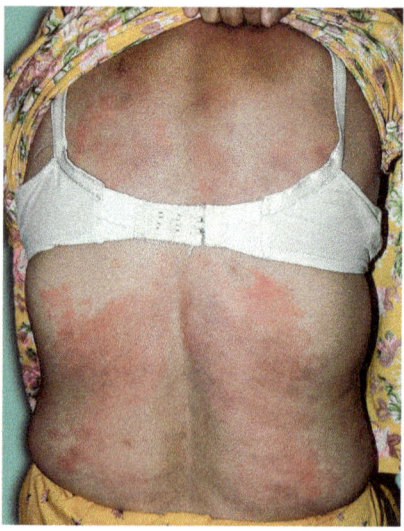

a. Widespread urticaria
b. Exanthematous rash
c. Erythroderma
d. Patch stage mycosis fungoides

502. This child is complaining of linear groove along the mid line in the frontal region for the last many years. There is no past history of injury. What is the clinical diagnosis?

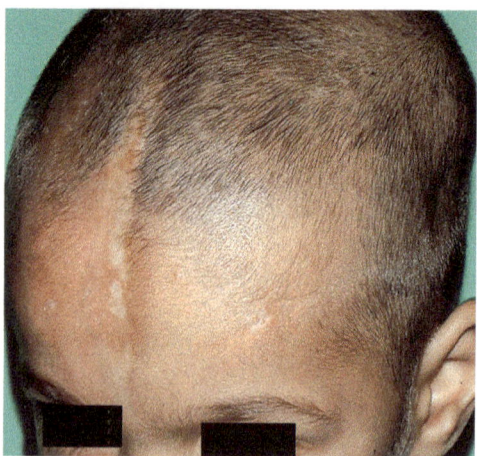

a. Lichen sclerosus et atrophicus
b. En coup de sabre
c. Scleredema
d. Dermatomyositis

503. This lady presented with small erythematous papules around her mouth sparing the lip margins. Which one of the following possibilities is closest for her?

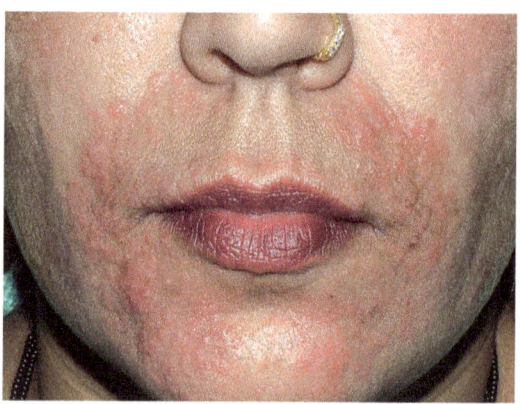

a. Gram negative folliculitis
b. Perioral dermatitis
c. Lupus miliaris disseminatus faciei (LMDF)
d. Acne rosaceà
e. Lip-lick cheilitis

504. This patient presented with various sized plaques on both shins. Plaques are having itching, oozing and crusting. What is the diagnosis?

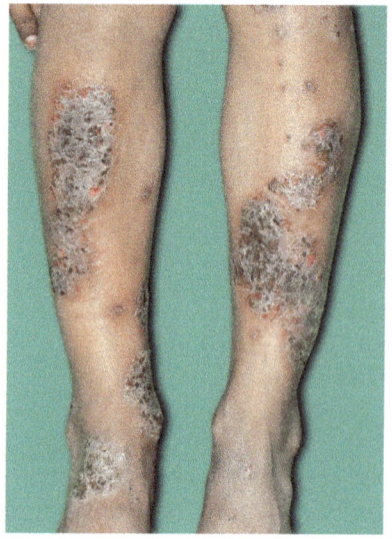

a. Psoriasis shins
b. Eczema shins
c. Lichen planus shins
d. Diabetic dermopathy

505. She presented with asymptomatic, shiny, red plaques on face, hands (for 476) and feet *(MCQ 479)*. Plaques are multiple, but still countable and have tendency to be symmetrical. What is the clinical diagnosis?

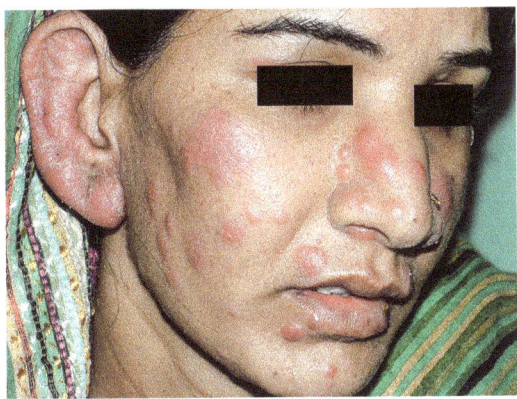

a. Lupus vulgaris
b. Borderline lepromatous leprosy
c. Sarcoidosis
d. Actinic lichen planus

507. This patient presented with multiple dry and crusted discoid plaques on the extremities. What is the closest clinical diagnosis?

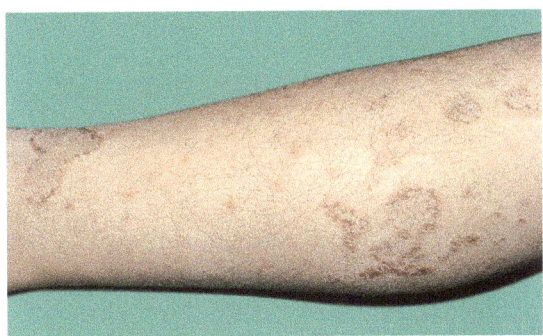

a. Pityriasis rosea
b. Dry discoid eczema
c. Parapsoriasis
d. Asteatotic eczema

506. This child is getting easy blistering of feet due to mild mechanical trauma since birth. Blisters heal without scarring. Hair, teeth and nails are normal. The family history of such a disease is positive. What is the clinical diagnosis?

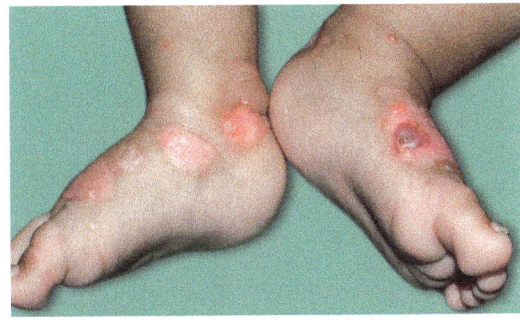

a. Epidermolysis bullosa simplex EB simplex
b. Chronic benign familial pemphigus
c. Epidermolysis bullosa acquisita EB acquisita
d. Cutaneous porphyria

508. What type of acne scars this patient is having on face?

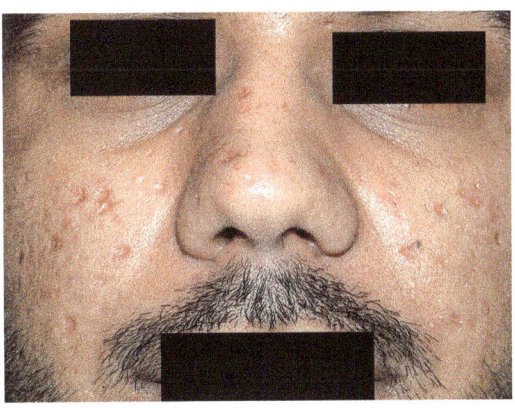

a. Macular scars
b. Anetoderma
c. Rolling scars
d. Boxcar scars

509. This patient presented with itching, papules and plaques with scaling on the buttocks extending to back of thigh and lower back. KOH smear from the lesions shows branching septate hyphae. What is the clinical diagnosis?

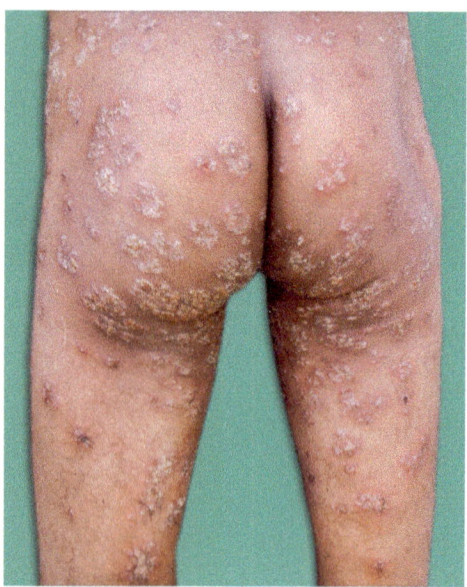

a. Tinea corporis
b. Tinea incognito
c. Pityriasis versicolor
d. Candidiasis

510. She presented with multiple, asymptomatic shiny umbilicated papules in the perineal region. What is the clinical diagnosis?

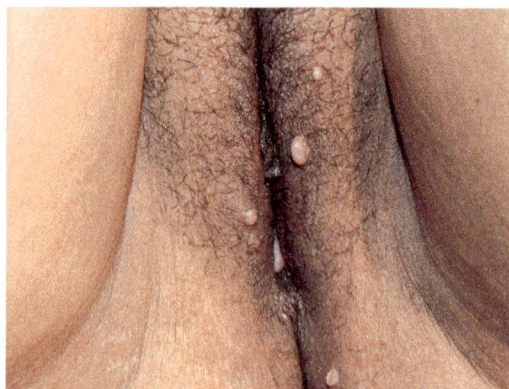

a. Genital warts
b. Molluscum contagiosum
c. Skin tags
d. Scabies

511. This patient presented with depigmentation of shins, feet and hands in a symmetrical manner. Which one of the following terms is most appropriate for him?

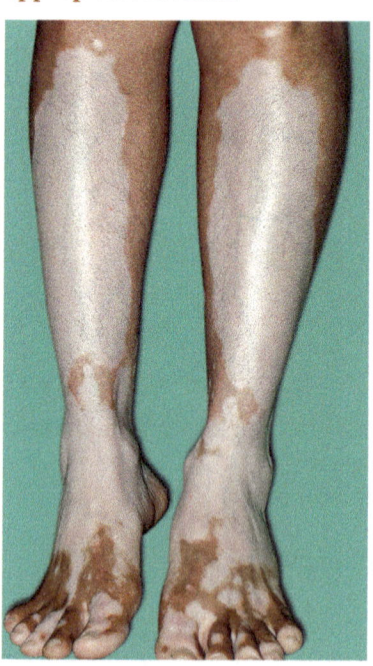

a. Leukoderma
b. Universal vitiligo
c. Vitiligo vulgaris
d. Segmental vitiligo

512. This patient is complaining of recurrent eruption of a group of tiny vesicles at varied intervals of time for the last 4 to 5 years. What is the clinical diagnosis?

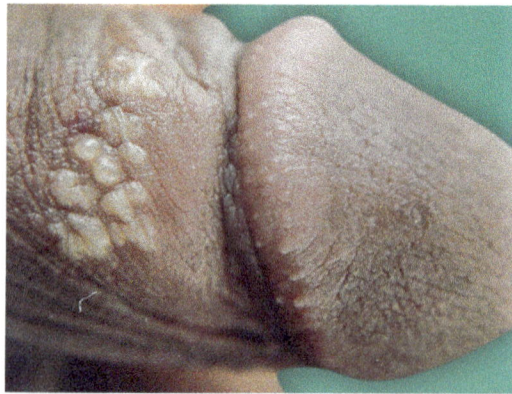

a. Fixed drug eruption (FDE)
b. Candidal balanoposthitis
c. Recurrent genital herpes
d. Lymphogranuloma venereum

513. This lady is complaining of itching, oozing and crusting of fingers of both hands. What is the clinical diagnosis?

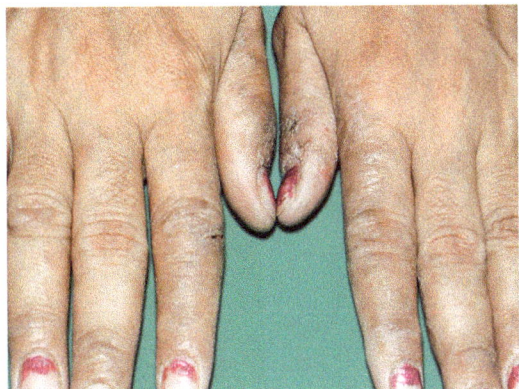

a. Dry type housewife dermatitis
b. Discoid eczema
c. Tinea manuum
d. Infective dermatitis

514. This patient complained of sharply defined punched out ulcers on toes covered with slough with minimal exudates. Pain is severe at night which improves with dependency. What type of ulcer is it?

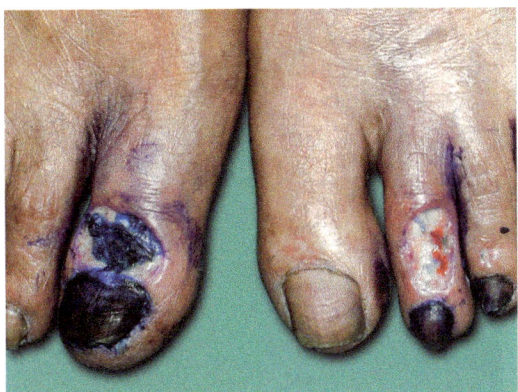

a. Tuberculous ulcer or chancre
b. Hypertensive ulcer
c. Venous ulcer
d. Arterial ulcer

515. She complained of single, red and well-defined plaque on her back for the last six months. On examination, sensations in the plaque were found to be diminished very significantly. What is the clinical diagnosis?

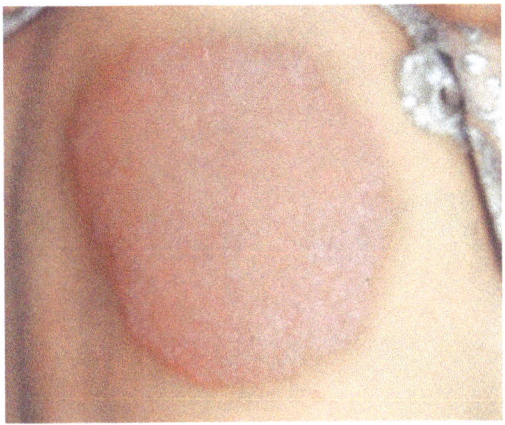

a. Lepromatous leprosy
b. Indeterminate leprosy
c. Lupus vulgaris
d. Tuberculoid leprosy

516. A 70-year-old patient complained of a single asymmetrical patch having irregular borders, varied color and 25 mm in diameter on his back for the last one year. What is the clinical diagnosis?

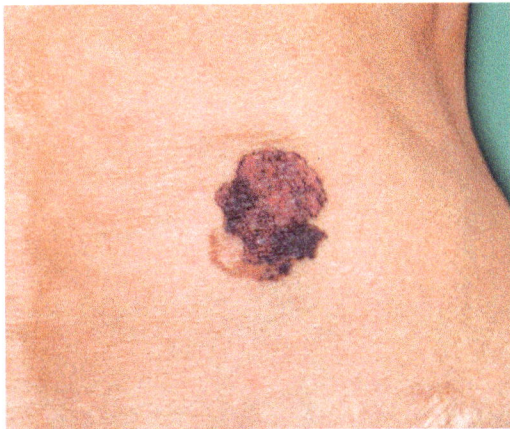

a. Mongolian spots
b. Superficial spreading melanoma (SSM)
c. Bowen's disease
d. Extramammary Paget's disease

517. A 16-year-old female presented with butterfly rash on her face. She also complained of increased loss of scalp hair. What is the clinical diagnosis?

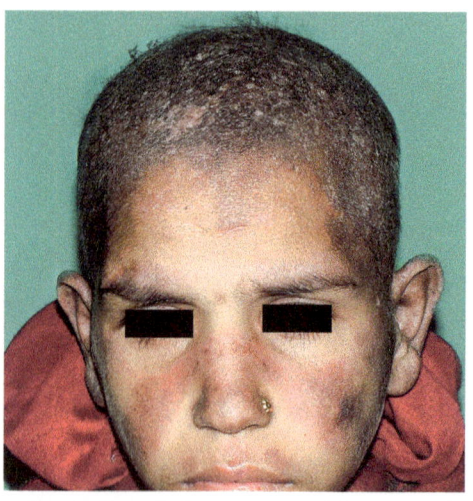

a. Butterfly rash due to systemic lupus erythematosus (SLE)
b. Dermatomyositis
c. Melanoma
d. Bilateral nevus of Ota

518. A 2-month-old baby was brought with a small red firm lesion at umbilicus. What is the clinical diagnosis?

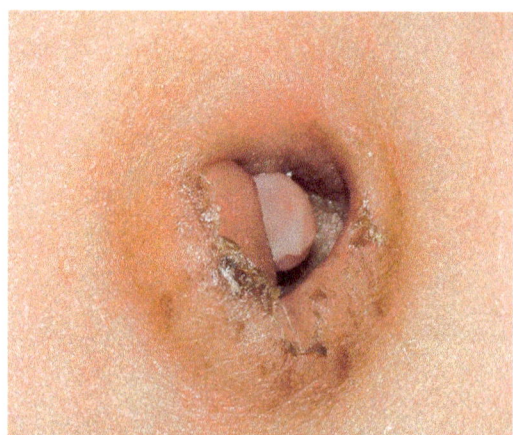

a. Umbilical granuloma
b. Umbilical hernia
c. Prolapsed patent vitellointestinal duct
d. Umbilical polyp

519. This patient presented with dystrophy of nail plates. What is the clinical diagnosis?

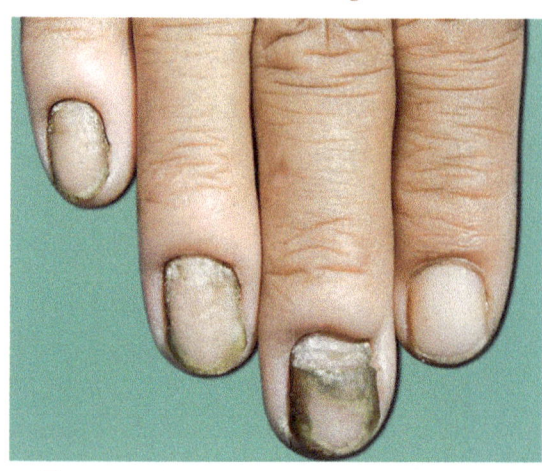

a. Tinea unguium
b. Chronic paronychia
c. Lichen planus
d. Psoriatic nails

520. Which one of the types of post-acne scars this patient is having?

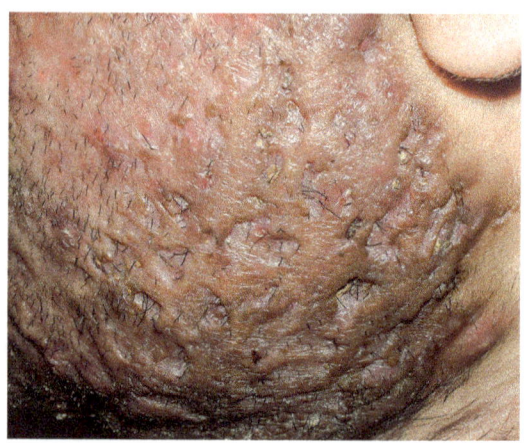

a. Anetoderma
b. Boxcar scars
c. Macular scars
d. Hypertrophic scars

521. This lady is having a red patch on left side of her forehead since birth. What is the clinical diagnosis?

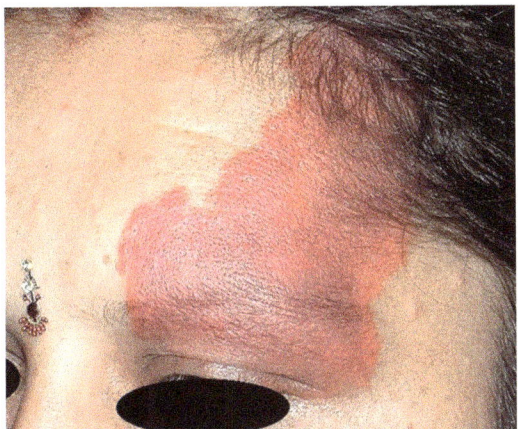

a. Strawberry hemangioma
b. Salmon patch
c. Port-wine stain
d. Cherry hemangioma

522. This patient complained of asymptomatic mottled hypo pigmentation on the back covered by fine dust like scales. KOH smear examination shows short coarse filaments together with spherical thick-walled spores. What is the clinical diagnosis?

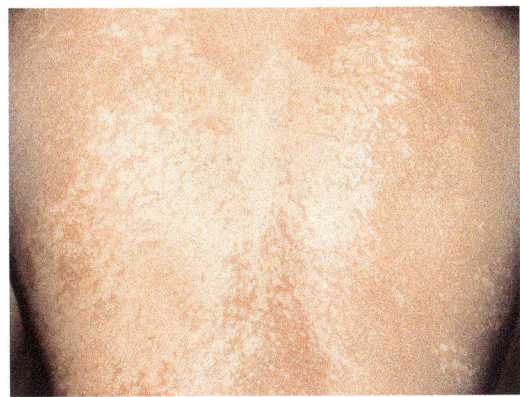

a. Tinea corporis
b. Pityriasis versicolor
c. Candidiasis
d. Pityriasis alba

523. A 70-year-old man presented with a single plaque on his cheek for the last three years. Its margins are thread like and center shows crusting at places. What is the clinical diagnosis?

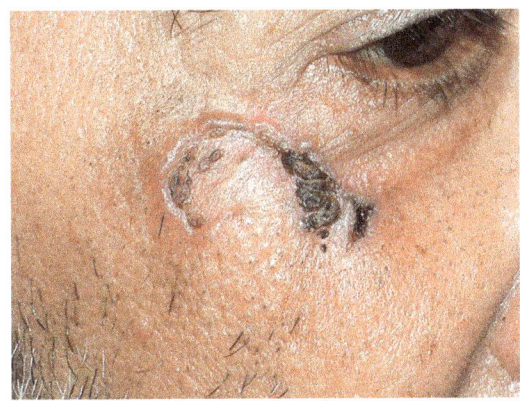

a. Basal cell carcinoma (BCC)
b. Squamous cell carcinoma (SCC)
c. Malignant melanoma (MM)
d. Actinic keratosis

524. This patient developed overnight multiple red patches in a linear pattern in the thoracic region with accompanying burning sensation. What is the clinical diagnosis?

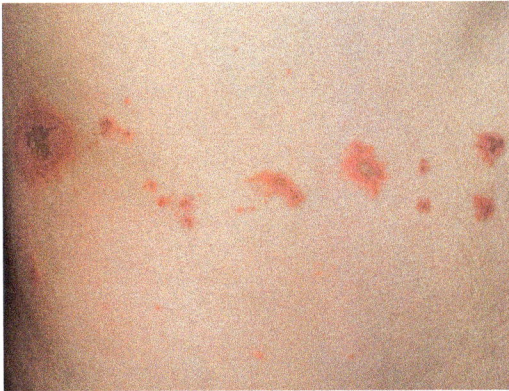

a. Herpes zoster
b. *Paederus dermatitis*
c. Petechiae and purpura
d. Palpable purpura

525. This patient complained of asymptomatic shiny papulonodular swelling of both ear lobules for the last one year. He also had multiple sinuses with discharge and crusting on both sides of body in the infra-auricular, cervical and inguinal regions *(MCQ 960)*. Which one of the followings is the closest clinical diagnosis for this patient?

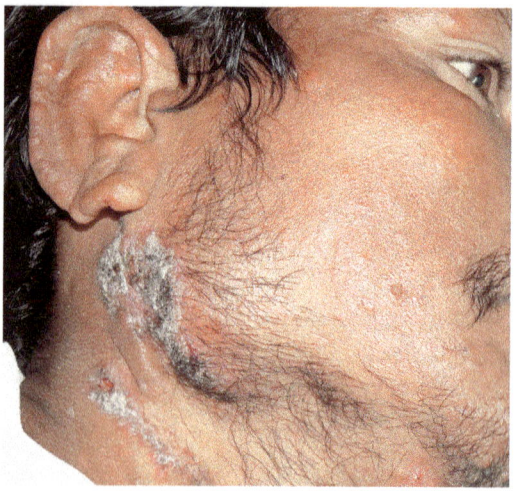

a. Lepromatous leprosy with hidradenitis suppurativa
b. Lepromatous leprosy with scrofuloderma
c. Chronic urticaria with scrofuloderma
d. Chronic urticaria with hidradenitis suppurativa

526. This patient presented with a group of asymptomatic, rough surfaced firm papules and nodules on the left wrist. What is the clinical diagnosis?

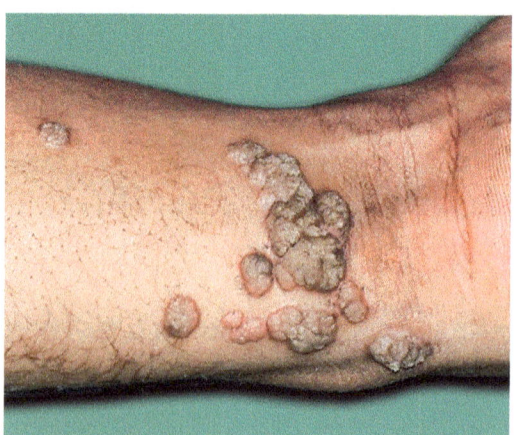

a. Common warts
b. Lichen planus hypertrophicus (LPH)
c. Tuberculosis verrucosa cutis (TVC)
d. Keloids

527. This patient presented with multiple 5 mm to 1 cm sized purpuric lesions on the legs. The lesions are non-blanchable and can be felt on palpation. What is the clinical diagnosis?

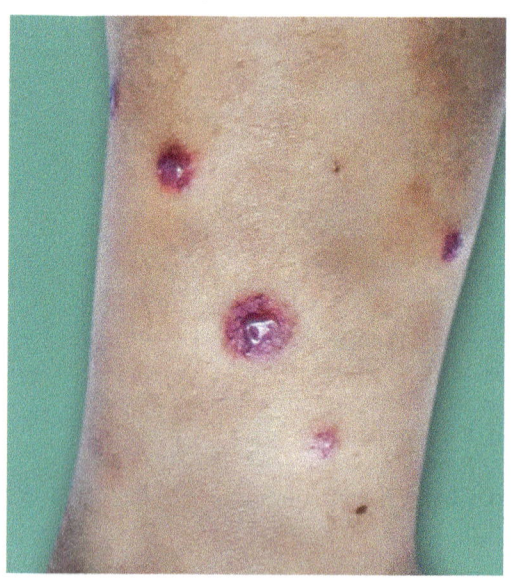

(Courtesy: Dr vijay singhal)

a. Henoch-Schonlein purpura (HSP)
b. Palpable purpura
c. Idiopathic thrombocytopenic purpura (ITP)
d. Thrombotic thrombocytopenic purpura (TTP)

528. This patient presented with exophytic, cauliflower like growth on his sole for the last 2 years. What is the closest diagnosis?

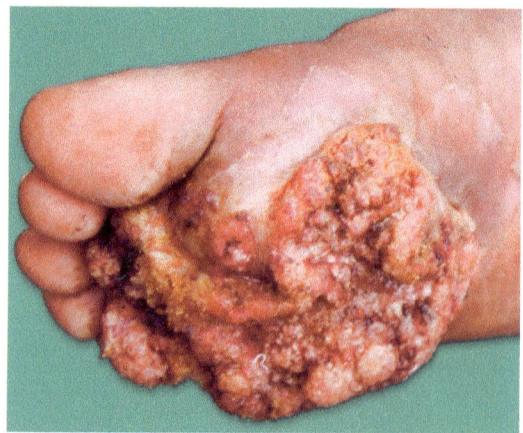

a. Tuberculosis verrucosa cutis (TVC)
b. Squamous cell carcinoma (SCC)
c. Basal cell carcinoma (BCC)
d. Madura foot

529. A 45-year-old farmer presented with ill defined, atrophic and scaly plaque on the lower lip for the last many years. What is the closest clinical diagnosis?

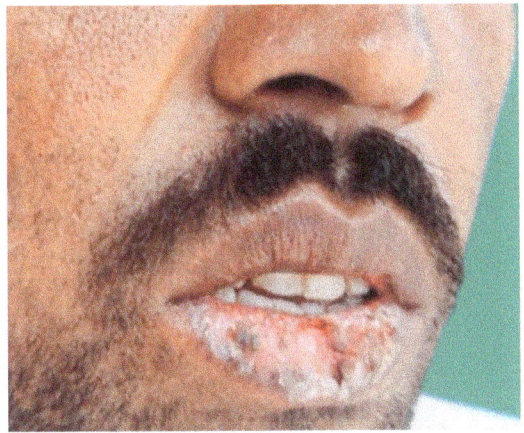

a. Lichen planus
b. Actinic cheilitis
c. Chronic cutaneous lupus erythematosus (CCLE)

530. This patient complained of fissuring of tongue. Which one of the following terms is used to describe it?

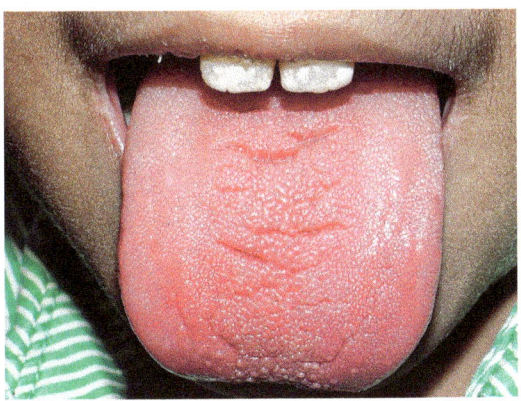

a. Scrotal tongue
b. Geographic tongue

531. This patient presented with multiple small shiny lesions on penile skin for the last three months. What is the clinical diagnosis?

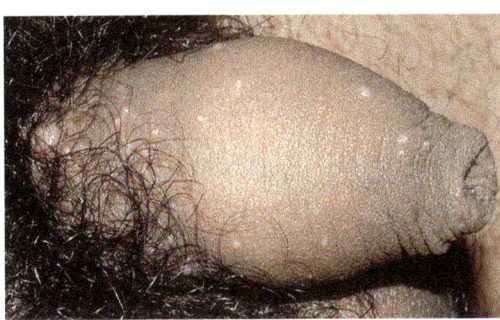

a. Pearly penile papules (PPP)
b. Scabies
c. Fordyce spots
d. Molluscum contagiosum
e. Lichen nitidus

532. What is the diagnosis of this patient?

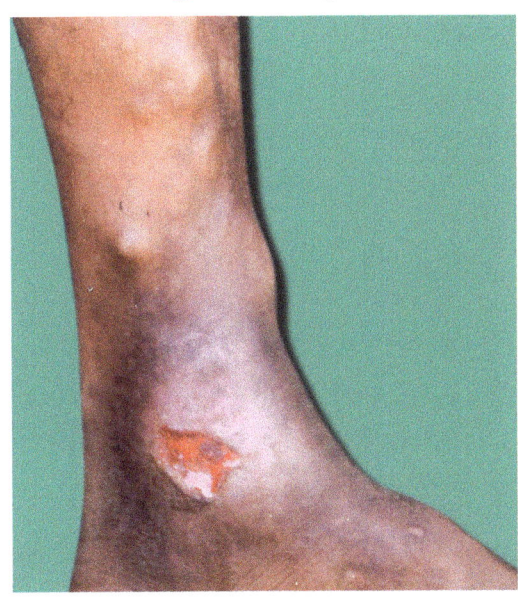

a. Varicose or venous ulcer
b. Arterial ulcer
c. Hypertensive ulcer
d. Tuberculous ulcer or chancre

533. Which one of the following acne scars this patient is having on his chest?

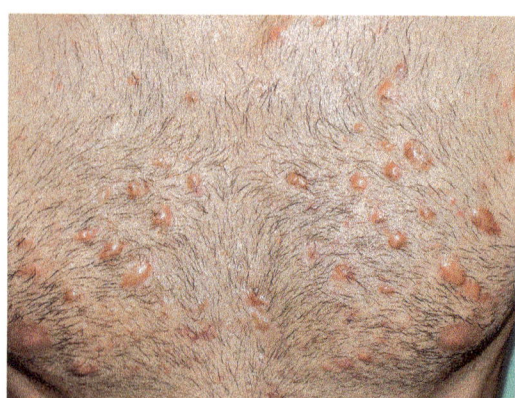

a. Hypertrophic scars
b. Anetoderma
c. Boxcar scars
d. Macular scars

534. This patient presented with a reddish brown, soft, gelatinous and psoriasiform plaque on the buttock for the last six months. What is the closest clinical diagnosis?

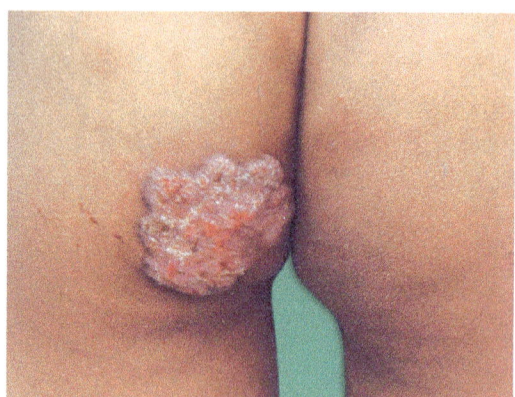

a. Lupus vulgaris
b. Psoriasis
c. Discoid lupus erythematosus
d. Cutaneous leishmaniasis

535. This patient is complaining of pigmentation studded with coarse terminal hairs on the left side of his abdomen for the last 5–6 years. What is the clinical diagnosis?

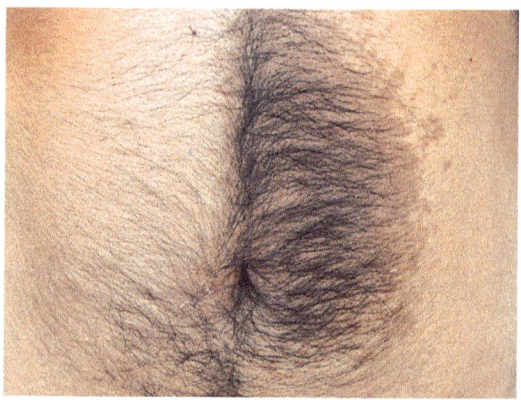

a. Becker's nevus
b. Localized hypertrichosis
c. Nevus of Ota

536. A 10-year-old child presented with pain and swelling of distal part of penile shaft. What is the clinical diagnosis?

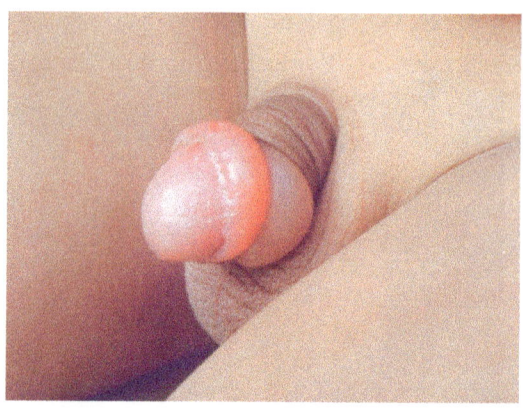

a. Phimosis
b. Paraphimosis
c. Balanoposthitis

537. This child presented with dark asymptomatic fish like scales. It started in the neonatal period. It is prominent on extensors and is sparing cubital fossae. What is the clinical diagnosis?

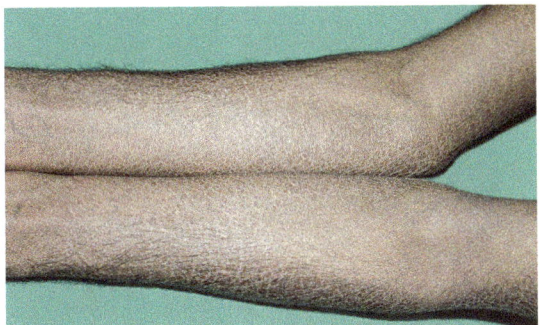

a. Ichthyosis vulgaris
b. X-linked recessive ichthyosis (XLRI)
c. Asteatotic eczema
d. Atopic dermatitis

538. This patient complained of gradual shortening of fingers. His skin over hands and forearms has bound down to underlying tissues. Skin has become stiff, indurated and is difficult to pinched off. There is no loss of sensations. What is the clinical diagnosis?

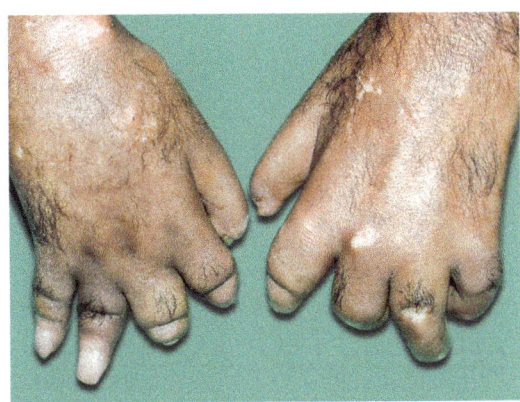

a. Lepromatous leprosy
b. Systemic sclerosis
c. Psoriatic arthritis
d. Parathyroidism

539. This lady presented with diffuse pigmentation of face and palmar creases. On examination, her buccal mucosa and palate *(MCQ 551)* were found to be pigmented. What is the closest clinical diagnosis?

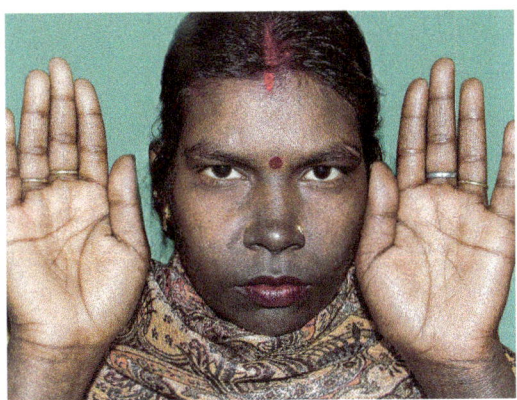

a. Addisonian pigmentation
b. Peutz-Jeghers syndrome
c. Cushing's disease
d. Drug-induced pigmentation

540. An 80-year-old patient presented with gangrenous changes in his foot. He is non-smoker, diabetic and hypertensive. What is the closest clinical diagnosis?

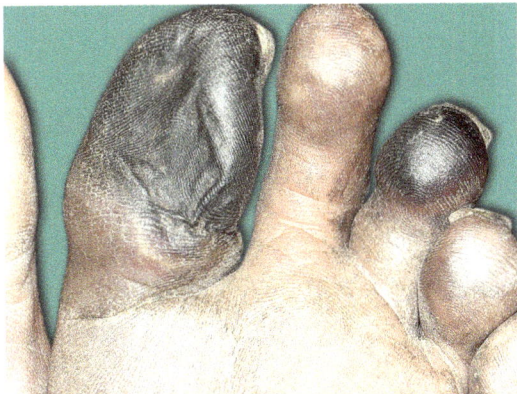

a. Buerger's disease
b. Atherosclerotic peripheral vascular disease
c. Due to metoprolol
d. Due to vasopressors

541. This boy presented with recurrent itching and swelling on upper lip for the last 5 days. There are no urticarial lesions on the other parts of body. What is the clinical diagnosis?

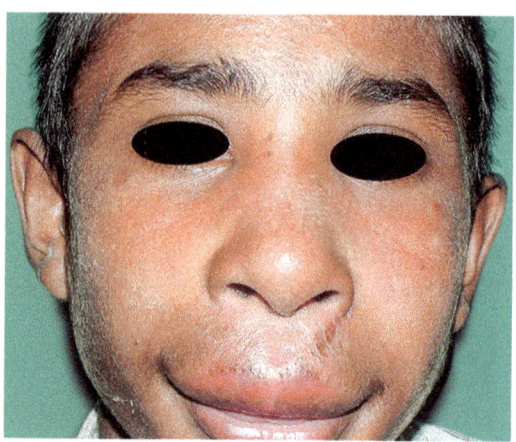

a. Acute urticaria
b. Angioedema
c. Cheilitis glandularis
d. Granulomatous cheilitis

542. A 38-year-old male presented with itchy, hyperkeratotic 5 mm-1.5 cm sized multiple lesions on scrotum, penis, adjacent part of thigh and perianal region for the last 5–7 years. The peripheral threadlike raised border observed in annular lesions on scrotum. Which one of the following options is correct?

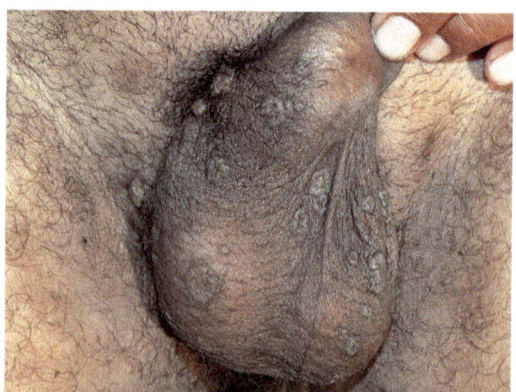

a. Genital warts
b. Genital porokeratosis
c. Condylomata lata
d. Molluscum contagiosum

543. Which one of the following acne scars this patient is having?

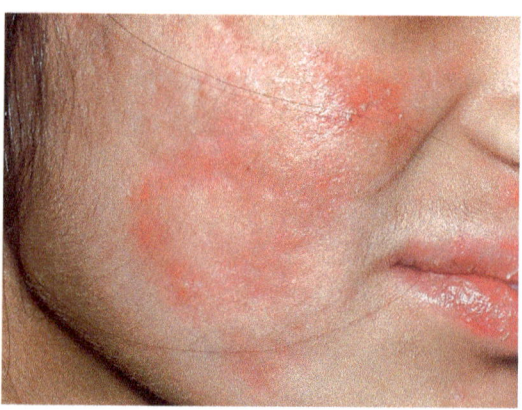

a. Macular scars
b. Hypertrophic scars
c. Anetoderma
d. Boxcar scars

544. An 18-month-old child presented with red-colored plaques on cheeks and extremities for the last five days. Mucosa and trunk were spared. No viscera were involved. What is the clinical diagnosis?

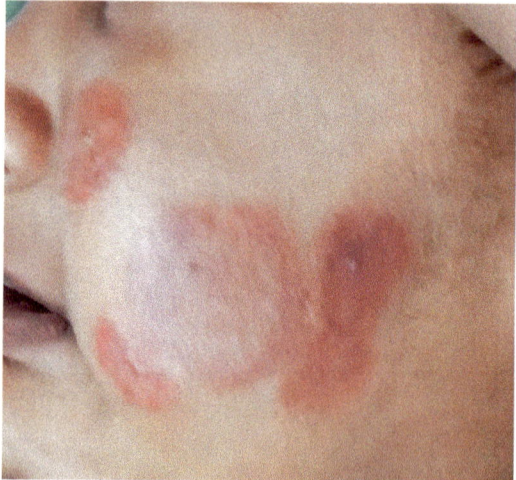

(*Courtesy:* Dr vijay singhal)

a. Henoch-Schonlein purpura
b. Acute hemorrhagic edema of infancy
c. Palpable purpura
d. Idiopathic thrombocytopenic purpura (ITP)

545. This patient presented with redness, superficial erosions and atrophic changes on glans and under surface of prepuce. He is applying some cream for last 5–6 months. What is the closest clinical diagnosis?

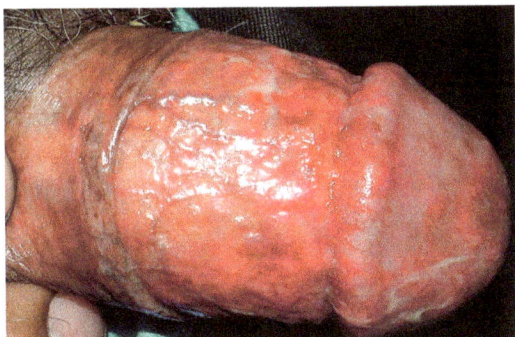

a. Fixed drug eruption (FDE)
b. Genital skin atrophy due to topical steroid cream
c. Candidal balanoposthitis
d. Secondary syphilis

546. This patient complained of severely restricted opening of mouth. He is a smoker and is in habit of betel quid chewing. What is the closest diagnosis?

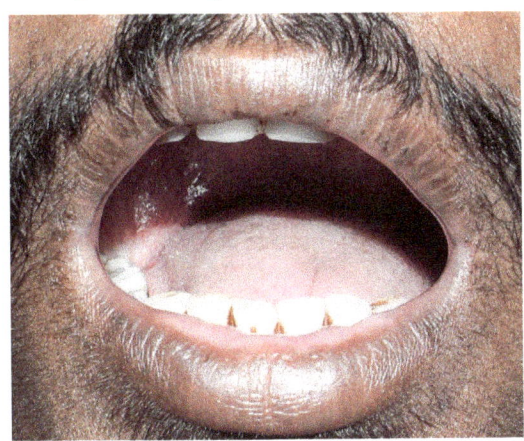

a. Scleroderma
b. Smoker's melanosis
c. Oral submucosal fibrosis

547. A 4-month-old child presented with grouped vesicular lesions on erythematous base on his right upper extremity for the last three days. What is the clinical diagnosis?

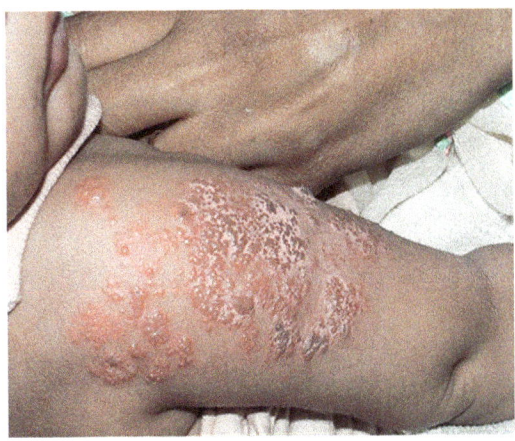

a. Herpes zoster
b. Chickenpox
c. *Paederus dermatitis*
d. Lymphangioma circumscriptum

548. A 3-year-old child presented with painful red swelling in the gluteal region for the last seven days. What is the clinical diagnosis?

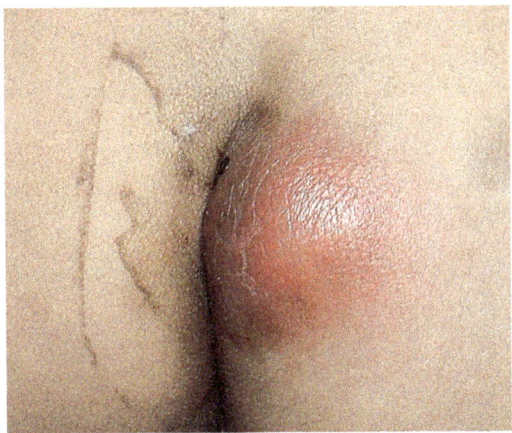

a. Sebaceous cyst
b. Gluteal abscess
c. Strawberry hemangioma
d. Cellulitis

549. A 7-year-old child presented with asymptomatic petechiae on both thighs for the last seven days. His platelet count is 17,000/mcL. What is the clinical diagnosis?

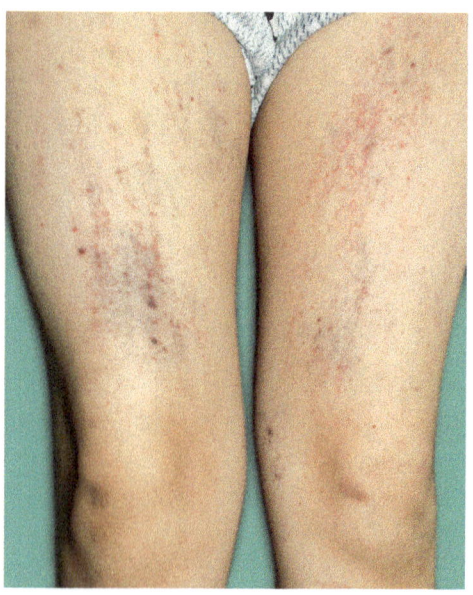

a. Idiopathic thrombocytopenic purpura (ITP)
b. Henoch-Schonlein purpura (HS Purpura)
c. Dermatitis artefacta
d. Thrombotic thrombocytopenic purpura (TPP)

550. This patient complained of absorption of fingers of both hands. Metacarpals and carpal bones are normal. It is accompanied by loss of sensations in both hands for the last many years. What is the possible cause of absorption of multiple fingers in this patient?

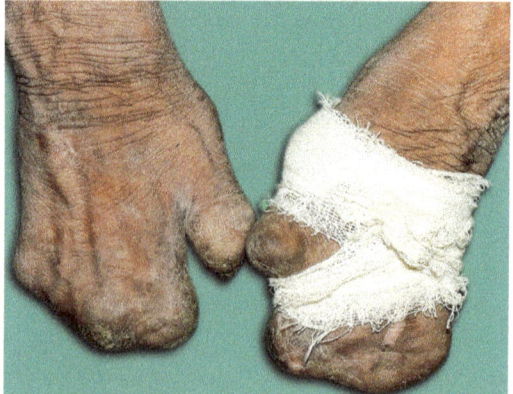

a. Lepromatous leprosy
b. Systemic sclerosis
c. Hyperparathyroidism
d. Psoriatic arthritis

551. A lady presented with pigmentation of face and palmar creases *(MCQ 539)*. On examination, her buccal mucosa and hard palate were found to be pigmented. What is the closest clinical diagnosis?

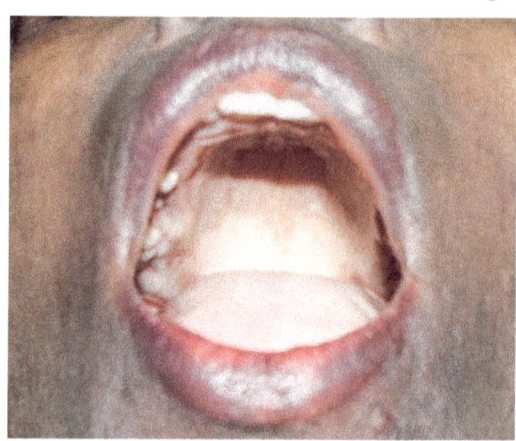

a. Peutz-Jeghers syndrome
b. Addisonian pigmentation

552. This patient complained of itching, redness and fine scaling in the beard region and scalp for last many years. What is the clinical diagnosis?

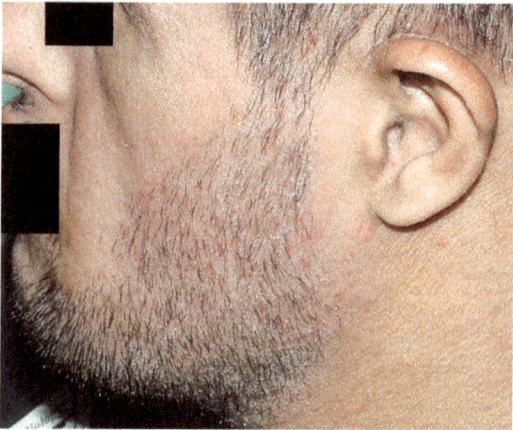

a. Atopic dermatitis
b. Seborrheic dermatitis
c. Tinea faciei
d. Psoriasis

553. This lady complained of red plaque studded with while scaling in the scalp for the last one year. What is the clinical diagnosis?

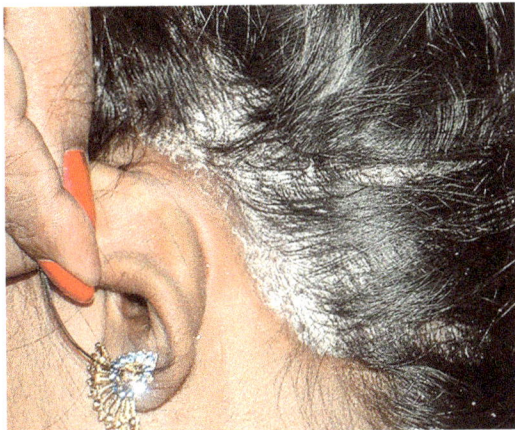

a. Pityriasis amiantacea
b. Seborrheic capitis
c. Scalp psoriasis
d. Tinea capitis

555. This patient presented with painful flat eroded malodorous plaques in both axillae for the last many years. It has characteristic fissured appearance and his sister is also suffering from the similar disease. What is the closest clinical diagnosis?

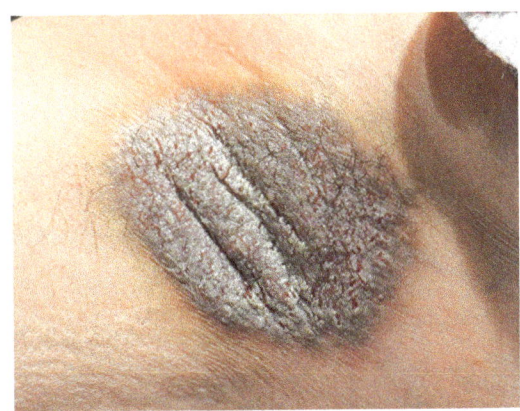

a. Hailey-Hailey disease
b. Candidal intertrigo
c. Discoid eczema

554. This child was brought with itching and rash in both groins. What is the clinical diagnosis?

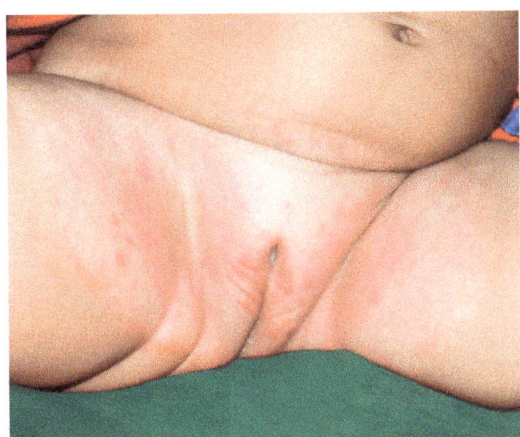

a. Seborrheic dermatitis
b. Diaper dermatitis
c. Candidiasis groins
d. Tinea cruris

556. This patient complained of itching, redness and scaling on buttocks for the last two months. What is the clinical diagnosis?

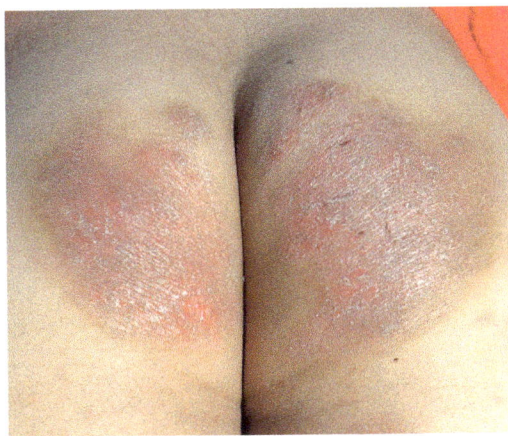

a. Psoriasis
b. Tinea corporis
c. Dermatitis buttocks
d. Candidiasis

557. This patient complained of red plaques studded with white scales on face. What is the clinical diagnosis?

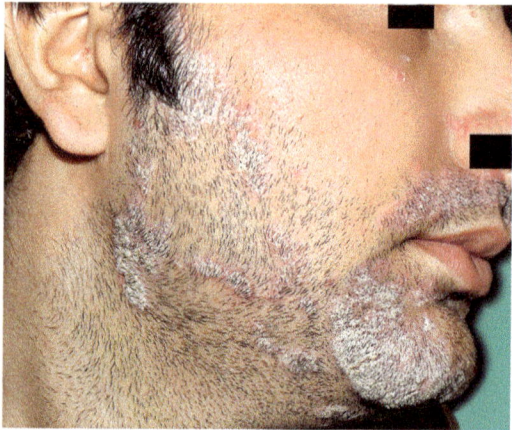

a. Psoriasis
b. Seborrheic dermatitis
c. Tinea faciei

558. This patient complained of a painful swelling with redness on the front of thigh. It is studded with multiple, pus discharging openings. What is the clinical diagnosis?

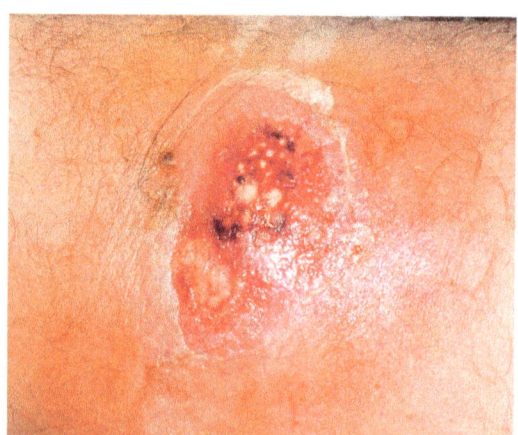

a. Superficial folliculitis
b. Boil
c. Carbuncle

559. This patient presented with a non-healing ulcer on the back of his arm. The ulcer has bluish margins and watery discharge. What is the clinical diagnosis?

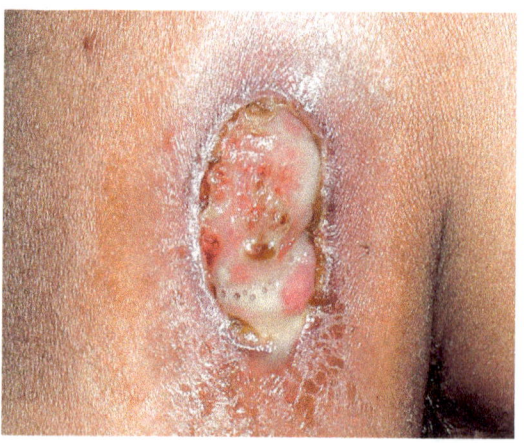

a. Scrofuloderma
b. Pyoderma gangrenosum
c. Trophic ulcer

560. This patient presented with itching and multiple crusted lesions on the back. What is the closest clinical diagnosis?

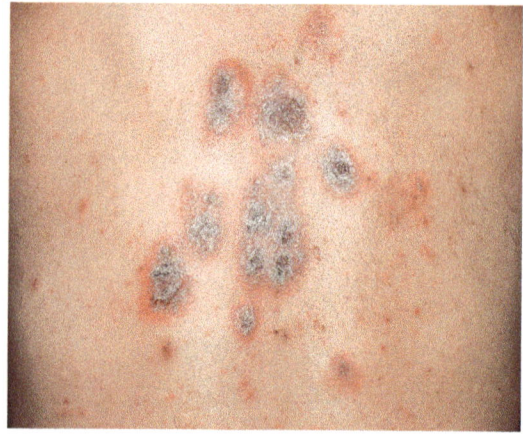

a. Discoid eczema back
b. Psoriasis back
c. Infected tinea corporis
d. Seborrheic dermatitis

561. This patient complained of itching and little oozing in groins and scrotal region for the last one year. What is the closest clinical diagnosis?

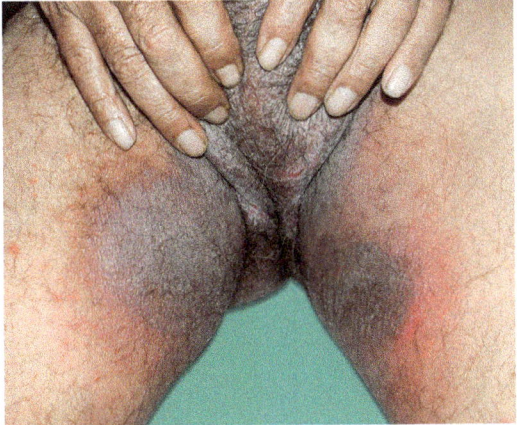

a. Intertrigo
b. Tinea cruris
c. Eczema groins
d. Candidiasis groins

562. A 40-year-old female presented with multiple asymptomatic dark coloured papules and nodules in the perineal region for the last six months. What is the clinical diagnosis?

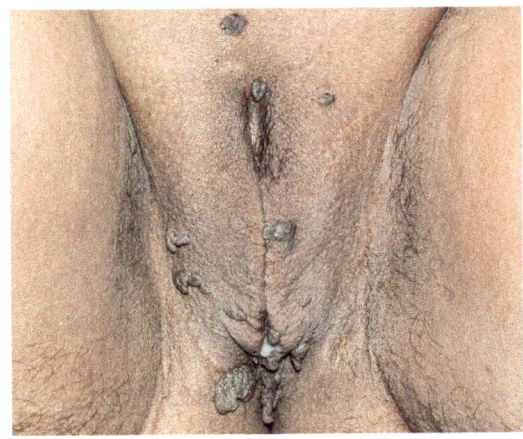

a. Skin tags
b. Perineal venereal warts
c. Molluscum contagiosum

563. This patient of leprosy having loss of sensations in feet, presented with a plantar ulcer opposite to the head of first metatarsal bone. What is the clinical diagnosis?

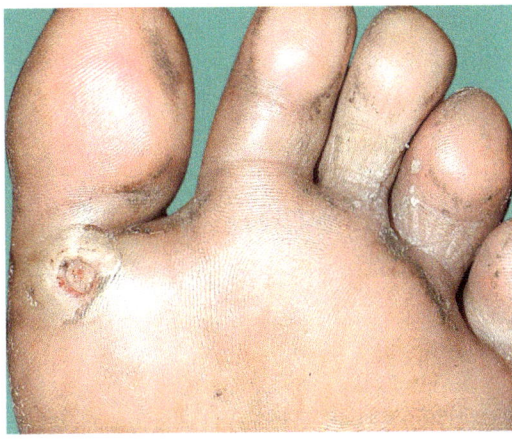

a. Trophic ulcer
b. Tropical ulcer
c. Arterial ulcer

564. This patient presented with a large asymptomatic hyperkeratotic brown and verrucous plaque involving the sole. It has developed in a span of 4 to 5 years and is showing white atrophic scaring in the centre. What is the closest diagnosis?

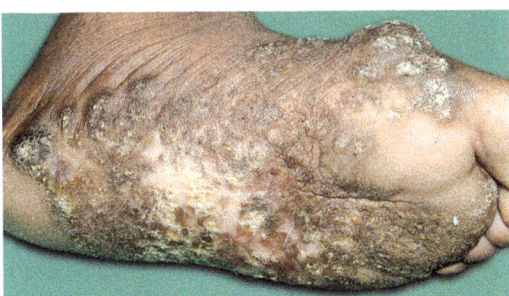

a. Plantar warts
b. Tuberculosis verrucosa cutis (TVC)
c. Lupus vulgaris
d. Madura foot

565. Which one of the following acne scars this patient is having?

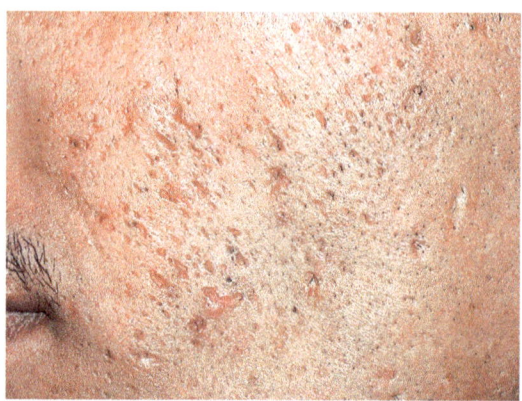

a. Anetoderma
b. Rolling scars
c. Macular scars
d. Boxcar scars

566. This patient complained of itching, whiteness and fine scaling in the beard region. What is the clinical diagnosis?

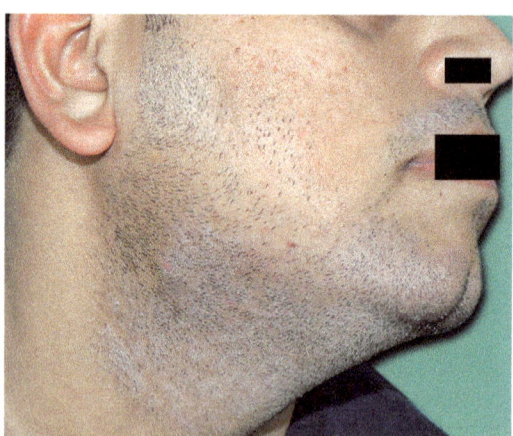

a. Psoriasis beard
b. Seborrheic dermatitis
c. Tinea faciei

567. This child presented with itching, pigmentation, thickening in the cervical region for the last many years. What is the closest clinical diagnosis?

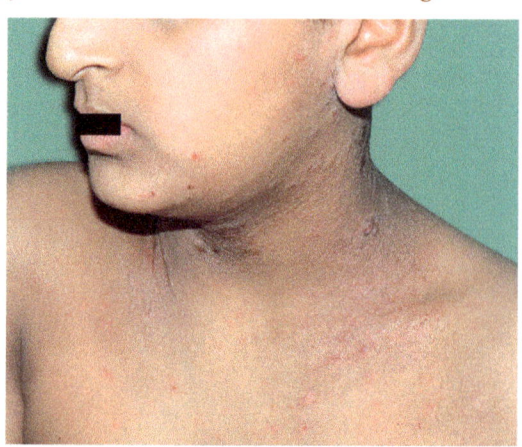

a. Acanthosis nigricans
b. Seborrheic dermatitis
c. Darier's disease
d. Atopic dermatitis

568. She complained of multiple rough papules in the anogenital region for the last six months. What is the closest clinical diagnosis?

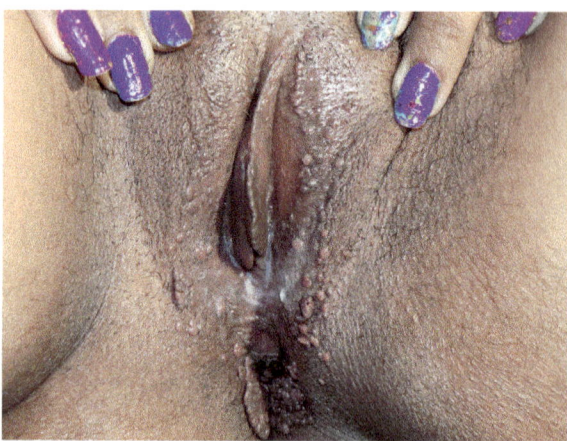

a. Condylomata lata
b. Condylomata acuminata
c. Molluscum contagiosum
d. Angiokeratoma of vulva

569. This child presented with multiple patches of hair loss. What is the possible diagnosis?

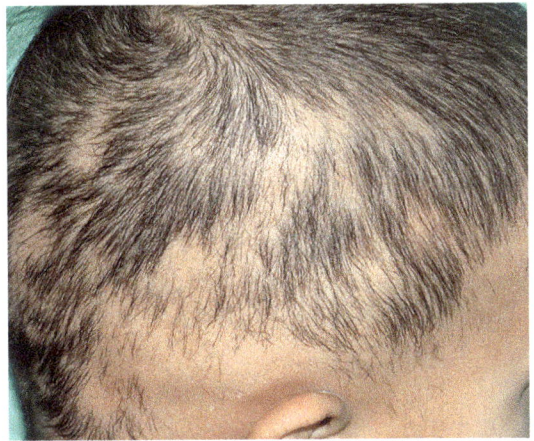

a. Tinea capitis
b. Trichotillomania
c. Alopecia areata
d. Telogen effluvium

571. She complained of red scaly plaques on both soles with insignificant itching. Scalp also shows similar plaques. What is the clinical diagnosis?

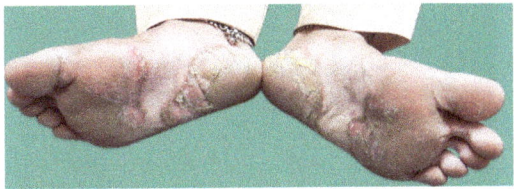

a. Hyperkeratotic eczema
b. Focal palmoplantar keratoderma
c. Psoriasis of soles
d. Tinea pedis

570. This patient complained of bluish discoloration of fingers on dipping in cold water. What is the clinical diagnosis?

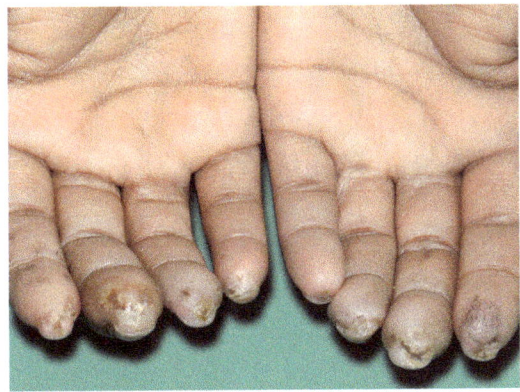

a. Raynaud's phenomenon
b. Chilblains
c. Buerger's disease

572. This patient was taking systemic steroids for bronchial asthma. She presented with white scaling on face, chest *(MCQ 595)* and extremities. What is the clinical diagnosis?

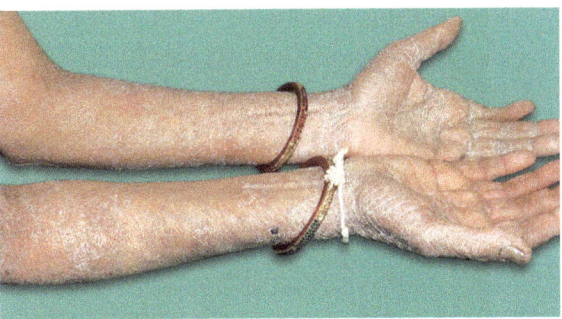

a. Tinea incognito
b. Psoriasis
c. Acquired ichthyosis
d. Asteatotic (senile) eczema

573. This patient complains of asymptomatic yellowish thickening of palms (*MCQ 486*) and soles since infancy. What is the clinical diagnosis?

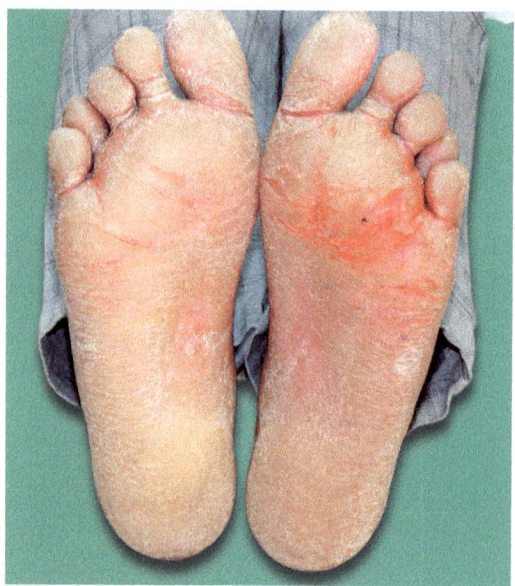

a. Palmoplantar keratoderma
b. Hyperkeratotic eczema

574. This patient is complaining of itching and scaling between two fingers of his right hand. What is the clinical diagnosis?

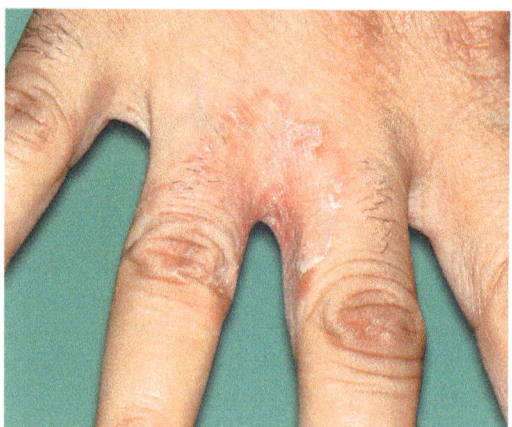

a. Candidiasis
b. Tinea manuum
c. Scabies
d. Discoid eczema

575. This patient complained of redness, irritation and white flakes on glans and prepuce. What is the most possible reason for this condition?

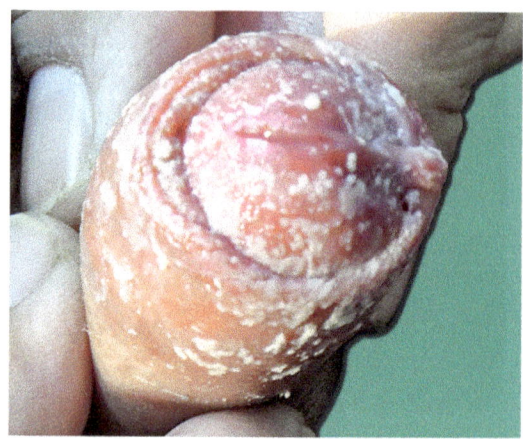

a. Smegma
b. Secondary syphilis
c. Prolonged use of topical steroid cream
d. Candidiasis due to diabetes mellitus

576. This patient complained of longitudinal bands in nail plates which end in V-shaped notch at free margin. On examination, multiple firm rough papules of skin or gray colored are seen in seborrheic areas *(MCQ 60)*. What is the clinical diagnosis?

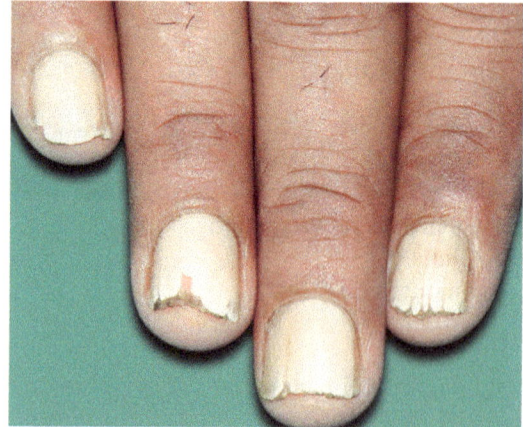

a. Lichen planus
b. Darier's disease
c. Seborrheic dermatitis
d. Pseudoacanthosis nigricans

577. This patient complained of a group of painful vesicles on erythematous base on the left side of back for the last five days. What is the clinical diagnosis?

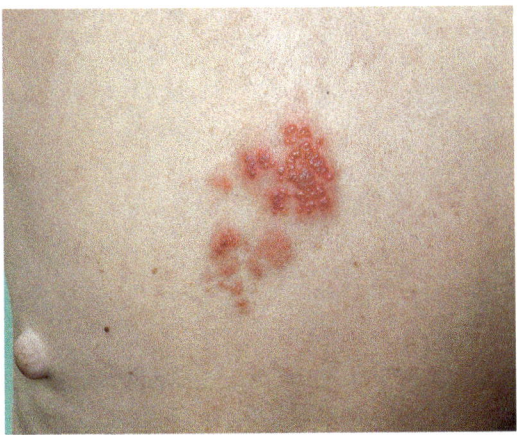

a. Herpes simplex
b. Dermatitis herpetiformis
c. *Paederus dermatitis*
d. Herpes zoster

579. This patient presented with multiple, sharply defined, deep seated and rough hyperkeratotic lesions on sole. What is the clinical diagnosis?

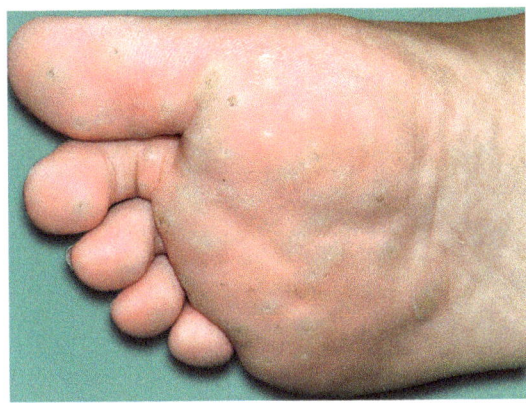

a. Corns
b. Superficial plantar warts
c. Deep plantar warts
d. Punctuate plantar keratoderma

578. This patient presented with whiteness of preputial skin along with few white macules on his wrist. What is the clinical diagnosis?

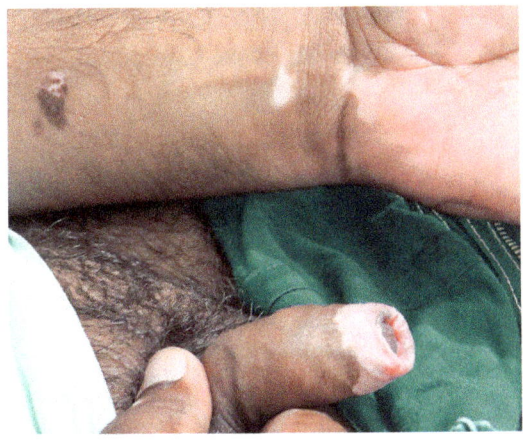

a. Vitiligo
b. Lichen sclerosus et atrophicus
c. Depigmentation due to steroid cream

580. This patient developed overnight multiple vesicles filled with clear fluid on his arm. There is no pain or itching. What is the clinical diagnosis?

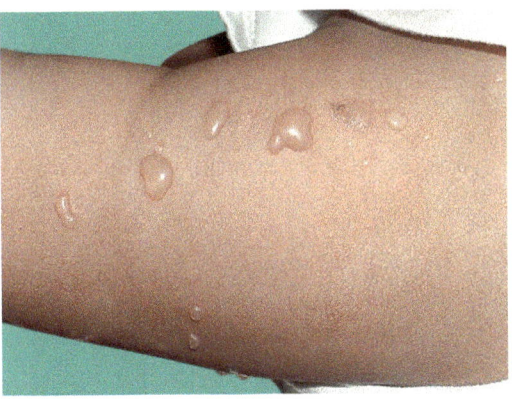

a. Chickenpox
b. Herpes zoster
c. *Paederus dermatitis*
d. Herpes simplex

581. This lady presented with a painful red swelling on her face for the last 10 days. What is the closest clinical diagnosis?

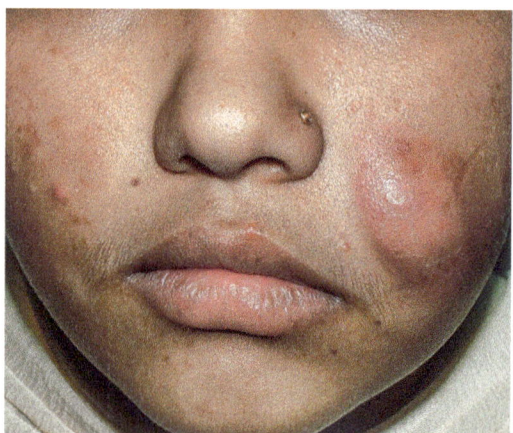

a. Sebaceous cyst
b. Acne cyst
c. Pyogenic abscess
d. Cold abscess

582. This patient complained of pain and swelling of both lower limbs accompanied by red patches for the last two months. The patches do not blanch on diascopy. What is the clinical diagnosis?

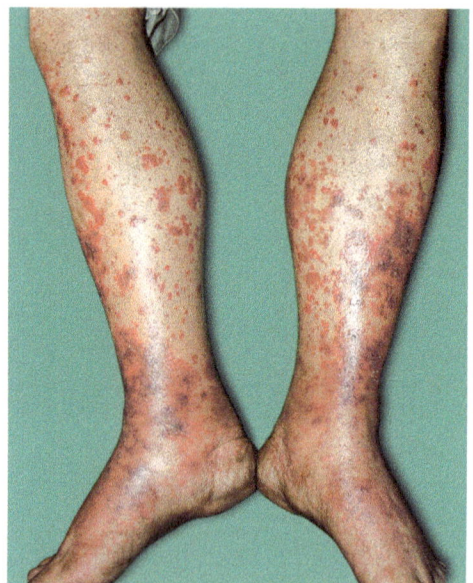

a. Henoch-Schonlein purpura
b. Cutaneous small vessel vasculitis (CSVV)
c. Idiopathic thrombocytopenic purpura (ITP)
d. Schamberg's disease

583. She complained of sparse and thin hair on the frontal and vertex regions of scalp in last 4–5 years. Hair from margins of scalp and occipital regions are spared. What is the clinical diagnosis?

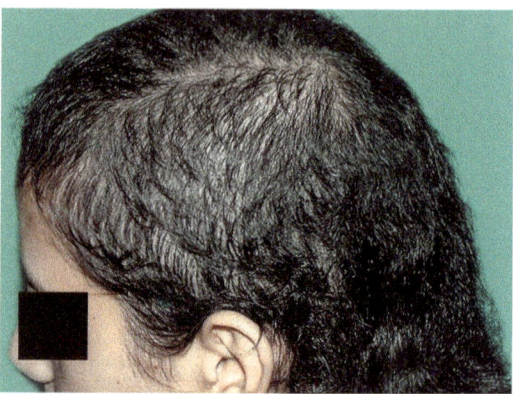

a. Androgenic alopecia
b. Telogen effluvium
c. Lupus hair of SLE
d. Trichotillomania

584. This patient is complaining of pain, swelling and redness with a pus discharging opening for the last one week. What is the clinical diagnosis?

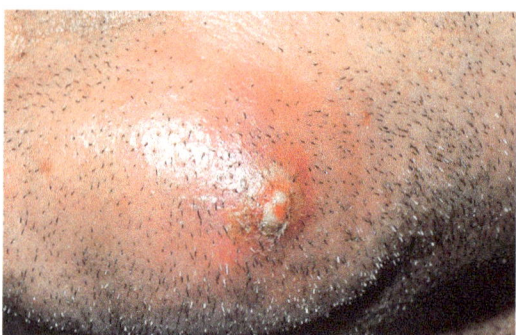

a. Boil
b. Folliculitis
c. Carbuncle

585. A 2-year-old child is having itching and crusting on finger for the last two months. What is the clinical diagnosis?

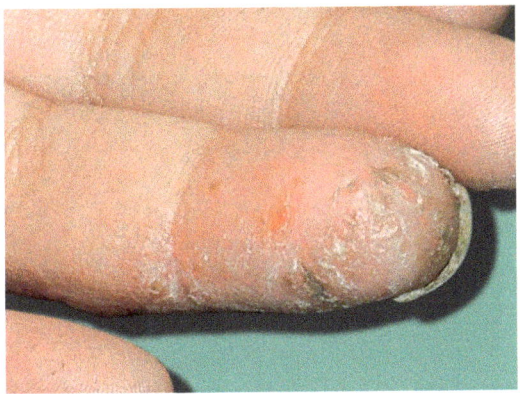

a. Psoriasis
b. Herpetic whitlow
c. Tinea manuum
d. Eczema of the finger

587. This patient developed overnight these multiple linear red lesions on trunk accompanied by burning sensation. What is the clinical diagnosis?

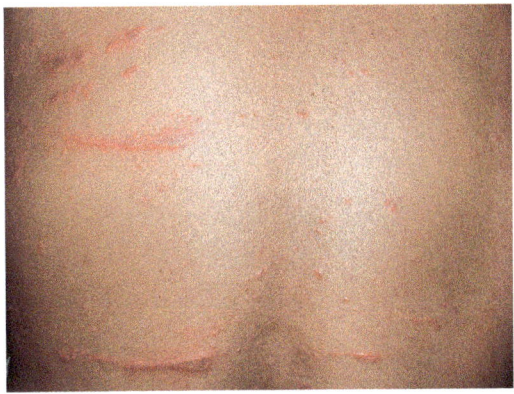

a. Dermatitis artefacta
b. *Paederus dermatitis*

586. This patient complained of loss of sensations in his right foot. On examination of dorsum of foot, a red plaque and thickening of a superficial cutaneous nerve were observed. What is the clinical diagnosis?

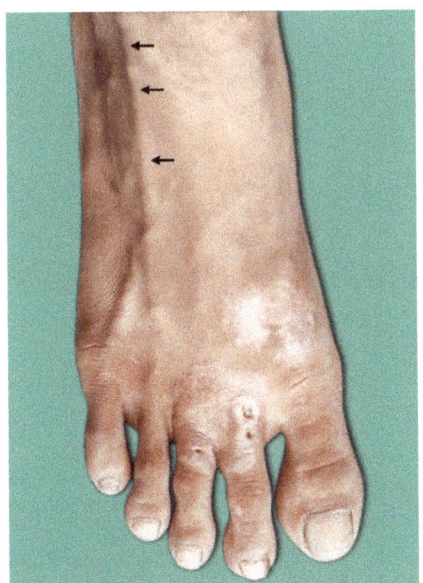

a. Tuberculoid leprosy
b. Lepromatous leprosy
c. Histoid leprosy
d. Indeterminate leprosy

588. A 10-year-old child presented with multiple, recurring, itchy, red, ill-defined plaques of various sizes on trunk and extremities. What is the clinical diagnosis?

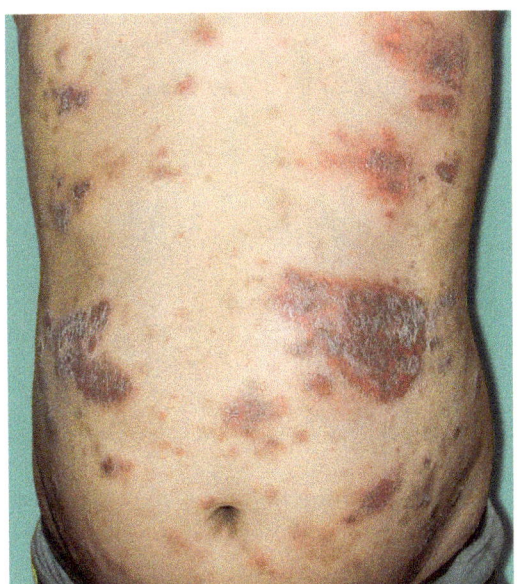

a. Psoriasis
b. Plaques of eczema
c. Tinea corporis

589. This lady presented with hair loss in the cervico-occipital region for the last six months. What is the clinical diagnosis?

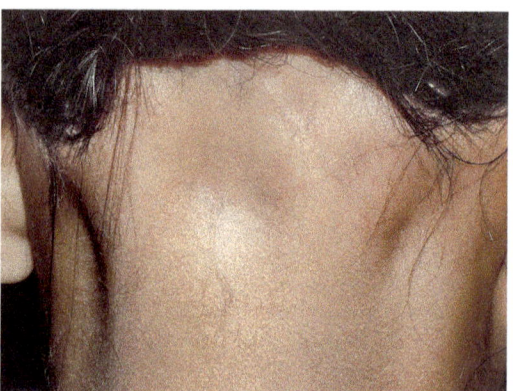

a. Trichotillomania
b. Androgenic alopecia
c. Alopecia areata
d. Telogen effluvium

590. This lady presented with roughness and dark coloration of nails. What is the clinical diagnosis?

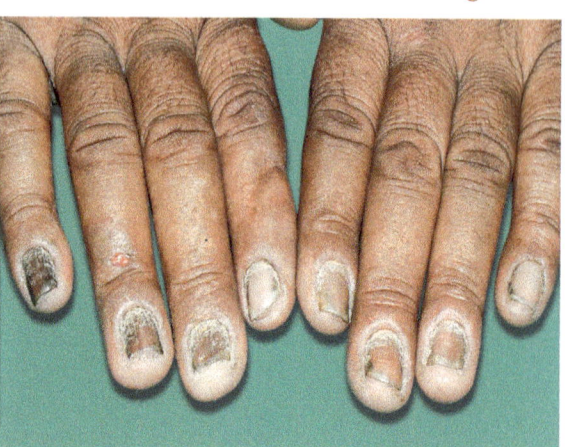

a. Tinea unguium
b. Chronic paronychia
c. Psoriasis of nails
d. Koilonychia

591. This patient presented with asymptomatic reddish-brown papules and plaques of various shapes and sizes on elbow for the last 4–5 years. There is no loss of sensations. What is the closest clinical diagnosis?

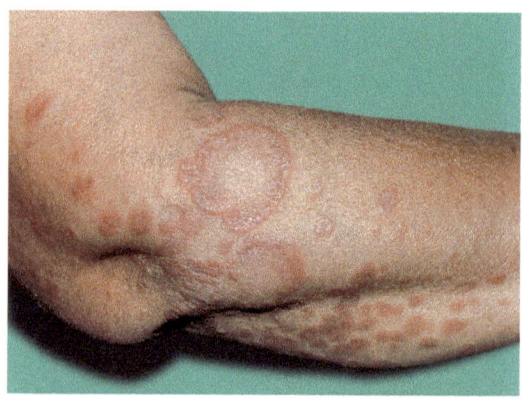

a. Psoriasis
b. Hansen's disease
c. Tinea corporis
d. Granuloma annulare

592. A 16-year-old child was brought by parents with short nails and habit of nail biting. What is the closest clinical diagnosis?

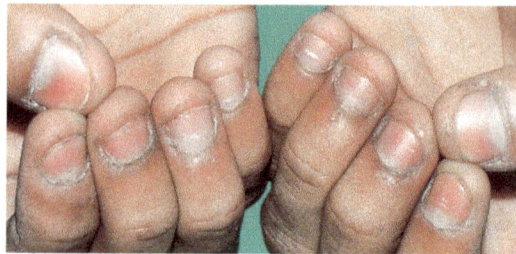

a. Lichen planus
b. Koilonychia
c. Onychophagia

593. This patient presented with multiple pustules on shin for last 10 days. What is the clinical diagnosis?

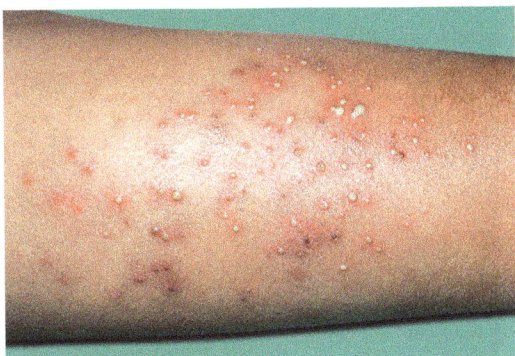

a. Boils
b. Superficial folliculitis
c. Carbuncle

595. She was taking systemic steroid for bronchial asthma. She presented with itching and scaling on face, chest and extremities *(MCQ 572)*. What is the clinical diagnosis?

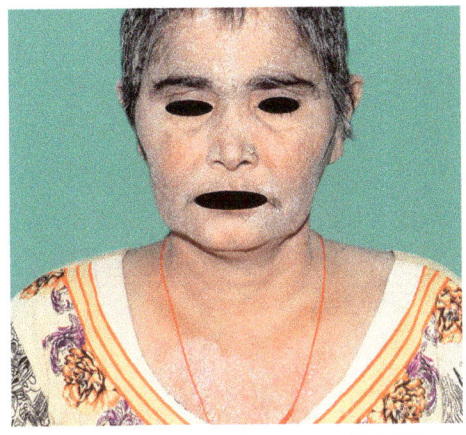

a. Airborne contact dermatitis (ABCD)
b. Polymorphous light eruption (PLE)
c. Tinea faciei with corporis
d. Seborrheic dermatitis (SD)

594. This patient developed overnight this red lesion having burning sensation. What is the clinical diagnosis?

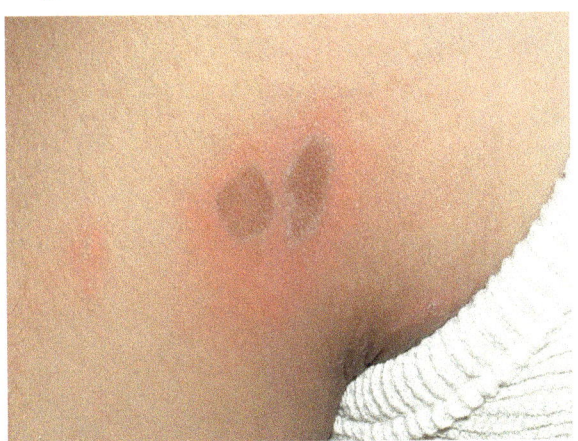

a. Herpes zoster
b. *Paederus dermatitis*

596. This patient presented with itching and thickening of skin of face and cervical region. On examination, similar changes were found in the cubital and popliteal fossae *(MCQs 401, 359)*. What is the clinical diagnosis?

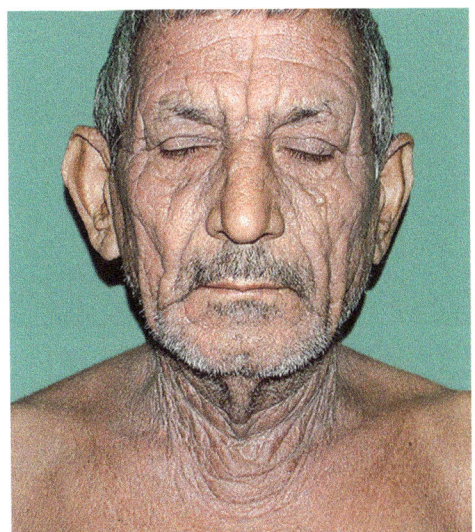

a. Seborrheic dermatitis
b. Adult phase atopic dermatitis
c. Airborne contact dermatitis (ABCD)
d. Chronic actinic dermatitis (CAD)

597. This lady presented with reddish brown soft gelatinous plaques, one on her face *(MCQ 26)* and two on her trunk. Plaques have active peripheral margin with trailing scar towards centre. There is no loss of sensations in the plaque. What is the closest clinical diagnosis?

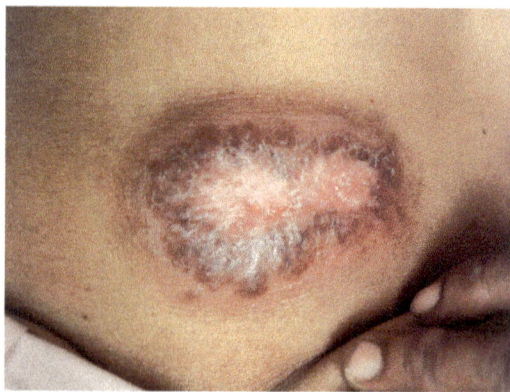

a. Lupus vulgaris
b. Psoriasis
c. Chronic cutaneous lupus erythematosus (CCLE)
d. Tuberculoid leprosy

598. This lady presented with brownish pigmentation for the last two years on both cheeks having irregular borders. What is the clinical diagnosis?

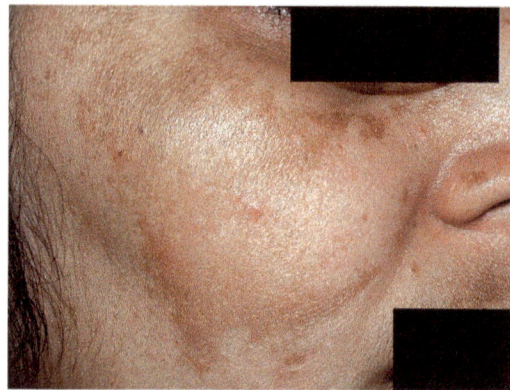

a. Butterfly rash due to SLE
b. Melasma
c. Bilateral nevus of Ota
d. Dermatomyositis

599. This patient complained of single, red infiltrated plaque on his forearm for the last six months. The sensations in the plaque were impaired and ulnar nerve was thickened. What is the diagnosis?

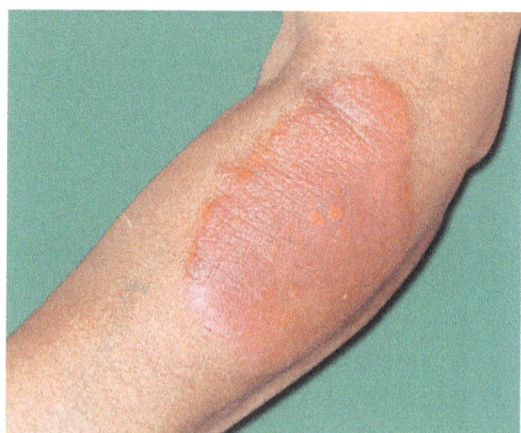

a. Tuberculoid leprosy
b. Lupus vulgaris
c. Lepromatous leprosy
d. Histoid leprosy

600. This patient presented with slowly evolving single reddish brown psoriasiform plaque on the elbow. Plaque has little scaling and polycyclic border with no loss of sensations. What is the closest clinical diagnosis?

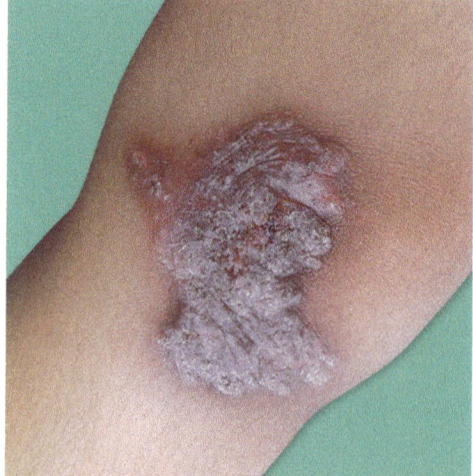

a. Lupus vulgaris
b. Psoriasis
c. Cutaneous leishmaniasis
d. Chronic cutaneous lupus erythematosus (CCLE)

601. This patient presented with red plaque studded with white scaling on the scalp and in the ear opening. There is no loss of sensations. What is the clinical diagnosis?

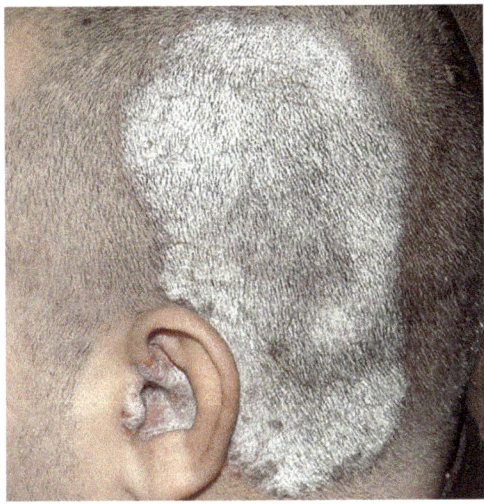

a. Tinea capitis
b. Tuberculoid leprosy
c. Psoriasis scalp
d. Lichen planus

602. This patient complained of itching and vesicular lesions in both palms for the last six months. What is the clinical diagnosis?

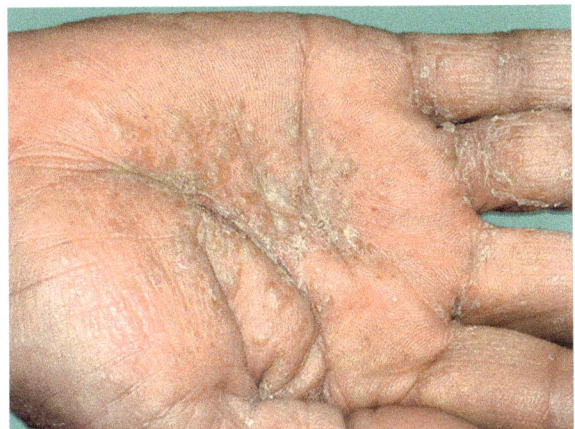

a. Tinea manuum
b. Pompholyx
c. Candidiasis
d. Contact dermatitis to cement

603. This patient complained of itching and scaling on the scalp. What is the closest clinical diagnosis?

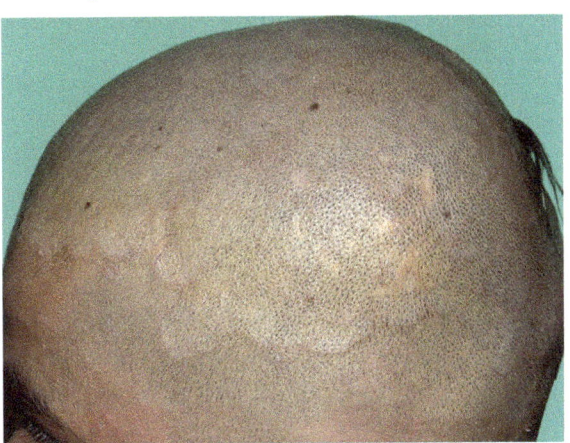

a. Tinea capitis
b. Psoriasis scalp
c. Seborrheic capitis

604. This lady presented with multiple erythematous plaques with little scaling under the breast and neighboring part of chest. Itching is little. What is the clinical diagnosis?

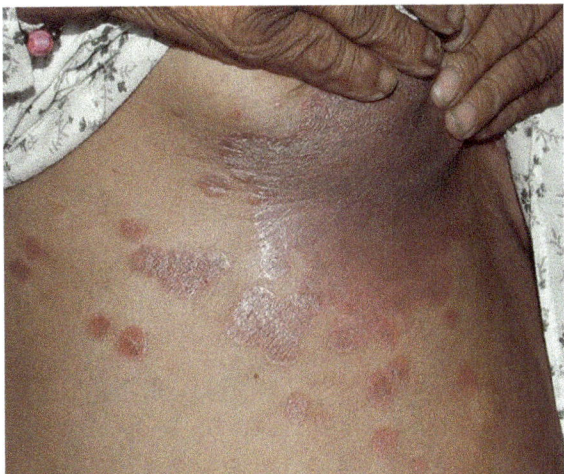

a. Flexural psoriasis
b. Tinea corporis
c. Intertrigo
d. Candidiasis

605. A one-month old child presented with deep red colored patch of many centimeters size on right side of face since birth. What is the closest clinical diagnosis?

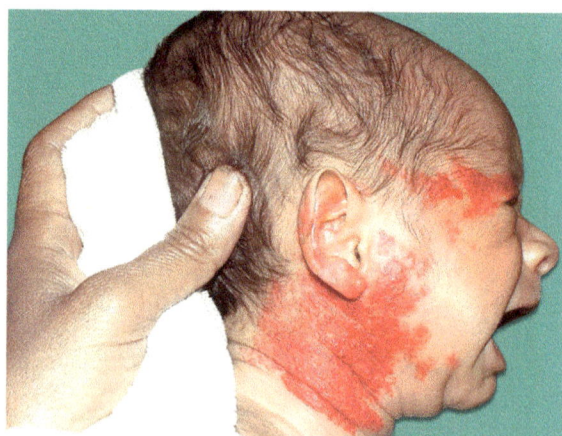

a. Salmon patch
b. Strawberry hemangioma
c. Port-wine stain
d. Cherry hemangiomas

606. This lady is having extensive tinea corporis during 3rd trimester of her pregnancy. Which one of the following systemic antifungal drugs is safest for her?

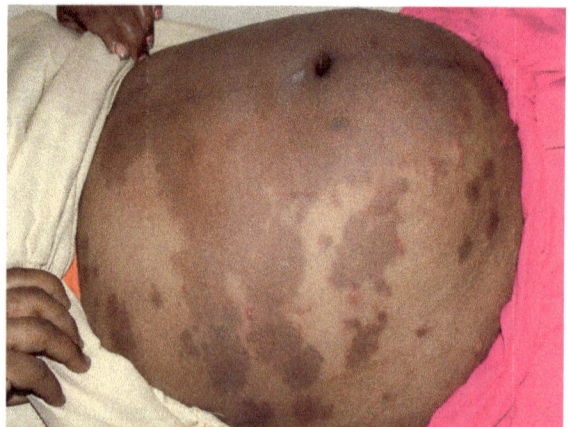

a. Griseofulvin
b. Ketoconazole
c. Itraconazole
d. Terbinafine

607. This lady presented with itching and redness in the groins and vulva. She also had increased frequency of micturition at night. What is the closest clinical diagnosis?

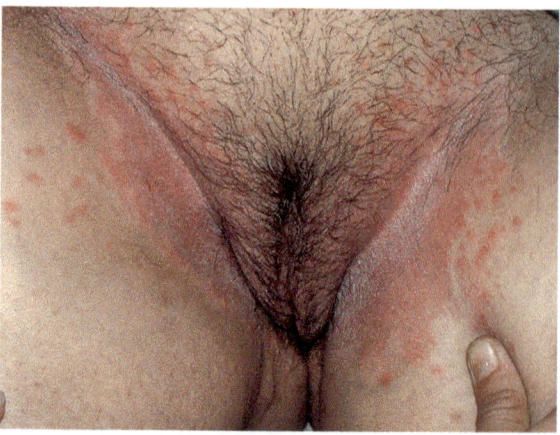

a. Tinea cruris
b. Intertrigo
c. Flexural psoriasis
d. Candidiasis groins and vulva

608. Five days after the unprotected sex with a commercial sex worker this man developed multiple painful ulcers at preputial orifice. What is the closest clinical diagnosis?

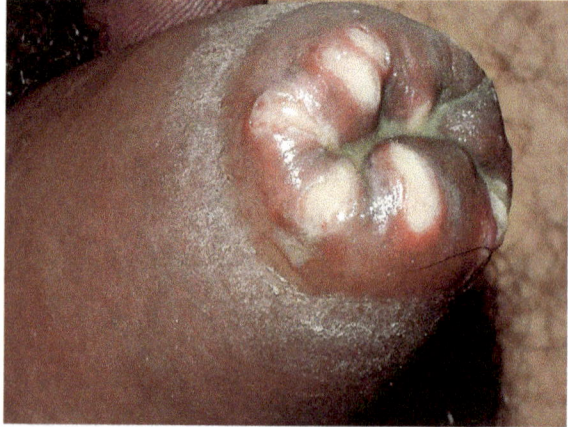

a. Primary syphilis
b. Chancroid
c. Donovanosis
d. Lymphogranuloma venereum

609. This patient presented with a single, circumscribed, slightly raised, velvety and waxy yellow plaque on scalp for the last many years. What is the closest clinical diagnosis?

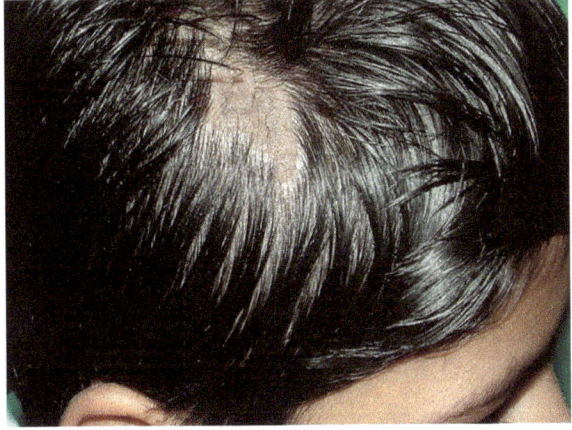

a. Warts
b. Sebaceous nevus
c. Tinea capitis
d. Psoriasis

610. This patient developed overnight severe burning sensation with accompanying redness in his left axilla. What is the clinical diagnosis?

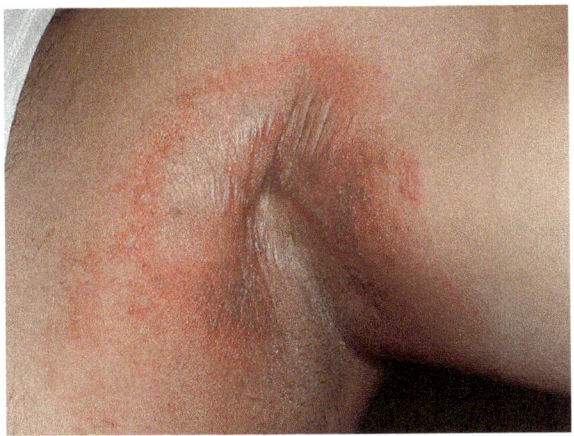

a. Herpes zoster
b. *Paederus dermatitis*

611. This patient developed multiple asymptomatic rough papules on the palmar aspect of fingers for the last six months. What is the closest clinical diagnosis?

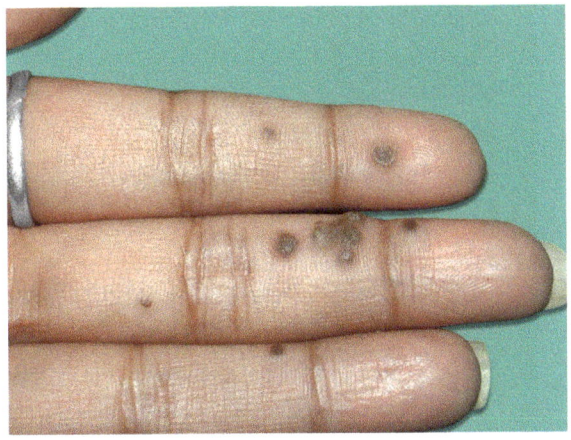

a. Lichen planus
b. Common warts
c. Molluscum contagiosum
d. Tuberculosis verrucosa cutis (TVC)

612. This lady came with chickenpox at 36 weeks of pregnancy with no complications. Which one of the following treatment options is most appropriate for her?

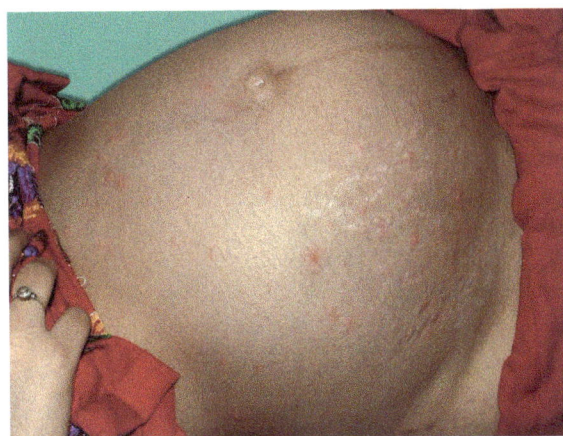

a. Only symptomatic treatments
b. Intravenous acyclovir
c. Oral acyclovir

613. She complained of multiple, well-defined, itchy red patches on shins. What is the closest clinical diagnosis?

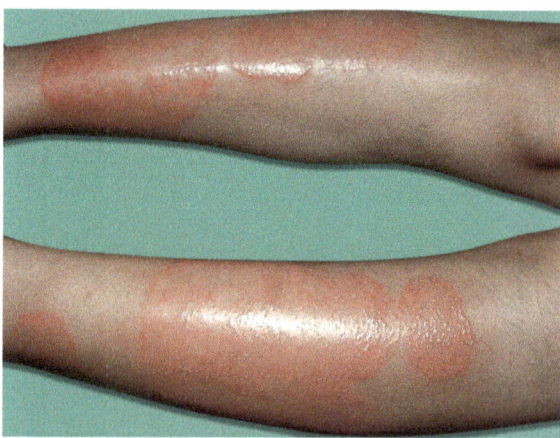

a. Psoriasis
b. Tinea corporis
c. Granuloma annulare
d. Discoid eczema

614. This patient complained of single, well-defined red plaque with loss of sensations. What is the clinical diagnosis?

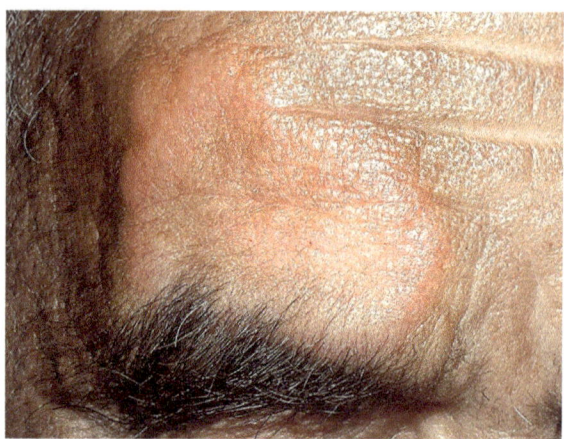

a. Lepromatous leprosy
b. Tuberculoid leprosy
c. Indeterminate leprosy
d. Histoid leprosy

615. This patient complained of a black multilobulated nodule with surrounding discoloration on his arm. What is the closest clinical diagnosis?

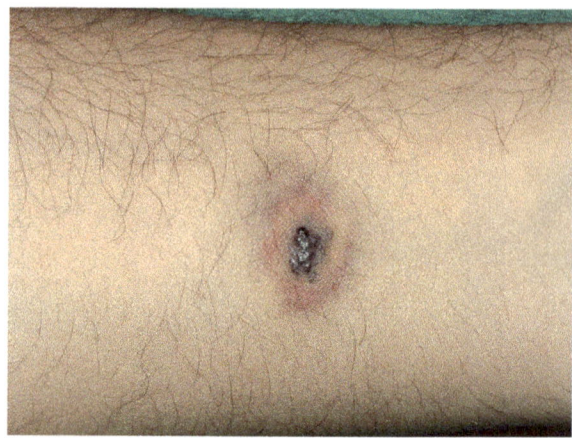

a. Compound nevus
b. Halo nevus
c. Nodular melanoma
d. Strawberry hemangioma

616. This obese patient complained of dark, velvety thickening of cervical skin with skin tags. What is the clinical diagnosis?

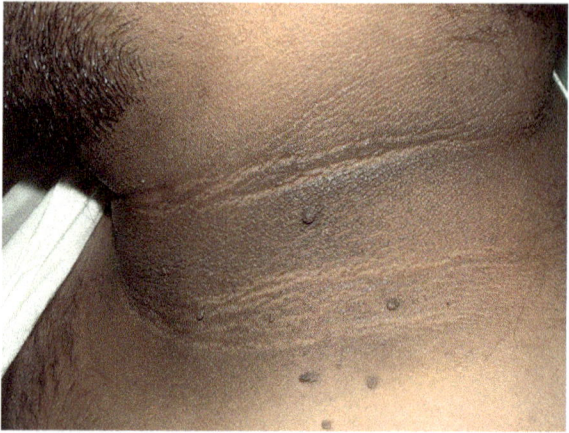

a. Darier's disease
b. Pseudoacanthosis nigricans
c. Acanthosis nigricans associated with malignancy

617. A 75-year-old patient complained of black comedones on the side of his nose. Which one of the following options is a correct diagnosis?

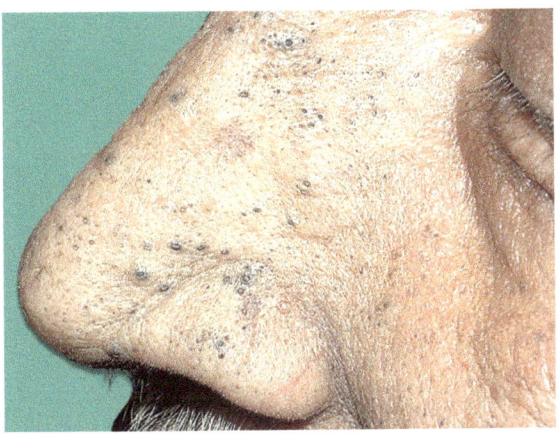

a. Acne comedones
b. Senile comedones
c. Drug-induced acne
d. Acne due to topical steroid

618. This patient presented with plaques on forearm. Plaques have hyperpigmented borders and adherent scales. Similar plaques are also present on face. What is the closest clinical diagnosis?

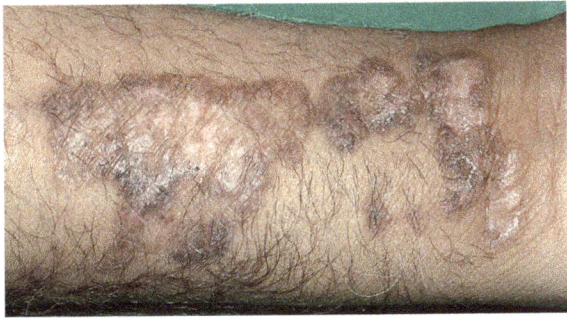

a. Chronic cutaneous lupus erythematosus forearm
b. Annular psoriasis
c. Lichen planus
d. Granuloma annulare

619. This child is having multiple small red papular lesions on face for the last many years. He is also having mental retardation and epilepsy. What is the clinical diagnosis?

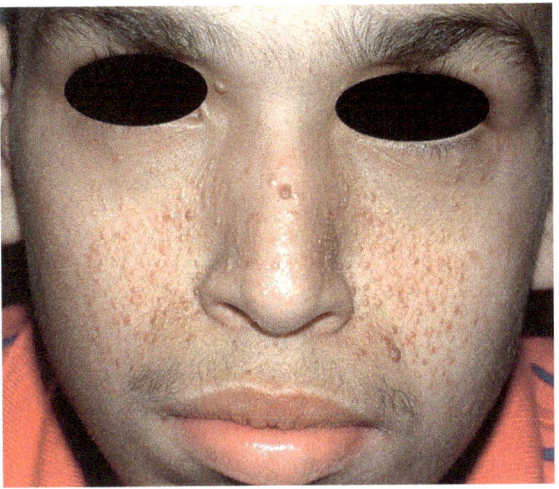

a. Acne vulgaris
b. Lupus miliaris disseminatus faciei (LMDF)
c. Tuberous sclerosis complex (TSC)
d. Drug-induced acne

620. This patient presented with slowly evolving hyperkeratotic verrucous asymptomatic plaque on the sole for the last two years. What is the closest clinical diagnosis?

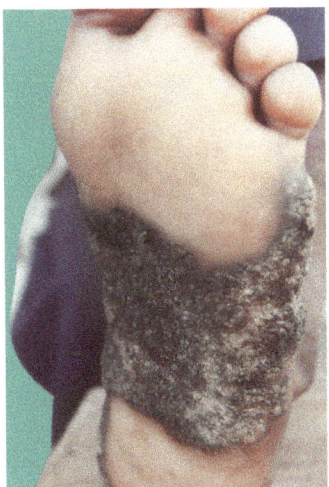

a. Tuberculosis verrucosa cutis
b. Squamous cell carcinoma (SCC)
c. Plantar wart
d. Madura foot

621. This patient presented with multiple, red plaques with white scaling on both soles. Similar plaques were also present on scalp and elbows. What is the clinical diagnosis?

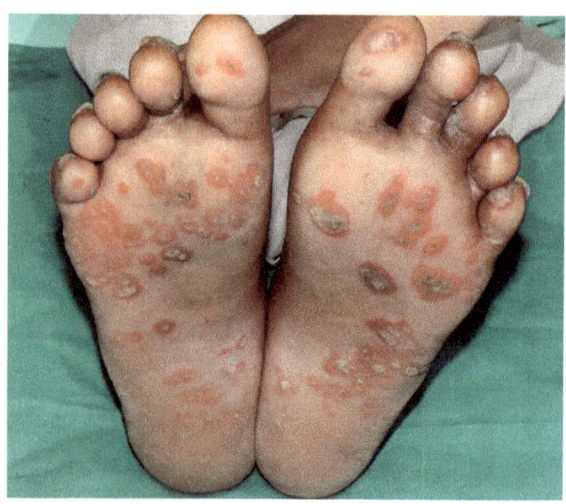

a. Lichen planus
b. Tinea pedis
c. Psoriasis
d. Hyperkeratotic eczema soles

622. This patient presented with a crop of red papular lesions with scaling and little itching all over the trunk and extremities for the last 1 month. What is the closest clinical diagnosis?

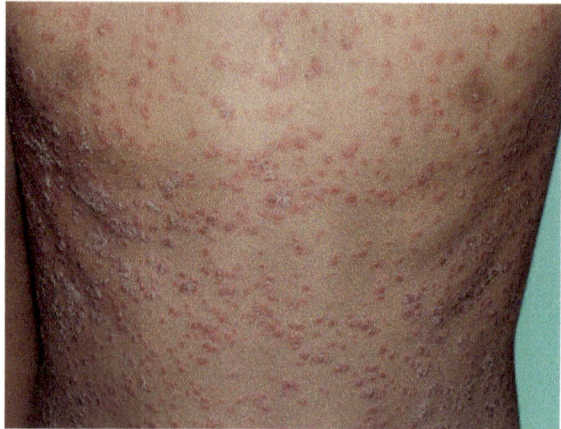

a. Guttate psoriasis
b. Lichen planus
c. Pityriasis rosea
d. Secondary syphilis

623. She developed herpes zoster during 37 weeks of her pregnancy. Which one of the following treatment options is most appropriate for her?

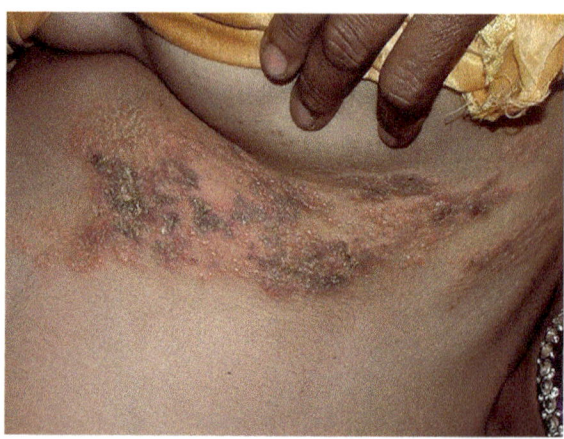

a. Systemic antiviral drugs + analgesics
b. Topical antiviral cream + analgesics
c. Calamine lotion + analgesics
d. Intravenous antiviral therapy + analgesics

624. She complained of itching and redness under both breasts. She is also having increased frequency of micturition at night. What is the clinical diagnosis?

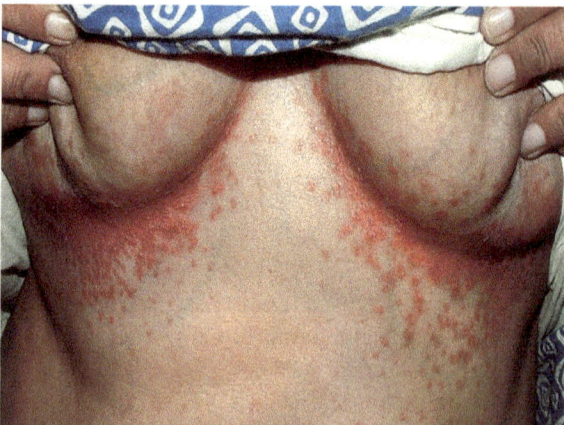

a. Tinea corporis
b. Flexural psoriasis
c. Candidiasis under breast
d. Intertrigo under breast

625. A 52-year-old patient having renal dysfunction with hyperuricemia has developed severe herpes zoster. Which one of the following options about recommendations of valacyclovir is correct for him?

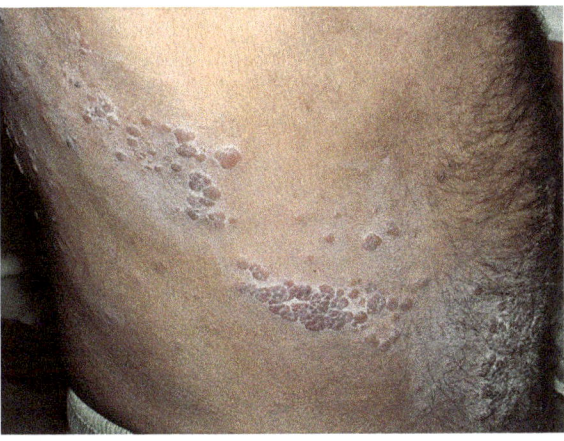

a. Cannot be given
b. Can be given in full dosage
c. Dosage adjustment is required

626. This lady developed chickenpox at 18 weeks of her pregnancy. Which one of following options is correct for her therapy?

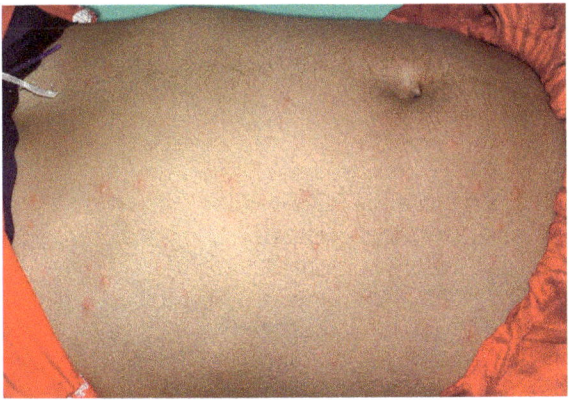

a. Intravenous acyclovir
b. Oral acyclovir
c. Only symptomatic treatments

627. She presented with pruritic brownish coloration with little thickening on upper back and limbs for the last three years. What is the closest clinical diagnosis?

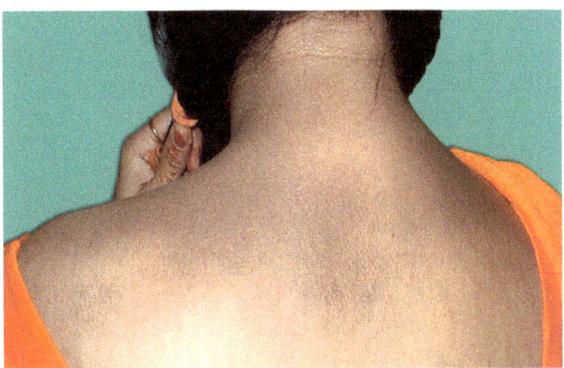

a. Pseudoacanthosis nigricans
b. Macular amyloidosis
c. Sun-induced delayed tanning
d. Addisonian pigmentation

628. After completing 10 days intake of ciprofloxacin, this patient complained of itching and erythema. Face, eyes, lips are spared. What is the clinical diagnosis?

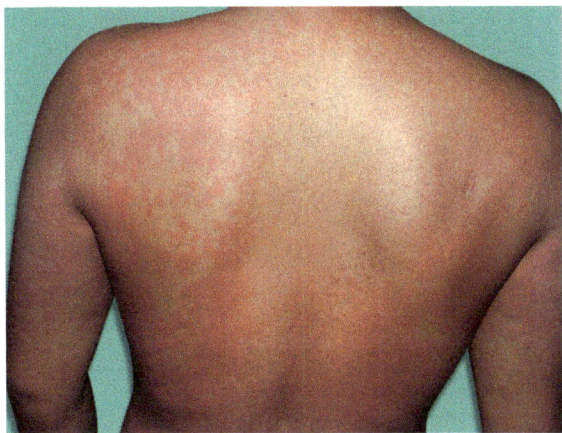

a. Exanthematous rash
b. Drug-induced urticaria
c. Miliaria rubra
d. Measles

629. This patient presented with pruritic, hyperkeratotic and linear lesion on his right hand since infancy. What is the clinical diagnosis?

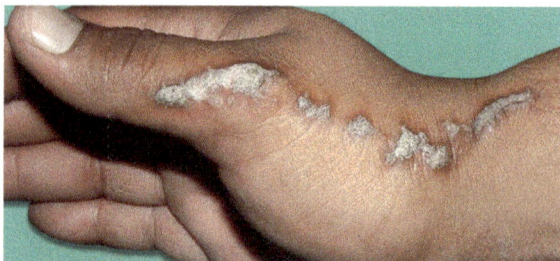

a. Tuberculosis verrucosa cutis (TVC)
b. Inflammatory linear verrucous epidermal nevus (ILVEN)
c. Nevus sebaceous
d. Common warts showing Koebner phenomenon

630. This patient presented with persistent, multiple, skin or gray colored, firm and rough papules in the seborrheic areas of body. Nails showed longitudinal bands which ended in V-shaped notch at free margin of nail *(MCQ 576)*. What is the clinical diagnosis?

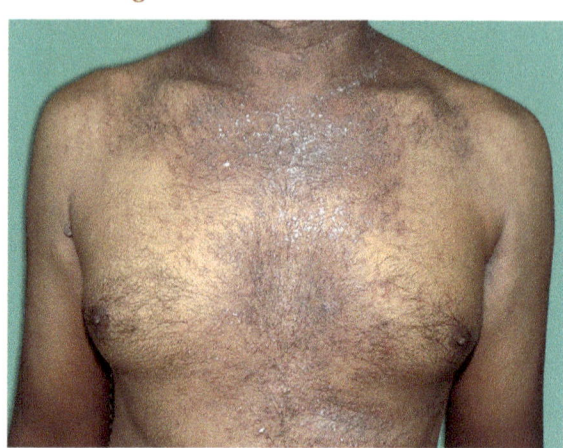

a. Seborrheic dermatitis
b. Darier's disease
c. Lichen planus

631. This patient complained of ulcers with surrounding pigmentation on the medial side of leg above the medial malleolus. What is the clinical diagnosis?

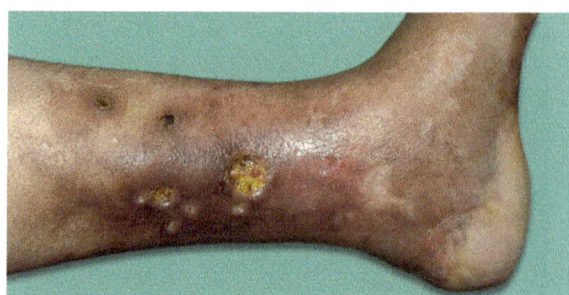

a. Trophic ulcer
b. Arterial ulcer
c. Burger's disease
d. Venous ulcer

632. A 60-year-old patient presented with multiple bullae on the flexural aspects of limbs. Bullae are tense and filled with clear fluid having no tendency to spread peripherally. Bullae remain intact for several days and contents became jelly like. Mucosae are not involved. What is the clinical diagnosis?

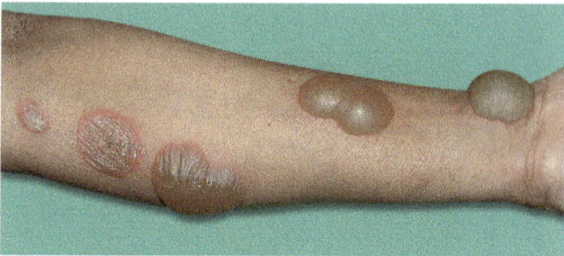

a. Pemphigus vulgaris
b. Bullous pemphigoid
c. Linear IgA dermatosis in adult
d. *Paederus dermatitis*

633. This patient presented with asymptomatic reticular pigmentation on both thighs for the last three years. What is the clinical diagnosis?

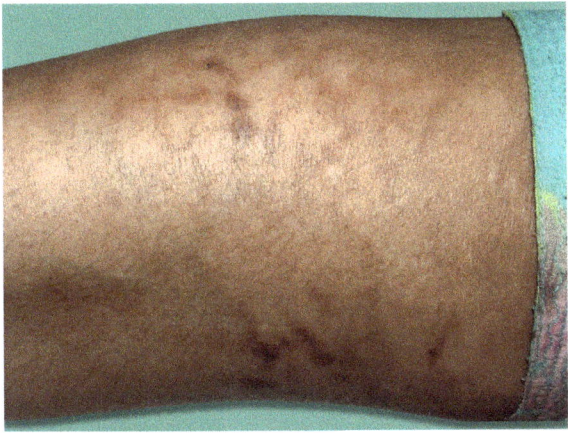

a. Lichen planus
b. Erythema ab igne
c. Livedo reticularis

634. This patient presented with a group of red hyperkeratotic and rough papules on scalp for the last two months. What is the clinical diagnosis?

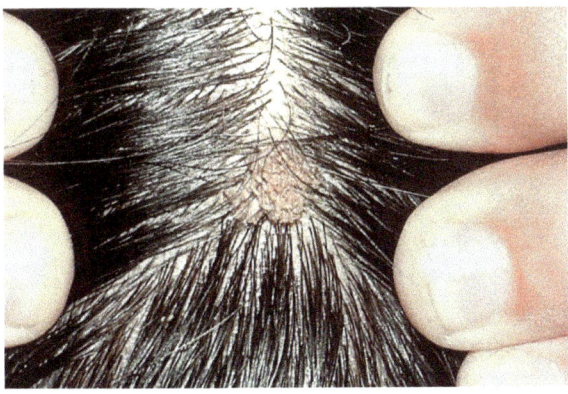

a. Nevus sebaceous
b. Warts scalp
c. Tinea capitis

635. This lady presented with multiple erythematous plaques on tongue. The plaques have well-defined white borders with loss of filiform papillae. What is the clinical diagnosis?

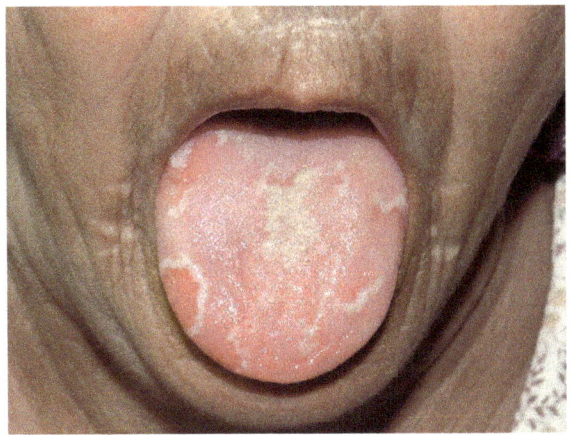

a. Lichen planus tongue
b. Sideropenic anemia
c. Scrotal tongue
d. Geographic tongue

636. Following is the diagrammatic representation of epidermal cell layers. What is the name of the cell layer with the question mark?

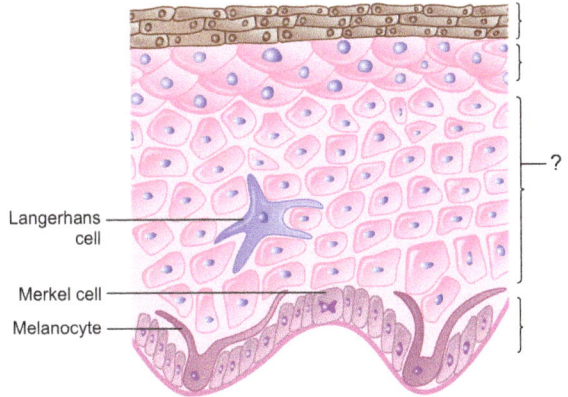

a. Stratum lucidum
b. Stratum granulosum
c. Stratum spinosum
d. Stratum corneum

637. A 40-year-old patient is showing patchy hair loss. At the periphery of the patch characteristic 'exclamation mark hairs' are seen which are short broken and easily pluckable. Which one of the following options is correct for him?

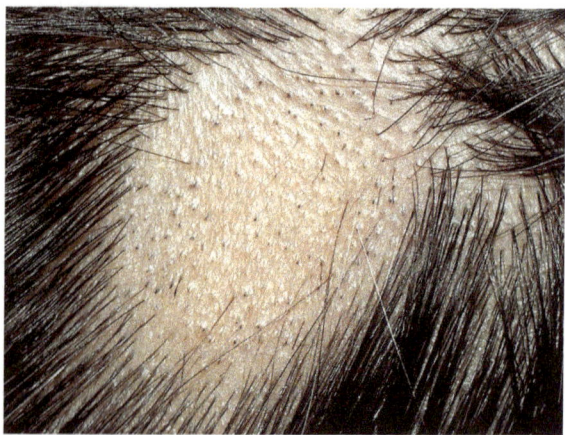

a. Trichotillomania
b. Alopecia areata
c. Ophiasis
d. Tinea capitis

638. She is having depigmentation involving about 90% of body surface. Face, chest, back, whole of upper and lower extremities are showing depigmentation. Which one of the following diagnosis is correct for her?

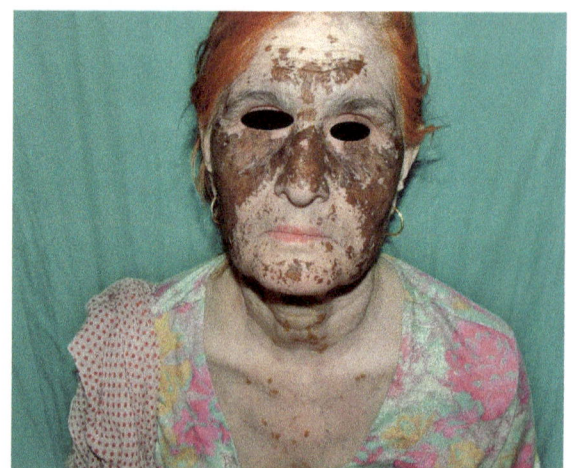

a. Generalized vitiligo
b. Universal vitiligo
c. Vitiligo vulgaris
d. Leukoderma

639. What type of inheritance is shown by the following diagram? One of the parents is heterozygous for the abnormal gene and 50% of the children are affected.

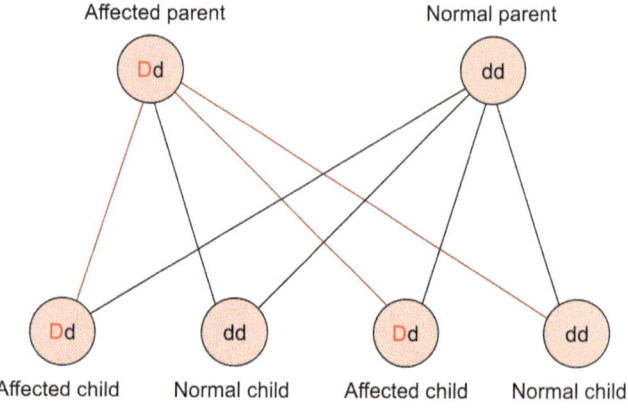

a. Autosomal recessive inheritance
b. Autosomal dominant inheritance
c. X-linked recessive inheritance
d. X-linked dominant inheritance

640. This patient presented with dry rough hyperkeratotic, asymptomatic warty plaques on his right palm for the last two years. What is the closest clinical diagnosis?

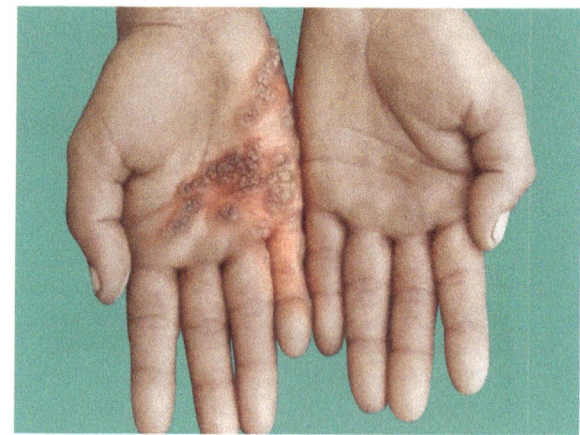

a. Palmar warts
b. Inflammatory linear verrucous epidermal nevus (ILVEN)
c. Tuberculosis verrucosa cutis (TVC)
d. Nevus sebaceous

641. This child presented with multiple small sized off white beads along the midline in the penoscrotal region for the last 3–4 years. What is the closest clinical diagnosis?

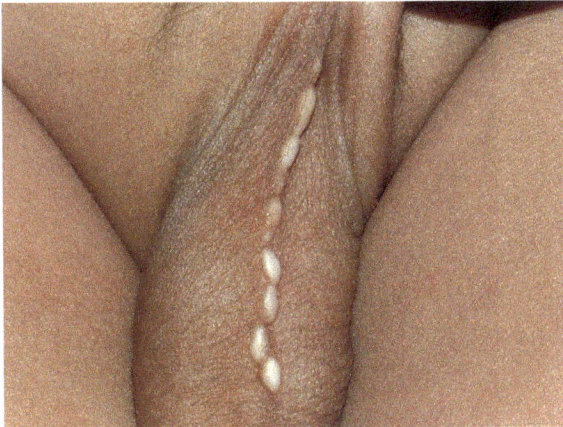

a. Molluscum contagiosum
b. Median raphe cysts
c. Steatocystoma multiplex
d. Urethral diverticulum

642. This 20-year-old patient presented with purulent discharge without any dysuria after an unprotected sex with a commercial sex worker. He had some tablets also. What is the closest clinical diagnosis?

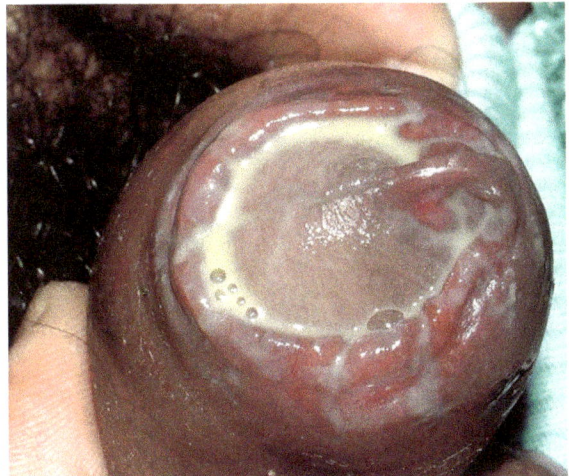

a. Candidal balanoposthitis
b. Fixed drug eruption
c. Urethral syndrome
d. Bacterial balanoposthitis

643. An adult was having multiple psoriatic lesions. An unqualified practitioner gave him multiple steroid injections. It was followed by eruption of enormous macropustules on the psoriatic plaques and on the neighboring skin. What is the clinical diagnosis?

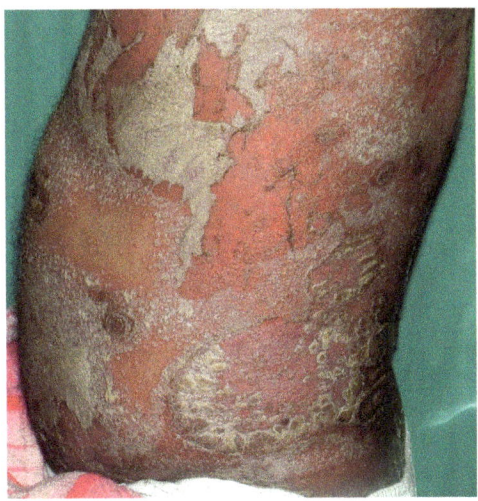

a. Psoriasis with secondary infection
b. Generalized pustular psoriasis
c. Acropustulosis
d. Impetigo herpetiformis

644. Which one of the following options is correct for the following microphotograph of a KOH smear examination?

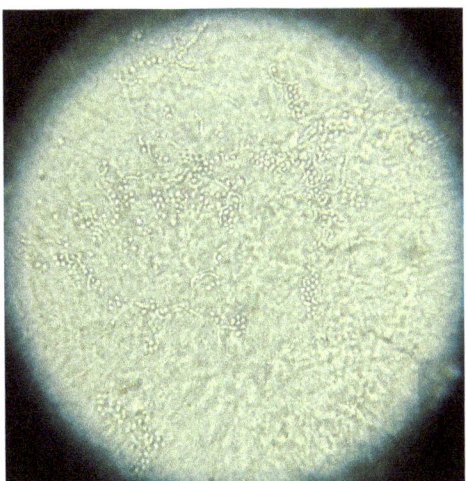

a. Candidiasis
b. Pityriasis versicolor
c. Dermatophytosis
d. Chromoblastomycosis

645. Following is the diagrammatic representation of epidermal cell layers. What is the name of the cell layer with the question mark?

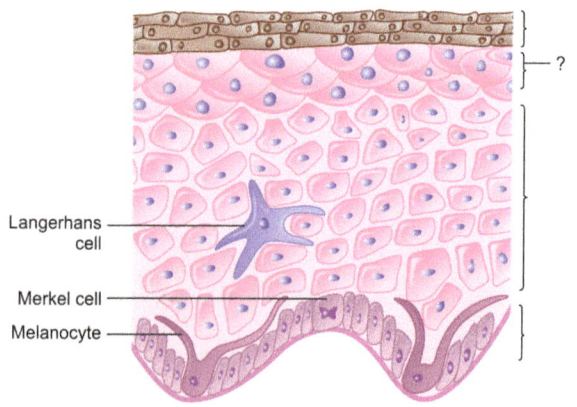

a. Stratum spinosum
b. Stratum granulosum
c. Stratum corneum
d. Stratum lucidum

646. A 3-year-old female presented with multiple pearly white shiny papular lesions in perineal and perianal region. What is the closest clinical diagnosis?

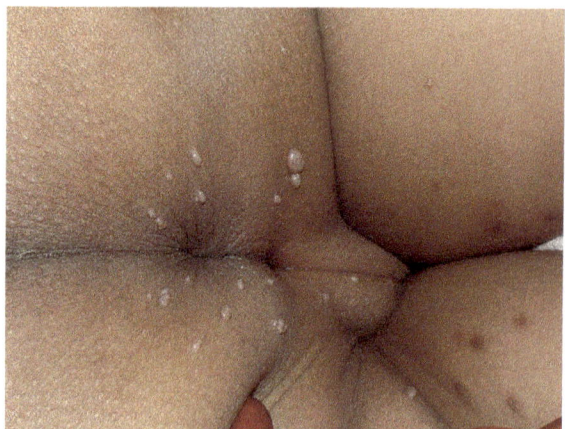

a. Median raphe cysts
b. Molluscum contagiosum
c. Condylomata acuminata

647. This old man presented with thick, warty, nonpruritic crusts on buttocks, arms and elbows *(MCQ 67)*. He is not responding to topical steroid creams. Few family members are suffering from itching. What is the clinical diagnosis?

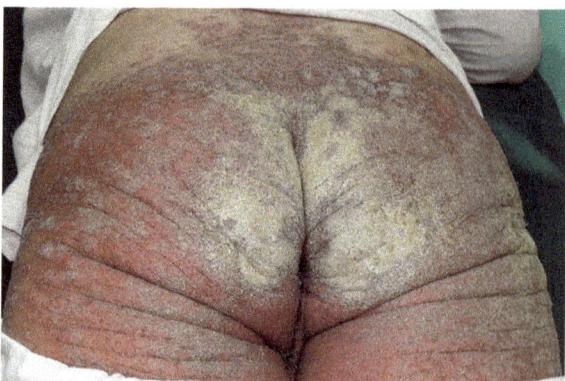

a. Psoriasis
b. Crusted scabies
c. Tinea corporis
d. Chromoblastomycosis

648. This patient presented with red, itchy and linear eruption on lower abdomen. Which one of the following options is the most appropriate for this patient?

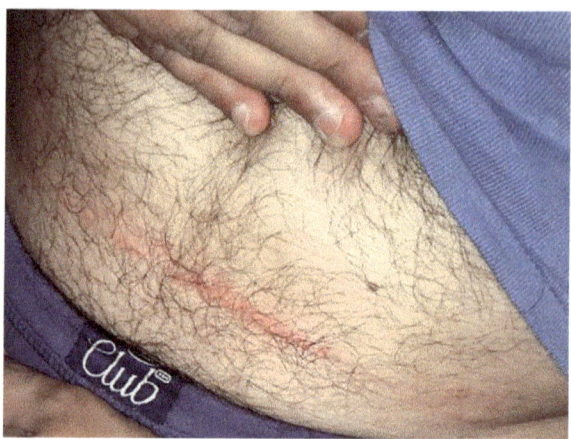

a. *Paederus dermatitis*
b. Tinea corporis
c. Pressure urticaria

649. This patient presented with itching and crusting on big toe. Which one of the following options is most appropriate for this patient?

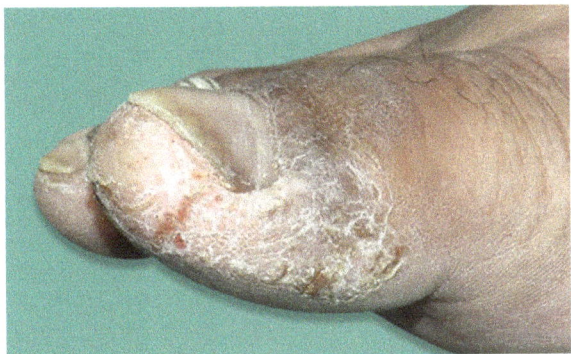

a. Ingrown toe nail with secondary infection
b. Tinea pedis
c. Eczema big toe
d. Tuberculosis verrucosa cutis big toe

651. An old man presented with non-pruritic, warty crusts on extremities. He was also having similar lesions on buttocks *(MCQ 647)*. KOH smear examination showed the following microscopic picture. What is the diagnosis?

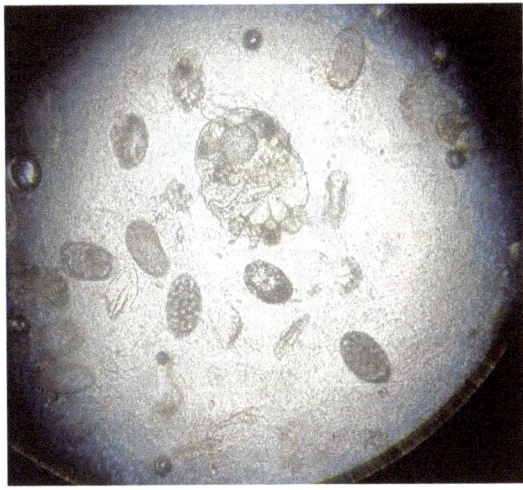

a. Pediculosis corporis
b. Sarcoptes scabiei in crusted scabies
c. Dermatophyte infection
d. Chromoblastomycosis

650. Following is the diagrammatic representation of cell cycle. Which one of the following options represents the interphase?

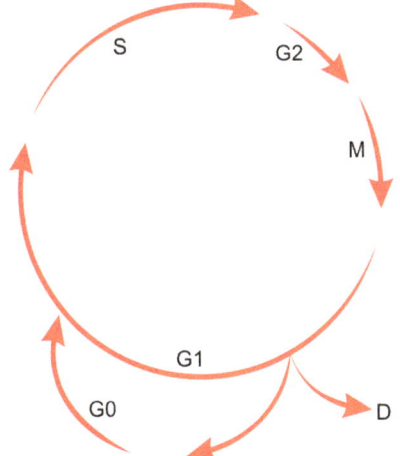

a. S
b. G-2
c. M
d. G-1

652. A 4-month-old baby presented with single, lobulated, scarlet red and round tumor on his arm since the age of two months. What is the clinical diagnosis?

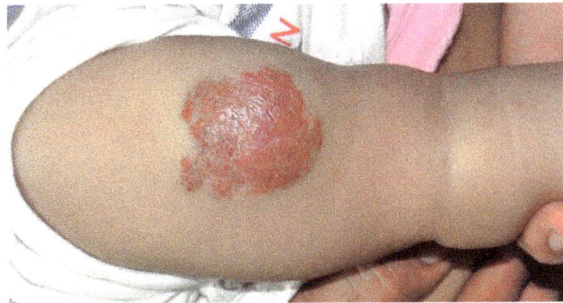

a. Deep or subcutaneous infantile hemangioma
b. Superficial infantile hemangioma
c. Salmon patch
d. Port-wine stain

653. This patient presented with a light red-colored nodule on the nail fold of his middle finger of his right hand for the last three months. What is the closest clinical diagnosis?

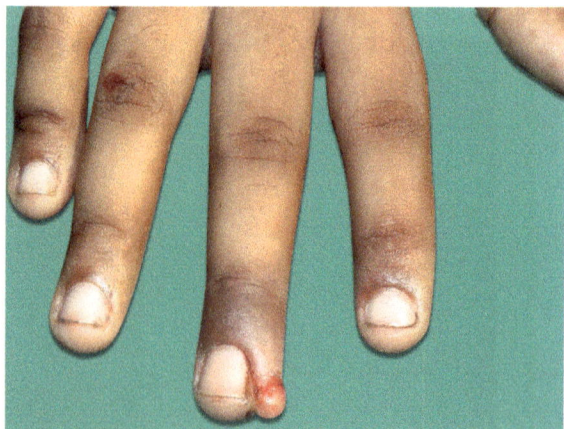

a. Glomus tumor
b. Herpetic whitlow
c. Pyogenic granuloma
d. Ingrown nail

655. Following is the diagrammatic representation of epidermal cell layers. What is the name of the unlabeled cell with question mark?

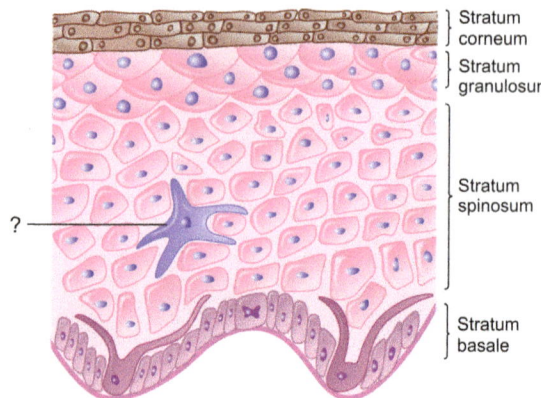

a. Langerhans cell
b. Merkel cell
c. Melanocyte
d. Parakeratotic epidermal cell

654. This patient complained of itching, redness in groins and lower abdomen. What is the closest clinical diagnosis?

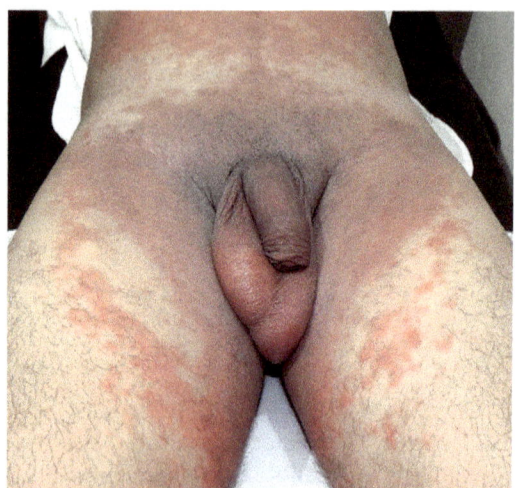

a. Tinea cruris
b. Flexural psoriasis
c. Intertrigo
d. Dermatitis groins
e. Candidiasis

656. A 55-year-old male presented with a varied-colored plaque on chest for the last four years. Which one of the followings is the closest option for him?

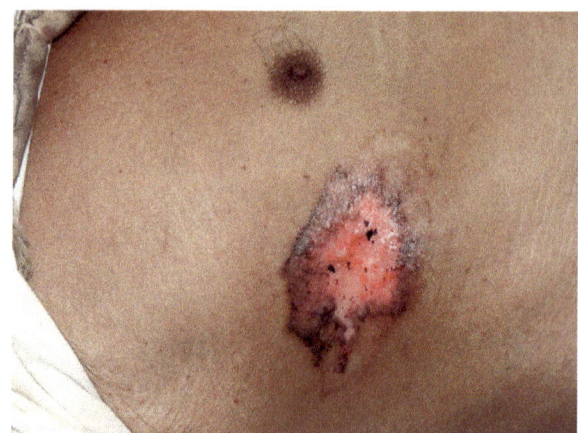

a. Squamous cell carcinoma (SCC)
b. Superficial spreading melanoma (SSM)
c. Basal cell carcinoma (BCC)
d. Bowen's disease

657. This patient presented with burning sensation and blistering on right side of neck and chest for the last three days. Which one is the closest diagnosis?

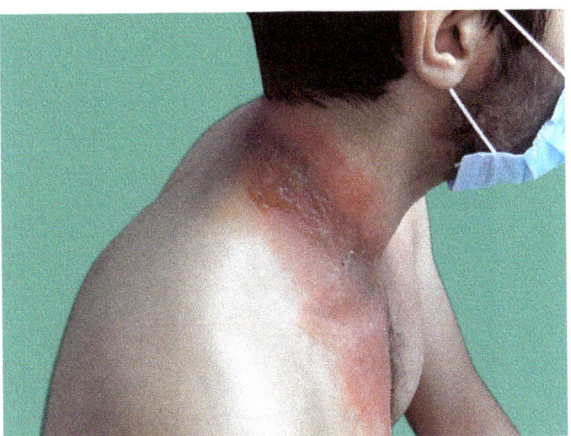

a. Herpes zoster
b. *Paederus dermatitis*
c. Contact irritant dermatitis

658. This lady presented with erythema, scaling, itching on trunk and extremities. Which one of the following options is closest clinical diagnosis?

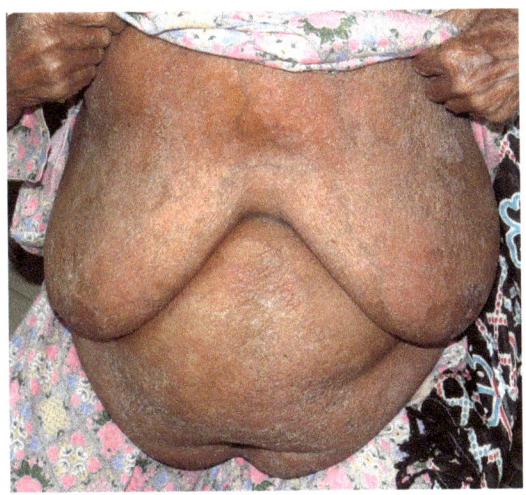

a. Senile eczema
b. Exfoliative dermatitis
c. Seborrheic dermatitis
d. Tinea corporis

659. She complained of excessive hair loss from scalp for the last many years. Which one of the following options is closest clinical diagnosis for her?

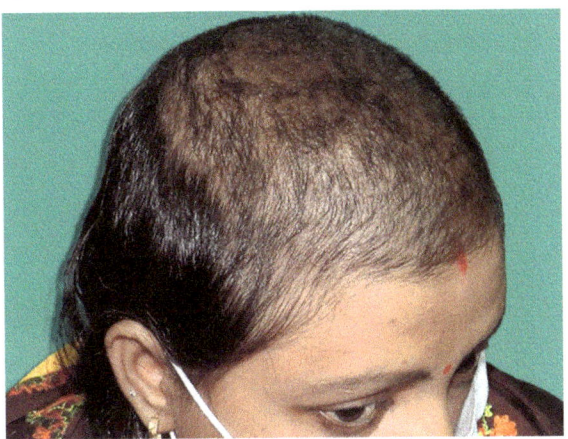

a. Androgenic alopecia
b. Alopecia areata
c. Telogen effluvium
d. Trichotillomania

660. Following is the diagrammatic representation of epidermal cell layers. What is the name of the unlabeled cell with the question mark?

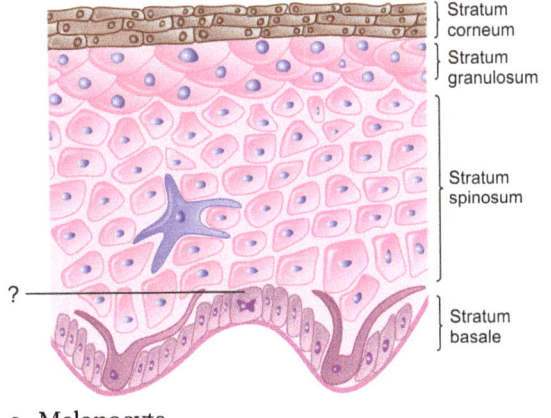

a. Melanocyte
b. Parakeratotic epidermal cell
c. Langerhans cell
d. Merkel cell

661. This patient presented with four erythematous plaques. Plaques have sharply defined and elevated border that slopes down to a flattened atrophic center. Sensations in the plaques are impaired. What is the closest clinical diagnosis?

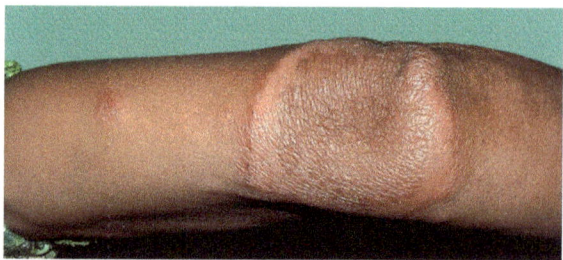

a. Tuberculoid leprosy
b. Lepromatous leprosy
c. Histoid leprosy
d. Mid-borderline leprosy

662. This patient complained of dry, rough, hyperkeratotic papules and nodules in the groins. What is the closest clinical diagnosis?

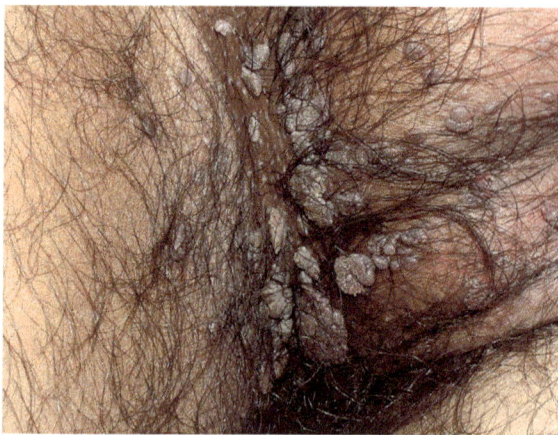

a. Condylomata lata
b. Condylomata acuminata

663. This patient presented as multiple, hard, yellowish brown finger like projections. What is the clinical diagnosis?

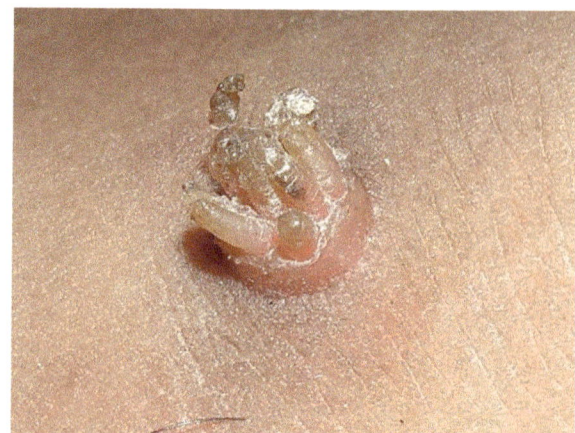

a. Filiform warts
b. Multiple cutaneous horns

664. When both parents are heterozygous and affects one out of four children. If one parent is affected and other is normal, then all the children are heterozygous and healthy. Which type of inheritance is shown by the following diagram?

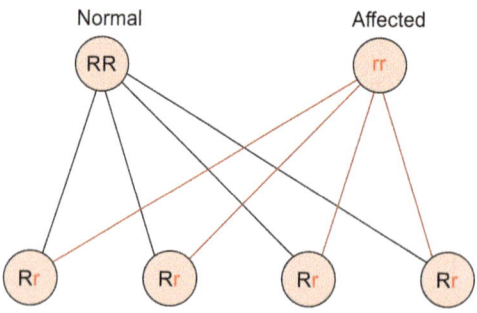

a. Autosomal dominant inheritance
b. Autosomal recessive inheritance
c. X-linked recessive inheritance
d. X-linked dominant inheritance

665. Following is the diagrammatic representation of epidermal cell layers. What is the name of unlabeled cell with the question mark?

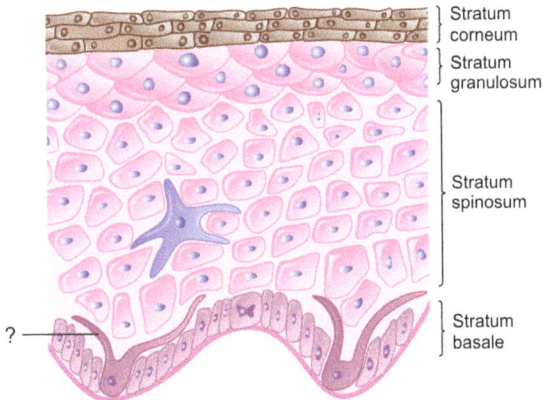

a. Parakeratotic epidermal cell
b. Langerhans cell
c. Melanocyte
d. Merkel cell

666. This patient complained of multiple, flesh colored, soft, flat topped sessile papules with oozing and macerations in the anal region. What is the closest clinical diagnosis?

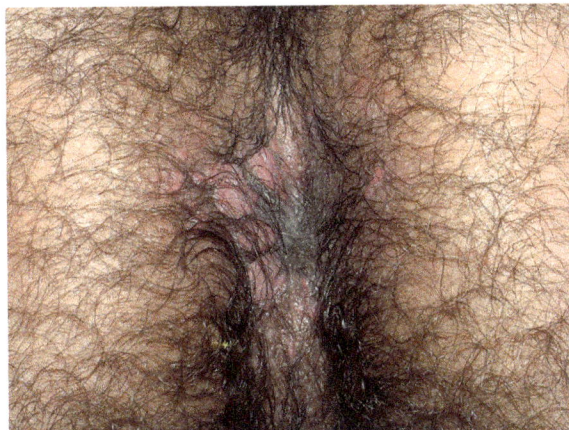

a. Condylomata acuminata
b. Skin tags
c. Condylomata lata

667. A 52-year-old male patient presented with multiple various sized red, non-scaly plaques on trunk. Plaques are studded with nodules and tumors. What is the closest clinical diagnosis?

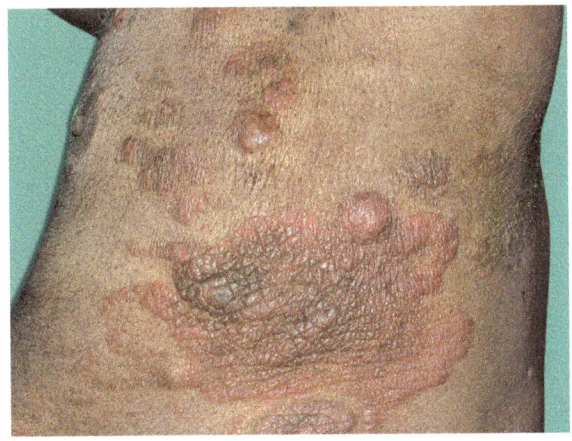

a. Psoriasis
b. Tumor stage cutaneous T-cell lymphoma
c. Large plaque parapsoriasis
d. Cutaneous B-cell lymphoma

668. Which one of the following options is most appropriate for the following patient?

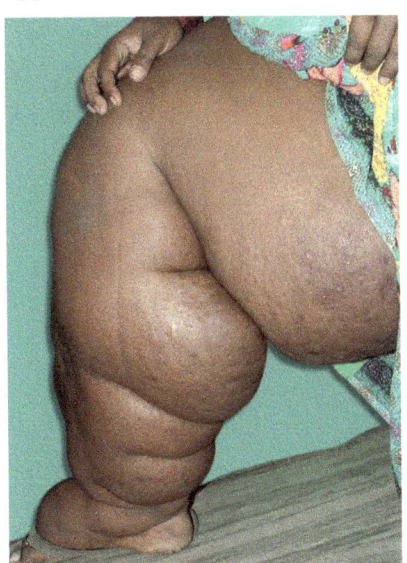

a. Esthiomene
b. Elephantiasis nostras verrucosa
c. Elephantiasis

669. A 70-year-old patient complained of growth at the angle of mouth for the last three years. What is the most appropriate option for him?

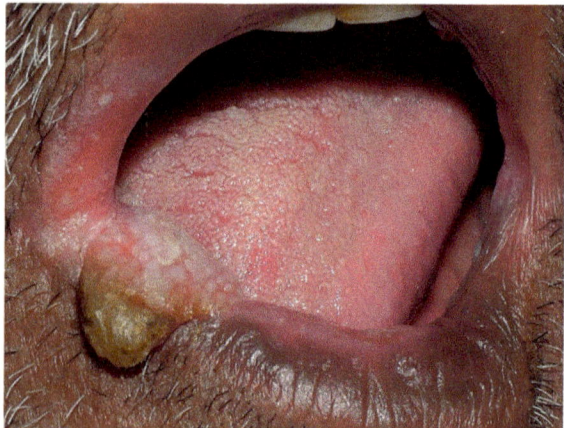

a. Digitate wart
b. Squamous cell carcinoma

670. Following is the diagrammatic representation of epidermal cell cycle. Which one of the following options represents resting phase?

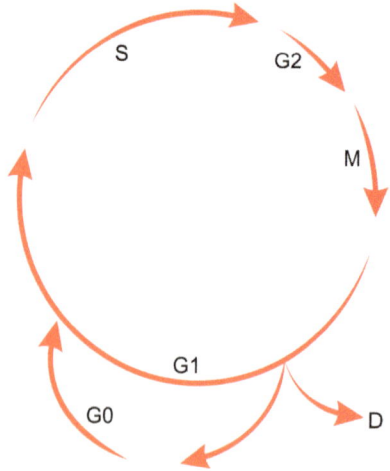

a. S
b. G2
c. M
d. G1

671. A 52-year-old man complained of itching and wheals on contact with water of any temperature. The wheals last for 30–60 minutes. In addition to hepatosplenomegaly, complete hemogram shows the following values. Which one of the following options is correct diagnosis for this patient?

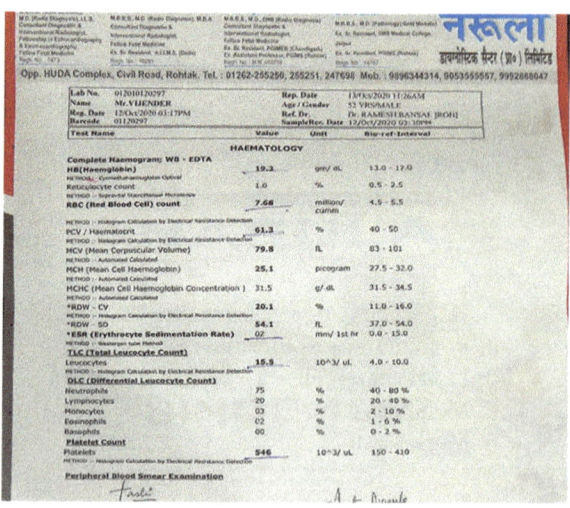

a. Chronic myeloid leukemia (CML)
b. Polycythemia vera
c. Essential thrombocytosis
d. Leukemoid reaction

672. This patient complained of a single, red, firm, uneven growth inside the external urinary meatus two months after an exposure to a commercial sex worker. What is the diagnosis?

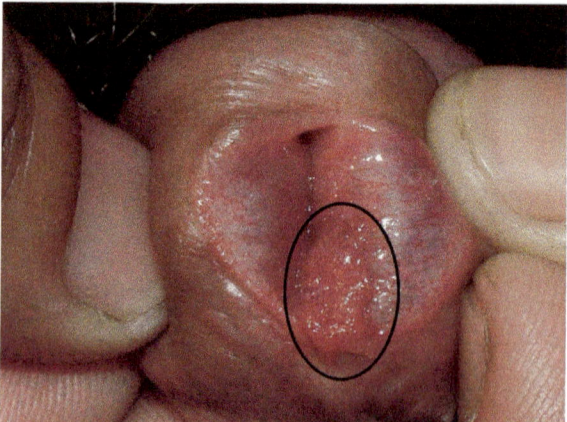

a. Pearly penile papules
b. Intrameatal wart

673. A 70-year-old man presented with single indurated plaque on right cheek for the last five years. What is the closest clinical diagnosis?

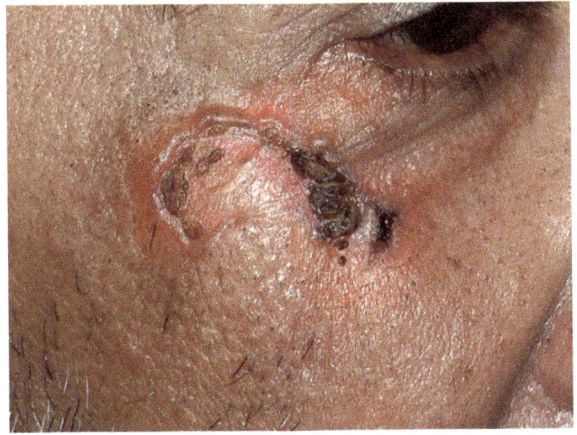

a. Basal cell carcinoma (BCC)
b. Superficial spreading melanoma (SSM)
c. Squamous cell carcinoma (SCC)
d. Old world cutaneous leishmaniasis

674. Which one of the following type of inheritance is shown by the diagram. If a healthy male marries a carrier female, then half of sons are affected. If a healthy female marries an affected male, then daughters will be carrier and males will be healthy.

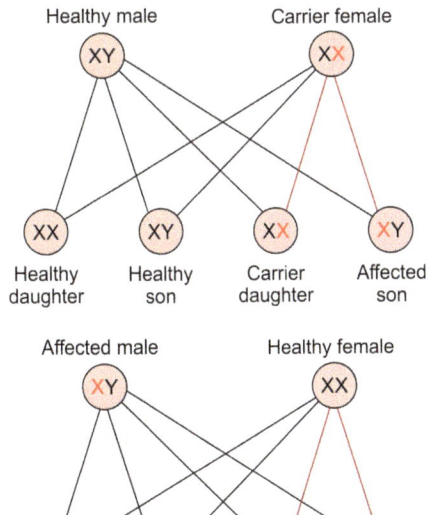

a. Autosomal dominant
b. X-linked recessive inheritance
c. Autosomal recessive
d. X-linked dominant inheritance

675. Following is the diagrammatic representation of epidermal cell layers. What is the name of the cell layer that has been shown in bracket?

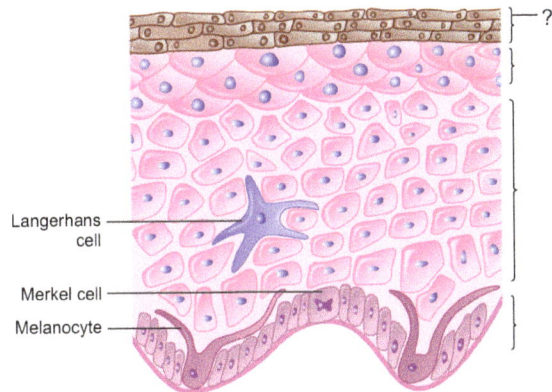

a. Stratum spinosum
b. Stratum basale
c. Stratum granulosum
d. Stratum corneum

676. A 75-year-old lady presented with a single firm flesh-colored plaque resembling eczema at paranasal site for the last two years. What is the closest clinical diagnosis?

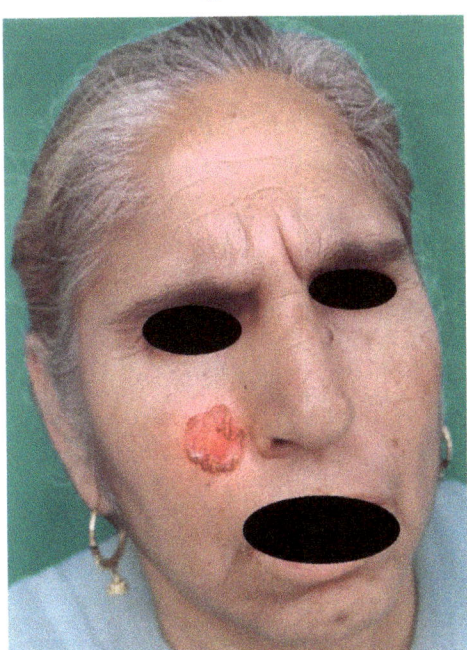

a. Squamous cell carcinoma
b. Basal cell carcinoma
c. Lupus vulgaris
d. Old world cutaneous leishmaniasis

677. Both hands this patient show separation of proximal part of nail plate from nail matrix and nail bed in all the nails. Which one of the following options is correct for this nail change?

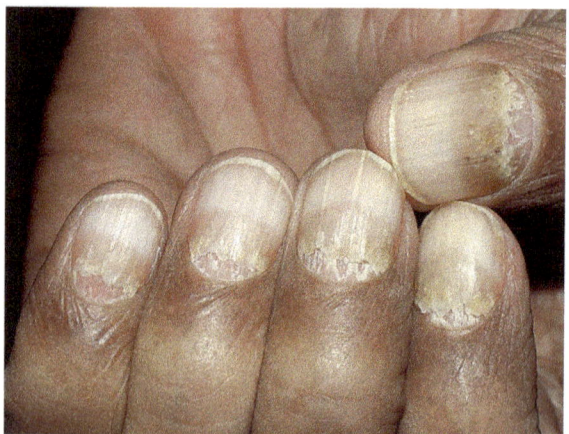

a. Onycholysis
b. Proximal subungual onychomycosis
c. Onychomadesis
d. Beau's lines

678. This patient presented with loss hair from his right eye brow in last three months. What is the closest clinical diagnosis?

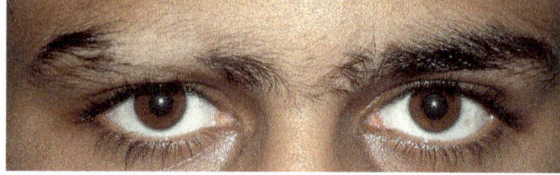

a. Hypothyroidism
b. Alopecia areata
c. Tinea barbae of eyebrow
d. Superciliary madarosis due to lepromatous leprosy

679. This patient presented with single asymptomatic black irregular macule on sole for the last one year. What is the most appropriate clinical diagnosis for this patient?

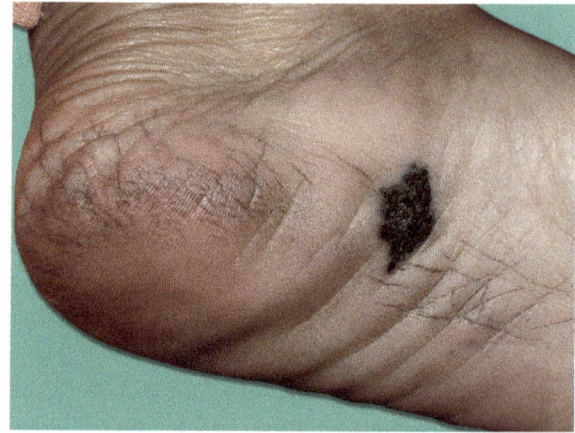

a. Lichen planus
b. Acral lentiginous melanoma
c. Junctional nevus

680. Following is the diagrammatic representation of dermoepidermal junction. What is the name of the layer with the question mark?

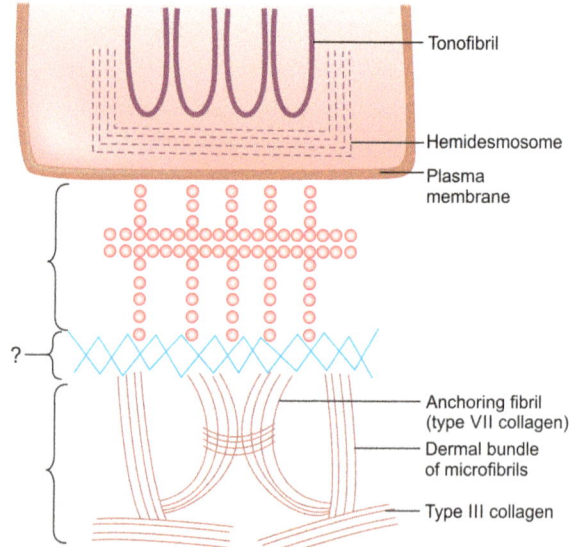

a. Lamina lucida
b. Sub basal dense plaques
c. Lamina densa
d. Lamina fibroreticularis

681. A middle-aged man presented with few, indolent non scaly red lumps on chest for the last 2–3 years. What is the closest clinical diagnosis?

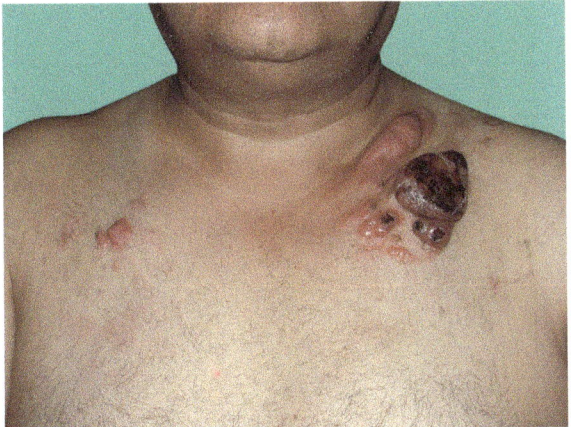

a. Tumor stage cutaneous T-cell lymphoma
b. Lupus vulgaris
c. Cutaneous B-cell lymphoma
d. Squamous cell carcinoma

682. Nails of this patient show yellow discoloration, coarse pitting and separation of distal part of nail plate. These changes are seen in which of the following disorders?

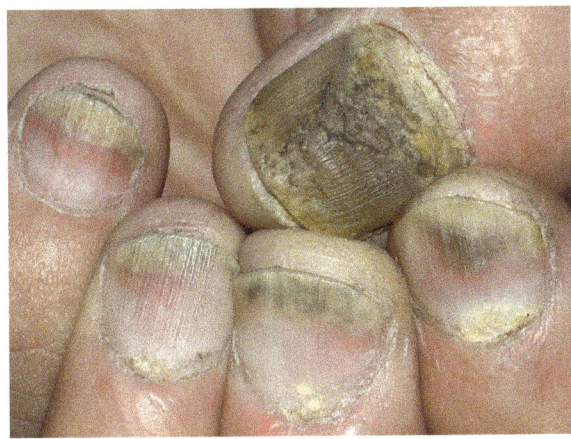

a. Lichen planus (LP)
b. Onychomycosis
c. Psoriasis
d. Darier's disease

683. This patient complained of recurrent itching and swelling of ear lobule with a circular red plaque on cheek for the last one week. What is most appropriate clinical diagnosis?

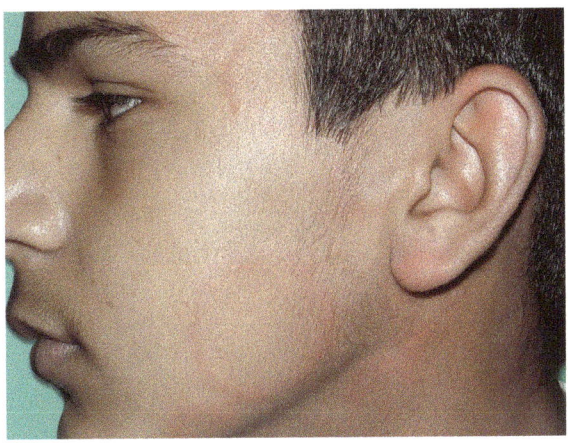

a. Chronic urticaria
b. Tinea faciei
c. Lepromatous leprosy
d. Acute urticaria

684. A 70-year-old man presented with multiple 1–6 mm sized, slightly elevated, circular, cherry red, firm papules on trunk for the last two years. What is the diagnosis?

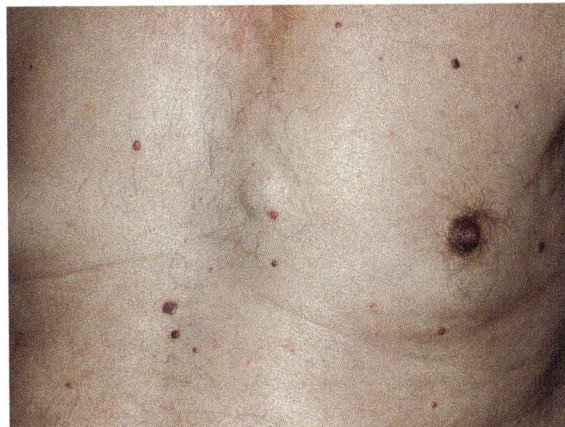

a. Strawberry hemangioma
b. Cherry angiomas
c. Pyogenic granuloma
d. Lymphangioma circumscriptum

685. Following is diagrammatic histopathological findings in a vesiculobullous disorder. Which one of the following options is correct diagnosis for a disorder showing suprabasal cleavage?

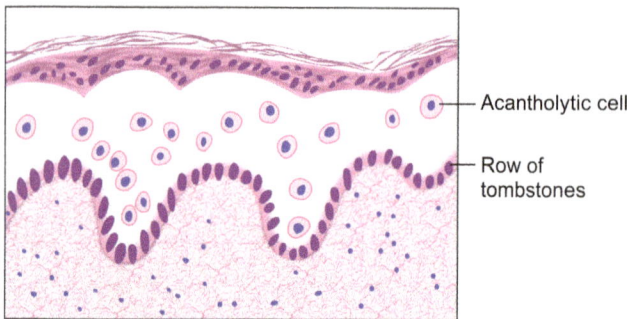

 a. Dermatitis herpetiformis (DH)
 b. Pemphigus vulgaris
 c. Bullous pemphigoid (BP)
 d. Pemphigus foliaceous (PF)

686. This patient is having non-pitting edema of legs with verrucous papules and nodules giving a cobble stone appearance. Which one of the following options is most appropriate for this patient?

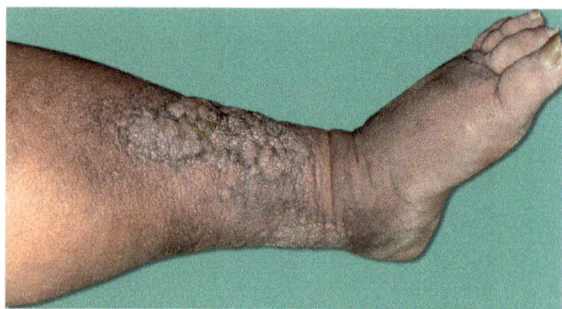

 a. Esthiomene
 b. Elephantiasis
 c. Elephantiasis nostras verrucosa

687. This patient complained of growth on nose with black pigmentation. What is the closest clinical diagnosis?

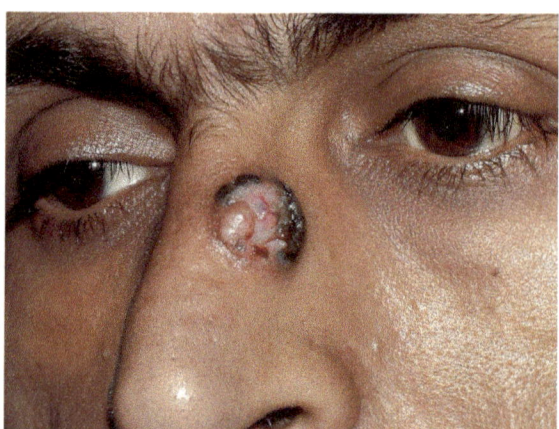

 a. Basal cell carcinoma
 b. Nodular melanoma
 c. Squamous cell carcinoma
 d. Keratoacanthoma

688. This patient complained of multiple, flesh colored soft, flat topped sessile papules with oozing and macerations in the groins and anal regions. What is closest clinical diagnosis?

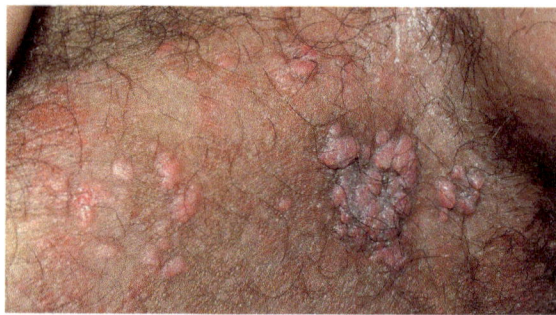

 a. Condylomata acuminata
 b. Condylomata lata
 c. Molluscum contagiosum

689. This patient presented with chronic plantar ulceration on the plantar surface of big toe. It is accompanied by loss of sensations in both feet, legs and hands. He is also having superciliary madarosis and nasal collapse. There is a h/o thickening of ear lobules. What is the cause of plantar ulceration?

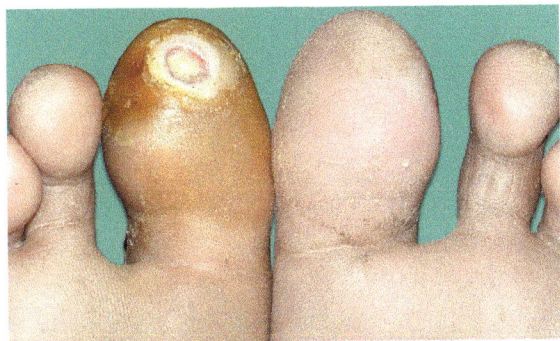

a. Buerger's disease
b. Diabetes mellitus
c. Lepromatous leprosy
d. Venous ulcer

690. Following is the diagrammatic representation of dermoepidermal junction. What is the name of the layer with question mark?

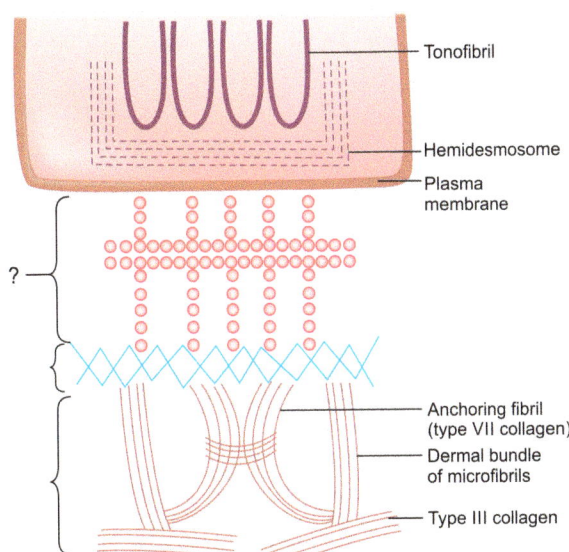

a. Lamina densa
b. Lamina lucida
c. Lamina fibroreticularis
d. Sub-basal dense plaques

691. Overnight this patient developed subpreputial discharge and dusky red coloration of prepuce with accompanying burning sensation. There is no history of sexual exposure. What is the clinical diagnosis?

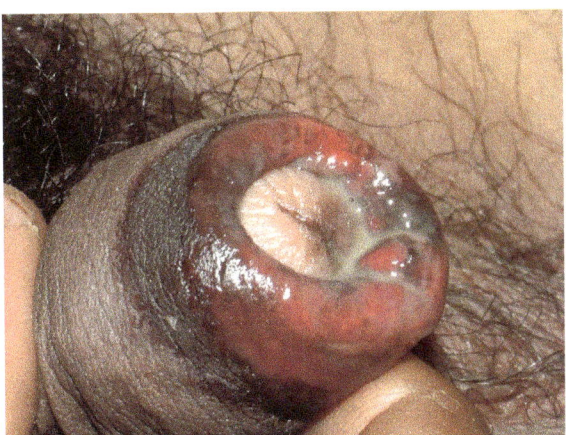

a. Secondary syphilis
b. Candidal balanoposthitis due to diabetes
c. Fixed drug eruption
d. Gonococcal urethritis

692. This lady presented with asymptomatic swelling of both ears and cheeks for the last one year. There was no remission in between. What is the closest clinical diagnosis for her?

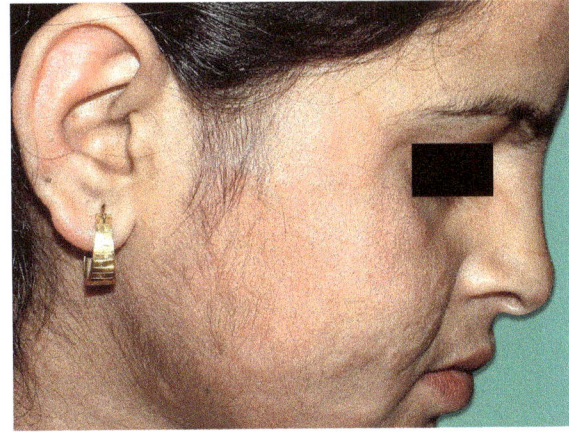

a. Chronic urticaria
b. Lepromatous leprosy
c. Post-kala-azar dermal leishmaniasis (PKDL)
d. Myxedema

693. This patient presented with redness and itching in groins, scrotum and preputial opening. He also complains of increased frequency of micturition at night. There is a no history of sexual exposure. What is the closest clinical diagnosis?

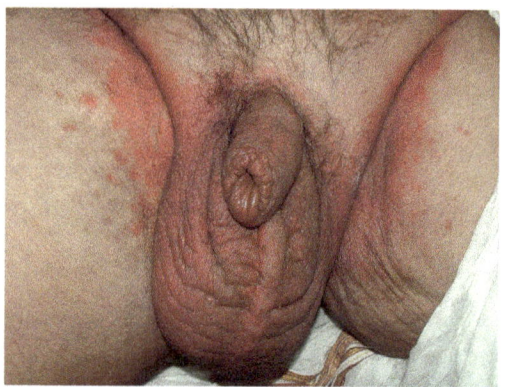

   a. Tinea cruris
   b. Candidal balanoposthitis with intertrigo
   c. Bacterial intertrigo in an obese patient
   d. Flexural psoriasis

694. If an affected hemizygous male marries with a normal female, then disease is transmitted to daughters but not to sons. If an affected female, marries with a normal male, then half of her sons and daughters are affected. What is the type of inheritance shown by the following diagram?

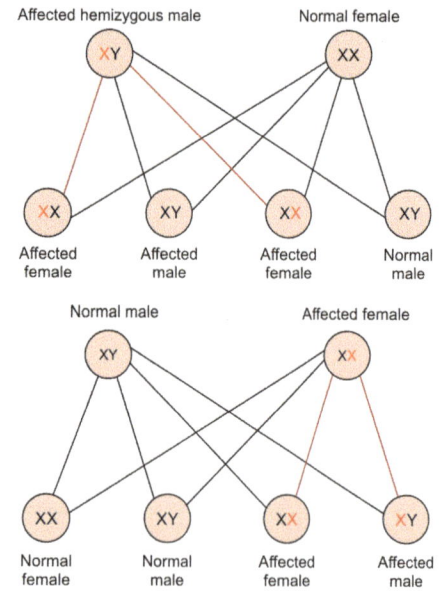

   a. Autosomal dominant inheritance
   b. X-linked recessive inheritance
   c. Autosomal recessive inheritance
   d. X-linked dominant inheritance

695. This lady is complaining of redness and itching in the groins and vulva. She is also having increased frequency of micturition at night. What is the closest clinical diagnosis?

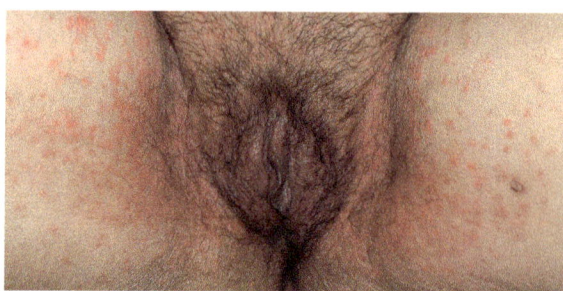

   a. Seborrheic dermatitis
   b. Tinea cruris
   c. Scabies
   d. Candidiasis

696. This patient complained of large erythematous plaque on face for the last one year. Plaque has well-defined margins and loss of sensations. What is the clinical diagnosis?

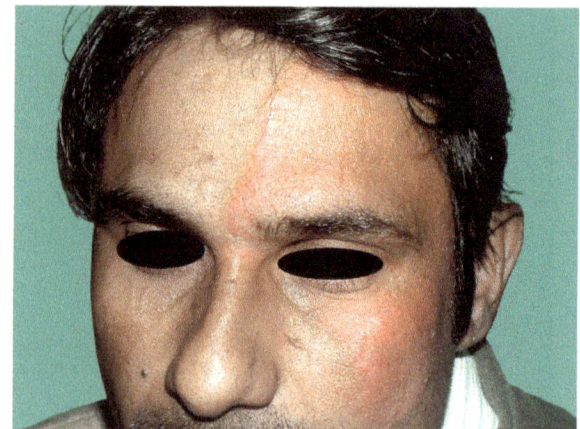

   a. Tinea faciei
   b. Tuberculoid leprosy
   c. Lepromatous leprosy
   d. Lupus vulgaris

697. This patient received many steroid injections for long time from an unqualified practitioner. He developed moon facies, muscle atrophy, striae. Which one of the following diagnosis is correct for him?

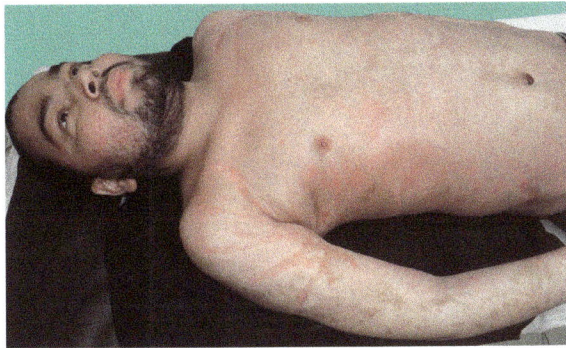

a. Cushing's syndrome
b. Cushing's disease
c. Pseudo-Cushing's syndrome

698. This patient developed over night multiple vesicles filled with clear fluid on shoulder and arm. It is accompanied by little burning sensation. What is the clinical diagnosis?

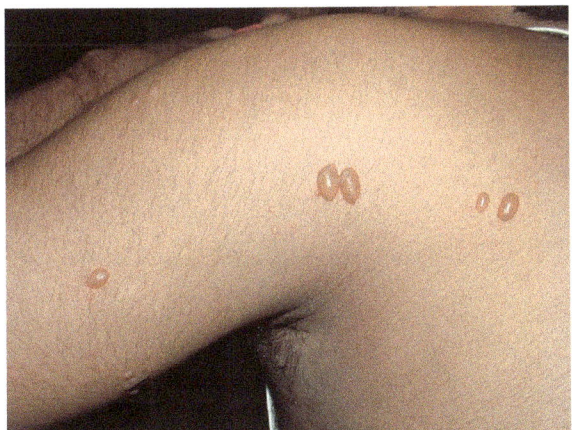

a. *Paederus dermatitis*
b. Herpes zoster
c. Chickenpox
d. Herpes simplex

699. This patient complained of painful eruption of grouped vesicles limited to left upper extremity for the last five days. What is the clinical diagnosis?

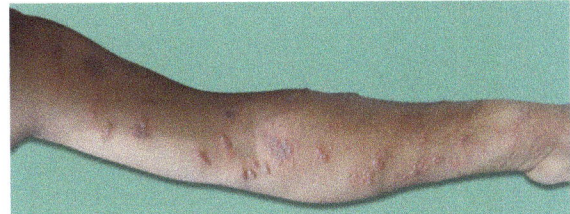

a. Herpes simplex
b. Dermatitis herpetiformis
c. *Paederus dermatitis*
d. Herpes zoster

700. Following is a diagrammatic representation of dermo-epidermal junction. What is the name of the layer with question mark?

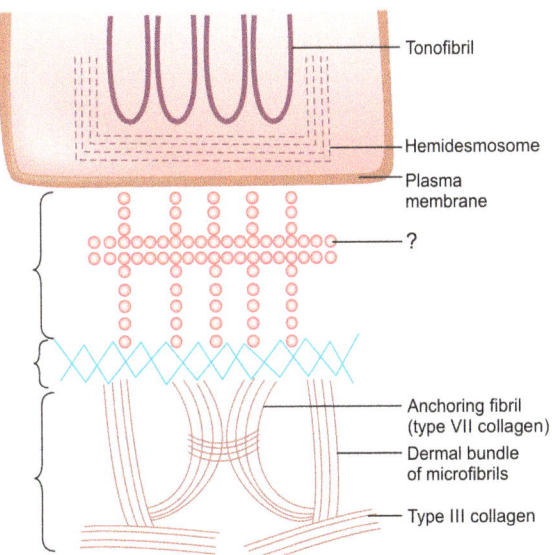

a. Lamia lucida
b. Lamina densa
c. Sub-basal dense plaques
d. Lamina fibroreticularis

701. A 6-year-old child developed overnight red linear lesions on both legs with accompanying pain and burning sensation. What is the closest clinical diagnosis?

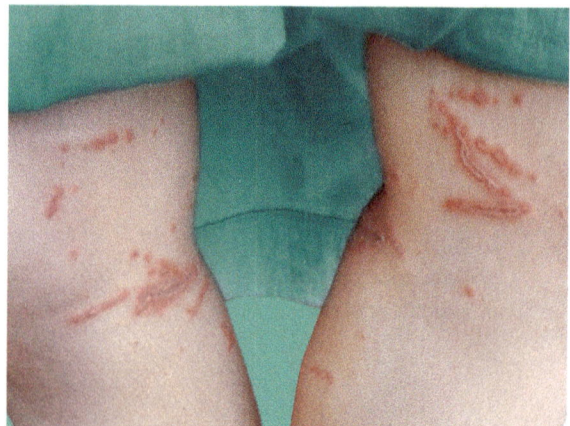

a. Papular urticaria
b. *Paederus dermatitis*
c. Scabies

702. A 40-year-old female presented with generalized hyperpigmentation, swelling of hands, sclerodactyly and binding down of forearm skin. Skin of upper chest and cervical region showed salt pepper dyschromatosis *(MCQ 714)*. There is a h/o blue coloration of hands on exposure to cold. What is the closest clinical diagnosis?

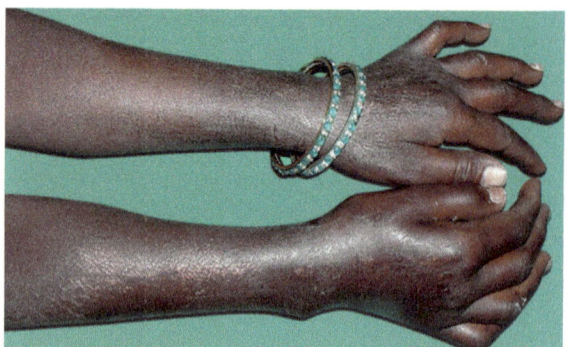

a. Generalized morphea
b. Systemic lupus erythematosus (SLE)
c. Systemic sclerosis
d. Addisonian pigmentation

703. A 14-year-old child presented with a patch of hair loss. Which one of the following options is closest clinical diagnosis for him?

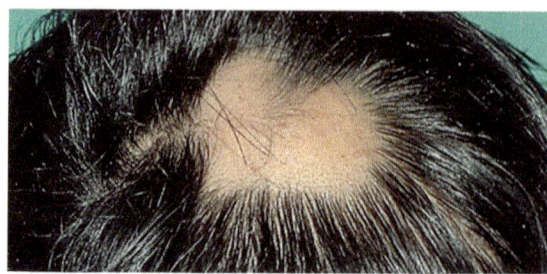

a. Trichotillomania
b. Tinea capitis
c. Alopecia areata
d. Cicatricial alopecia

704. This patient complained of multiple dry of rough, hyperkeratotic papules in the anal region for the last three months. What is the closest clinical diagnosis?

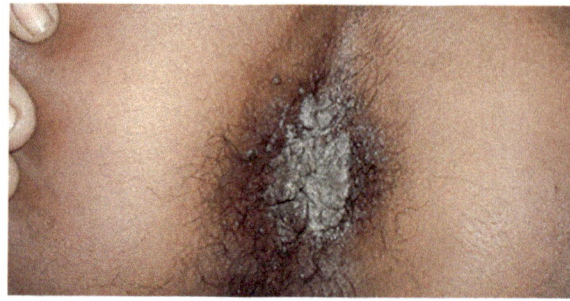

a. Condylomata lata
b. Condylomata acuminata

705. Following picture shows diagrammatic histological findings in a vesiculobullous disorder. It is showing subcorneal cleft. Which one of the following options is correct for this?

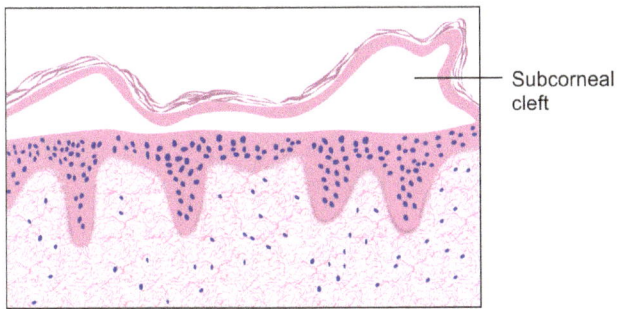

a. Pemphigus foliaceous
b. Dermatitis herpetiformis (DH)
c. Bullous pemphigoid
d. Pemphigus vulgaris

706. This lady presented with erythematous, dry and thick plaques on lower lip and chest region. What is the closest clinical diagnosis?

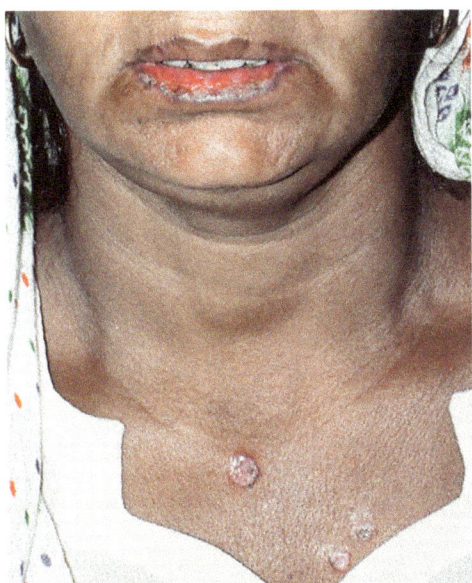

a. Systemic lupus erythematosus (SLE)
b. Lichen planus
c. Chronic cutaneous lupus erythematosus (CCLE)
d. Actinic cheilitis

707. This patient presented with a big patch of hair loss after a burn injury. Which one of the following options is correct for him?

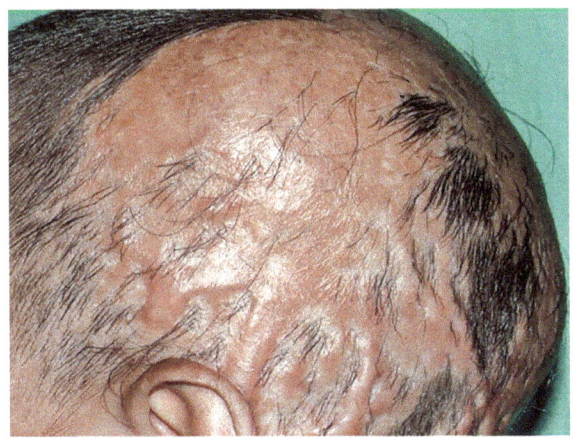

a. Telogen effluvium
b. Alopecia areata
c. Alopecia totalis
d. Cicatricial alopecia

708. A 58-year-old lady developed excessive hairs on cheeks, upper lip and forehead during the last five months with no virilizing features. Which one of the followings is most probable cause in her?

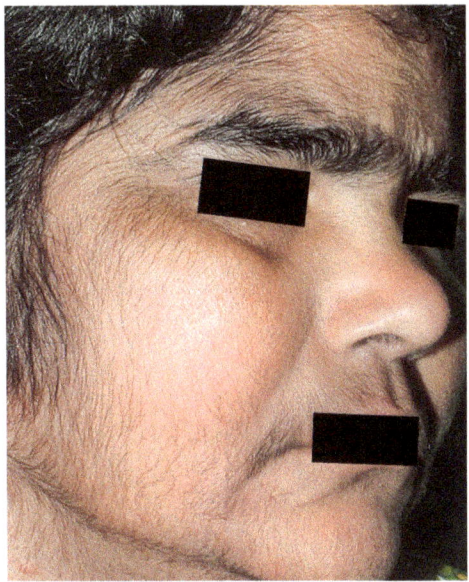

a. Idiopathic hirsutism
b. Androgen secreting tumor
c. Systemic corticosteroids
d. Polycystic ovarian syndrome (PCOS)

709. A 50-year-old male slowly developed multiple red, non-scaly plaques and tumors on chest, axillae and abdomen *(MCQ 408)*. What is the closest clinical diagnosis?

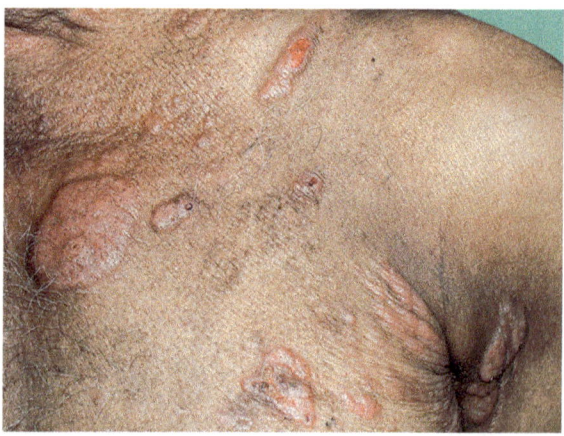

a. Mycosis fungoides
b. Psoriasis
c. Cutaneous B-cell lymphoma
d. Lupus vulgaris

710. This patient developed overnight multiple red patches on the front of the thigh with accompanying burning sensation. What is the possible diagnosis?

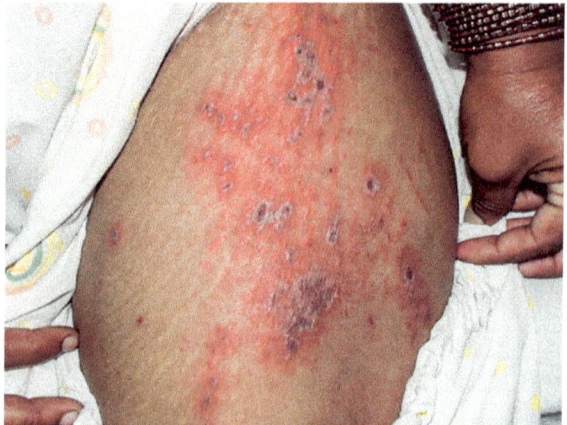

a. Herpes zoster
b. *Paederus dermatitis*
c. Dermatitis artefacta

711. Following is the diagrammatic representation of various levels of cleavages in some vesiculobullous disorders. What is the level of cleavage in dystrophic epidermolysis bullosa?

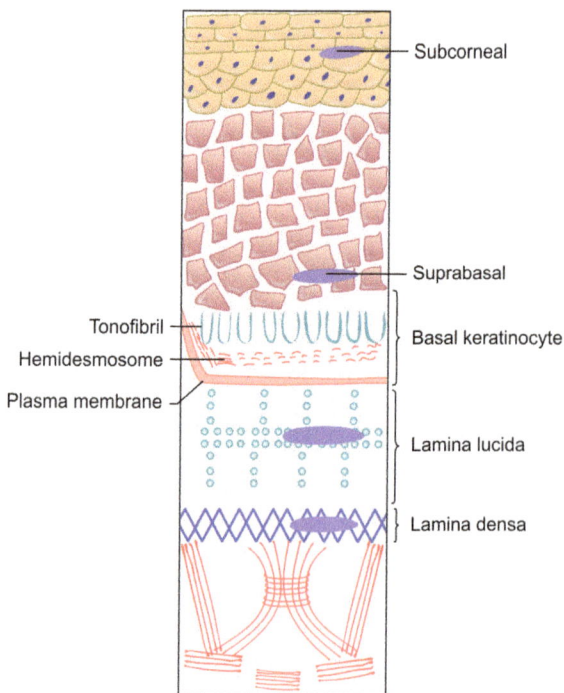

a. Lamina densa
b. Suprabasal
c. Subcorneal
d. Lamina lucida

712. This patient gave a history of development of grouped fluid filled vesicles in lower abdominal skin since infancy. On excision, there is a recurrence of similar lesions in the neighboring skin of excision scar. What is the closest clinical diagnosis?

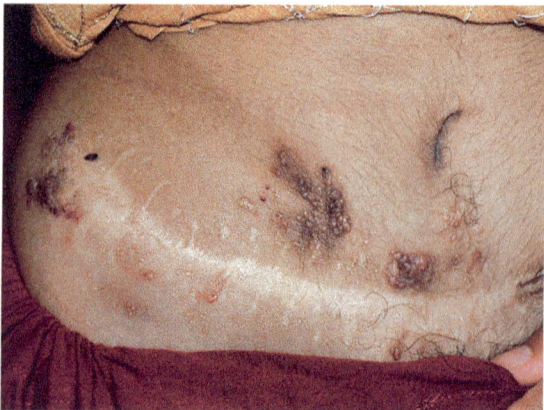

a. Herpes simplex
b. Lymphangioma circumscriptum
c. Dermatitis herpetiformis

713. A 70-year-old man presented with a firm dark-colored rough circumscribed plaque on the frontal region on his scalp. In addition, there is a development of verrucous cauliflower like growth on it. What is the closest clinical diagnosis?

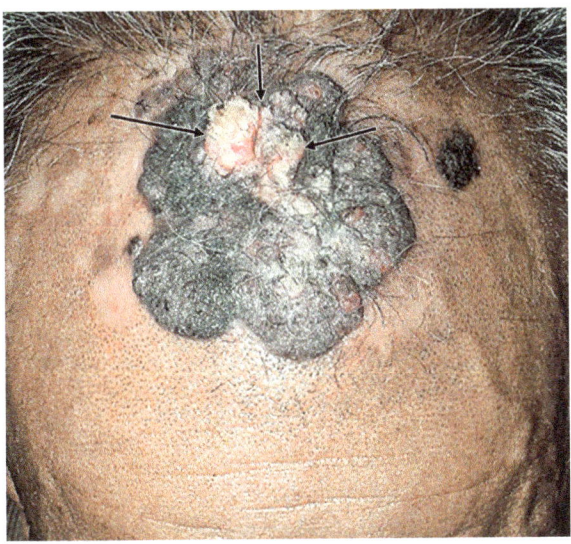

a. Basal cell carcinoma (BCC)
b. Squamous cell carcinoma (SCC)
c. Keratoacanthoma

714. A 40-year-old female presented with generalized hyperpigmentation. Skin of upper chest and cervical region showed salt pepper dyschromatosis. She had swelling of hands, sclerodactyly and binding down of forearm skin *(MCQ 702)*. There is a h/o blue coloration of hands on exposure to cold. What is the closest clinical diagnosis?

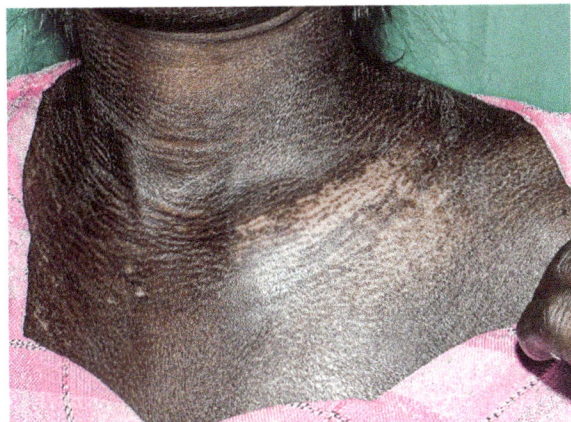

a. Systemic sclerosis
b. Generalized morphea
c. Systemic lupus erythematosus

715. Following is a diagrammatic representation of various cutaneous receptors. What is the name of the receptor with question mark?

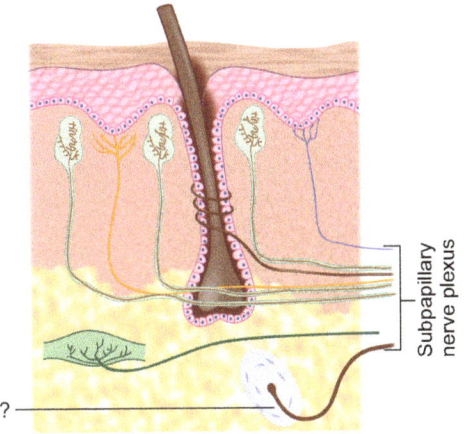

a. Merkel's receptor
b. Ruffini's corpuscle
c. Pacinian corpuscle
d. Meissner's corpuscle

716. A 45-year-old female presented with red plaques on nose, lips and cheeks for the last two years. What is the closest clinical diagnosis?

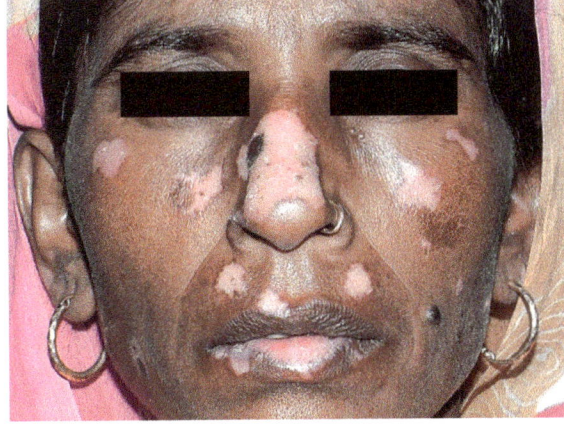

a. Chronic cutaneous lupus erythematosus (CCLE)
b. Vitiligo
c. Systemic lupus erythematosus (SLE)
d. Lichen planus

717. This patient started developing red, soft, verrucous papules and nodules on his decades old burn scar on his heel. What is the closest clinical diagnosis?

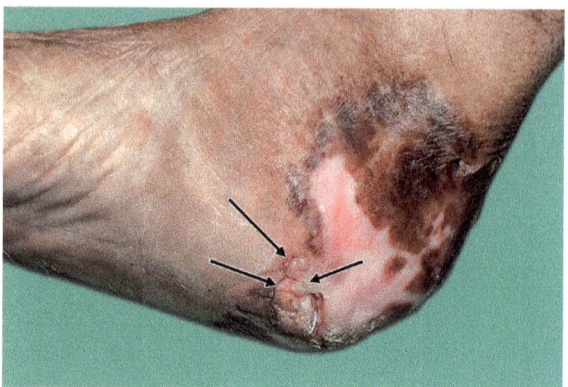

a. Marjolin's ulcer
b. Scar sarcoid
c. Scar tuberculosis

718. What is the diagnosis of this patient who complains of depigmentation on his elbow only?

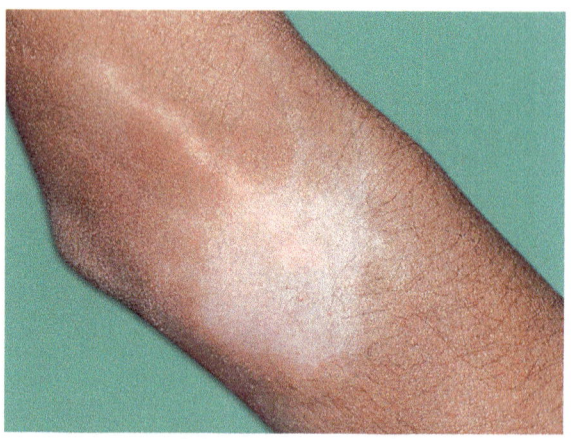

a. Segmental vitiligo
b. Focal vitiligo
c. Depigmentation due to intraarticular triamcinolone

719. This patient complained of itching, burning and diffuse redness of dorsa of fingers of both hands. What is the clinical diagnosis?

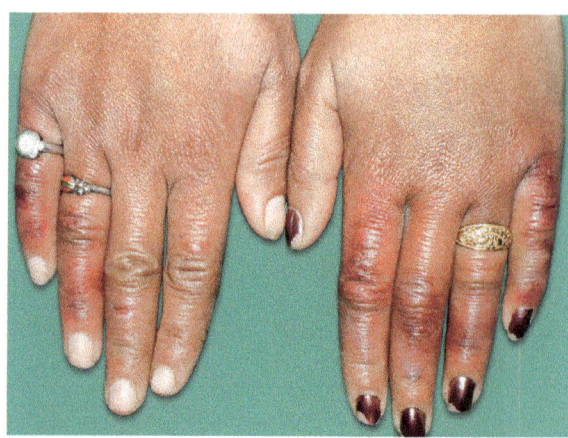

a. Chilblains
b. Raynaud's phenomenon
c. Livedo reticularis

720. Following is a diagrammatic representation of histopathological findings in a vesiculobullous disorder. It is showing subepidermal cleft and inflammatory infiltrate in superficial dermis. Which one of the following options is correct for this patient?

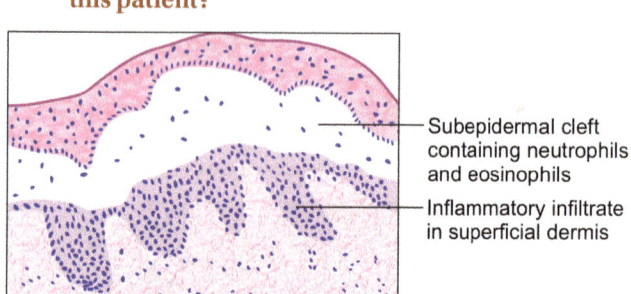

a. Pemphigus vulgaris
b. Pemphigus foliaceus
c. Bullous pemphigoid
d. Dermatitis herpetiformis

721. A 2-year-old child was brought with dry rough, hyperkeratotic and asymptomatic papules in the anal region. What is the closest clinical diagnosis?

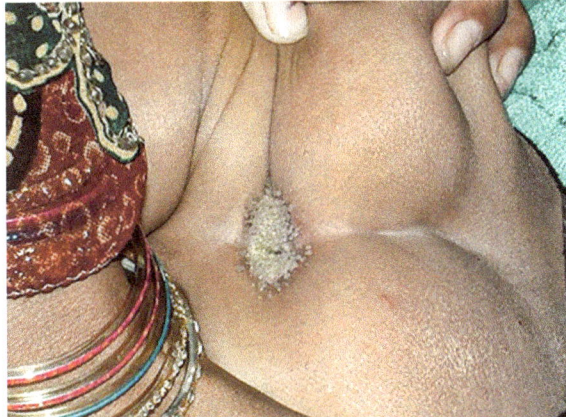

a. Condylomata acuminata
b. Condylomata lata

722. This patient presented with a single, circumscribed, thickened waxy, looking plaque on the trunk for the last one year. The surface is shiny, smooth with absence of hairs. There is no loss of sensations. What is the closest clinical diagnosis?

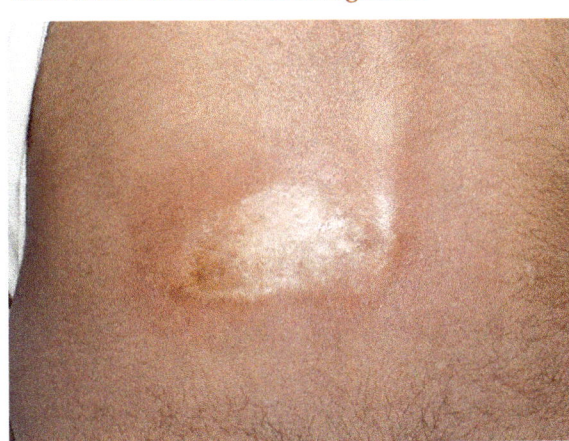

a. Lupus vulgaris
b. Tuberculoid leprosy
c. Circumscribed morphea
d. Localized vitiligo

723. A 60-year-old female developed dark-colored nodules on her heel for the last 6 months. She also had 2–3 satellites lesions in the surroundings area. What is the closest clinical diagnosis?

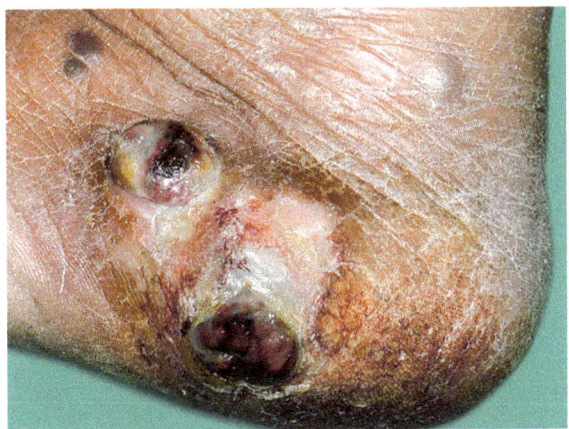

a. Nodular melanoma
b. Squamous cell carcinoma (SCC)
c. Mycosis fungoides
d. Lichen planus hypertrophicus (LPH)

724. An 18-year-old boy complained of eruption of 1–3 mm sized monomorphic wheals on trunk and extremities on taking spicy food or after taking severe exercise. The episodes are usually accompanied by sweating. What is the clinical diagnosis?

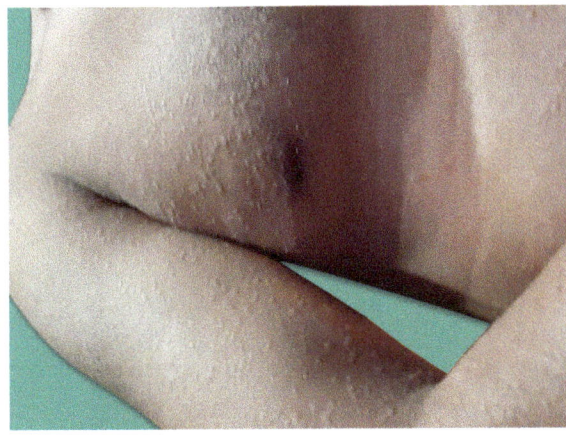

a. Aquagenic pruritus
b. Cholinergic urticaria
c. Contact urticaria
d. Ordinary acute urticaria

725. Following is a diagrammatic representation of various cutaneous receptors. What is name of the receptor with question mark?

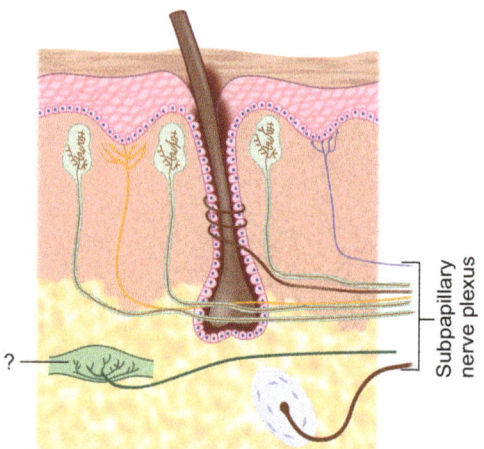

a. Meissner's corpuscle
b. Merkel's receptor
c. Pacinian corpuscle
d. Ruffini's corpuscle

726. Following figure shows the magnified views of axilla of a patient. This patient had transient vesiculobullous lesions in axillae and back. Oral mucosa was not involved. What is the clinical diagnosis?

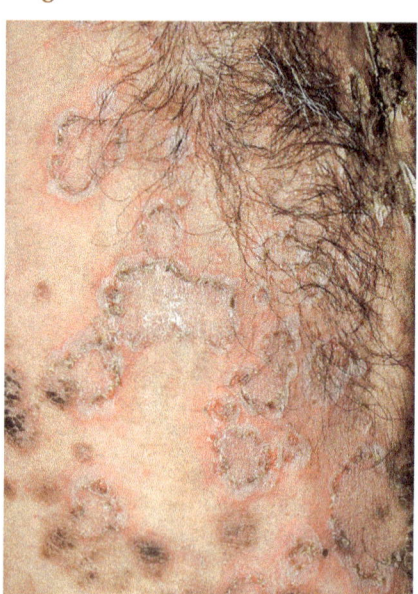

a. Pemphigus vulgaris
b. Pemphigus foliaceous
c. Benign chronic familial pemphigus
d. Linear IgA disease of adult

727. She complained of gray color pigmentation of both cheeks since her infancy. What is the clinical diagnosis?

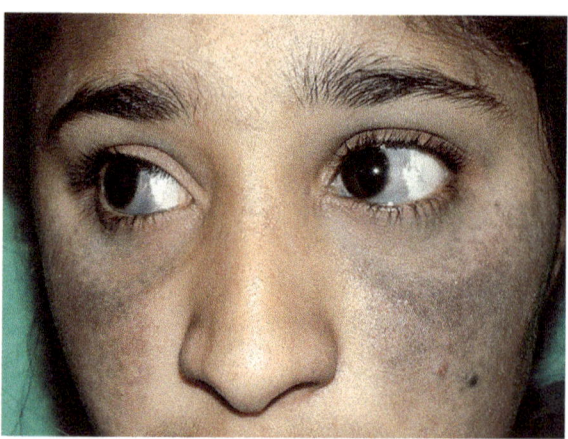

a. Melasma
b. Butterfly rash of SLE
c. Bilateral nevus of Ota

728. Within 4–5 days after fever and herpes simplex infection at angle of mouth, this child developed monomorphic rash on face, extremities and trunk *(MCQ 744)*. He was having blood-stained saliva and cervical lymphadenopathy. What is the closest diagnosis?

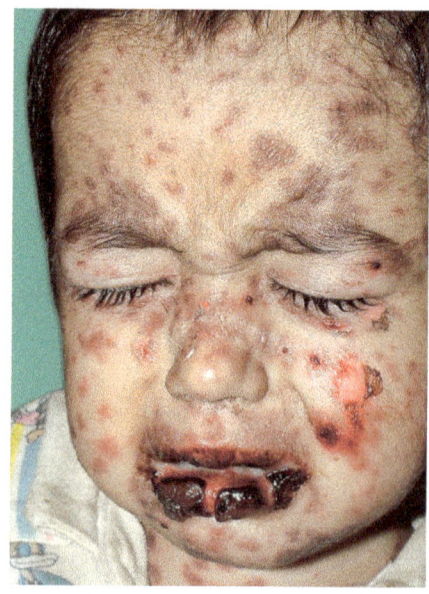

a. Erythema multiforme major (EMM)
b. Stevens Johnson syndrome (SJS)
c. Toxic epidermal necrolysis (TEN)

729. A 8-year-old child developed red plaques with white scaling on buttocks, scalp and other parts of body. What is the clinical diagnosis?

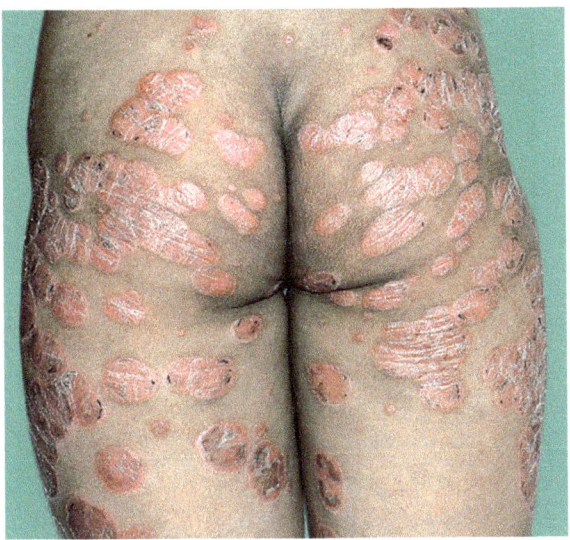

a. Psoriasis
b. Dermatophytosis
c. Dermatitis buttocks

730. This lady developed overnight burning sensation and erythema on the front of the chest. What is the clinical diagnosis?

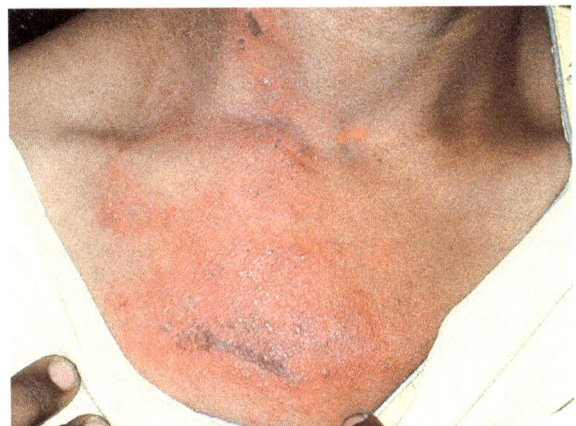

a. Dermatitis artefacta
b. *Paederus dermatitis*
c. Herpes zoster

731. Following is the diagrammatic representation of various levels of cleavages in some vesiculobullous disorders. What is the level of cleavage in bullous pemphigoid?

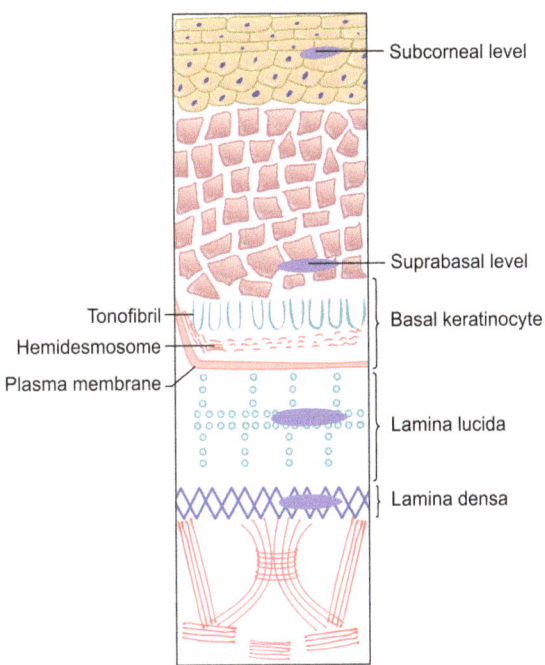

a. Just below lamina densa
b. Subcorneal
c. Suprabasal
d. Lamina lucida

732. An old female presented with red hyperkeratotic plaques on nose and lips for the last three years. Scales are adherent to the plaques. What is the closest clinical diagnosis?

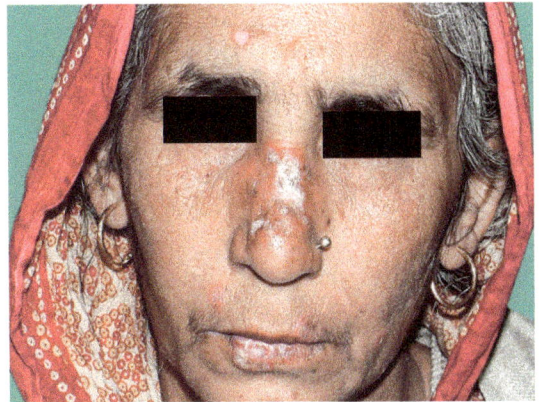

a. Psoriasis
b. Actinic lichen planus
c. Actinic keratosis
d. Chronic cutaneous lupus erythematosus

733. What is the diagnosis for the following patient?

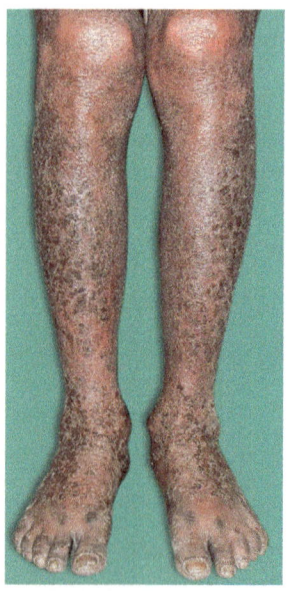

a. Psoriasis
b. Eczema
c. Tinea corporis

734. An 8-year-old child developed red plaques with white scaling on face and other parts of body. What is the clinical diagnosis?

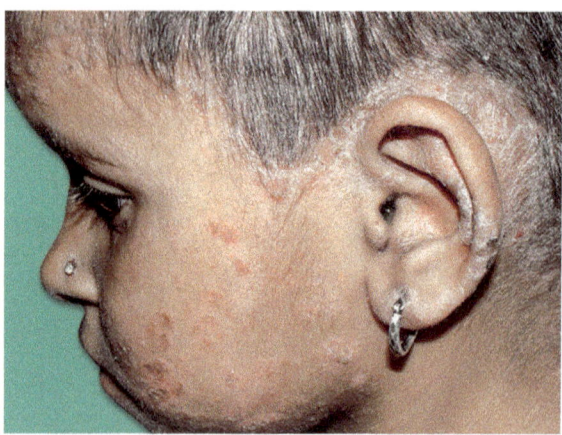

a. Tinea infection
b. Seborrheic dermatitis
c. Psoriasis

735. Following is the diagrammatic representation of various cutaneous receptors. What is the name of the receptor with question mark?

a. Merkel's receptor
b. Pacinian corpuscle
c. Meissner's corpuscle
d. Ruffini's corpuscle

736. This patient presented with red plaques with white scaling. What is the diagnosis of this patient?

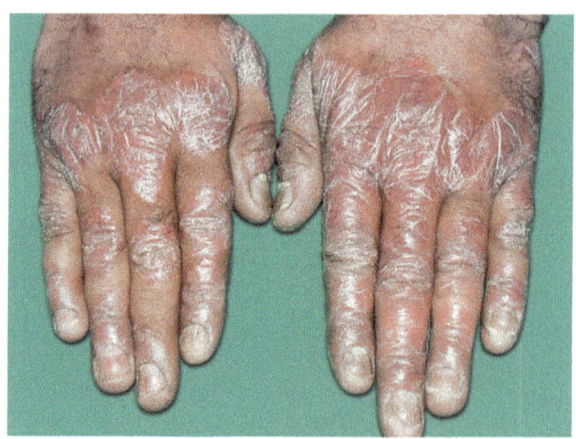

a. Tinea manuum
b. Psoriasis
c. Eczema hands
d. Lichen planus

737. This patient complained of asymptomatic exfoliation and scaling both palms. What is the closest clinical diagnosis?

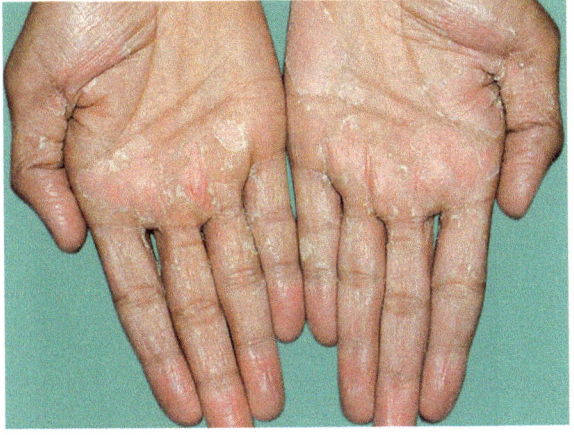

a. Tinea manuum
b. Keratolysis exfoliativa
c. Dermatitis palms

738. What is the most appropriate option of clinical diagnosis for this patient complaining of thick hyperkeratotic lesions between 4th and 5th toes?

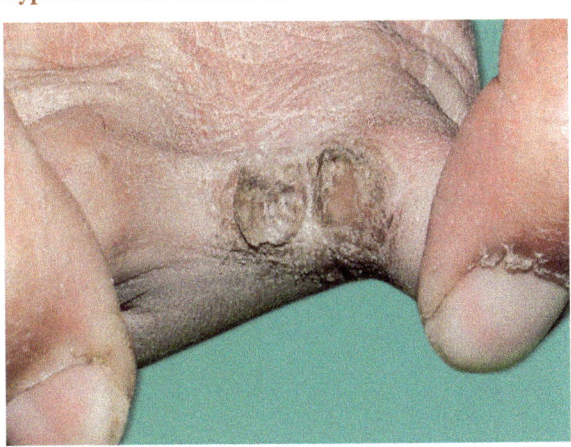

a. Callus
b. Soft corn
c. Warts

739. A 10-year-old child presented with a patch on scalp showing fine white scaling and partial hair loss. What is the closest clinical diagnosis?

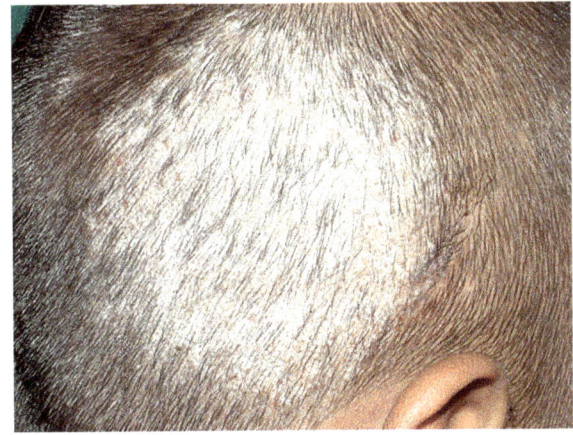

a. Scalp psoriasis
b. Tinea capitis
c. Seborrheic capitis
d. Alopecia areata

740. Following is the diagrammatic histopathological findings in a vesiculobullous disorder. It is showing subepidermal vesiculation and papillary collection of neutrophils and eosinophils. Which one of the following options is correct for this patient?

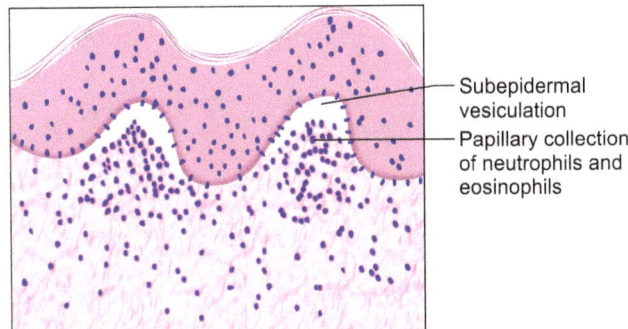

a. Pemphigus foliaceous
b. Dermatitis herpetiformis
c. Pemphigus vulgaris
d. Bullous pemphigoid

741. Next day after intercourse patient complained of penile swelling and bluish coloration of suprapubic region and scrotum. What is the clinical diagnosis?

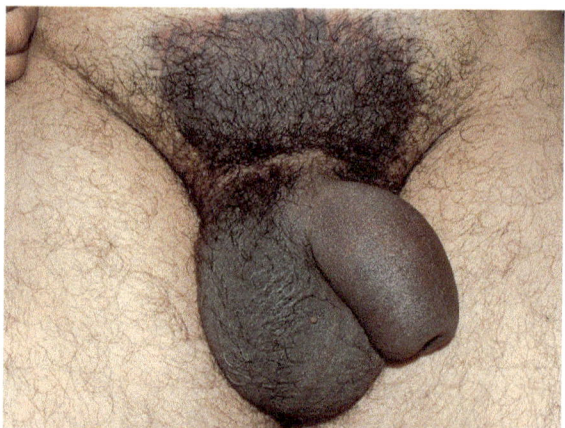

a. Contact irritant dermatitis to condom
b. Fracture penis
c. Idiopathic thrombocytopenic purpura (ITP)

743. This patient complained of itching and thickening of both soles. What is the closest clinical diagnosis?

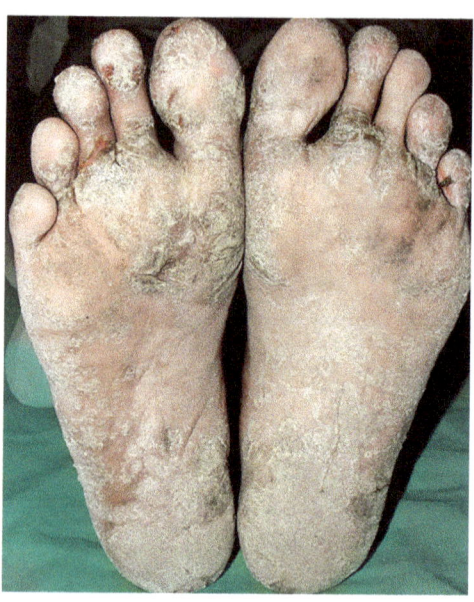

a. Psoriasis soles
b. Hyperkeratotic eczema soles
c. Tinea pedis
d. Diffuse plantar keratoderma

742. This patient complained of white fine scaling on her right palm only. The involvement was extending on to the dorsal side also. What is the clinical diagnosis?

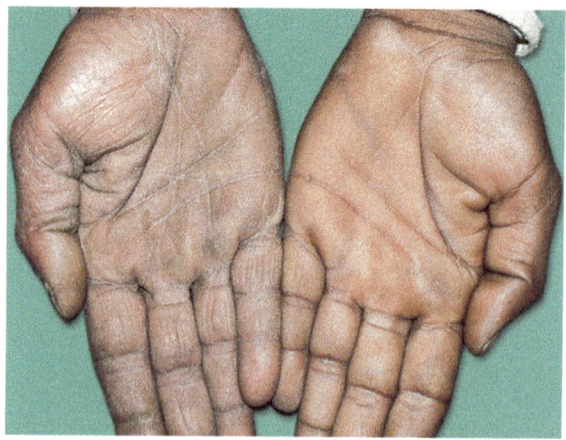

a. Candidiasis
b. Housewife's contact dermatitis
c. Tinea manuum

744. Within 4–5 days after fever and herpes simplex infection at the angle of his month, this child developed monomorphic rash on his trunk, extremities and face *(MCQ 728)*. He was also having blood-stained saliva and cervical lymph adenopathy. What the closest clinical diagnosis?

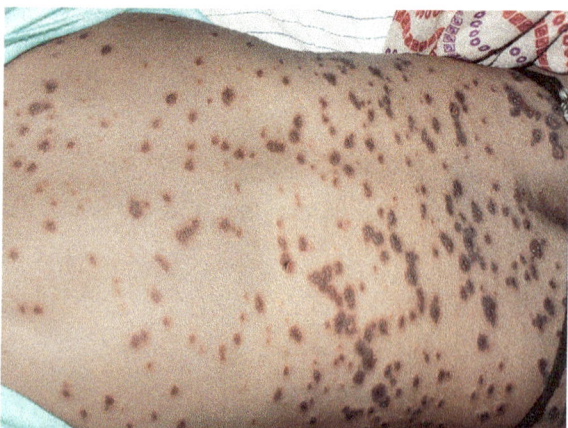

a. Stevens Johnson Syndrome (SJS)
b. Toxic epidermal necrolysis (TEN)
c. Erythema multiforme major (EMM)

745. Following is the diagrammatic representation of direct immunofluorescence showing fish-net pattern in a vesiculobullous disease. Which one of the following options is correct for this?

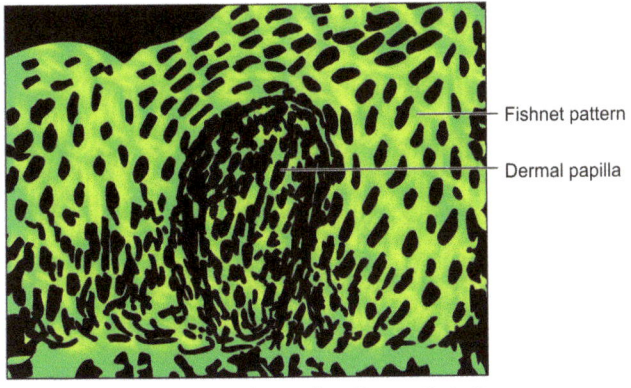

a. Bullous pemphigoid or linear IgA disease
b. Erythema multiforme
c. Pemphigus vulgaris or pemphigus foliaceous.
d. Epidermolysis bullosa simplex

746. A 70-year-old patient complained of painful grouped vesicles on erythematous base. He was also having discrete and scattered vesicles on the neighboring area of his trunk. What is the clinical diagnosis?

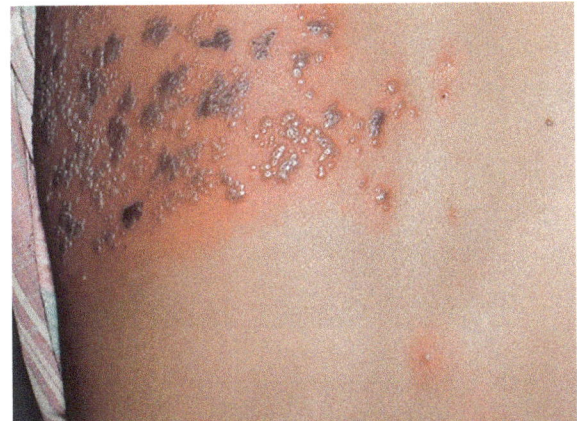

a. Herpes zoster with dissemination
b. Herpes zoster with chickenpox
c. Kaposi's varicelliform eruption

747. What is the appropriate name of the type of vitiligo in this child?

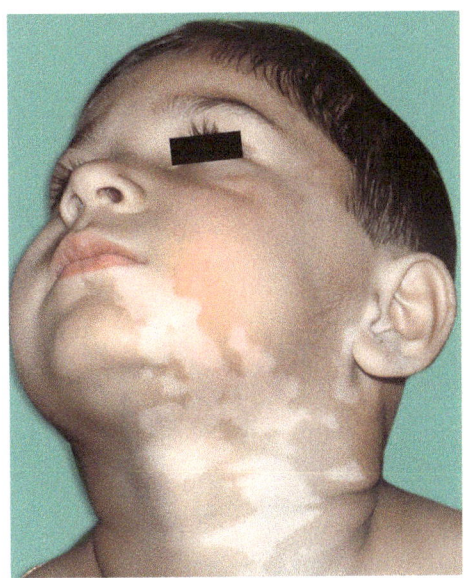

a. Vitiligo vulgaris
b. Focal vitiligo
c. Segmental vitiligo

748. A 8-month-old child presented with raw areas in perioral region. He was also having psoriasiform scaly patches in perianal region *(MCQ 763)*. He was weaned off few weeks back. What is the most appropriate clinical diagnosis?

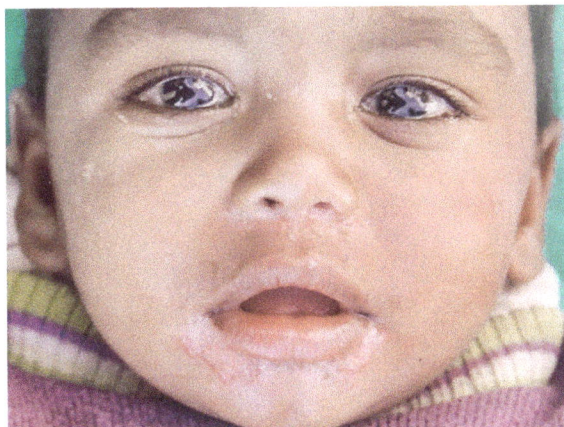

a. Impetigo contagiosa
b. Acrodermatitis enteropathica
c. Atopic dermatitis

749. This patient complained of redness, burning and itching on face for the last many months. She is applying some cream for the last 1 year. Which one of following creams is she most probably applying?

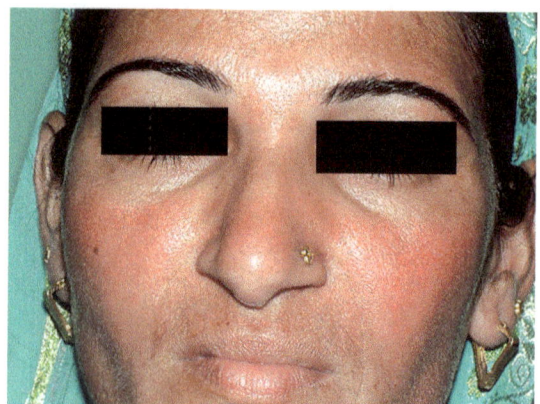

a. Corticosteroid cream
b. Sunscreen
c. Emollient cream
d. Face wash

750. Following is the diagrammatic representation of levels of cleavages in various vesiculobullous disorders. What is the level of cleavage in pemphigus foliaceous?

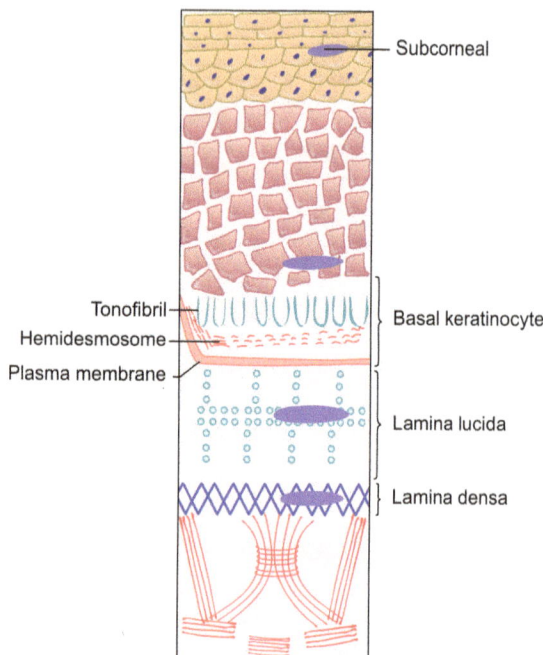

a. Lamina lucida
b. Lamina densa
c. Subcorneal
d. Suprabasal

751. A newly married man had pain and bleeding during sexual intercourse. Which one of the following is incorrect for him for management?

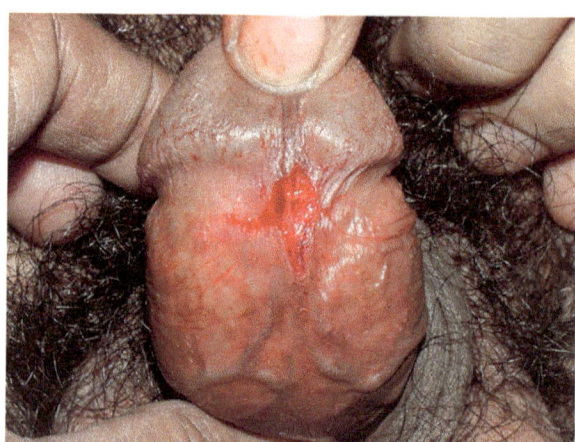

a. Requires reassurance
b. Requires immediate suturing
c. Symptomatic treatment
d. Abstinence till healing

752. A 8-year-old child presented with single inflammatory boggy swelling on scalp with partial hair loss for the last 5 months. It was accompanied by lymphadenitis also. What is the closest clinical diagnosis?

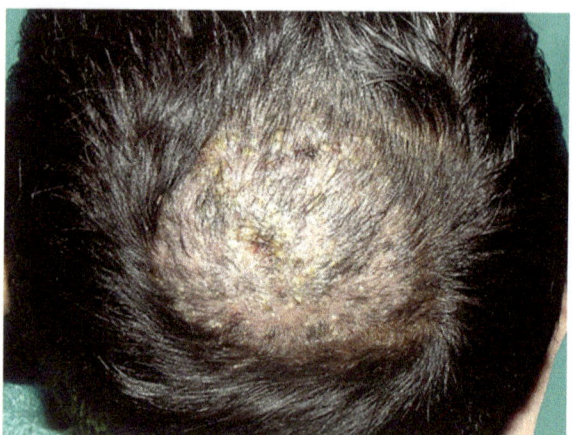

a. Sebaceous nevus
b. Pyogenic abscess
c. Tinea capitis (kerion)

Chapter 4 ✦ MCQs of Dermatology, Venereology and Leprology

753. This patient came with crusted lesions of varicella on his face. Which one of the following statements is incorrect for him?

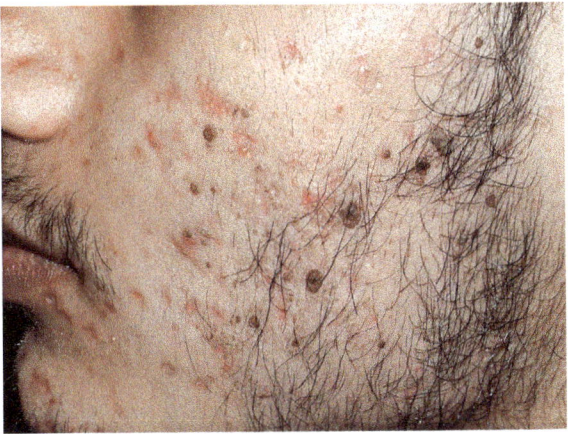

a. He is highly infectious
b. He needs no antiviral therapy
c. He is not infectious

754. A 9-year-old female child came with a patch of vitiligo on her upper eyelid. Which one of the following treatment options is most appropriate?

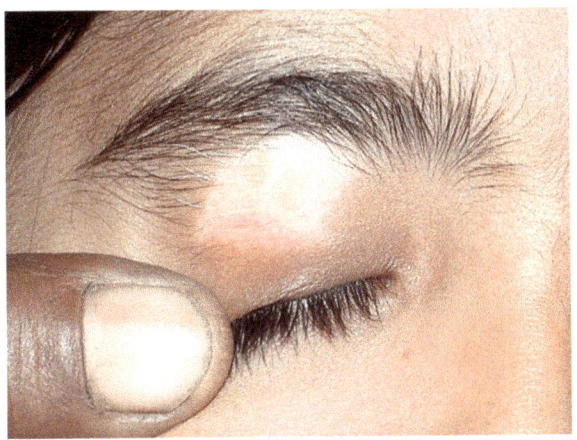

a. Corticosteroid cream
b. Tacrolimus cream
c. Systemic PUVA therapy
d. Systemic PUVA therapy + corticosteroid cream

755. Following is a diagrammatic representation of histopathological findings in a vesiculobullous disease. It is showing dilapidated brick wall appearance of epidermal changes. Which one of the following options is correct for this?

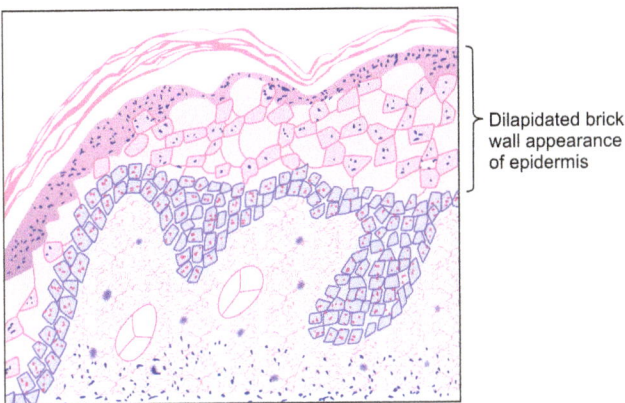

a. Pemphigus foliaceous (PE)
b. Pemphigus vulgaris (PV)
c. Hailey-Hailey disease
d. Bullous pemphigoid (BP)

756. This patient of acne is having cheilitis. Which one of the following anti-acne systemic drugs can cause cheilitis?

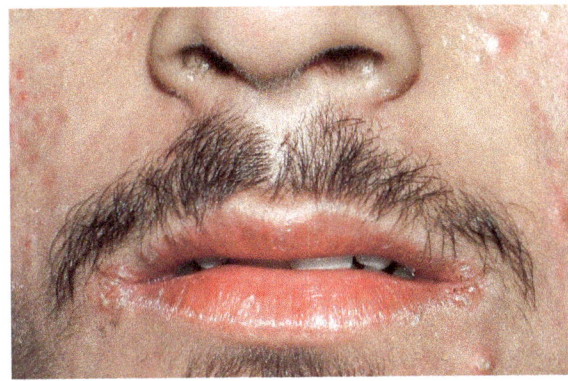

a. Tetracycline
b. Isotretinoin
c. Azithromycin
d. Minocycline

757. Which type of post-acne scar this patient is having?

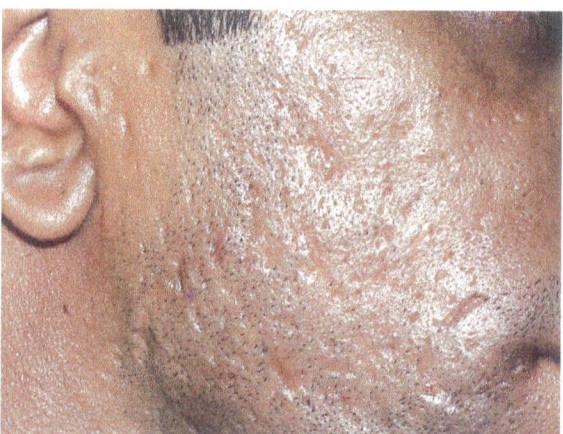

a. Anetoderma
b. Box scar
c. Ice pick scar
d. Rolling scar

759. This patient presented with atrophic striae after prolonged use of some cream. Which one of the following creams has he applied?

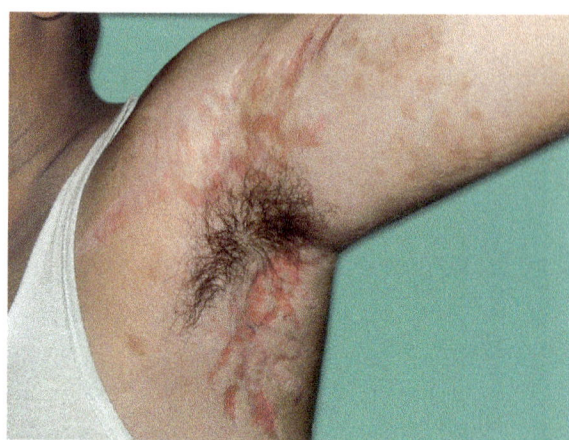

a. Potent corticosteroid cream
b. Luliconazole cream
c. Nadifloxacin cream
d. Fusidic acid cream

758. This patient complained of multiple red discrete plaques on his scalp having white scales. What is the closest clinical diagnosis?

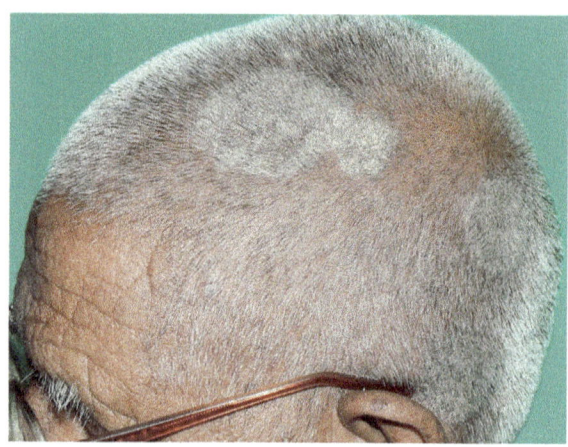

a. Tinea capitis
b. Seborrheic capitis
c. Scalp psoriasis
d. Lichen planus

760. Following is the diagrammatic representation of various cutaneous receptors. What is the name of the receptor with question mark?

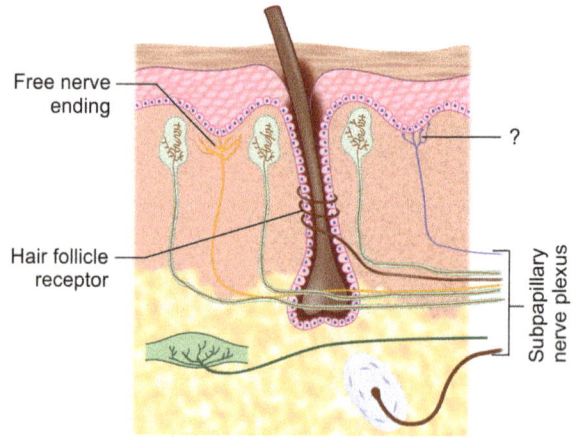

a. Merkel's receptor
b. Meissner's corpuscle
c. Ruffini's corpuscle
d. Pacinian corpuscle

761. Following vitiligo patient developed redness and blistering during treatment. Which one of the following treatments is a cause for these blisters?

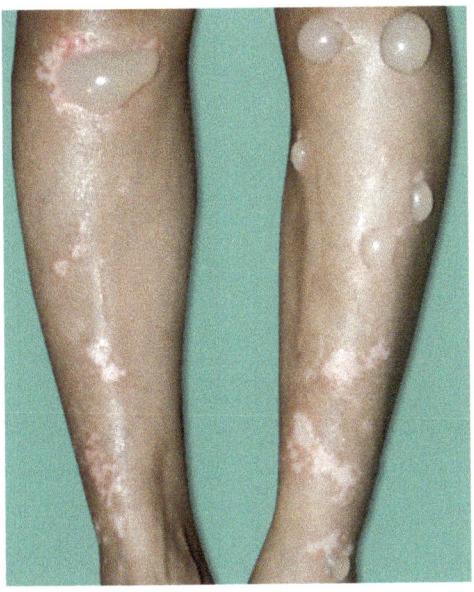

a. Systemic PUVA therapy
b. Narrow band phototherapy
c. Topical PUVA therapy
d. Tacrolimus ointment 1%

762. This patient complained of hoarseness of voice, puffiness of face, eyelids and hands for the last one year. What is the closest option of clinical diagnosis for him?

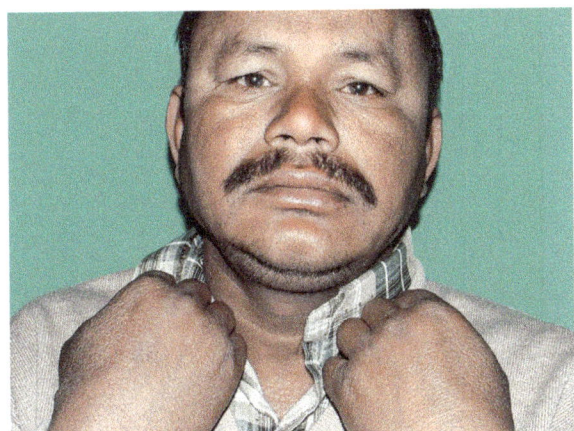

a. Chronic urticaria
b. Myxedema
c. Lepromatous leprosy
d. Systemic sclerosis

763. A 6-month-old baby developed psoriasiform lesions on buttocks and lower extremities just after weaning. Perioral region is also affected *(MCQ 748)*. What is the closest clinical diagnosis?

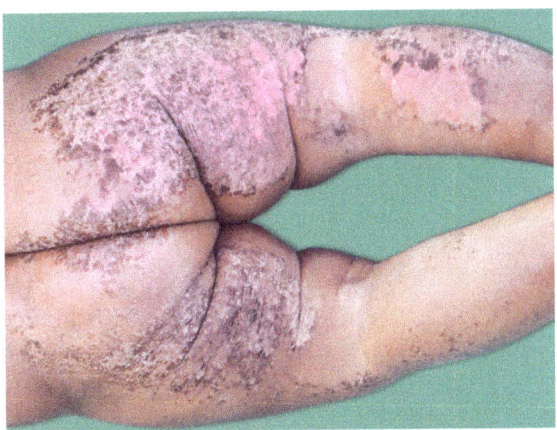

a. Impetigo contagiosa
b. Atopic dermatitis
c. Acrodermatitis enteropathica (ADE)
d. Psoriasis

764. This infant was brought with swelling face with excessive growth of hair on forehead and checks. It was found that he had been taking a drug for the last many months from an unqualified practitioner. Which one of the followings is that drug?

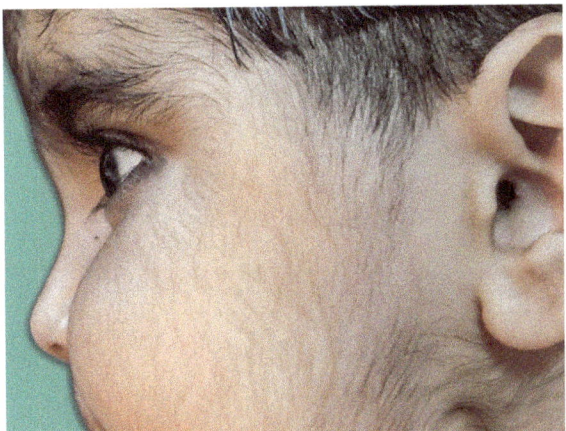

a. Systemic corticosteroids
b. B-complex syrup
c. Iron syrup
d. Vitamin D drops

765. Following is the diagrammatic representation of an arthropod. Which one of the following options is correct for this diagram?

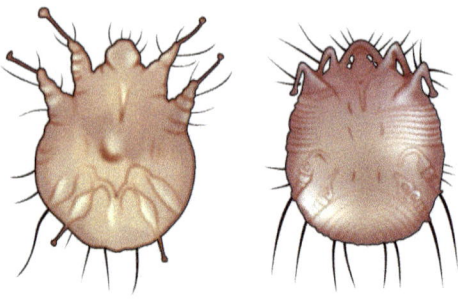

Male   Female

a. Pediculus humanus capitis (Head louse)
b. Sarcoptes scabiei male and female
c. Pediculus humanus corporis (body/clothing louse)
d. *Phthirus pubis* or crab louse

766. This patient complained of a thick, well-defined red plaque in front of his left ear for the last three years. What is the most appropriate option for clinical diagnosis?

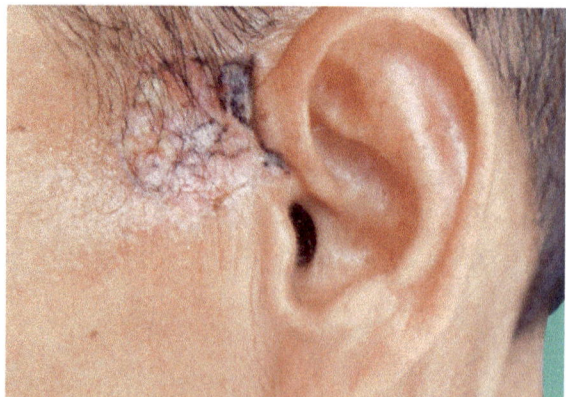

a. Squamous cell carcinoma
b. Basal cell carcinoma
c. Chronic cutaneous lupus erythematosus (CCLE)
d. Lupus Vulgaris

767. Which one of the following systemic drugs has led to worsening of tinea and appearance of striae on the abdominal wall?

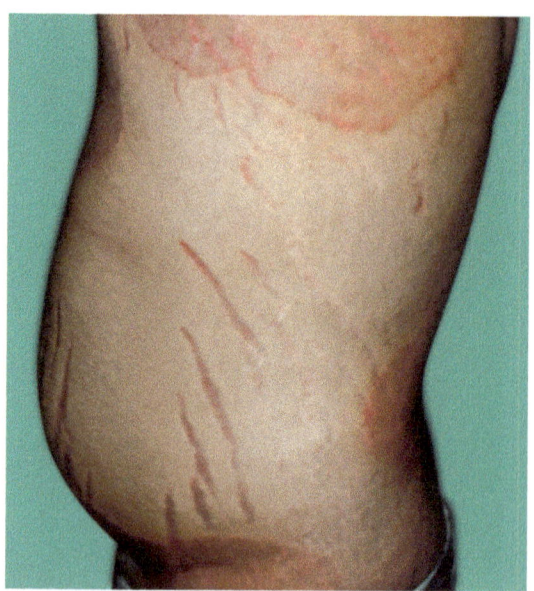

a. Antiepileptic drugs
b. Systemic corticosteroids
c. Antitubercular drugs
d. Isotretinoin

768. A 3-year-old child presented with darkening and thickening of his hands and feet which started at the age of 10 days. Similar changes are also present around neck, knees and other parts of body. Hair and nails are normal. What is the clinical diagnosis?

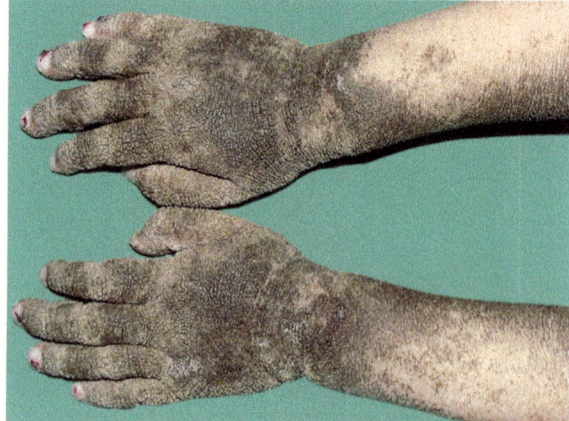

a. Malignancy associated acanthosis nigricans (AN)
b. Congenital acanthosis nigricans
c. Pseudo-acanthosis nigricans

769. A 5-year-old child presented with itchy, violaceous papules on both soles. What is the closest clinical diagnosis?

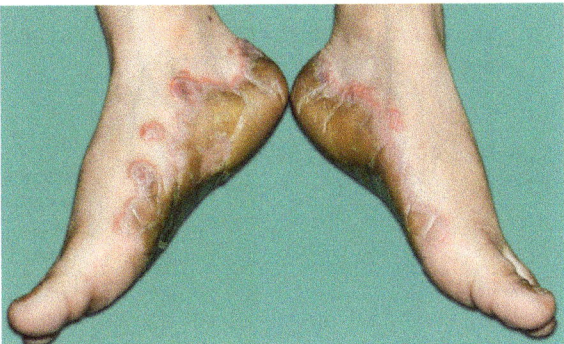

a. Psoriasis
b. Lichen planus
c. Eczema soles

770. Following is the diagrammatic representation of levels of cleavages in various vesiculobullous disorders. What is the level of cleavage in pemphigus vulgaris?

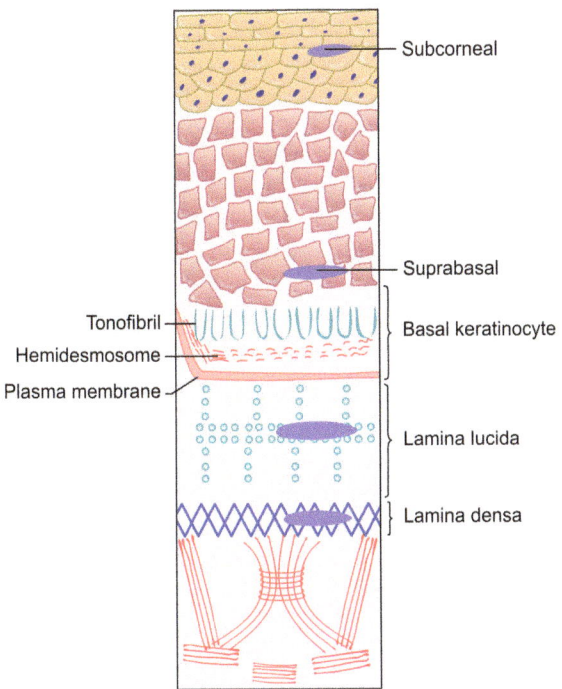

a. Subcorneal
b. Lamina lucida
c. Suprabasal
d. Just below lamina densa

771. This patient complained of intense itching and tingling sensation in a hyperpigmented patch in the middle of his back for the least 2–3 years. What is the closest clinical diagnosis?

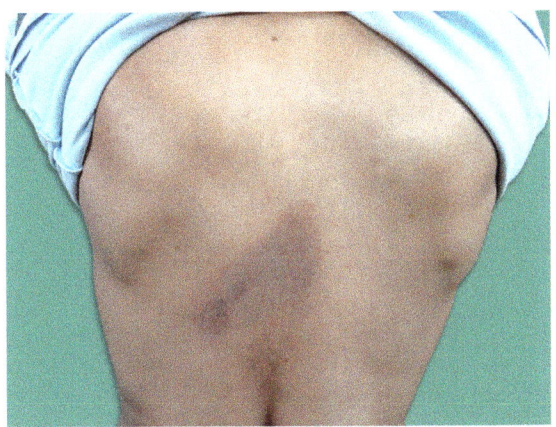

a. Macular amyloidosis
b. Notalgia paresthetica
c. Lichen simplex chronicus

772. This patient complained of severe itching and scaling in both palms for last one year with no other skin lesions on other parts of body. What is the closest clinical diagnosis?

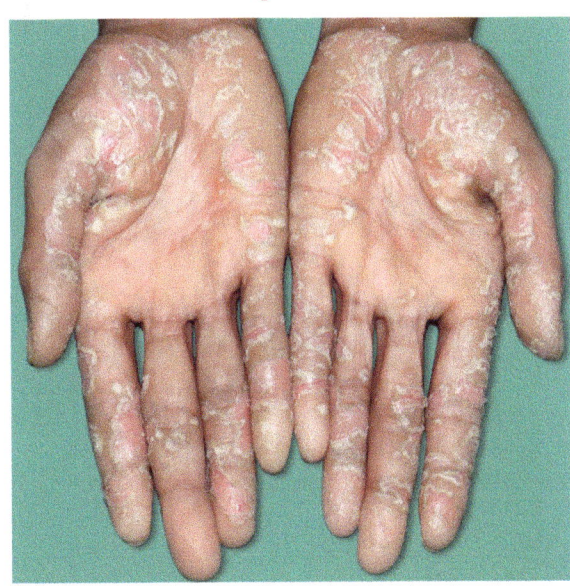

a. Psoriasis of palms
b. Hyperkeratotic eczema of palms
c. Dermatophytosis palms
d. Palmar keratoderma

773. This patient presented with red scaly itchy patches on buttocks. What is the closest clinical diagnosis?

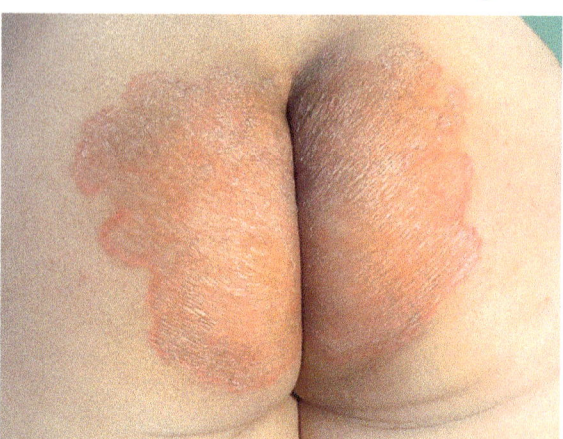

a. Tinea corporis
b. Psoriasis
c. Dermatitis buttocks

774. This patient presented with thick and white scales on scalp limited to hair line. Eyebrows also showed similar involvement. What is the closest clinical diagnosis?

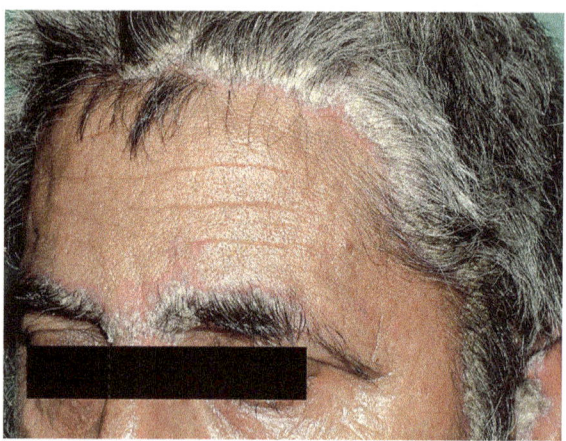

a. Psoriasis
b. Seborrheic dermatitis

775. Following is the diagrammatic representation of an intraepidermal vesicle. Peripheral to the vesicle in the adjoining epidermis, there is a reticular degeneration with the presence of multinucleate giant cells. Inside the nucleus, inclusion bodies are also seen. What is the diagnosis?

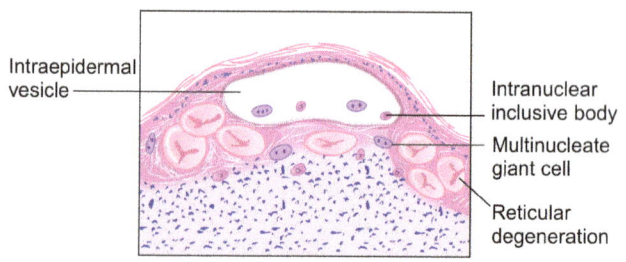

a. Varicella or herpes simplex
b. Pemphigus foliaceous
c. Pemphigus vulgaris
d. Hailey-Hailey disease

776. A 70-year-old female presented with a single, slowly developed, rough pigmented plaque. What is the closest clinical diagnosis?

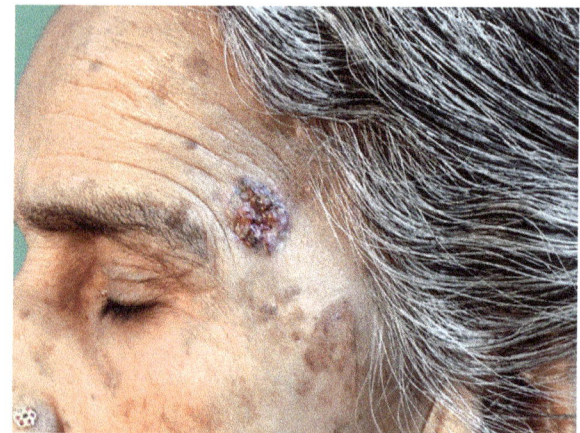

a. SCC on photodamaged skin
b. Basal cell carcinoma (BCC)
c. Chronic cutaneous lupus erythematosus (CCLE)
d. Actinic keratosis

777. She presented with three psoriasiform plaques on trunk and face for the last one year. Plaques showed an advancing peripheral border and trailing scar in the center. There is no loss of sensations in the plaques. What is the clinical diagnosis?

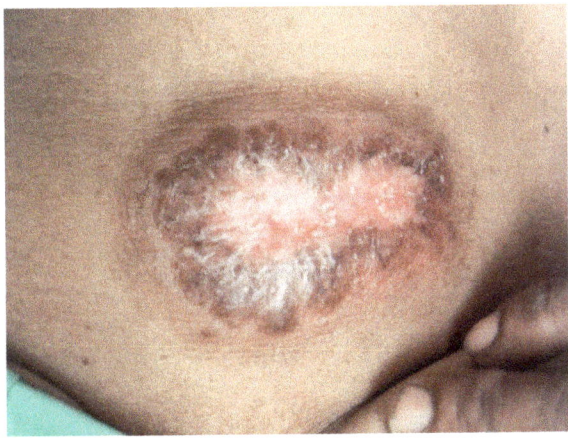

a. Tuberculoid leprosy
b. Psoriasis
c. Lupus vulgaris
d. Chronic cutaneous lupus erythematosus (CCLE)

778. This lady presented with multiple, rough, hyperkeratotic papules on dorsum of hands only. What is the clinical diagnosis?

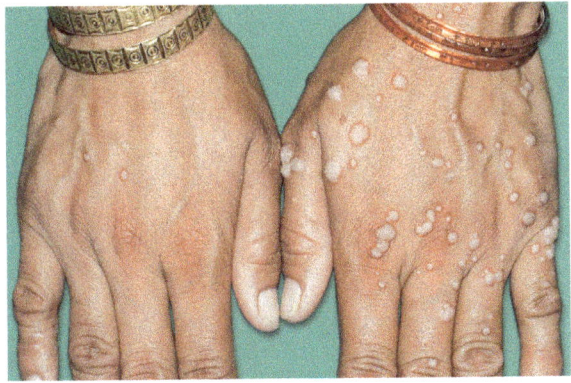

a. Common warts
b. Lichen planus

779. Following figure is the magnified picture of lesions on back. These lesions have developed four days after fever. What is the diagnosis?

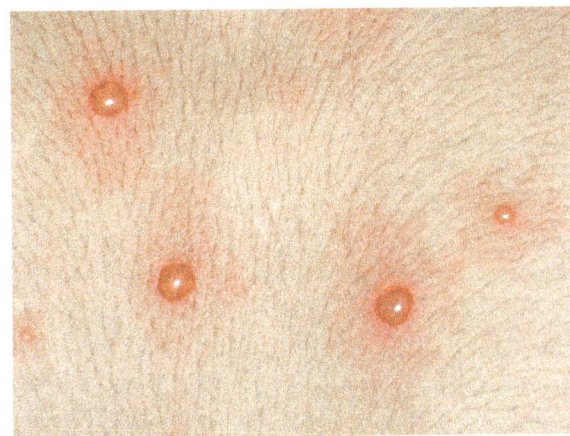

a. Chickenpox (varicella)
b. Molluscum contagiosum
c. Lichen planus

780. Following is the diagrammatic representation of a Tzanck smear made from a vesicle. It is showing multinucleate giant cells and intranuclear inclusion bodies. What is the diagnosis?

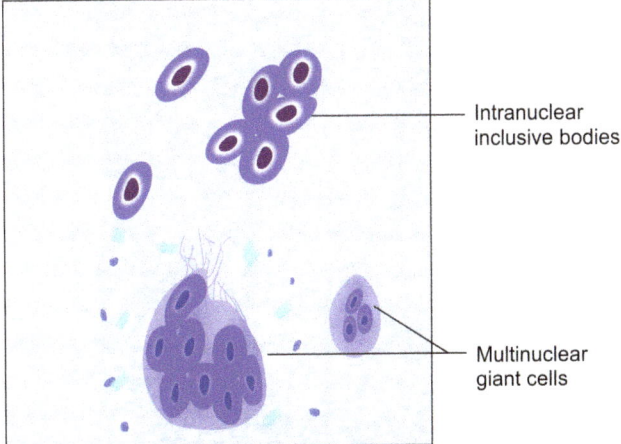

a. Pemphigus vulgaris or foliaceous
b. Herpes simplex or varicella zoster virus infection
c. Bullous pemphigoid
d. Chronic bullous dermatosis of childhood (CBDC)

781. This patient complained of multiple violaceous papules on the undersurface of prepuce for the last one year. What is the clinical diagnosis?

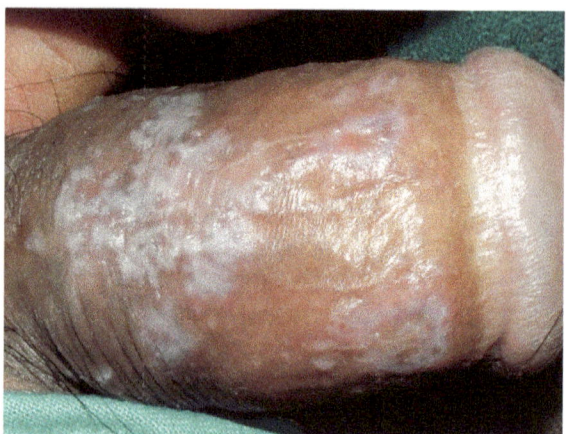

a. Lichen planus
b. Psoriasis on glans
c. Fixed drug eruption (FDE)
d. Venereal warts

782. For this patient of acne which antiacne systemic drug is most appropriate?

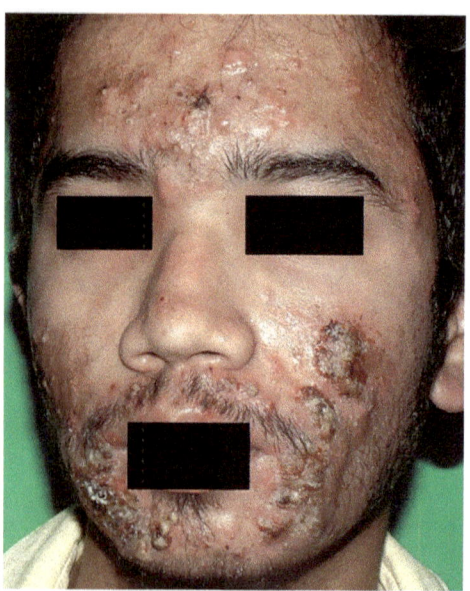

a. Tetracycline
b. Doxycycline
c. Minocycline
d. Isotretinoin

783. This patient complained of multiple painless small vesicles on upper lip only for the last four days. What is the most appropriate clinical diagnosis?

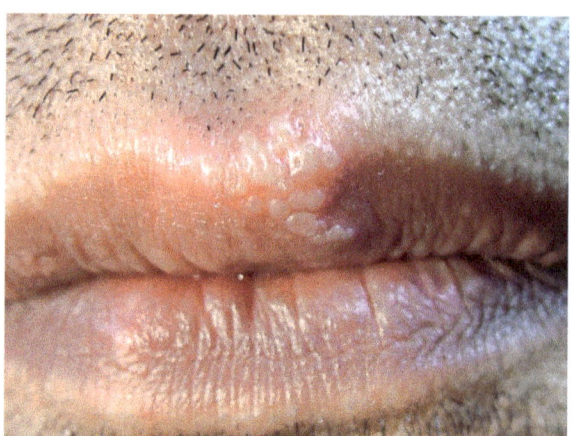

a. Fixed drug eruption (FDE)
b. Herpes simplex labialis
c. Herpes zoster

784. This patient came with striae on his abdominal wall after the prolonged use of some systemic drug. Which one of the followings is that systemic drug?

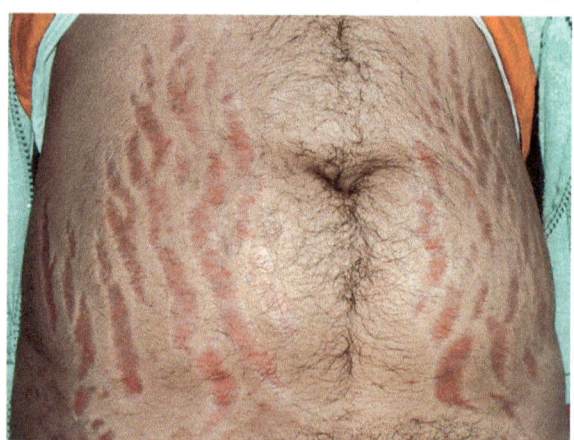

a. Systemic corticosteroids
b. Antitubercular drugs
c. Antiepileptic drugs
d. Vitamin A

Chapter 4 ✦ MCQs of Dermatology, Venereology and Leprology

785. Following is the diagrammatic representation of an autosomal dominant condition. It is showing grains[1] in horny layer, corps ronds[2] in the stratum spinosum and suprabasal cleft. Which one of the following options is correct for this?

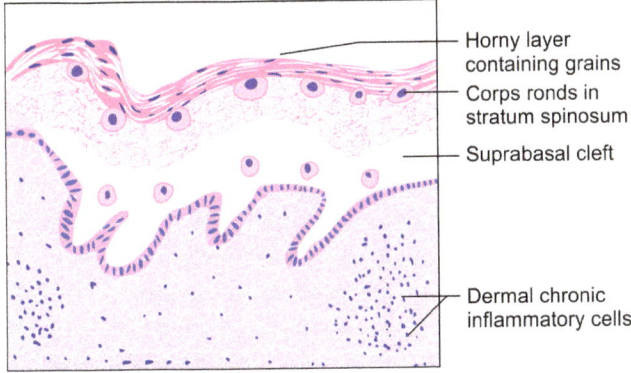

  a. Epidermolysis bullosa
  b. Darier's disease
  c. Hailey-Hailey disease
  d. Pemphigus vulgaris

786. This patient presented with multiple, dry, rough, hyperkeratotic papules and nodules in the anal region. What is the closest clinical diagnosis?

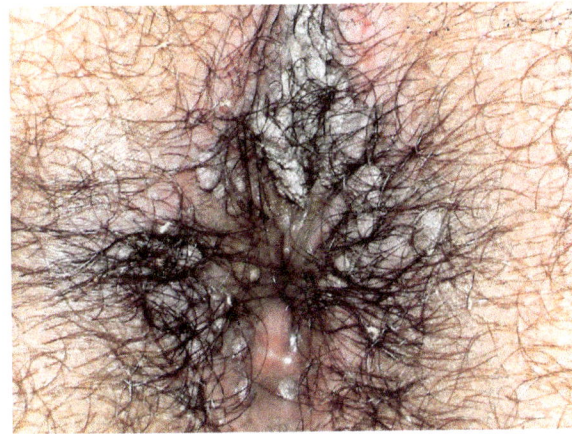

  a. Condylomata lata
  b. Condylomata acuminata

787. This patient presented with multiple small well-defined, itchy papulosquamous lesions on the dorsum of right hand. Involvement also extends on to the palmar surface. What is the closest clinical diagnosis?

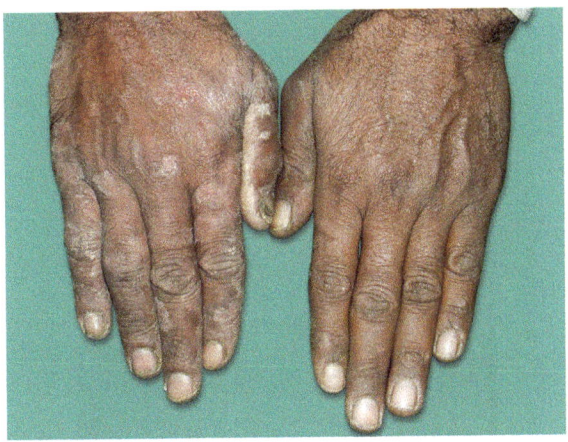

  a. Tinea manuum
  b. Dermatitis or eczema
  c. Psoriasis

788. This man presented with multiple, asymptomatic, smooth, slightly elevated plane topped, rounded or polygonal, 1–5 mm sized skin-colored papules on face. What is the clinical diagnosis?

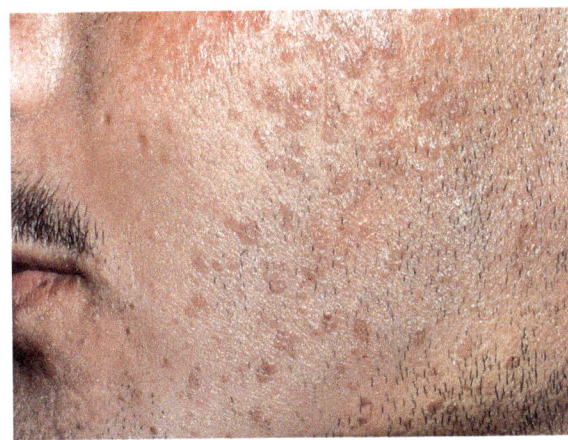

  a. Actinic keratosis
  b. Acne vulgaris
  c. Plane warts

---

[1]**Grains:** They resembles parakeratotic cells. Their nuclei are elongated looking grain like.
[2]**Corps ronds:** They have central homogeneous and basophilic nucleus surrounded by a clear halo.

789. Two days after fever, a 25-year-old male developed these lesions on trunk, extremities and face. What is the clinical diagnosis?

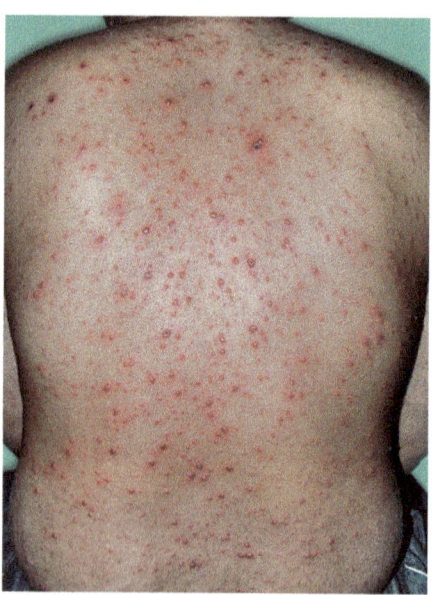

a. Drug-induced acne
b. Chickenpox
c. Morbilliform rash
d. Exanthematous rash

790. A 10-year-old child presented with many groups of grouped vesicles on left side of forehead, nose and temporal region for the last four days. It was accompanied by severe pain. What is the clinical diagnosis?

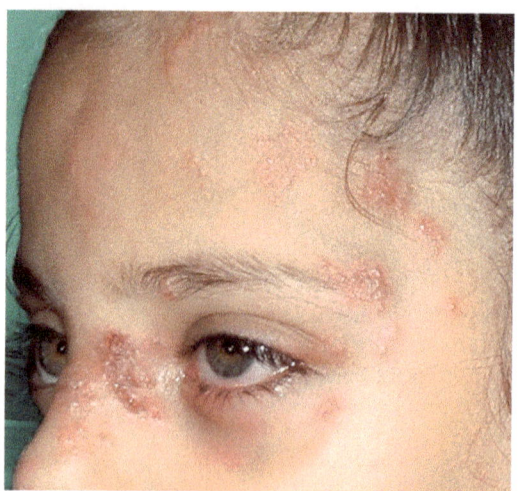

a. Herpes simplex
b. Herpes zoster
c. *Paederus dermatitis*

791. This patient presented with asymptomatic, hyperkeratotic, indurated papules and plaques affecting his right sole only for the last one year. What is the closest clinical diagnosis?

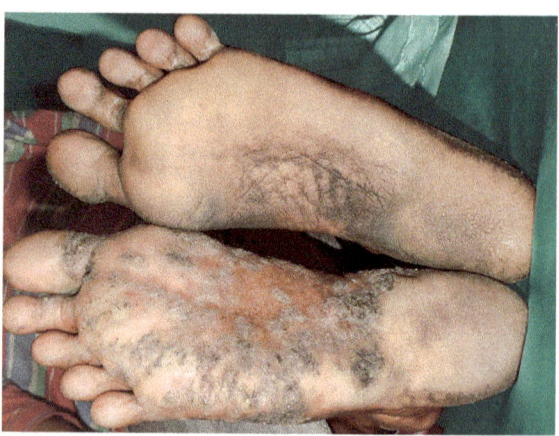

a. Superficial plantar warts
b. Plantar psoriasis
c. Tuberculosis verrucosa cutis (TVC)
d. Plantar eczema

792. A 6-year-old child presented with a well-defined red patch of hair loss studded with tiny pustules. What is the closest clinical diagnosis?

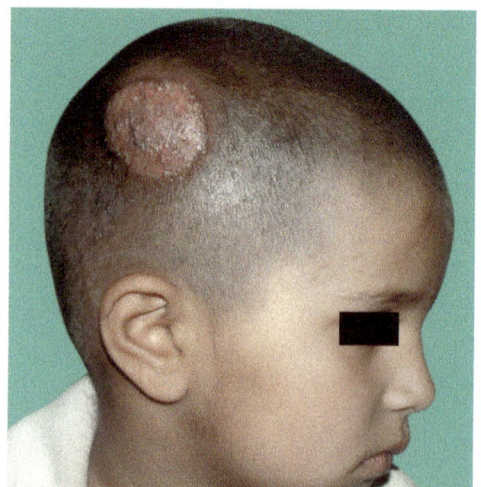

a. Alopecia areata
b. Trichotillomania
c. Tinea capitis

793. A young girl having psoriasis received many injections of steroids from an unqualified practitioner. It has led to appearance of minute pustules on the psoriatic plaques. What is the most appropriate clinical diagnosis for her?

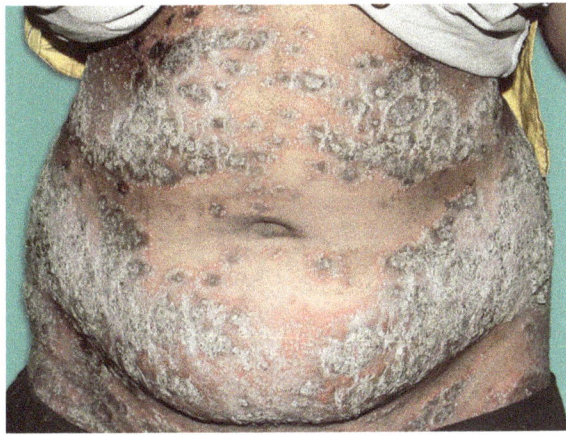

a. Generalized psoriasis with secondary infection
b. Generalized pustular psoriasis
c. Impetigo herpetiformis
d. Acropustulosis

794. Following is the diagrammatic representation of direct immunofluorescence findings in a vesiculobullous disease. It is showing a linear pattern. Which one of the following options is correct for this patient?

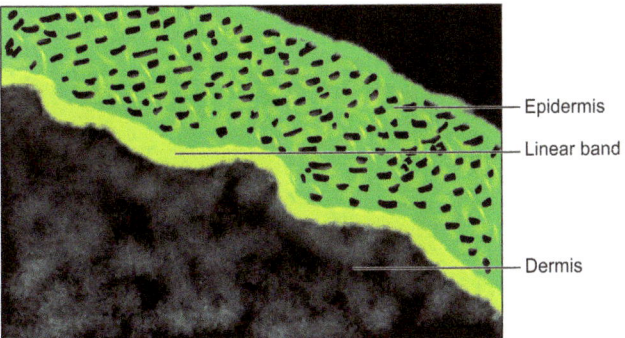

a. Pemphigus vulgaris or pemphigus foliaceous
b. Bullous pemphigoid or linear IgA disease
c. Epidermolysis bullosa simplex
d. Erythema multiforme

795. This patient complained of burning, itching and diffuse redness of dorsa of toes of both feet. It is recuring every winter for the last 3-4 years. What is the diagnosis?

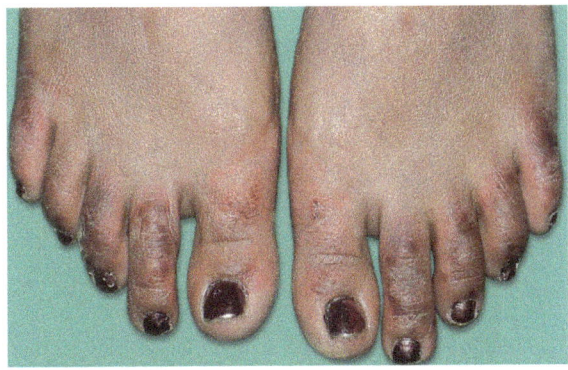

a. Raynaud's phenomenon
b. Chilblains
c. Livedo reticularis

796. This patient complained of the development of hypertrophic, verrucous fleshy growth on the dorsum of big toe in the last six months. What is the closest clinical diagnosis?

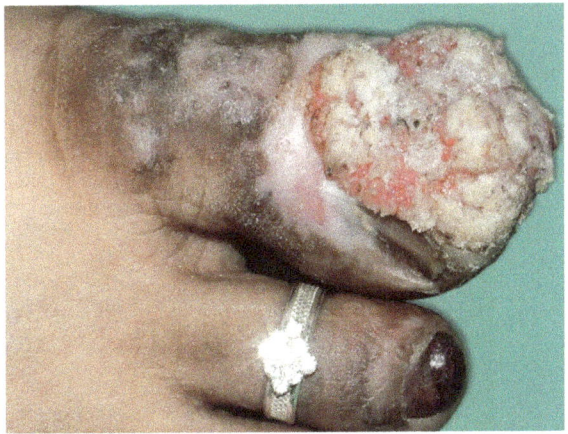

a. Tuberculosis verrucosa cutis (TVC)
b. Pyogenic granuloma
c. Squamous cell carcinoma

797. This patient complained of redness, soreness, irritation, tiny papules, pustules and collarette of white papules and pustules on glans. There is no history of sexual exposure. What is the closest clinical diagnosis?

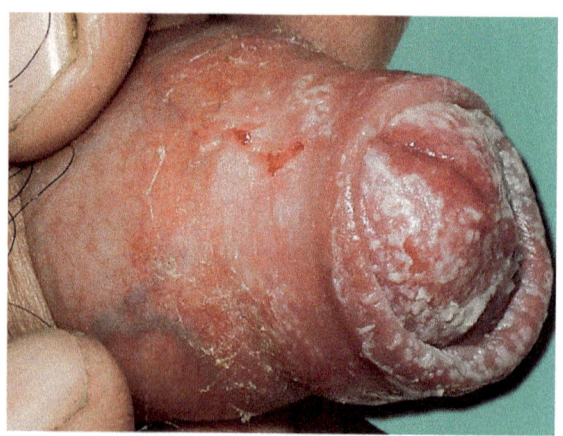

a. Genital skin atrophy due to prolonged use of steroid cream
b. Candidal balanoposthitis due to underlying diabetes
c. Fixed drug eruption (FDE)
d. Secondary syphilis

798. Following in the diagrammatic representation of dermoepidermal junction. What is the name of the layer with question mark?

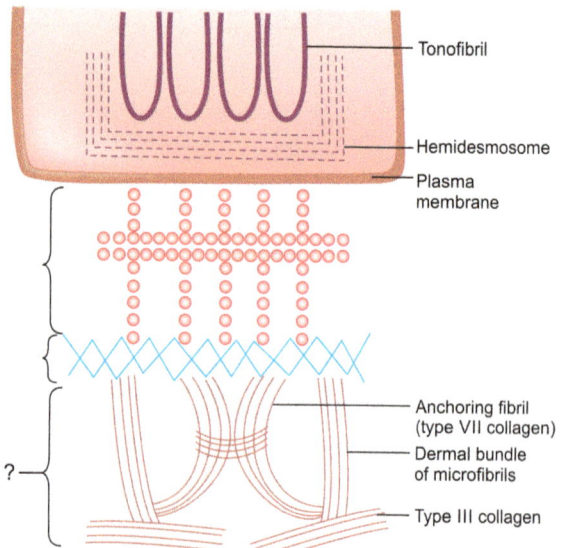

a. Lamina fibroreticularis
b. Sub-basal dense plaques
c. Lamina densa
d. Lamina lucida

799. This lady presented with itching and redness in the groins accompanied by polydipsia and polyuria. What is the clinical diagnosis?

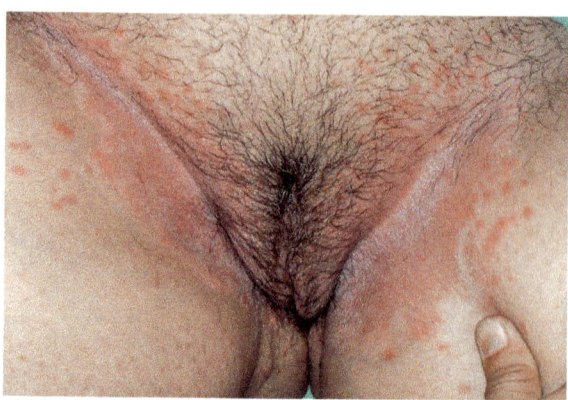

a. Tinea cruris
b. Candidiasis groins
c. Intertrigo
d. Flexural psoriasis

800. Following is the diagrammatic representation of histopathology showing elongated rete ridges pointing towards center and presence of koilocytotic cells in granular cell layer. Epidermal cells have dense clumps of basophilic keratohyalin granules. What is the diagnosis?

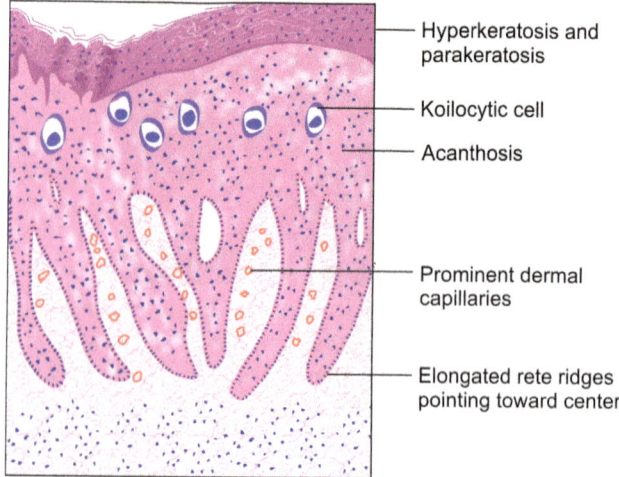

a. Psoriasis
b. Lichen planus
c. Wart
d. Molluscum contagiosum

801. This patient complained of red plaques in both groins. He also had red plaques on other parts of body. What is the closest clinical diagnosis?

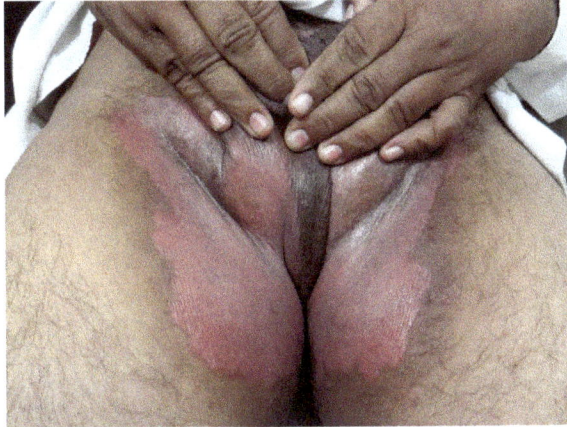

a. Tinea cruris
b. Candidiasis groins
c. Flexural psoriasis
d. Intertrigo groins

802. A 6-year-old child presented with multiple itchy plaques on shins. What is the closest clinical diagnosis?

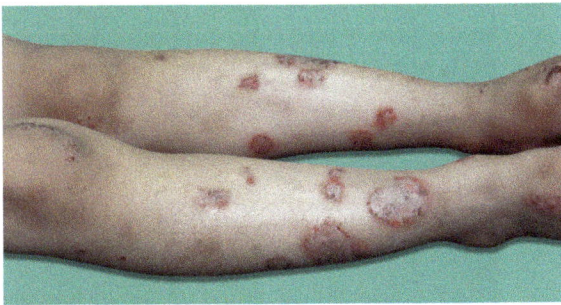

a. Infected tinea corporis
b. Discoid eczema
c. Psoriasis

803. This patient complained of asymptomatic dark macules studded with scales on both palms, soles, forearms and trunk. What is the closest clinical diagnosis?

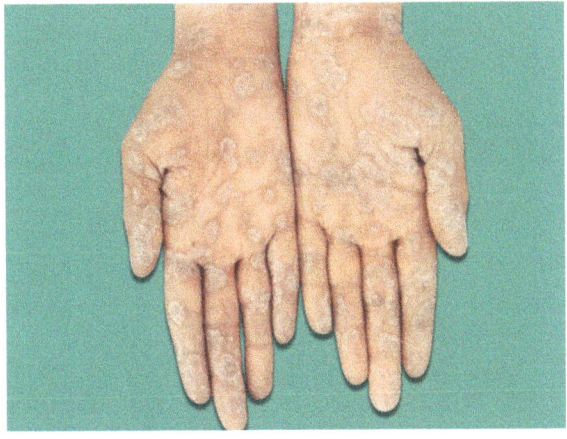

a. Lichen planus
b. Secondary syphilis
c. Hyperkeratotic eczema
d. Keratolysis exfoliativa

804. This patient complained of pin head sized asymptomatic papules on the coronal margin for the last 3–4 years. There is a h/o sexual exposure with a commercial sex worker about one year back. What is the clinical diagnosis?

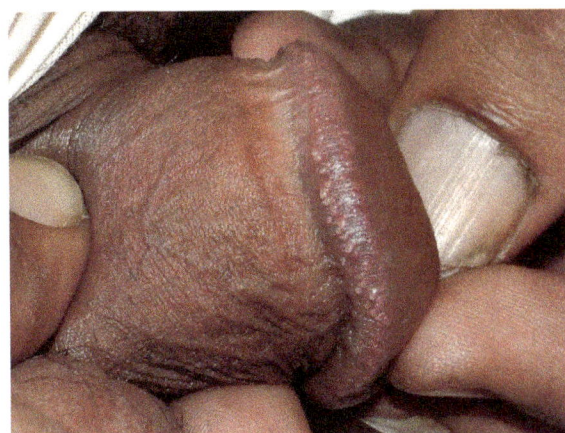

a. Genital warts
b. Pearly penile papules
c. Secondary syphilis
d. Herpes genitalis

805. Following diagrammatic histopathology is showing (i) Hyperkeratosis and parakeratosis. (ii) Aggregations of neutrophils in parakeratotic layer (Munro's microabscesses) and in upper spinous layer (spongiform pustules of Kogoj). (iii) Granular layer is absent. (iv) Elongated rete ridges show clubbing in lower portions. What is the diagnosis?

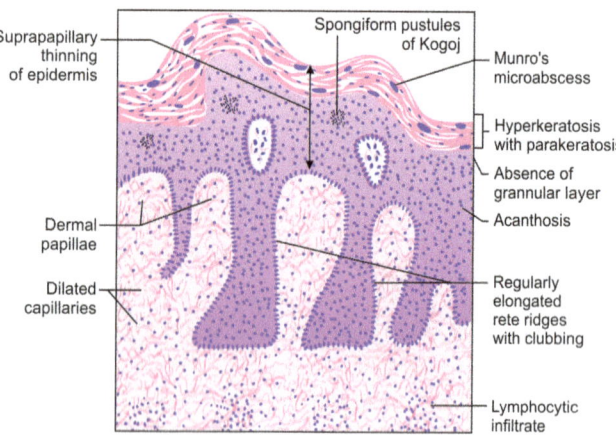

a. Lichen planus
b. Warts
c. Psoriasis
d. Molluscum contagiosum

806. She complained of redness and itching on face. She is applying a cream for the last 1½ years. Which of the following creams she is applying?

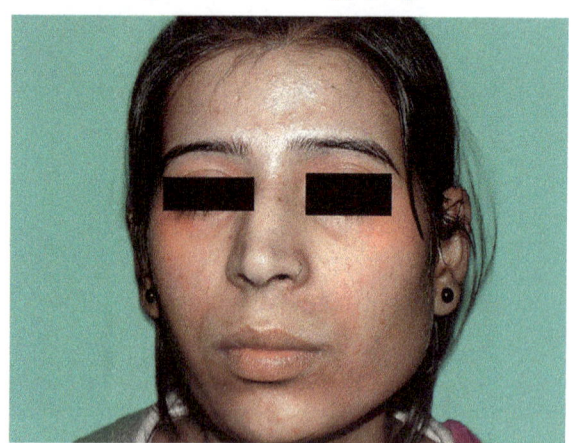

a. Corticosteroid cream
b. Adapalene 1%
c. Moisturizing cream
d. Sunscreen cream

807. A middle-aged man presented with an indolent, asymptomatic, moist, shiny, well-demarcated red patch on glans and adjoining inner surface of prepuce.

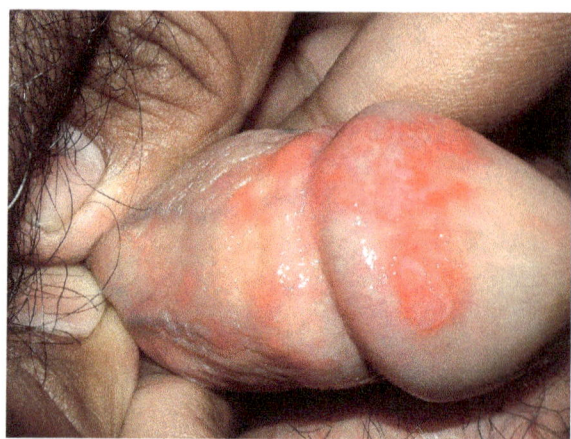

a. Candidal balanitis
b. Psoriasis
c. Zoon's balanitis
d. Erythroplasia of Queyrat

808. She complained of depigmentation in front of her ankle joint. There is no depigmentation on other parts of body. What is most appropriate diagnosis for her?

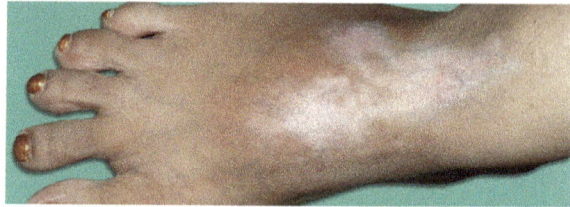

a. Focal vitiligo
b. Depigmentation following intralesional steroid
c. Prolonged use of tacrolimus 1% ointment

809. A 10-year-old child presented with rough, hyperkeratotic and follicular papules on the skin of knees and elbows for the last two years. What is the closest clinical diagnosis?

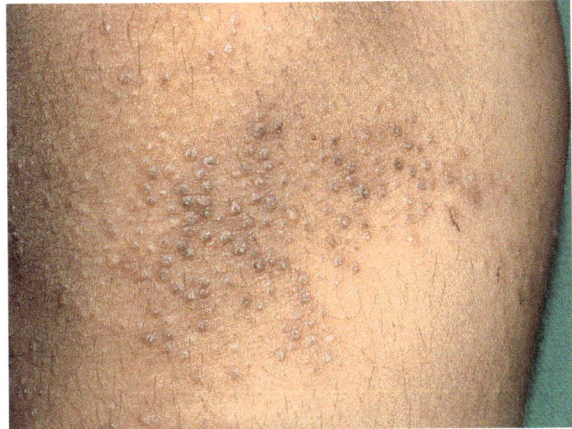

a. Follicular lichen planus
b. Phrynoderma (hypovitaminosis A)
c. Keratosis pilaris

810. Following is a diagrammatic histopathology of a plaque on face. It is showing (i) Basal cell layer liquefaction degeneration. (ii) Immediately below the epidermis there are connective tissue degenerative changes, i.e., hyalinization, edema and fibrinoid change. (iii) Patchy dermal infiltrate around dermoepidermal junction and appendages. What is the diagnosis?

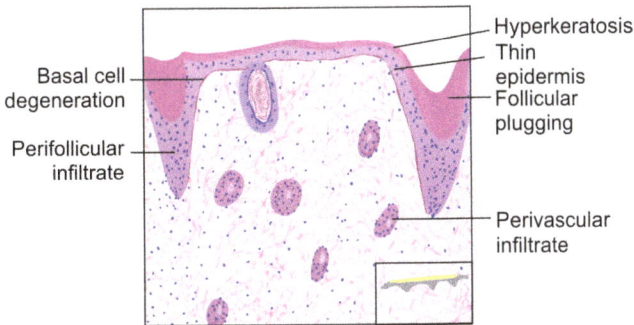

a. Psoriasis
b. Lichen planus
c. Lupus erythematosus
d. Wart

811. This patient complained of asymptomatic yellowish thickening of plantar surface of forefeet for the last many years. What is the clinical diagnosis?

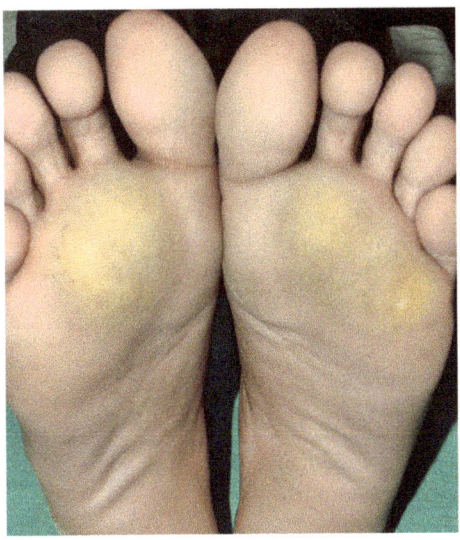

a. Focal plantar keratoderma
b. Callus (tylomata)

812. This patient presented with thick, hypertrophic and itchy lesion on chest for the last four years. It has developed several months after a minor injury and is not regressing with time. What is the clinical diagnosis?

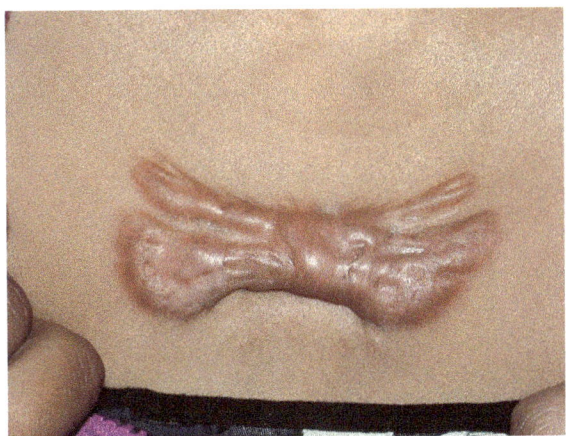

a. Keloid
b. Hypertrophic scar

813. This patient presented with highly pruritic, closely placed papules on shins. What is the diagnosis?

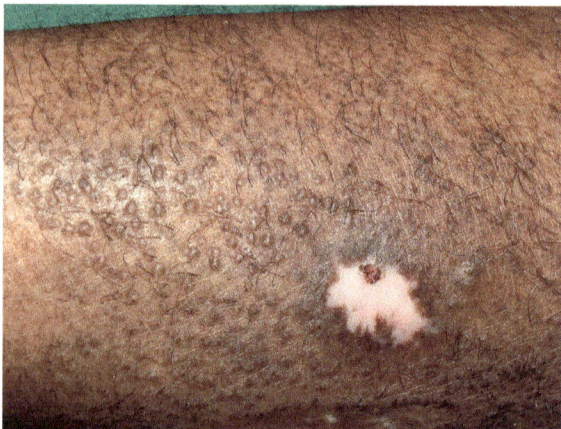

a. Lichen planus
b. Lichen amyloidosis
c. Prurigo nodularis

814. This patient gradually developed multiple tumors on his face in the last five years. Similar lesions are also present on the back *(MCQ 823)*. What is the clinical diagnosis?

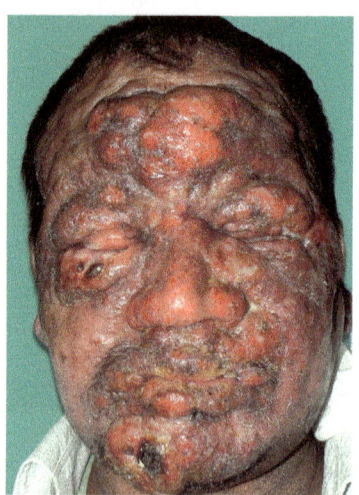

a. Lepromatous leprosy
b. Tumor stage mycosis fungoides
c. Chronic actinic dermatitis (CAD)

815. In the following diagram, what is the name of the area just above the bulb of the follicle?

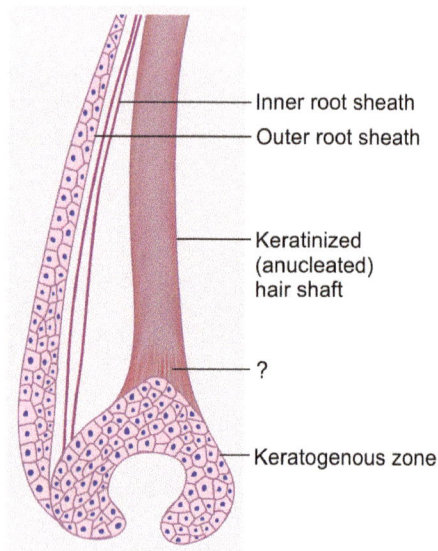

a. Isthmus of the follicle
b. Stem cells
c. Adamson's fringe
d. Suprabulbar part

816. One month old child presented with easy blistering of feet due to mild mechanical trauma. Hair, nails and mucosa are normal. His father is also suffering from similar disorder. What is the closest clinical diagnosis?

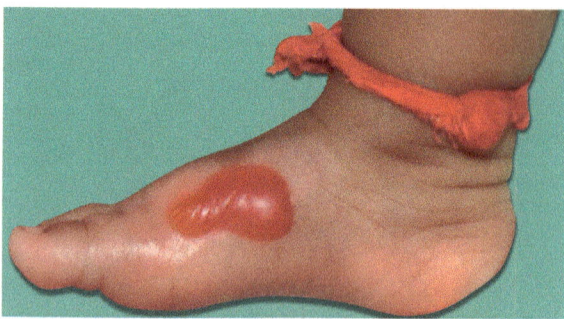

a. Epidermolysis bullosa simplex
b. Chronic benign familial pemphigus

817. A 50-year-old female presented with annular patches on her elbow with no inflammation, scaling, itching or loss of sensations. What is the clinical diagnosis?

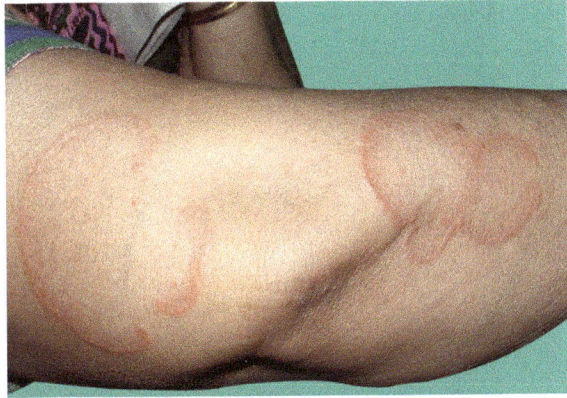

a. Annular psoriasis
b. Mid-borderline leprosy
c. Tinea incognito
d. Granuloma annulare

818. An uncircumcised man presented with an indolent, asymptomatic moist, shiny, well demarcated red patch on glans and opposing inner surface of prepuce. What is the clinical diagnosis?

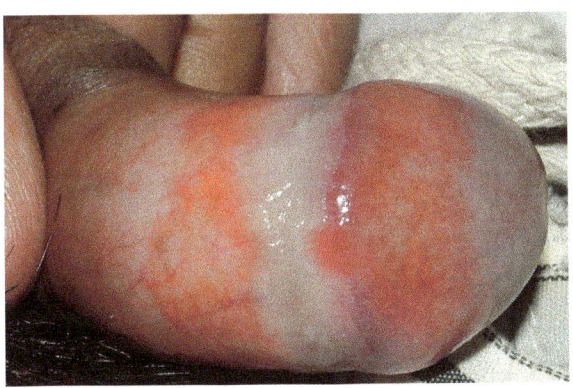

a. Secondary syphilis
b. Erythroplasia of Queyrat
c. Zoon's balanitis
d. Candidal balanitis

819. A 9-month-old child was brought with a circumscribed, scarlet red, smooth and lobulated single tumor or his cheek which appeared in first month of life. What is the clinical diagnosis?

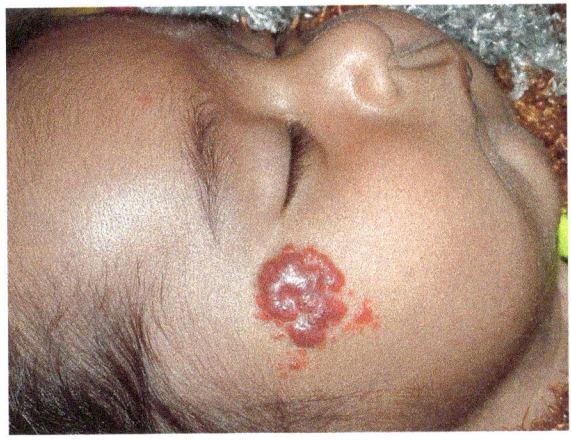

a. Strawberry hemangioma
b. Port-wine stain
c. Salmon patch

820. What is the name of the structure with question mark in the following diagram?

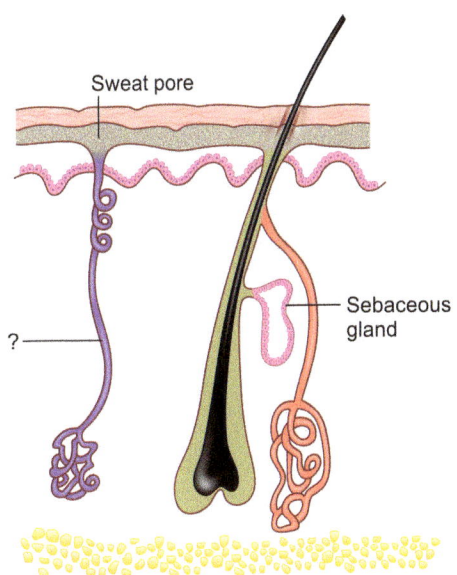

a. Sebaceous gland
b. Eccrine sweat gland
c. Apocrine sweat gland
d. Adamson's fringe

821. A 2-month-old baby presented with abnormal asymptomatic yellowish thickening of soles. His father is also having abnormal thickening of palms *(MCQ 486)* and soles *(MCQ 192)*. What is the clinical diagnosis?

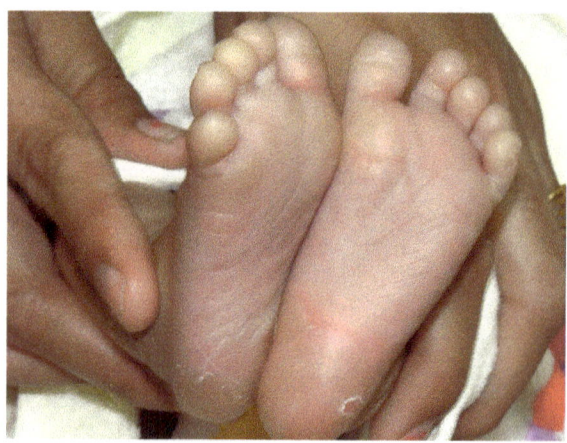

a. Diffuse plantar keratoderma
b. Tylosis

822. This patient complained of extremely itchy cutaneous nodules on lower extremities. What is the clinical diagnosis?

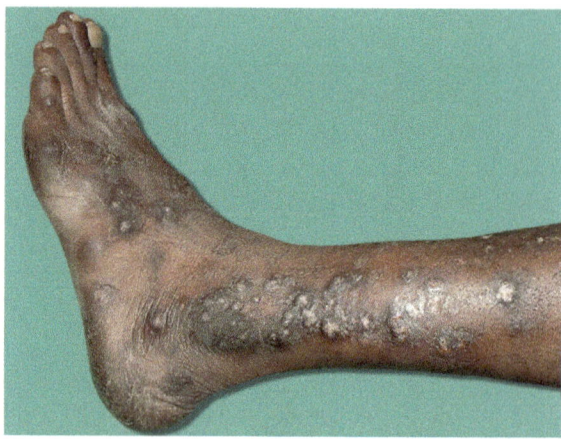

a. Lichen planus
b. Prurigo nodularis
c. Lichen amyloidosis

823. This patient presented with a slowly developed tumor on his back. Similar tumors developed on his face also *(MCQ 814)*. What is the closest clinical diagnosis?

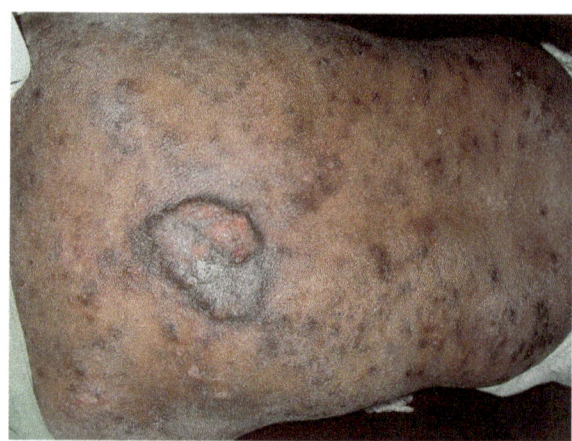

a. Squamous cell carcinoma (SCC)
b. Mycosis fungoides tumor stage
c. B-cell cutaneous lymphoma

824. A diabetic patient had a sexual exposure with a commercial sex worker. After taking some tablets, he developed redness and discharge. What is closest clinical diagnosis?

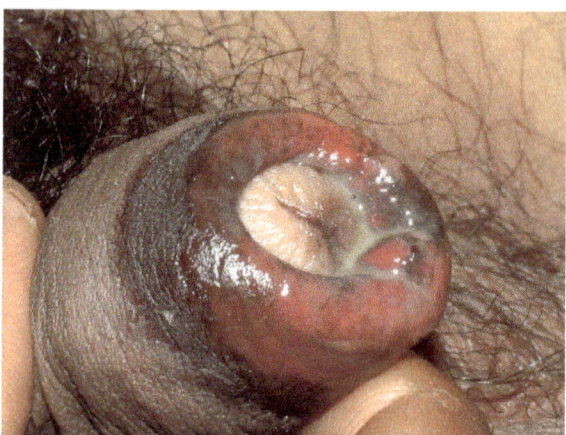

a. Candidal balanoposthitis
b. Secondary syphilis
c. Fixed drug eruption

825. Following is the diagram of structure of nail unit. What is the name of the structure in deep brown color with question mark?

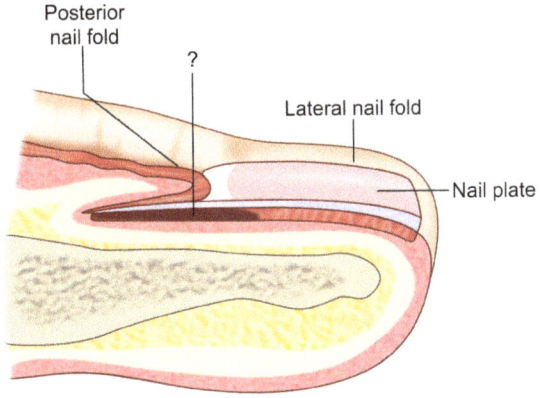

a. Hyponychium
b. Nail matrix
c. Nail bed
d. Cuticle

826. A nonsmoker patient presented with a painless, slowly penetrating ulcer opposite to the head of first metatarsal. Ulcer is circular, punched out with surrounding callosity. Sensations in the feet are impaired. The pulsations of dorsalis pedis artery on dorsum of foot are not felt. Which is the closest clinical diagnosis?

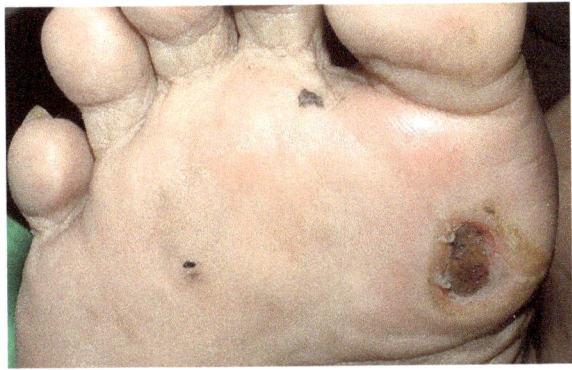

a. Tropical ulcer
b. Diabetic trophic ulcer
c. Leprotic trophic ulcer
d. Buerger's disease

827. A 2-year-old child was brought with an asymptomatic large hypopigmented patch. What is the clinical diagnosis?

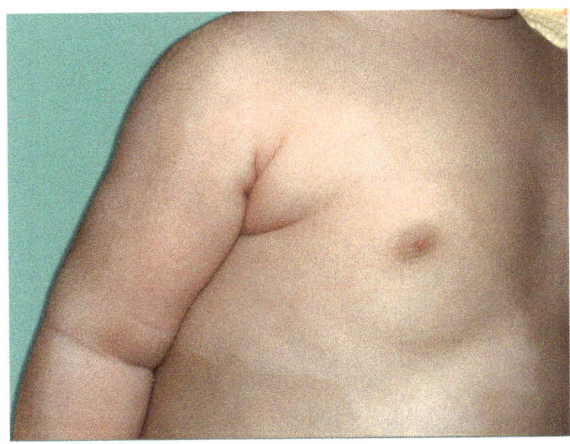

a. Nevus anemicus
b. Nevus depigmentosus
c. Focal vitiligo
d. Tuberous sclerosis

828. During chemotherapy for breast cancer, she complained of dark pigmented macules of various parts of body. What is it?

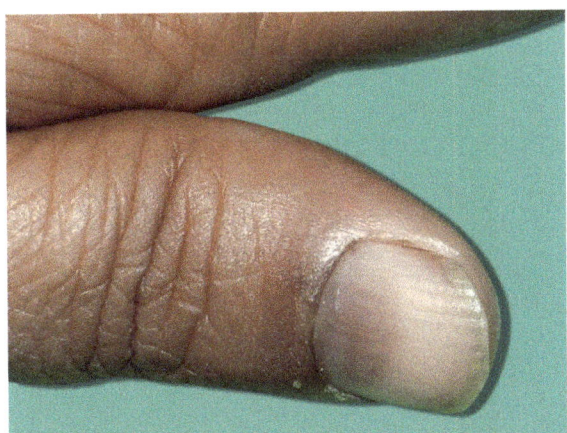

a. Hutchinson's sign
b. Pseudo-Hutchinson's sign

829. This patient presented with 1–3 mm sized, firm and erythematous papules on trunk and extremities without any discomfort or itching. What is the clinical diagnosis?

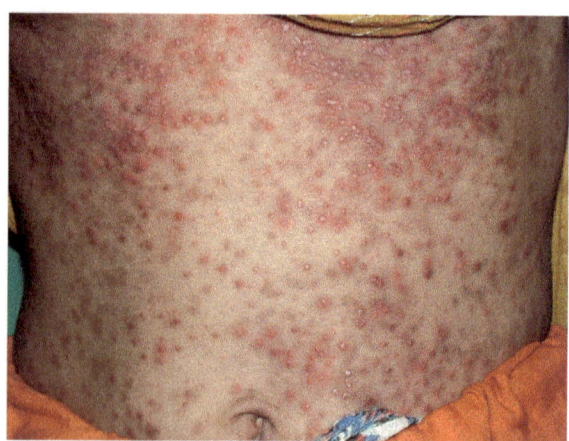

a. Miliaria rubra
b. Miliaria profunda
c. Miliaria crystallina

830. Following is the diagrammatic representation of a skin cancer. It is showing (i) Thinning of epidermis (ii) Round and multilobular tumor masses in the dermis. Masses show palisading arrangement in their peripheral part. (iii) Connective tissue stroma around tumor masses contracts to form peritumoral lacunae. What is the diagnosis?

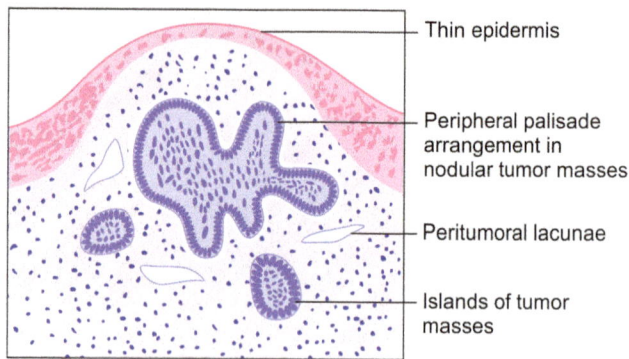

a. Squamous cell carcinoma (SCC)
b. Basal cell carcinoma (BCC)
c. Paget's disease
d. Cutaneous T-cell lymphoma (CTCL)

831. This patient complained of depigmented macules on dorsal aspects of hands, finger tips and perioral region. What is name of this type of vitiligo?

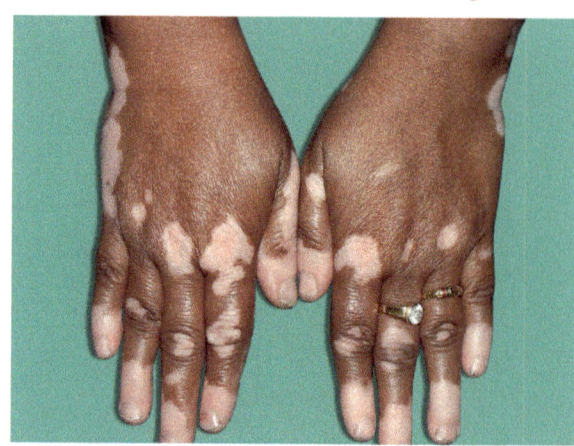

a. Focal vitiligo
b. Segmental vitiligo
c. Acrofacial or lip and tip vitiligo

832. A 25-year-old female complained of amenorrhea, hirsutism and facial acne lesions. Serum testosterone levels are mildly raised. Ovarian volumes on ultrasonography are 8 cc and 3 cc. What is the diagnosis of this patient?

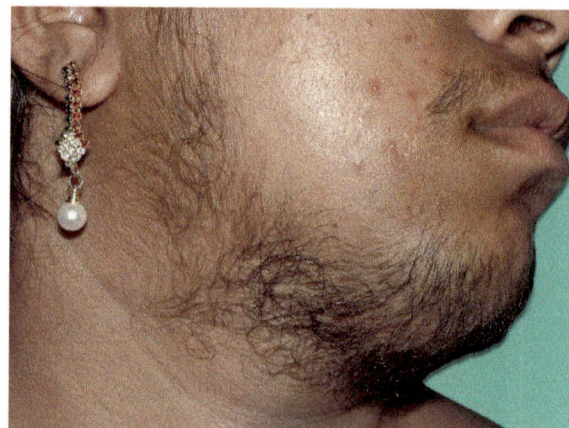

a. Idiopathic hirsutism
b. Polycystic ovarian syndrome (PCOS)
c. Late onset congenital adrenal hyperplasia (LO-CAH)
d. Androgen secreting tumor

Chapter 4 ✦ MCQs of Dermatology, Venereology and Leprology

833. This adult female presented with excessive hair loss on scalp. What is the clinical diagnosis?

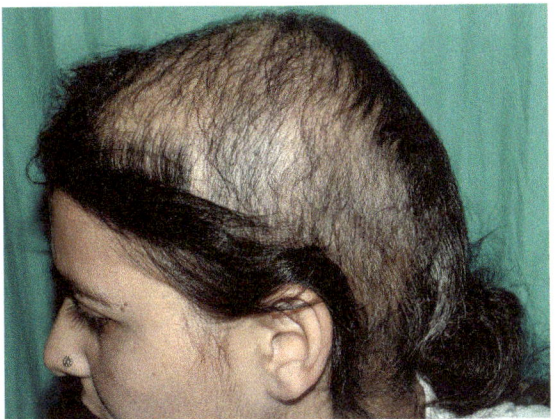

a. Telogen effluvium
b. Androgenic alopecia
c. Trichotillomania
d. Alopecia areata

834. This patient complained of episodic bluish discolorations of fingers on exposure to cold. No underlying cause is found. What it is called?

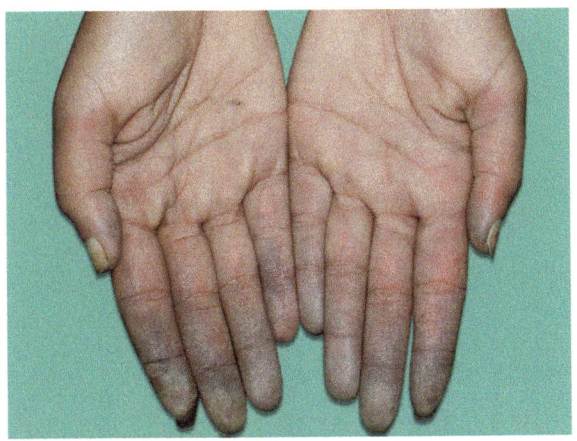

a. Chilblains
b. Raynaud's phenomenon
c. Raynaud's disease

835. Following is the diagram of structure of nail unit. What is the name of the structure in light brown color with question mark?

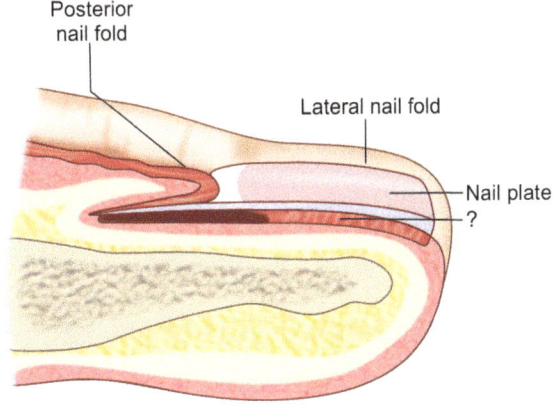

a. Nail matrix
b. Hyponychium
c. Nail bed
d. Cuticle

836. This patient complained of unbearable pinpricking and burning sensation on back. Back showed uniformly minute red papules. What is the clinical diagnosis?

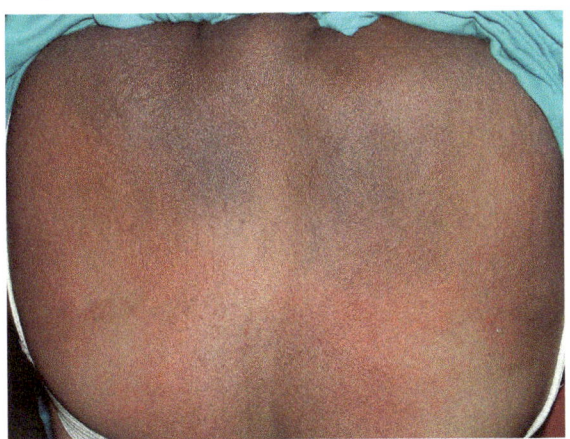

a. Miliaria crystallina
b. Miliaria rubra
c. Exanthematous rash

837. She complained of extensive hair loss on scalp. What is the clinical diagnosis?

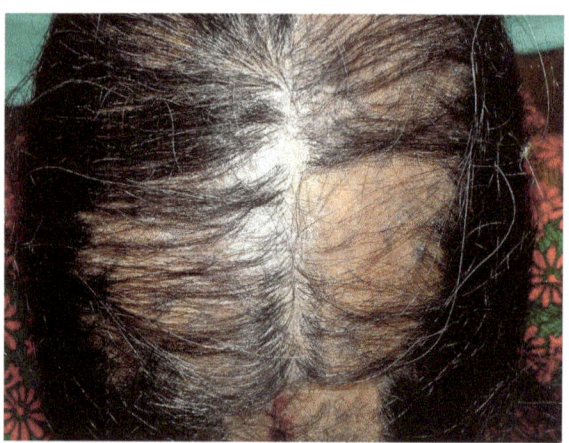

a. Androgenetic alopecia (central parting)
b. Telogen effluvium
c. Cicatricial alopecia
d. Alopecia areata

838. This patient presented with 2-4 mm sized, reddish brown and monomorphic papules distributed symmetrically on face. What is the clinical diagnosis?

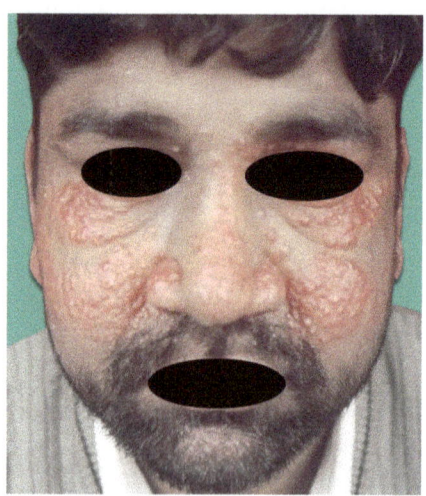

a. Acne vulgaris
b. Lupus miliaris disseminatus faciei
c. Acne rosacea
d. Acneiform eruption

839. An adolescent girl complained of erythema of posterior nail folds. In which of the following disorders is it seen?

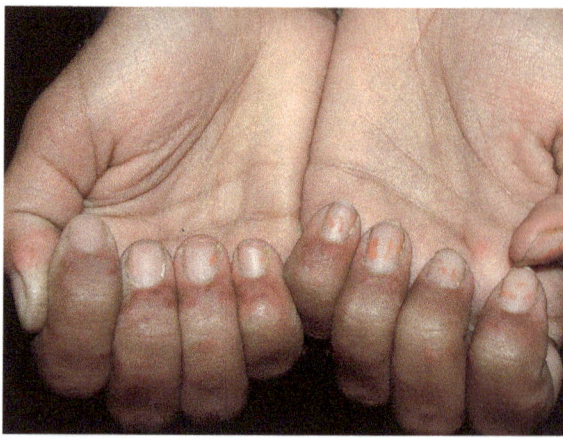

a. Morphea
b. Chronic cutaneous lupus erythematosus (CCLE)
c. Systemic lupus erythematosus (SLE)
d. Systemic sclerosis

840. What is the name of the structure with question mark in the following diagram?

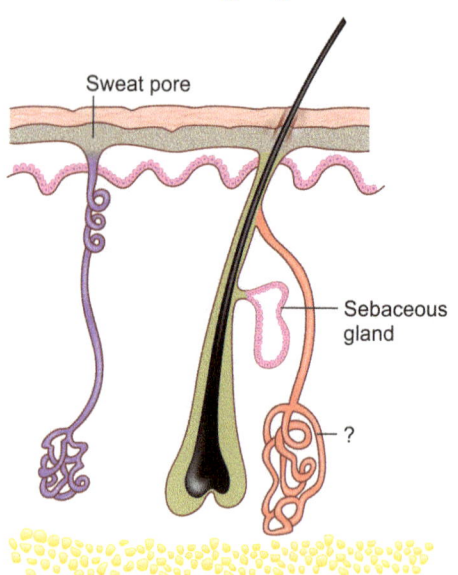

a. Apocrine sweat gland
b. Adamson's fringe
c. Eccrine sweat gland
d. Sebaceous gland

841. This patient complained of discomfort, redness, papules and pustules in the beard region having curly hairs. What is the clinical diagnosis?

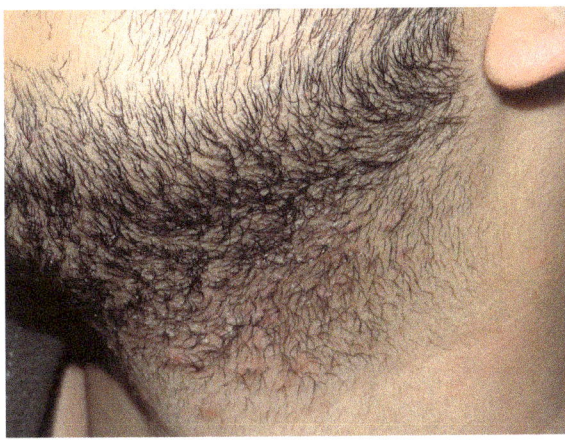

a. Sycosis barbae
b. Pseudofolliculitis
c. Tinea barbae

842. On the second day of fever, he took some treatment and developed red plaque on his lip. What is the clinical diagnosis?

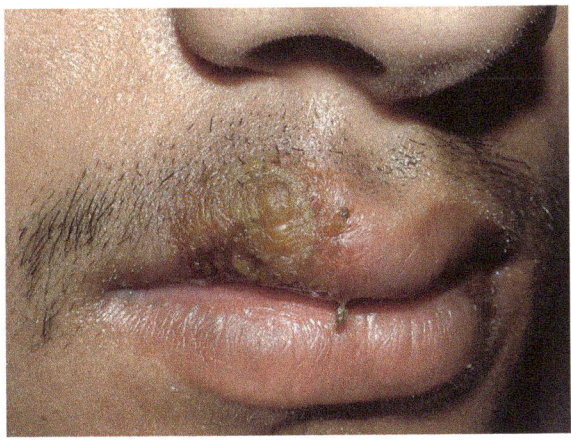

a. Fixed drug eruption
b. Herpes simplex labialis

843. She complained of depigmentation limited to toes and fingers around the nail plates. What is closest clinical diagnosis?

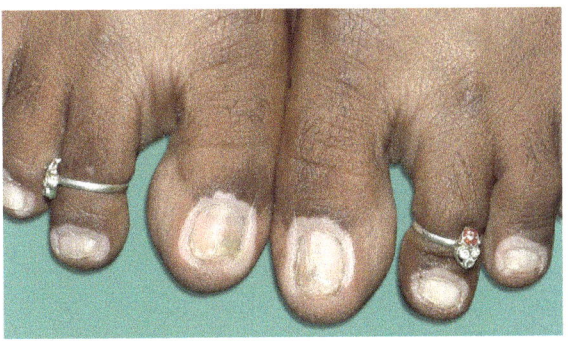

a. Focal vitiligo
b. Leukoderma due to nail polish
c. Acrofacial vitiligo

844. This patient complained of acne, hirsutism with no apparent menstrual irregularities. On ultrasonography, ovarian sizes are 15 cc and 18 cc volumes. Testosterone levels are also raised. LH/FSH ratio is 1.1. What is the diagnosis?

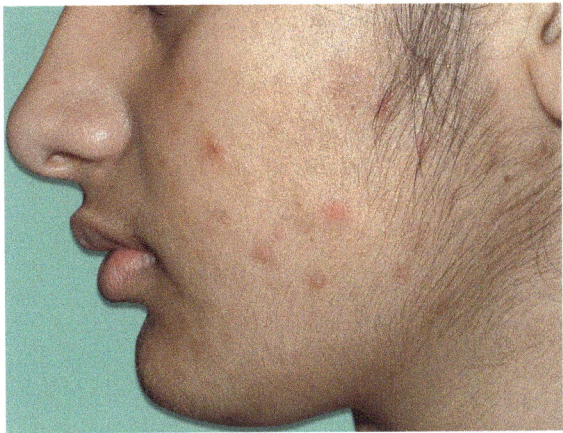

a. Idiopathic hirsutism
b. Polycystic ovarian syndrome (PCOS)
c. Late onset-congenital adrenal hyperplasia (LO-CAH)

845. Following is the diagram of nail unit structure. What is the name of the structure with question mark?

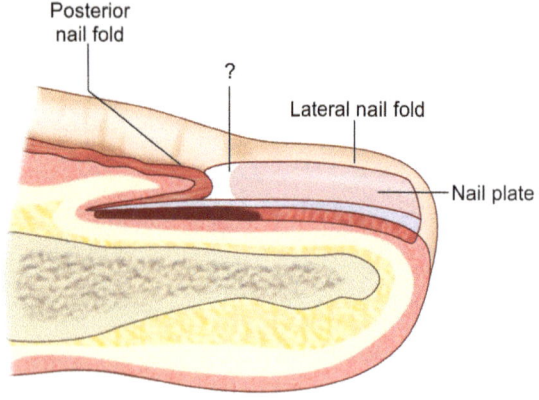

a. Cuticle
b. Nail bed
c. Hyponychium
d. Nail matrix

846. This lady presented with erythematous scaly plaques on nose and cheek for the last two years. What is the closest clinical diagnosis?

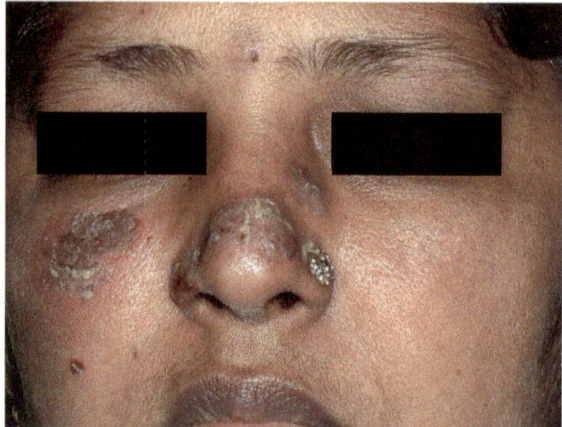

a. Chronic cutaneous lupus erythematosus (CCLE)
b. Systemic lupus erythematosus
c. Lupus vulgaris

847. This child presented with well-defined discoid lesions on hand and face. Lesions have deep hyperpigmented center and violaceous thread like edge. What is the clinical diagnosis?

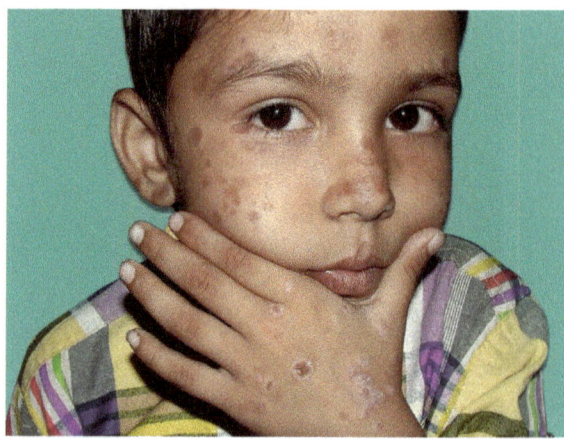

a. Actinic lichen planus
b. Plane warts

848. This patient presented with asymptomatic, symmetrically distributed, discrete, oval-shaped macules covered with fine scales on the back for the last 20 days. Lesions tend to be clear is the center and form collar at the margin. What is the clinical diagnosis?

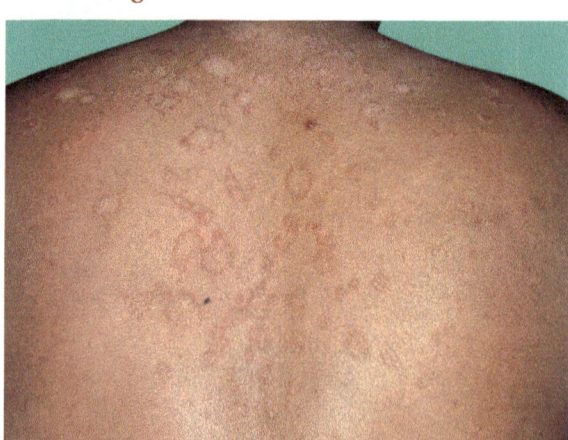

a. Secondary syphilis
b. Pityriasis rosea
c. Exanthematous rash

849. A 65-year-old female presented with redness and white scaling on whole scalp. What is the clinical diagnosis?

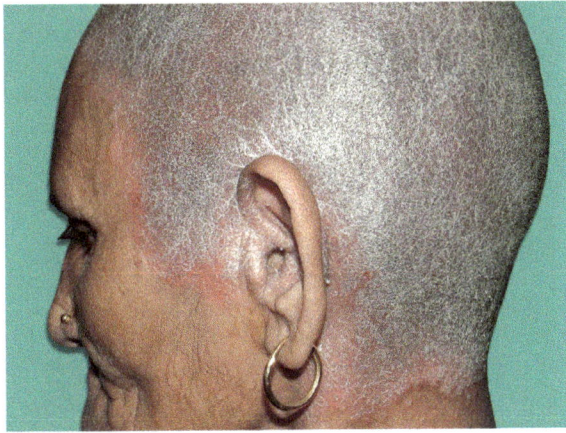

a. Seborrheic dermatitis
b. Psoriasis scalp
c. Tinea capitis

850. Following is the diagrammatic representation of skin cancer. It is showing (i) Irregular masses of proliferating and descending strands of epidermal keratinocytes. (ii) The extension of atypical keratinocytes beyond the basement membrane zone into the dermis. (iii) Presence of foci of concentric rings of parakeratotic squamous cells called horny pearls.

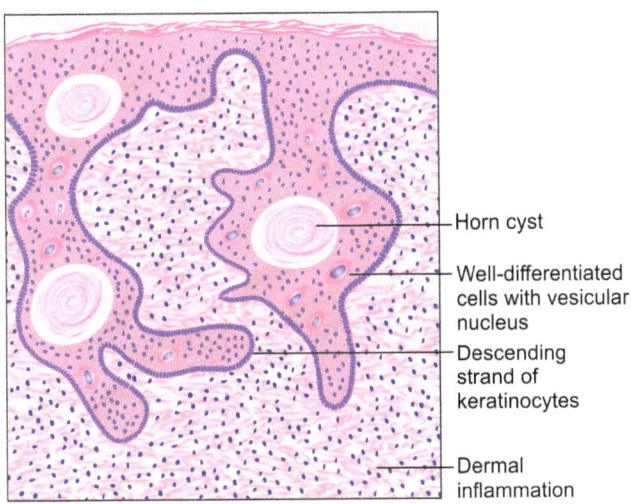

a. Basal cell carcinoma (BCC)
b. Paget's disease
c. Cutaneous T-cell lymphoma (CTCL)
d. Squamous cell carcinoma (SCC)

851. It is a magnified photograph of a hyperpigmented patch on the forehead of a 70-year-old female for the last two years. What is the closest clinical diagnosis?

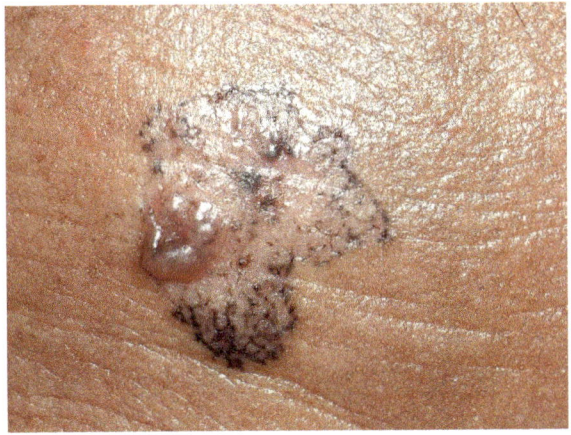

a. Superficial spreading melanoma (SMM)
b. Basal cell carcinoma (BCC)
c. Squamous cell carcinoma (SCC)

852. What is the closest clinical diagnosis for this patient who is having this lesion for the last three days?

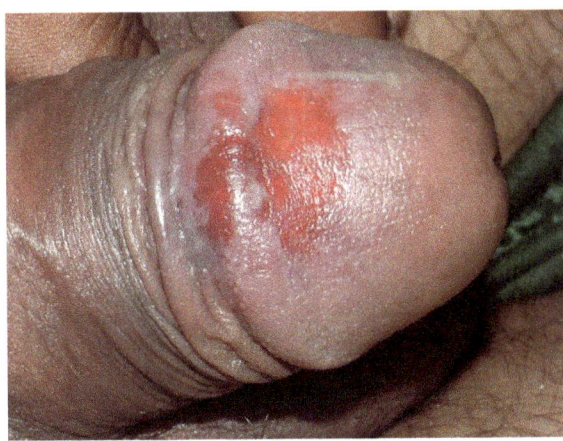

a. Lichen planus
b. Psoriasis
c. Fixed drug eruption
d. Herpes genitalis

853. A middle-aged female presented with papules, pustules and redness on chin and paranasal area. What is the diagnosis?

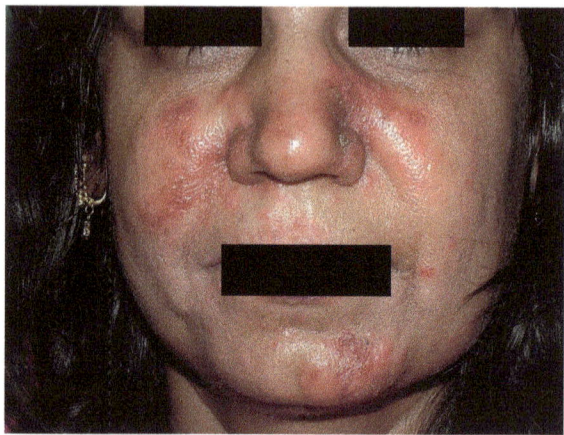

a. Acne vulgaris
b. Acne rosacea
c. Lupus miliaris disseminatus faciei (LMDF)
d. Drug induced acne

854. This lady complained of rash on her face and chest. What is the closest clinical diagnosis?

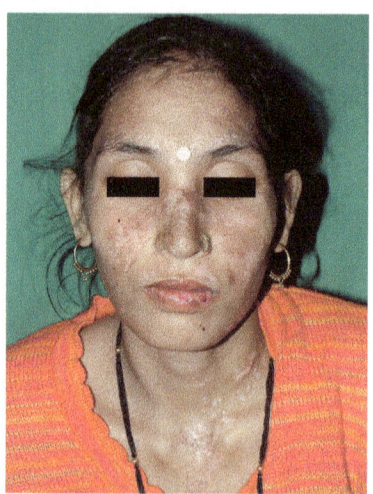

a. Chronic cutaneous lupus erythematosus (CCLE)
b. Systemic lupus erythematosus (SLE)

855. Following is the diagrammatic histopathology of a condition caused by the acid-fast bacillus. It is showing (i) Compact granuloma eroding the basal layer of normal epidermis. (ii) Granulomas consisting large epithelioid cells with dense peripheral rim of lymphocytes. (iii) Langhans giant cells are absent. What is the diagnosis?

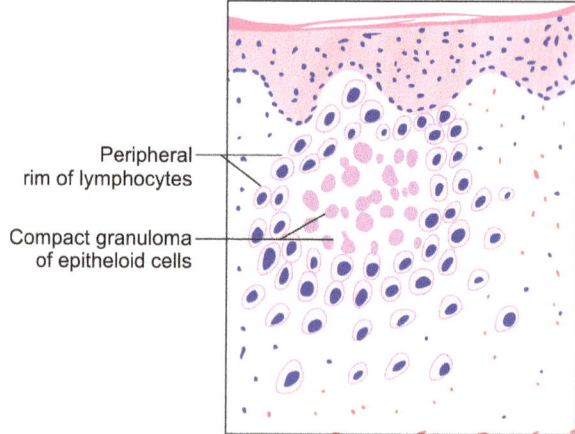

a. Lepromatous leprosy
b. Tuberculoid leprosy
c. Tuberculosis verrucosa cutis

856. Which one of the following terms is used to describe this nail change?

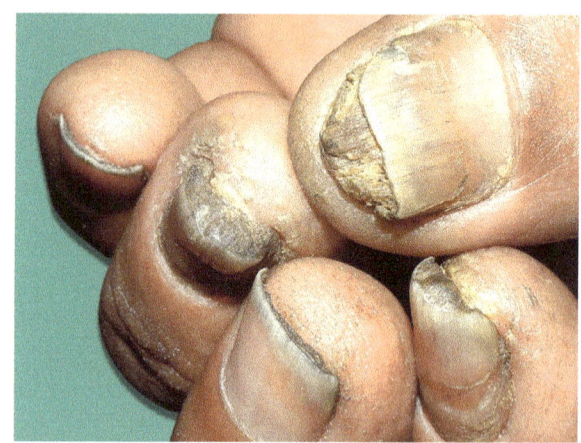

a. Onychomadesis
b. Onychogryphosis
c. Onycholysis
d. Subungual hyperkeratosis
e. Onychorrhexis

857. This lady presented with multiple asymptomatic erythematous plaques with white scales on trunk and extremities. The lesions show central clearing with no loss of sensations. What is the clinical diagnosis?

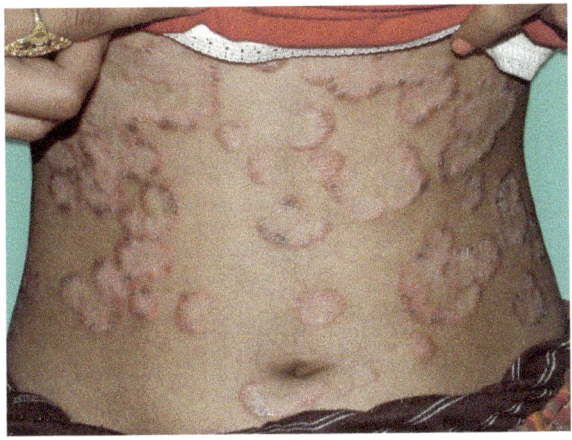

a. Annular plaques of mid borderline leprosy
b. Annular psoriasis
c. Annular lesions of granuloma annulare
d. Tinea corporis

858. This patient presented with hyperkeratotic plaques with white scales on both soles. Red plaques with white scaling are present on other parts of body also. What is the clinical diagnosis?

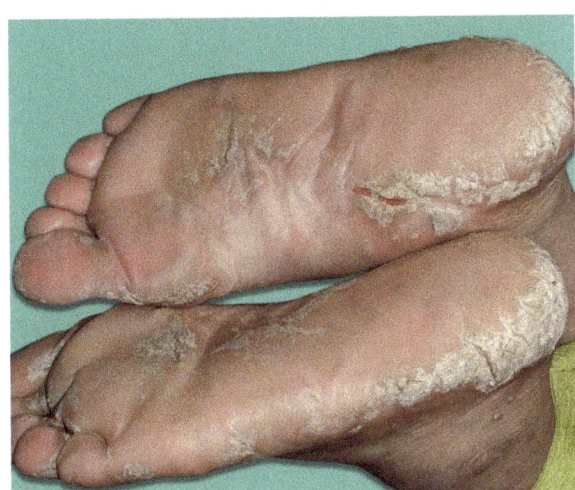

a. Focal keratoderma
b. Lichen planus soles
c. Psoriasis on soles
d. Tinea pedis
e. Hyperkeratotic eczema

859. This patient complained of extreme pruritus on shoulders, extensors of upper limbs, natal cleft and buttocks. Close examination *(MCQ 261)* showed group of small vesicles. Mucosae and genitals were not involved. What is the closest clinical diagnosis?

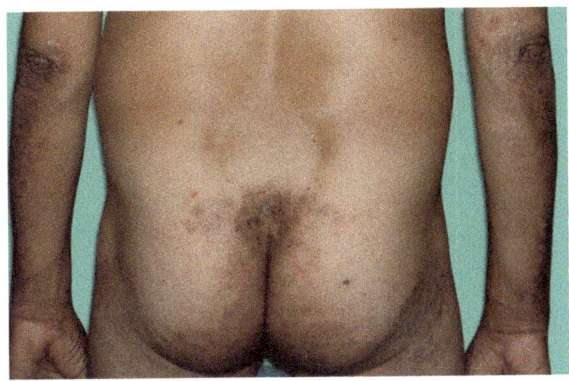

a. Dermatitis herpetiformis
b. Scabies
c. Pemphigus foliaceous
d. Linear IgA dermatosis

860. Following diagram shows the wavelengths of various equipments used in dermatology. What is name of the equipment having wavelength 810 nm?

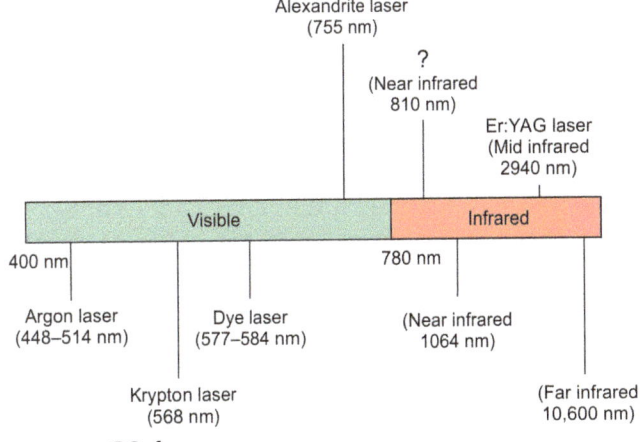

a. CO_2 laser
b. Nd: YAG-laser
c. Diode laser
d. Narrow band UVB chamber

861. A 60-year-old female presented on back with a single nonpruritic, persistent, thin and red plaque. It has well-defined irregular borders with overlying scale and resembles psoriasis.

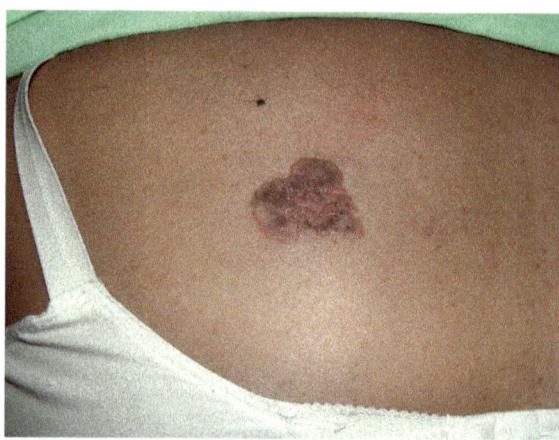

a. Squamous cell carcinoma
b. Malignant melanoma
c. Bowen' disease

862. A 1-month old baby was brought having many minute papules on cheeks, forehead and chin. What is the clinical diagnosis?

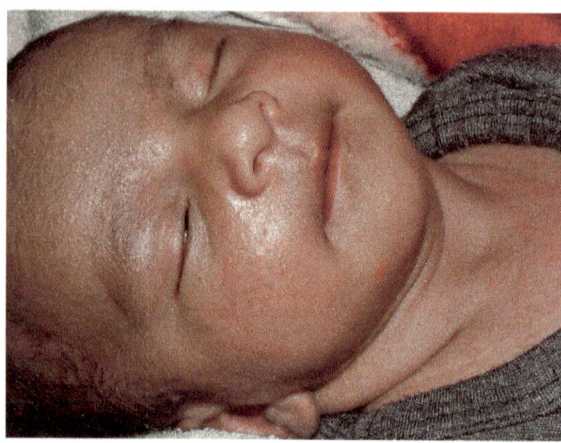

a. Erythema toxicum neonatorum (ETN)
b. Neonatal acne
c. Milia neonatorum
d. Miliaria crystallina

863. This patient presented with red well-defined plaques with white scaling on both palms. Similar red plaques with white scaling are also present on other parts of body. What is the clinical diagnosis?

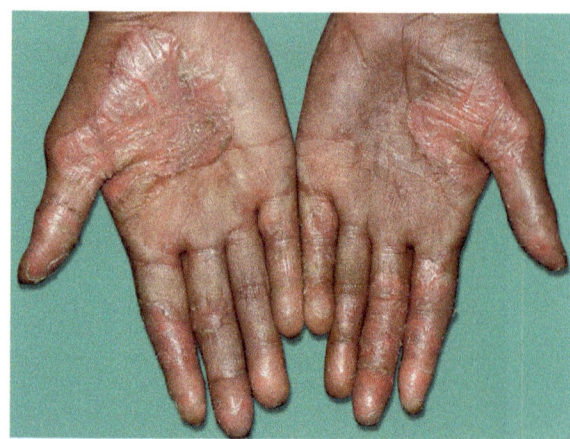

a. Lichen planus
b. Chronic cutaneous lupus erythematosus (CCLE)
c. Psoriasis
d. Hyperkeratotic eczema

864. This patient complained of multiple flaccid blisters on trunk and extremities without any mucosal involvement. What is closest clinical diagnosis?

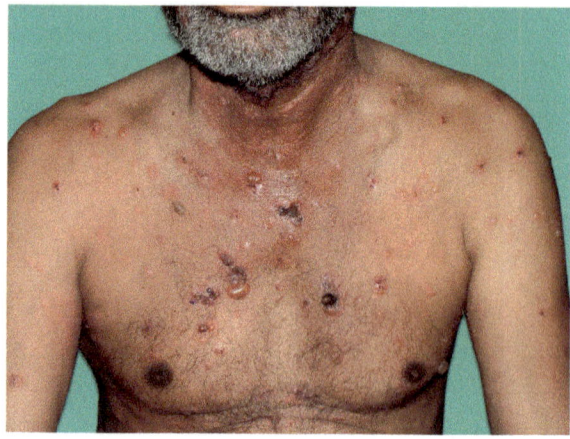

a. Pemphigus vulgaris
b. Pemphigus foliaceous
c. Dermatitis herpetiformis
d. Linear IgA dermatosis

865. Following is the diagrammatic structure of a single stranded RNA virus having two layered structure. Which one of the following viruses it belongs to?

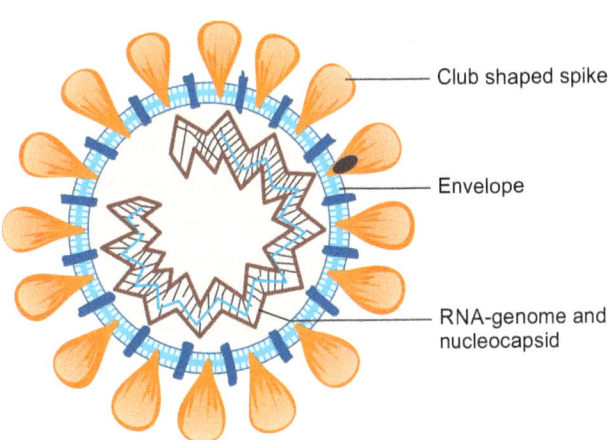

a. HIV
b. Corona virus

866. This patient complained of generalized redness and scaling all over body for the last 4–5 months. What is the clinical diagnosis?

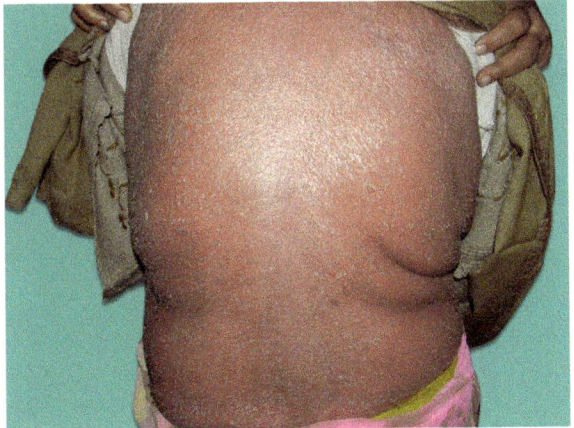

a. Erythroderma due to endogenous eczema.
b. Erythroderma due to psoriasis
c. Senile dermatitis
d. Exanthematous rash

867. Ten days after burn injury with silencer of bike, this patient developed itching and oozing around the injury. What is the diagnosis?

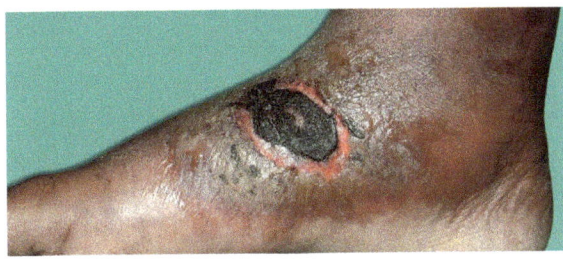

a. Infective dermatitis
b. Infected eczema
c. Id-eruption

868. A 6-year-old child having epilepsy and mental retardation presented with multiple, asymptomatic, red brown, discrete firm papules on face. What is the clinical diagnosis?

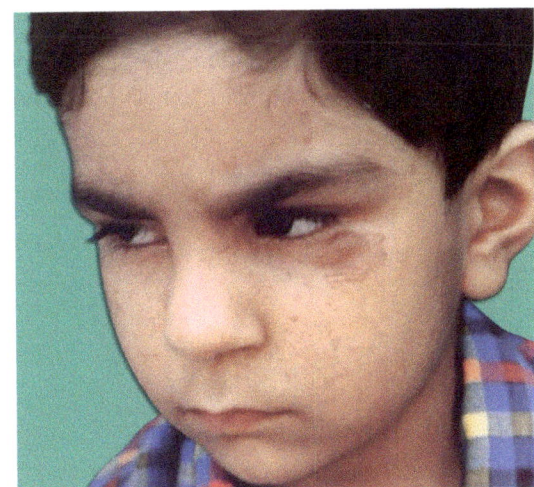

a. Tuberous sclerosis complex (TSC)
b. Plane warts
c. Lupus miliaris disseminatus faciei (LMDF)

869. This patient complained of itching, oozing and crusting of both soles. What is the clinical diagnosis?

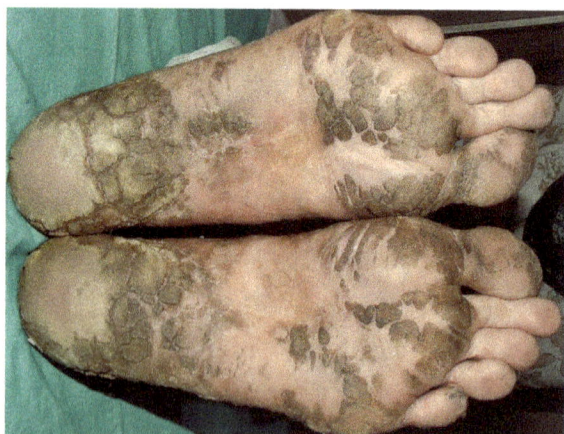

a. Plantar keratoderma
b. Psoriasis soles
c. Hyperkeratotic eczema

870. Following diagrammatic histopathology is showing (i) Hyperkeratosis without parakeratosis (ii) Irregular thickening of granular cell layer. (iii) Irregular lengthening of rete ridges giving a saw tooth appearance. (iv) Band-like dermal infiltrate in close approximation to epidermis. (v) Presence of hyaline colloid bodies. What is the diagnosis?

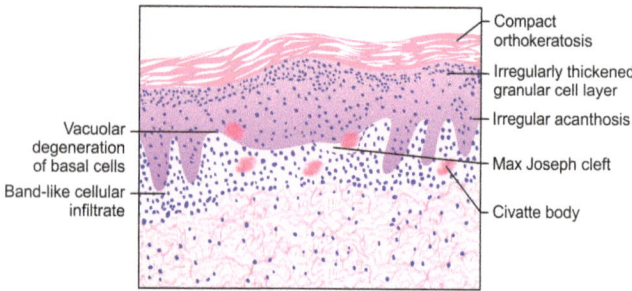

a. Psoriasis
b. Lichen planus
c. Wart
d. Molluscum contagiosum

871. She complained of itching, redness and swelling of eyelids and neighboring skin for the last two weeks. What is the closest clinical possibility for her?

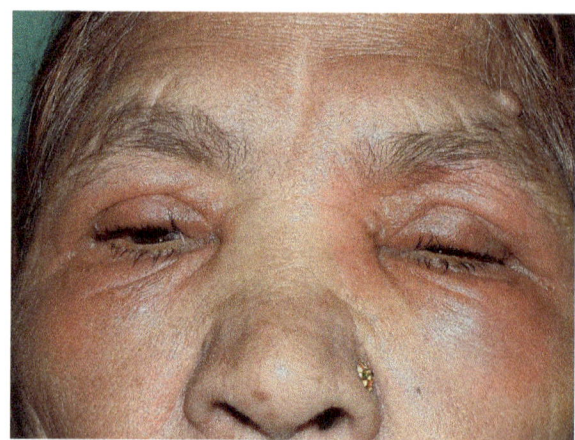

a. Airborne contact dermatitis (ABCD)
b. Allergic dermatitis due to hair dye
c. Allergic dermatitis due to eye drops

872. What is the diagnosis of this patient complaining of severe itching?

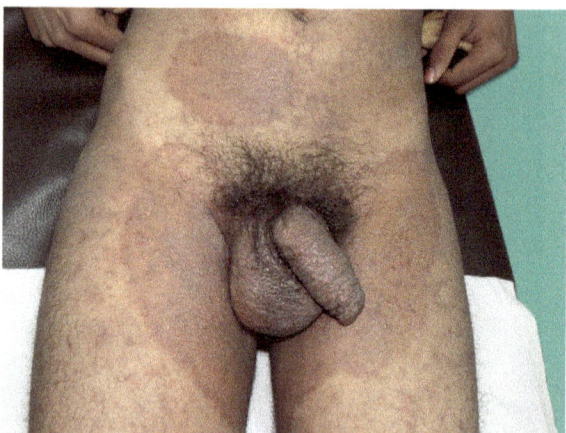

a. Tinea cruris
b. Tinea cruris with scabies
c. Flexural psoriasis with scabies
d. Scabies with tinea cruris and corporis

873. This man presented with a big itchy patch on his face with fine white scaling. What is the clinical diagnosis?

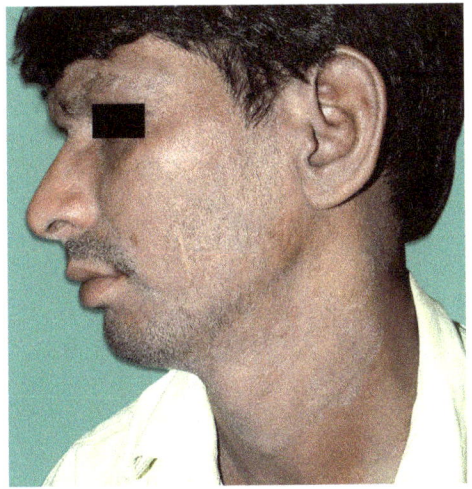

a. Pityriasis versicolor
b. Tinea faciei
c. Seborrheic dermatitis

874. She presented with severe itching for the last one year. What is the closest clinical diagnosis?

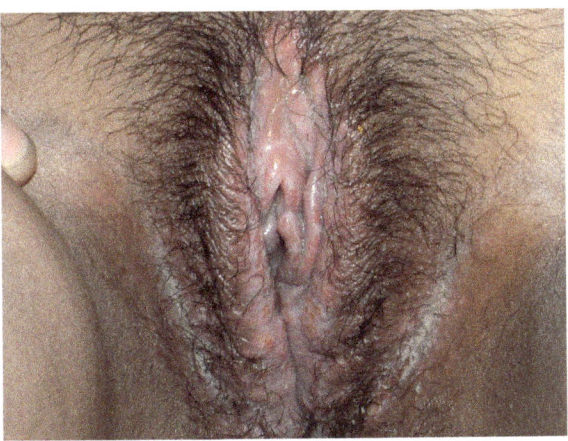

a. Lichen simplex chronicus (LSC)
b. Secondary syphilis
c. Lichen sclerosus et atrophicus
d. Vulvovaginal candidiasis

875. Following in the diagrammatic structure of a single stranded RNA virus consisting of three-layered structure. To which one of the following viruses it belongs to?

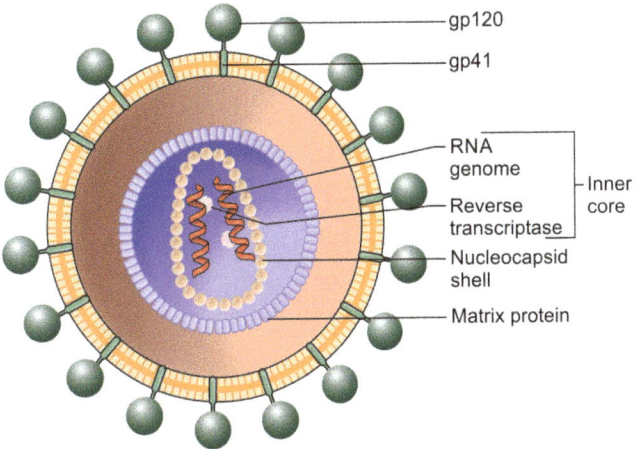

a. Human immune deficiency virus
b. Corona virus

876. A 9-year-old child presented with itching, oozing, fissuring and crusting in the perineal and suprapubic region for the last many years. She was also having involvement of scalp, post auricular region and nasolabial folds (next). What is the clinical diagnosis?

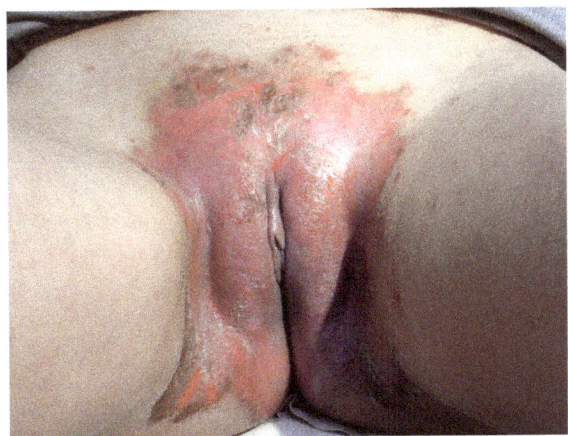

a. Atopic dermatitis with secondary infection
b. Flexural psoriasis
c. Seborrheic dermatitis with secondary infection
d. Hailey-Hailey disease

877. A 9-year-old female child presented with itching, oozing crusting behind the ears, external auditory meatus and nasolabial folds. She was also having similar involvement in perineal and suprapubic regions (previous MCQ). What is the clinical diagnosis?

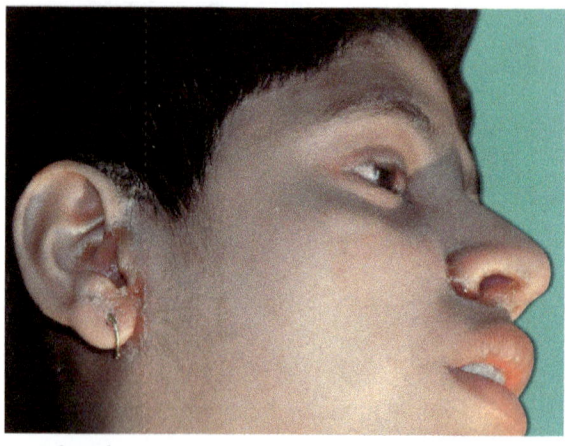

a. Seborrheic dermatitis with secondary infection
b. Atopic dermatitis with secondary infection
c. Infective eczematoid dermatitis (IED)

878. A milk vendor presented with itching between fingers. What is the clinical diagnosis?

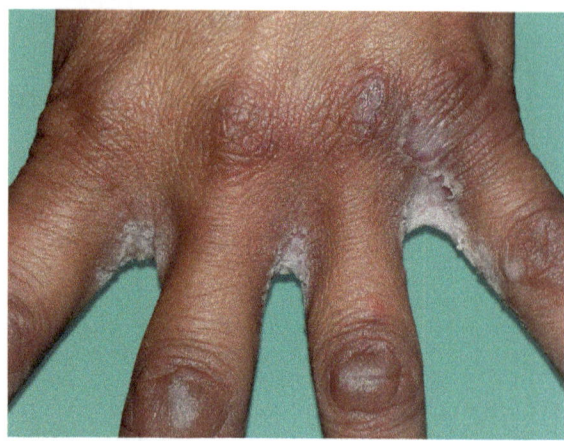

a. Candidiasis
b. Tinea manuum
c. Scabies
d. Household contact dermatitis

879. This patient of severe herpes zoster was also having disseminated vesicular lesions on rest of the trunk. Which one of the following statements is true about this patient?

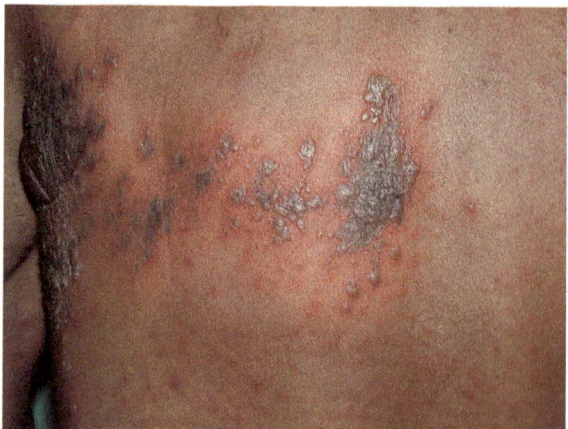

a. It can occur in diabetics
b. It can occur in patients on systemic steroids
c. It is not alarming and is quite common
d. It is alarming

880. Following is the diagrammatic histopathology of a condition caused by acid fast bacillus. It is showing (i) Diffuse granuloma formed by histiocytes and foamy macrophages packed with AFBs. (ii) Huge number of AFBs are seen singly or in clumps. (iii) Infiltrate is separated from thin and flattened epidermis by narrow grenz zone of normal collagen. What is the diagnosis?

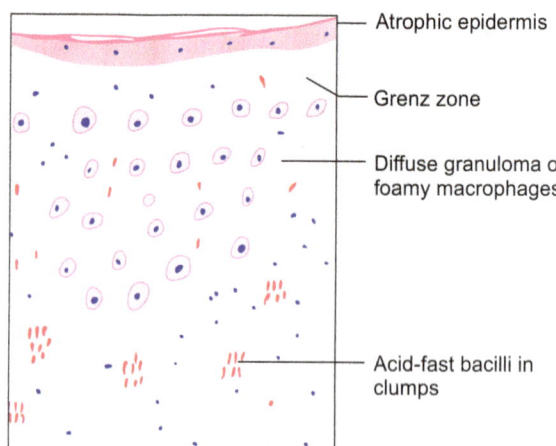

a. Tuberculoid leprosy
b. Lepromatous leprosy
c. Tuberculosis verrucosa cutis

Chapter 4 ✦ MCQs of Dermatology, Venereology and Leprology

881. This patient presented with multiple, hyperkeratotic growths with broad base on glans penis for the last 1 year. Inguinal lymph nodes are enlarged. What is the closest clinical diagnosis?

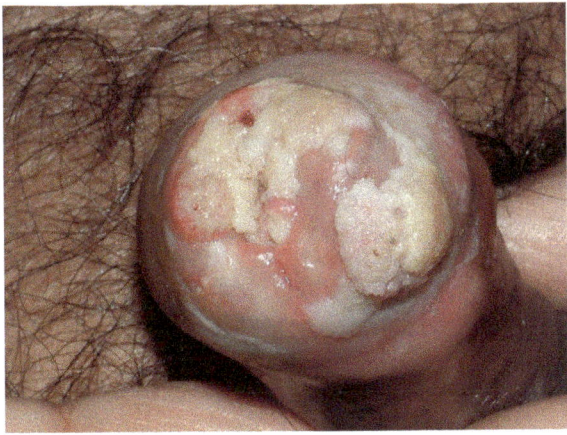

a. Venereal warts
b. Squamous cell carcinoma (SCC)

882. This man presented with a big size deep red-colored patch on left side of his face since birth. What is clinical diagnosis?

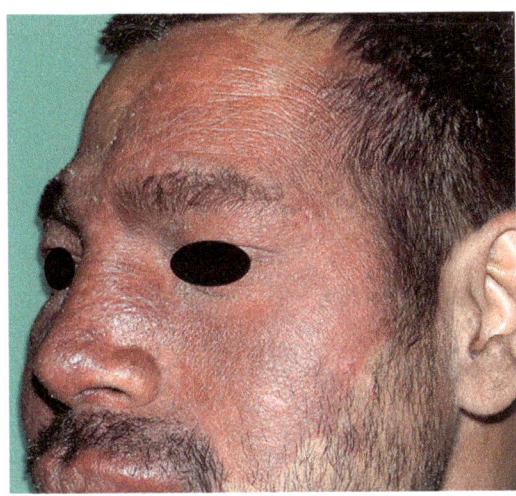

a. Strawberry hemangioma
b. Port-wine stain
c. Salmon patch

883. A household servant complained of redness and itching in both hands. What is the clinical diagnosis?

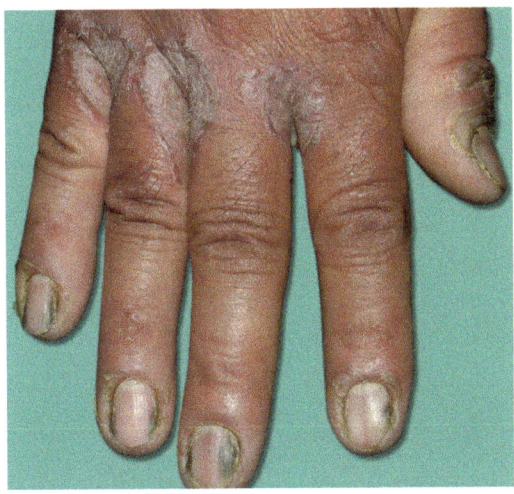

a. Tinea manuum
b. Candidal intertrigo and paronychia
c. Household contact dermatitis

884. This patient presented with extreme pruritus on shoulders, natal cleft and buttocks *(MCQ 859)*. On close examination *(MCQ 261)*, group of small tiny vesicles were observed. Mucosae were not involved. What is the closest clinical diagnosis?

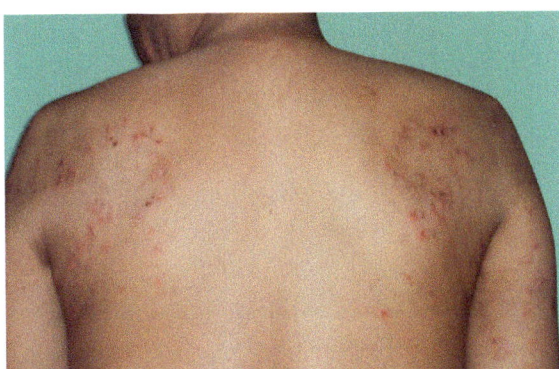

a. Linear IgA dermatosis
b. Scabies
c. Pemphigus foliaceous
d. Dermatitis herpetiformis

885. Following is the diagram of histopathology of skin cancer. It is showing (i) Hyperkeratosis, parakeratosis with papillomatosis. (ii) Presence of large round cells with ample cytoplasm and large nucleus with prominent nucleolus. (iii) These characteristic cells are seen in prickle cell layer and epithelium of hair follicles. What is the diagnosis?

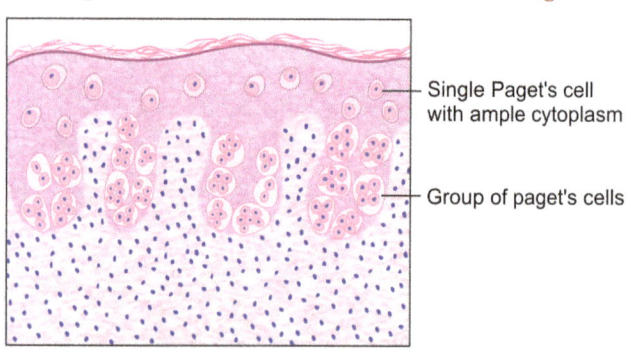

a. Squamous cell carcinoma (SCC)
b. Basal cell carcinoma (BCC)
c. Paget's disease
d. Cutaneous T-cell lymphoma (CTCL)

886. What is the diagnosis of this patient?

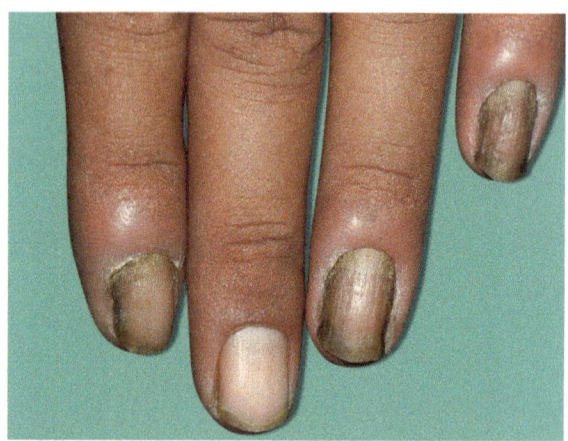

a. Tinea unguium
b. Chronic paronychia
c. Acute paronychia
d. Onychomycosis

887. A 3-year-old child presented with multiple hypopigmented macules on face. What is the clinical diagnosis?

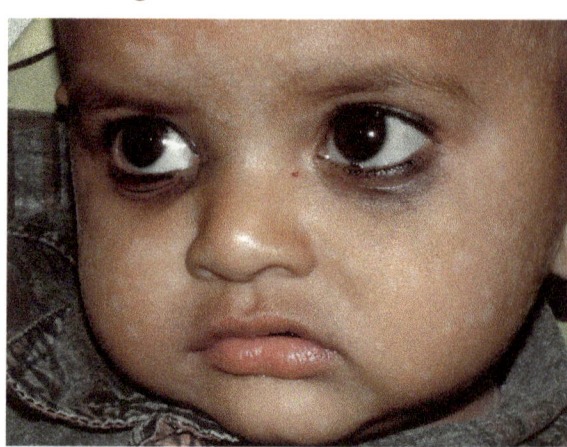

a. Pityriasis alba
b. Pityriasis versicolor
c. Vitiligo

888. This patient presented with multiple papules on eyelids. What is the clinical diagnosis?

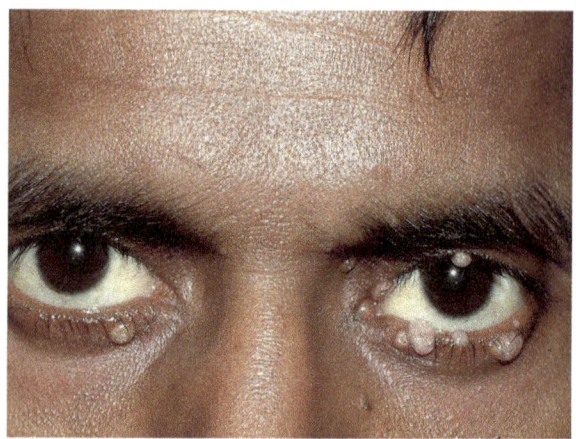

a. Common warts
b. Milia
c. Molluscum contagiosum

889. This lady came with itchy red patch on her face. What is the clinical diagnosis?

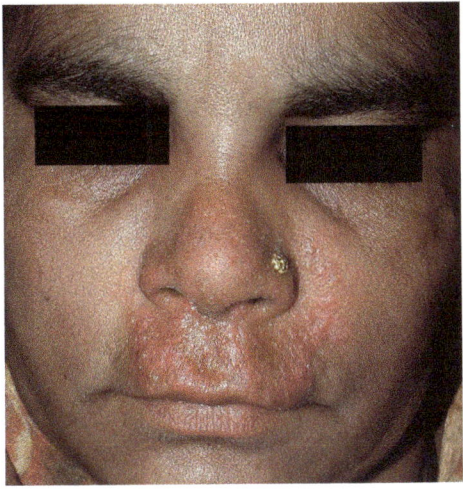

a. Acne rosacea
b. Psoriasis
c. Tinea faciei

890. Following is the diagram of structure of nail unit. What is the name of the structure with question mark?

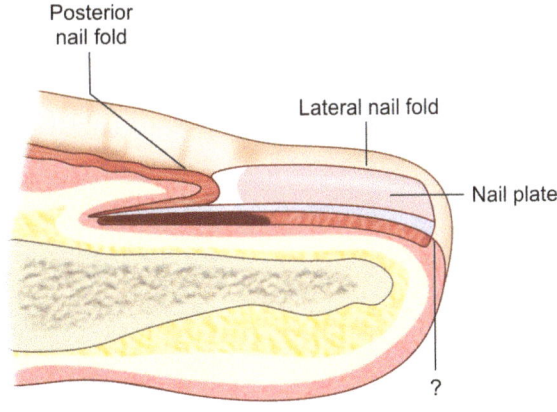

a. Nail matrix
b. Hyponychium
c. Cuticle
d. Nail bed

891. This child presented with a big patch of alopecia in temporal region. What is the clinical diagnosis?

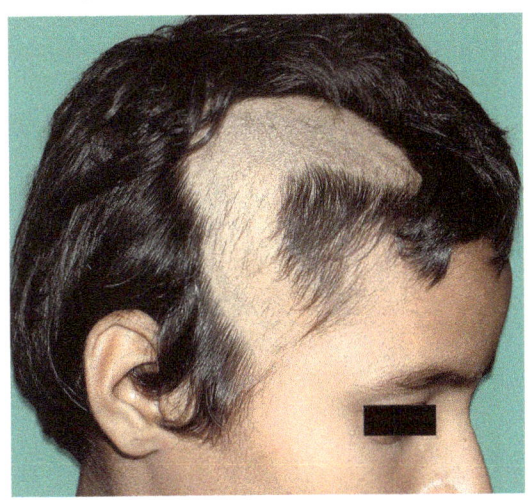

a. Alopecia areata
b. Trichotillomania
c. Telogen effluvium

892. This patient presented with severe itching, redness and thickening on face. What is the clinical diagnosis?

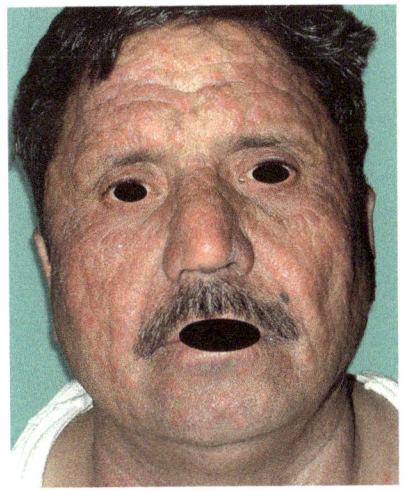

a. Polymorphous light eruption (PLE)
b. Chronic actinic dermatitis (CAD)
c. Airborne contact dermatitis (ABCD)

893. This patient presented with axillary freckling which comprises of multiple, various sized, sharply defined light brown macules, i.e., cafe-au-lait spots (CLSs). Which one of the following statements is not true?

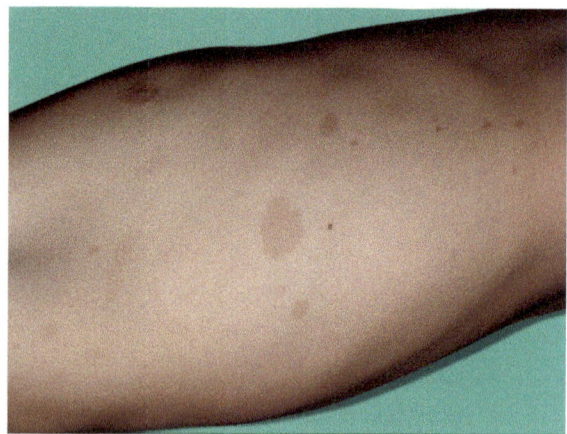

a. It is earliest feature of neurofibromatosis 1
b. 1–5 CLSs can be seen in 10% normal persons
c. It is one of the criteria for diagnosis of neurofibromatosis 1
d. CLSs are also common in neurofibromatosis 2

894. This patient presented with multiple, asymptomatic, discrete, oval and scaly macules on trunk for the last 25 days. Lesions have clear center and scales form peripheral collar. Lesions are distributed symmetrically on trunk. Palms and soles are not involved. What is the diagnosis?

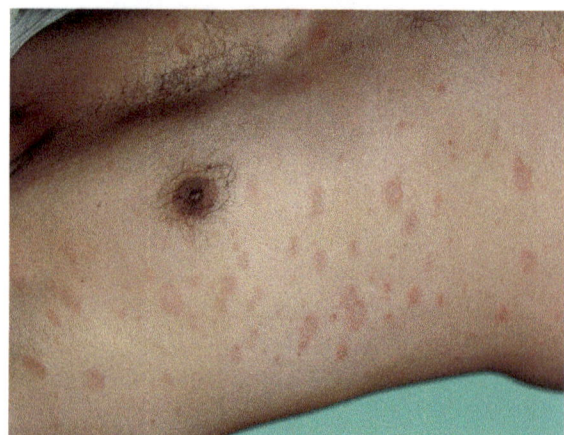

a. Secondary syphilis
b. Pityriasis rosea
c. Exanthematous rash

895. Following diagrammatic histopathology is showing (i) Formation of lobule which are compressing the papillae into thin septae. (ii) Epidermal cells have large inclusion bodies. (iii) Dermis shows little or no inflammatory change. What is the diagnosis?

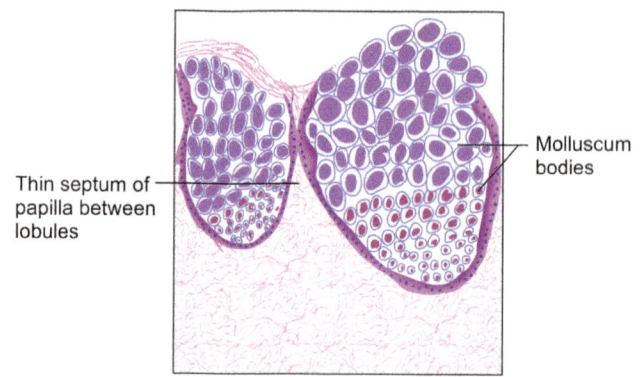

a. Wart
b. Psoriasis
c. Lichen planus
d. Molluscum contagiosum

896. A 20-year-old male presented with single large depigmented patch on back since birth and is not crossing the midline. What is the clinical diagnosis?

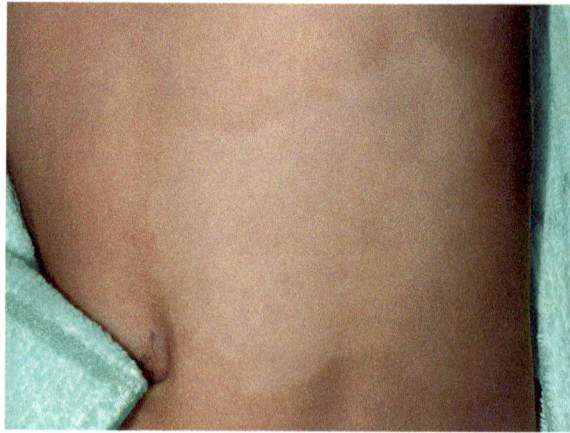

a. Nevus depigmentosus
b. Nevus anemicus
c. Focal vitiligo

897. This patient complains of redness, itching and burning sensation of ear lobule during extreme cold. Similar changes are observed in fingers and toes. What is the clinical diagnosis?

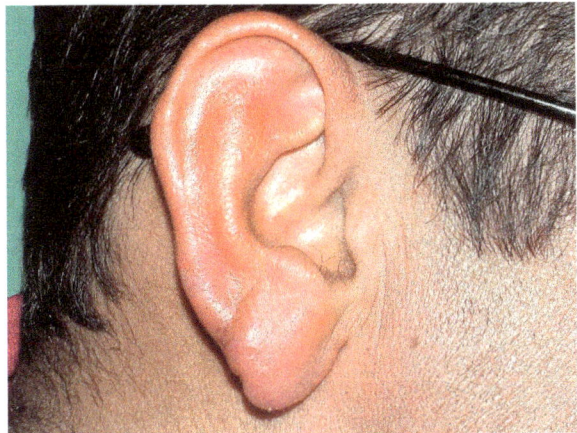

a. Perniosis (chilblains)
b. Lepromatous leprosy
c. Acute urticaria

898. Few hours after intake of some drug, this patient had itching and burning sensation with appearance of following lesions. Mucosae were normal. What is the clinical diagnosis?

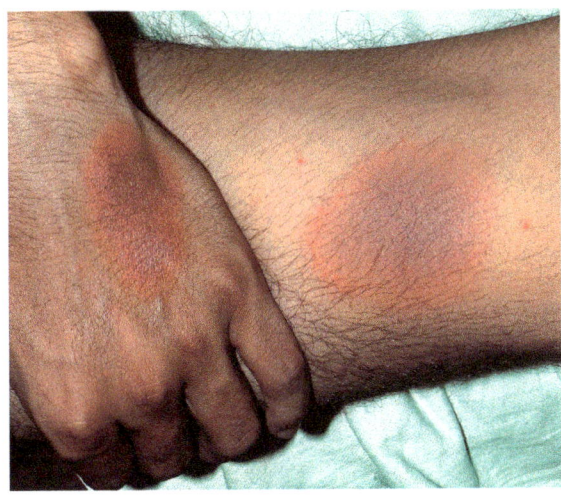

a. Fixed drug eruption
b. Target lesions of erythema multiforme

899. This lady presented with black-colored plaque with few dark-colored papules in the surrounding skin for the last six months. What is the closest clinical diagnosis?

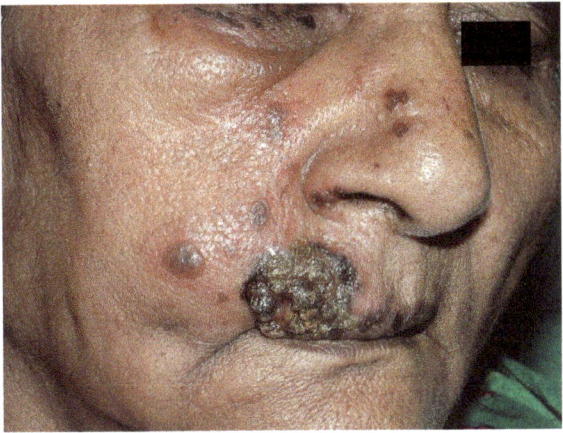

a. Squamous cell carcinoma (SCC)
b. Malignant melanoma with satellite lesions
c. Basal cell carcinoma (BCC)

900. A 15-year-old boy presented with recurrent lesions and scarring on his face. What is the clinical diagnosis?

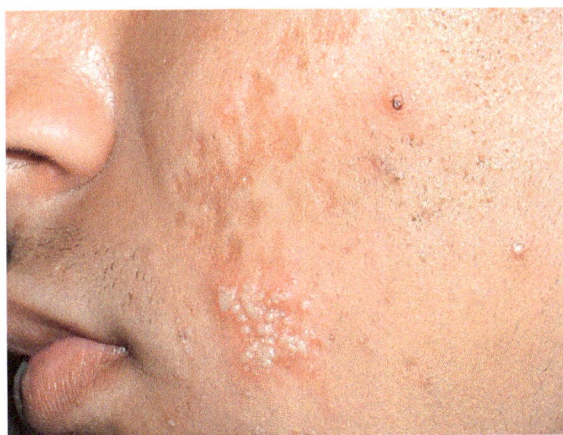

a. Acne vulgaris
b. Herpes labialis
c. Herpes zoster

901. This patient presented with a nonhealing ulcer in the groin with watery discharge for the last six months. What is the clinical diagnosis?

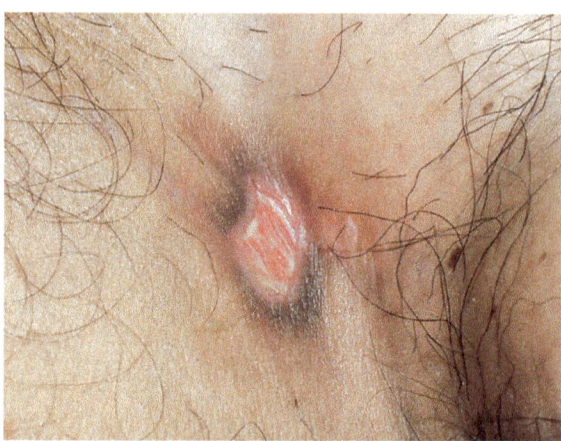

a. Pyoderma gangrenosum
b. Carbuncle
c. Scrofuloderma

902. This patient complained of itchy, flesh colored, migrating thread like eruption forming bizarre serpentine pattern on lower abdomen. It advances at the rate of few cm/day. What is the diagnosis?

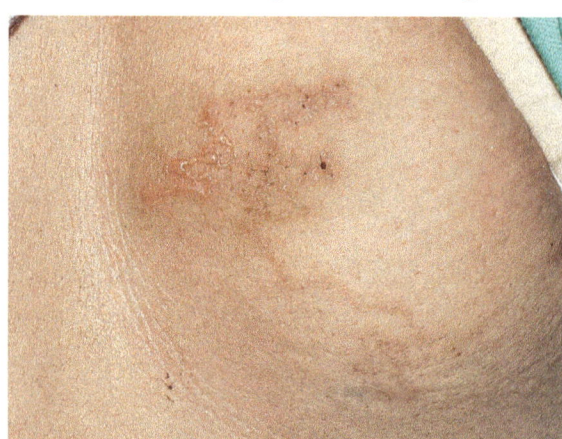

a. Larva migrans
b. Tinea corporis

903. This old man presented with redness, itching and scaling on scalp. What is the clinical diagnosis?

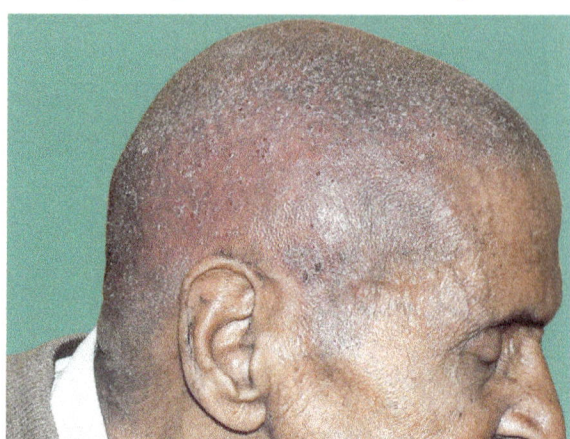

a. Psoriasis scalp
b. Seborrheic dermatitis
c. Tinea capitis

904. This lady complained of chronic, intractable vulval pruritus. What is the clinical diagnosis?

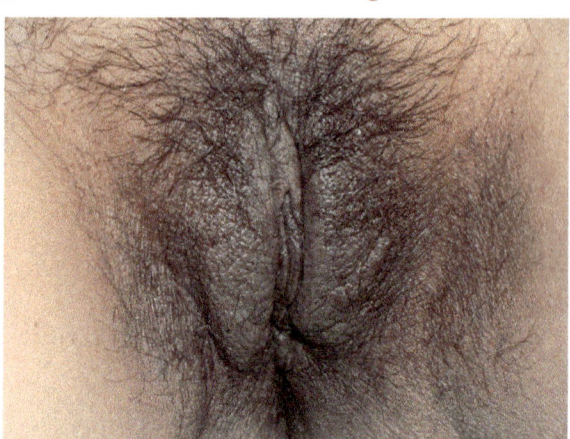

a. Lichen simplex chronicus
b. Candidiasis vulva
c. Angiokeratoma labia majora

905. This lady presented with itching and red plaques on her face for the last three days. What is the clinical diagnosis?

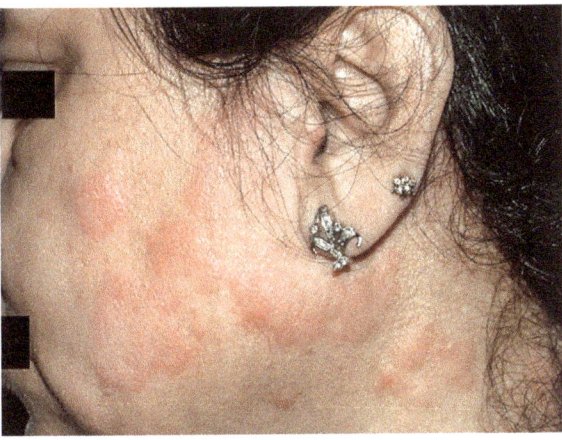

a. Lepromatous leprosy
b. Tinea faciei
c. Acute urticaria

906. This patient complained of long-standing severe itching on his shin. What is the clinical diagnosis?

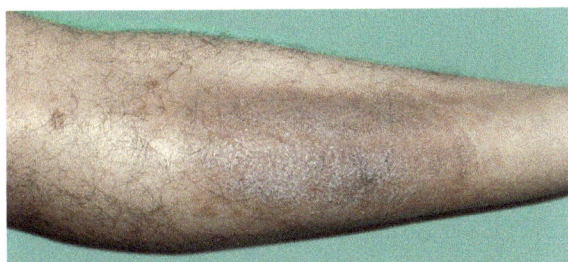

a. Psoriasis
b. Lichen simplex chronicus
c. Lichen planus hypertrophicus
d. Lichen amyloidosis

907. This child was brought with loss of eye lashes and eyebrows. What is the clinical diagnosis?

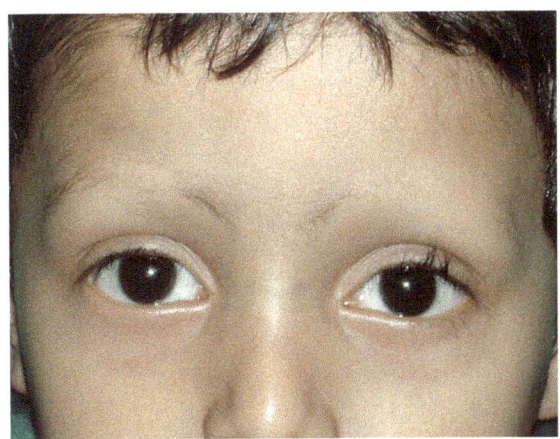

a. Alopecia areata
b. Seborrheic dermatitis
c. Tinea infection
d. Trichotillomania

908. This patient presented with itching and red plaque without any loss of sensation in axillae for the last seven days. What is the closest clinical diagnosis?

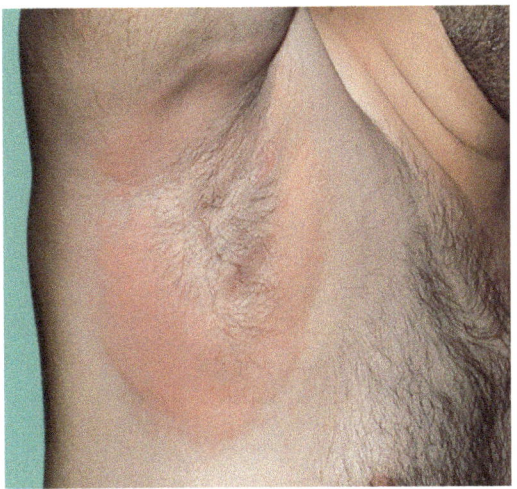

a. Tinea corporis
b. Contact irritant dermatitis
c. Acute urticaria

909. A 13-year-old child presented with an ill-defined hypo pigmented patch on face for the last one year. What is the clinical diagnosis?

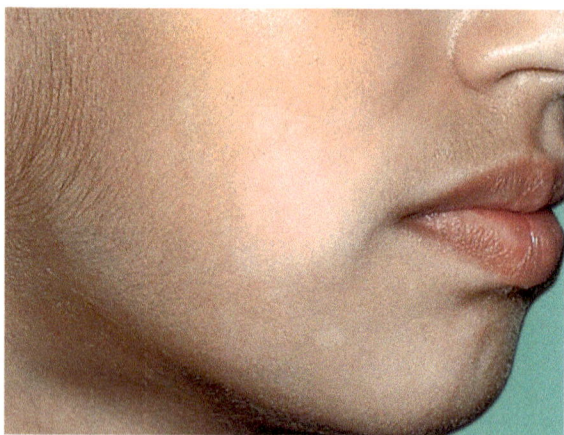

a. Pityriasis alba
b. Vitiligo
c. Nevus depigmentosus

910. This patient presented with itchy and violaceous papules on dorsum of hands and wrists. What is the closest clinical diagnosis?

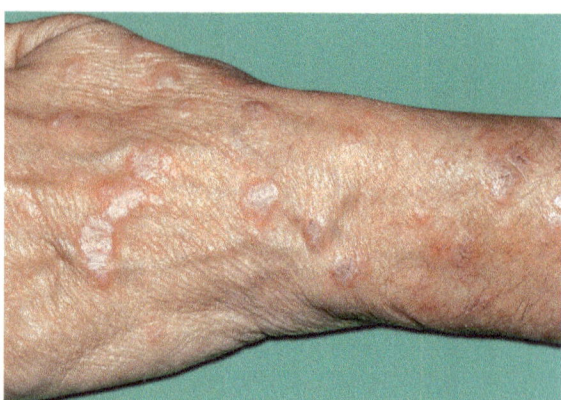

a. Chronic cutaneous lupus erythematosus
b. Psoriasis
c. Common warts
d. Prurigo nodularis
e. Lichen planus

911. This patient complains of pain and burning sensation of left side of his forehead for the last four days. What is the clinical diagnosis?

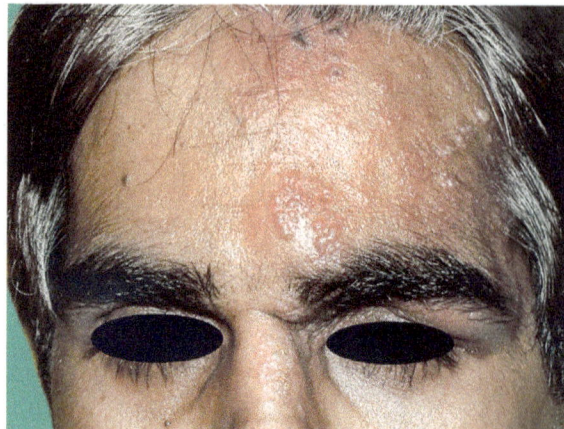

a. *Paederus dermatitis*
b. Herpes zoster ophthalmicus
c. Herpes simplex

912. This patient complained of depigmentation after prolonged application of a cream. Which one of the following creams has caused depigmentation?

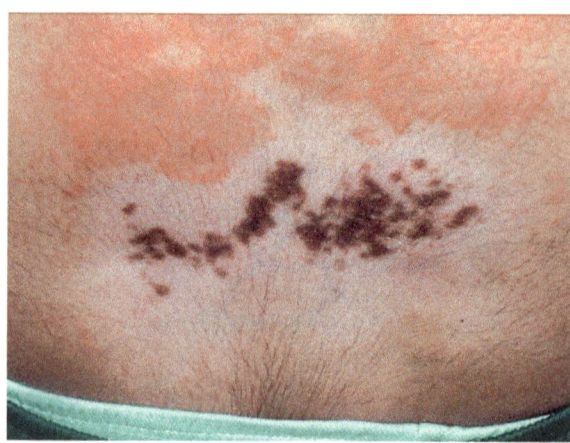

a. Corticosteroid cream
b. Tacrolimus ointment
c. Calcipotriol cream
d. Dapsone cream

913. This patient complained of red macules with mild scaling on trunk without significant itching for the last 15 days. Palms and soles are normal. What is the closest clinical diagnosis?

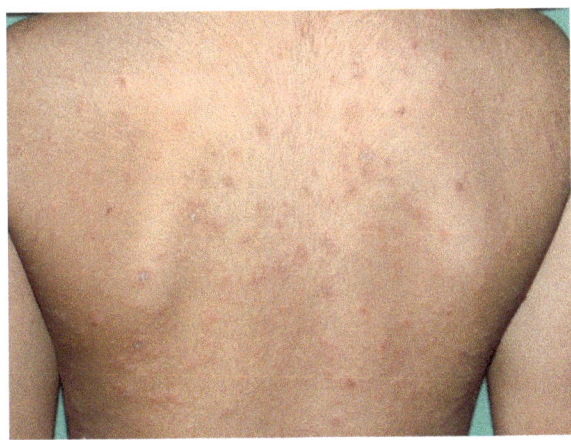

a. Secondary syphilis
b. Morbilliform or exanthematous rash
c. Pityriasis rosea
d. Psoriasis

914. She presented with a single red plaque on her face for the last one year. There is loss of sensation in the plaque. What is the clinical diagnosis?

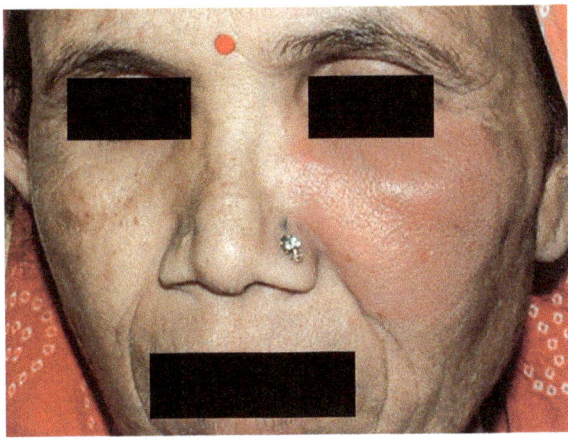

a. Tuberculoid leprosy
b. Lepromatous leprosy
c. Indeterminate leprosy
d. Histoid leprosy

915. A 70-year-old female presented with geometric shaped, dark purplish patches on her forearms. What is the clinical diagnosis?

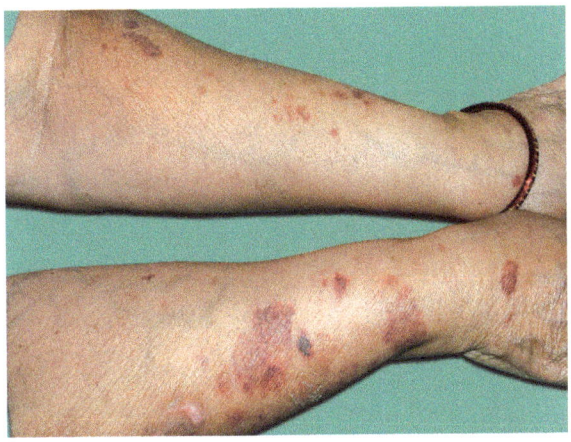

a. Idiopathic thrombocytopenic purpura (ITP)
b. Henoch–Schonlein purpura (HSP)
c. Senile Purpura
d. Palpable purpura

916. This patient complains of itching and crusting in his right palm. What is the clinical diagnosis?

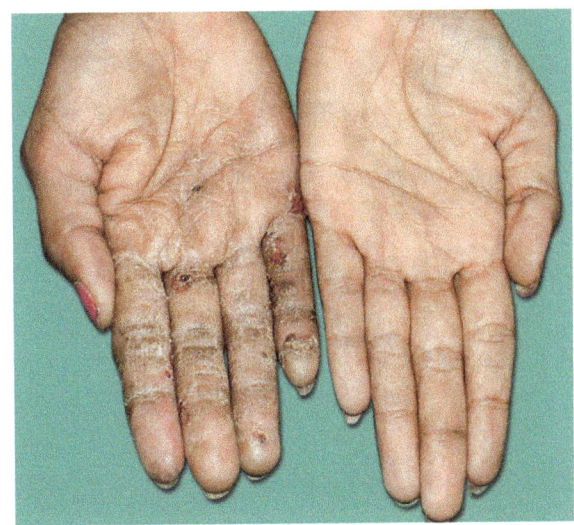

a. Tinea manuum
b. Tuberculosis verrucosa cutis (TVC)
c. Eczema of palm

917. This patient complained of red plaques with white scaling on dorsa of hand and wrists with no loss of sensations. What is the clinical diagnosis?

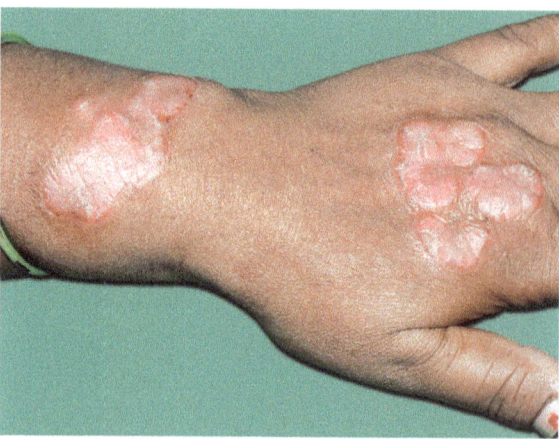

a. Psoriasis
b. Discoid eczema
c. Tuberculoid leprosy
d. Chronic cutaneous lupus erythematosus (CCLE)

918. This patient complained of itchy circular lesions on forearm. What is the clinical diagnosis?

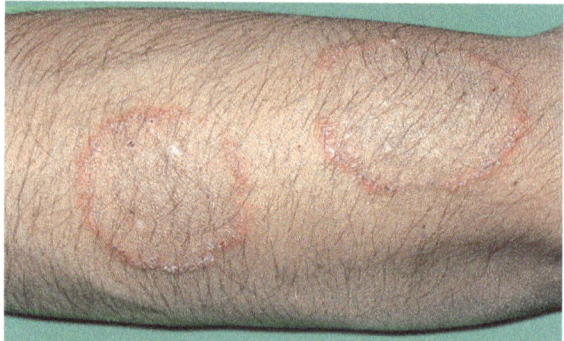

a. Granuloma annulare
b. Discoid eczema
c. Mid borderline leprosy
d. Annular psoriasis
e. Tinea corporis

919. This patient complained of increase in appetite and swelling of face with crop of monomorphic red papular lesions on forehead, cheeks and chin. What is the clinical diagnosis?

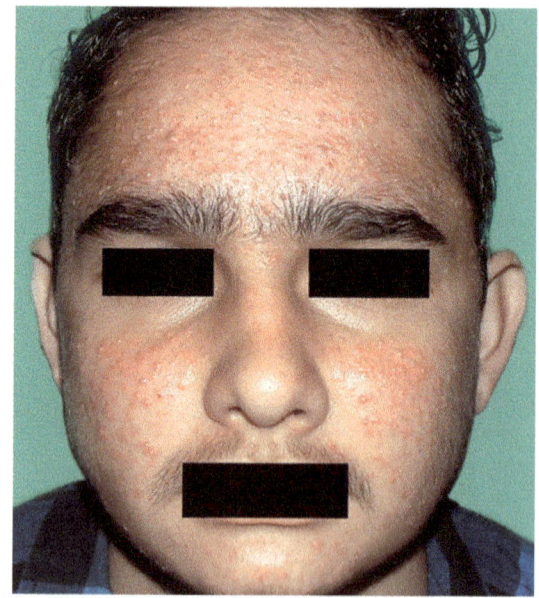

a. Drug-induced acne
b. Acne vulgaris
c. Lupus miliaris disseminated faciei
d. Acne rosacea

920. This patient complained of itchy patches on forearm. What is the clinical diagnosis?

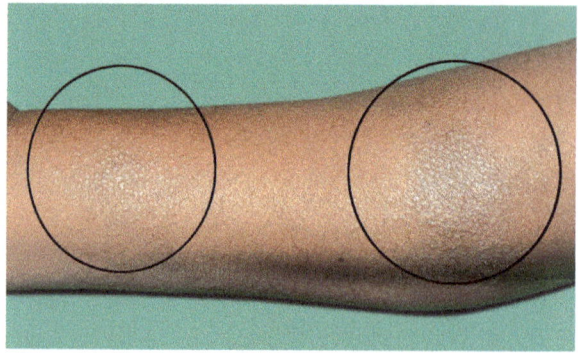

a. Psoriasis
b. Discoid eczema
c. Lichen planus
d. Tinea corporis

921. This child presented with fever, itching, erythema on face for the last 3–4 days. What is the clinical diagnosis?

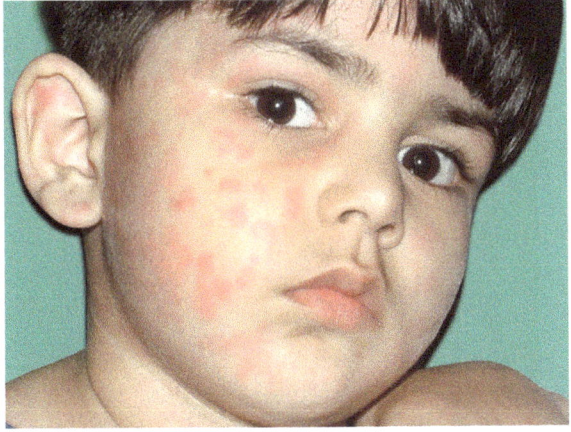

a. Acute urticaria
b. Measles
c. Exanthematous rash

922. This patient presented with red plaques with scaling on shaft of penis. What is the clinical diagnosis?

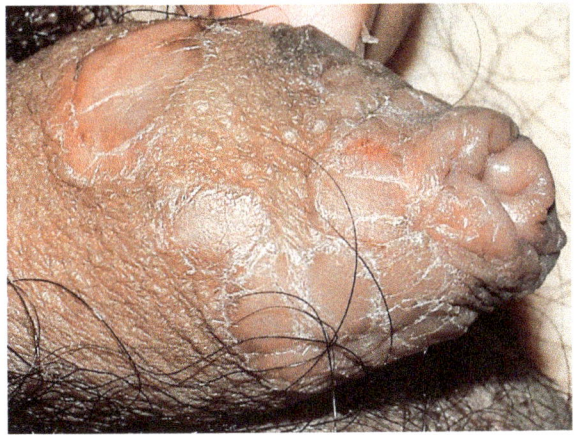

a. Lichen planus
b. Psoriasis
c. Lichen nitidus
d. Tinea
e. Scabies

923. A 3-year-old child presented with a painful swelling in the cervical region for the last seven days. What is the clinical diagnosis?

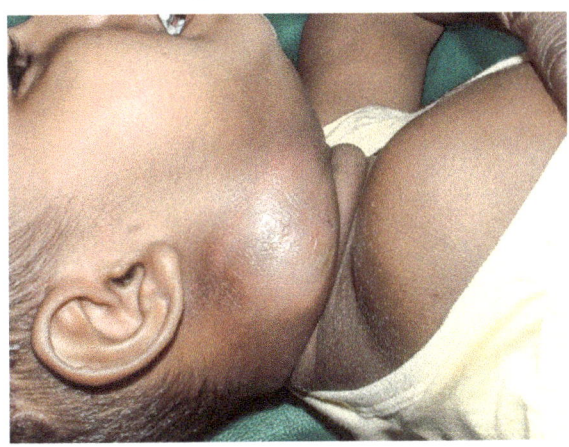

a. Cold abscess
b. Pyogenic abscess
c. Matted lymph nodes
d. Subcutaneous hemangioma

924. This patient presented with intractable itching of scrotal skin for the last 2–3 years. What is the clinical diagnosis?

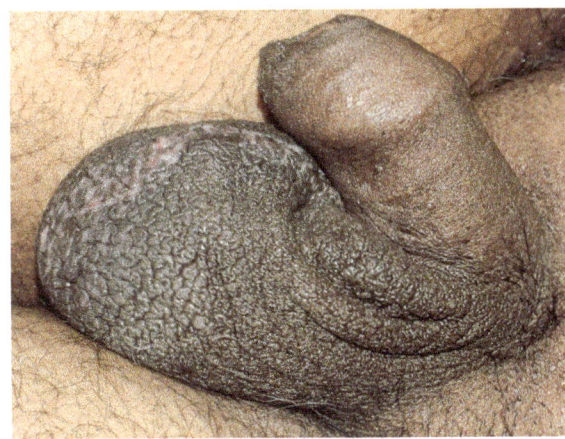

a. Red scrotum syndrome (RSS)
b. Circumscribed neurodermatitis scrotum
c. Angiokeratoma scrotum

925. A 40-year-old female presented with reddish brown papules and nodules about 4–5 in number on trunk and extremities. Levels of angiotensin converting enzyme is raised. X-ray chest showed bilateral hilar lymphadenopathy. What is clinical diagnosis?

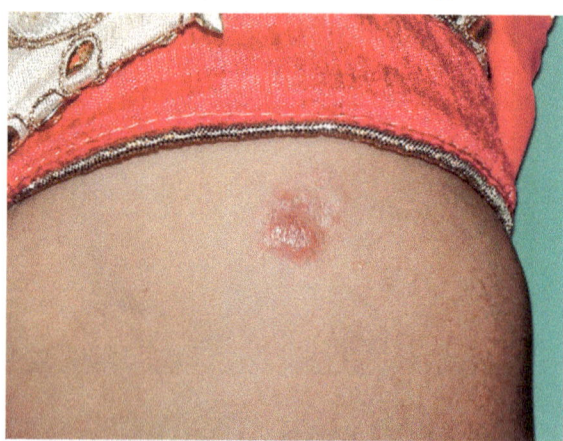

a. Tuberculosis
b. Sarcoidosis

926. This patient presented with multiple, deep seated papular lesions in right sole only. What is the clinical diagnosis?

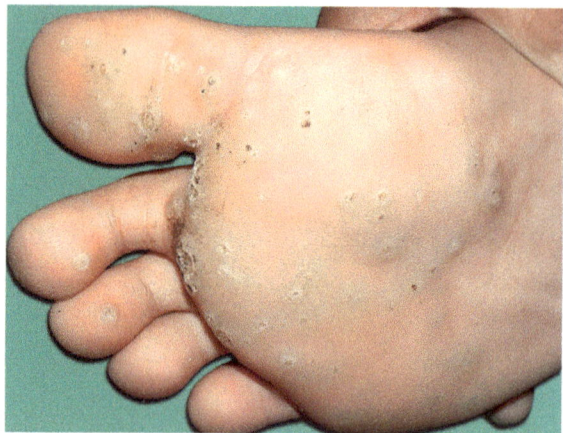

a. Tinea pedis
b. Deep plantar warts
c. Pitted keratolysis
d. Pompholyx

927. This patient presented with group of vesicles on undersurface of prepuce without any significant pain. He had similar lesions six months back also. What is the clinical diagnosis?

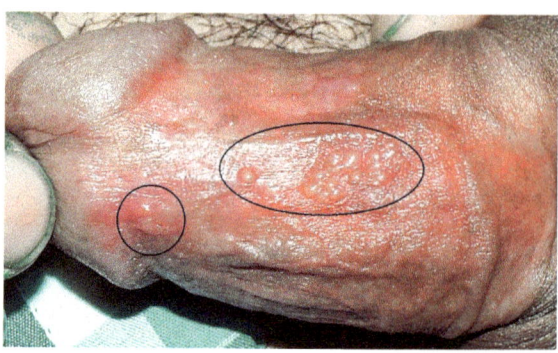

a. Herpes zoster
b. Recurrent herpes genitalis
c. Fixed drug eruption

928. One week after a sexual contact with a commercial sex worker, this man complained of burning and increased frequency of micturation with dirty yellow thick urethral discharge. What is the clinical diagnosis?

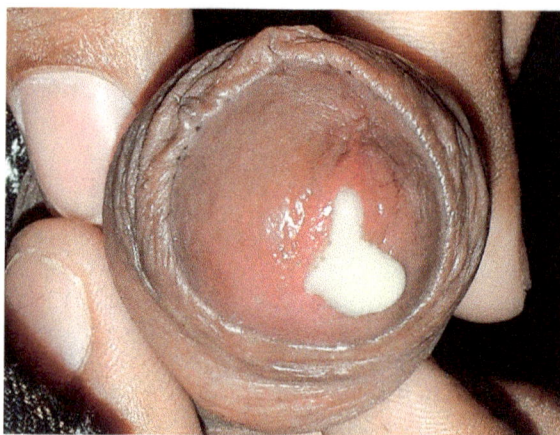

a. Candidal balanitis
b. Urethral syndrome
c. Reiter's syndrome

929. This patient presented with non-healing ulcer on wrist joint. It is not adherent to underlying bone which is normal. What is the clinical diagnosis?

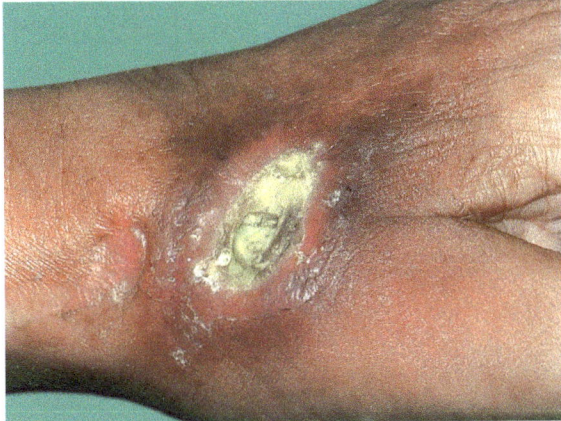

a. Chronic osteomyelitis
b. Scrofuloderma

930. A 14-year-old boy complained of hypopigmented patches on face. What is the closest clinical diagnosis?

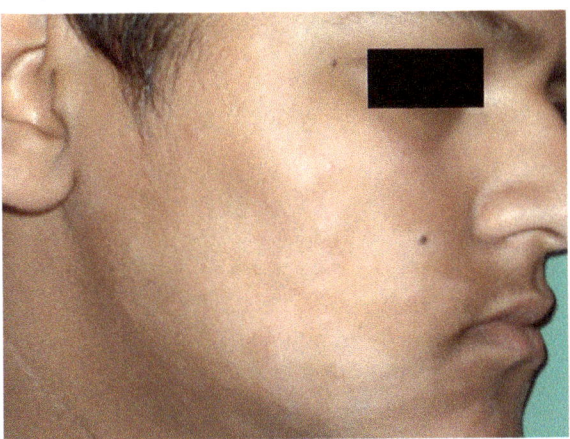

a. Segmental vitiligo
b. Pityriasis alba
c. Worm infestation
d. Calcium deficiency

931. This patient presented with redness and itching on front and back of his trunk for the last one week. There is a no h/o fever. What is the closest clinical diagnosis?

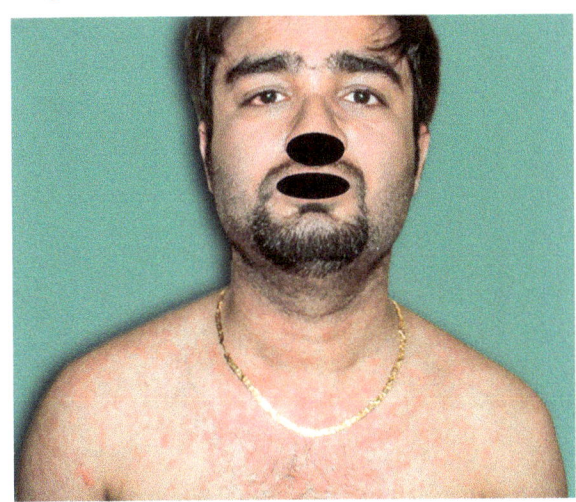

a. Acute urticaria
b. Measles
c. Drug-induced exanthematous rash
d. Morbilliform rash

932. This patient complained of itching in the groins. What is the clinical diagnosis?

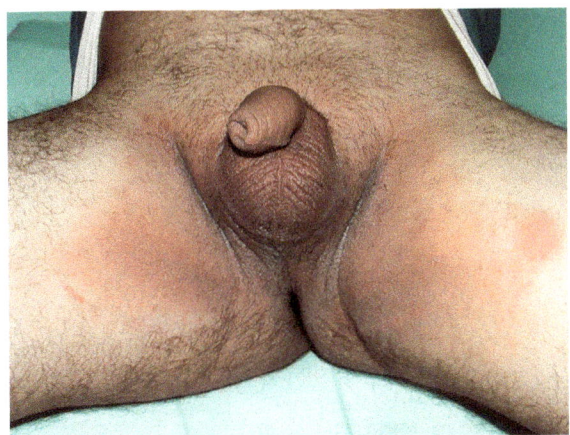

a. Intertrigo groins
b. Tinea cruris
c. Dermatitis groins
d. Candidiasis groins

933. This child presented with itchy red papules on face and extremities for the last 4–5 months. What is the clinical diagnosis?

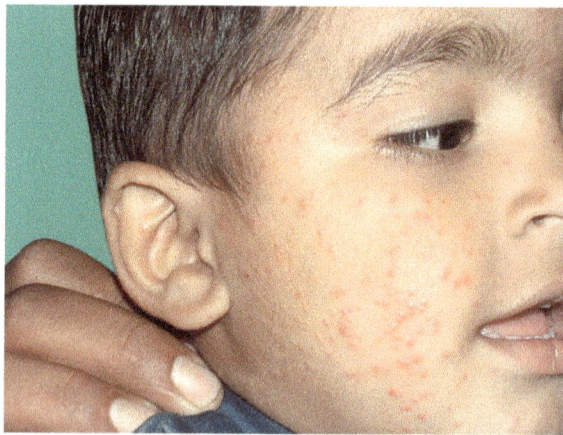

a. Insect bite hypersensitivity
b. Measles
c. Drug-induced exanthematous rash

934. This child presented with redness and itching in the groins. Similar involvement is also seen in cervical folds. What is the clinical diagnosis?

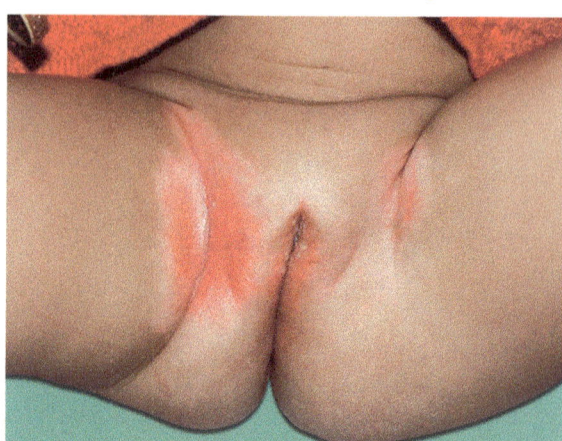

a. Napkin rash (diaper dermatitis)
b. Candidal intertrigo
c. Seborrheic dermatitis

935. This patient presented with rough, asymptomatic and hyperkeratotic lesions in both groins. What is the clinical diagnosis?

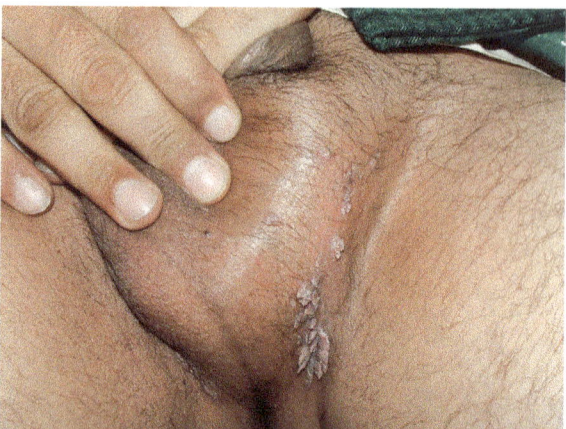

a. Condylomata lata
b. Condylomata acuminata

936. This child was brought with erythema and itching of both cheeks for the last one month. What is the clinical diagnosis?

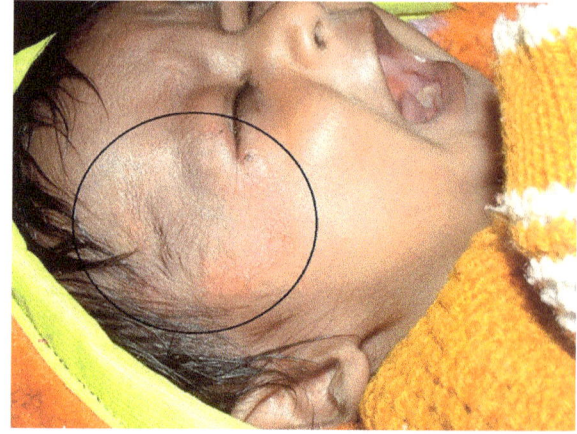

a. Atopic dermatitis
b. Seborrheic dermatitis
c. Tinea faciei

937. This patient of psoriasis received many injections of dexamethasone from an unqualified practitioner. It was followed by appearance of many small pustules on the psoriatic lesions. What is the clinical diagnosis?

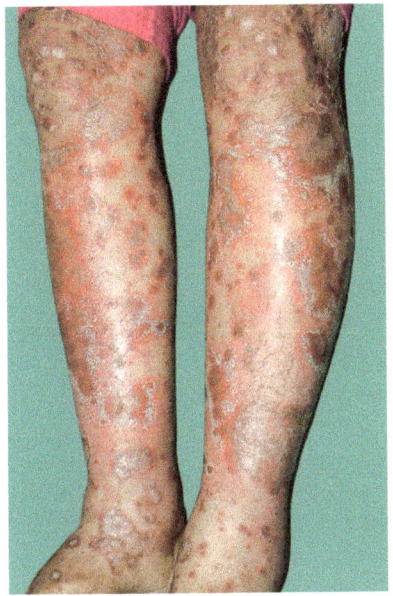

a. Generalized pustular psoriasis (GPP)
b. Acropustulosis
c. Psoriasis with secondary infection
d. Impetigo herpetiformis

938. This patient developed on his back a painful and tender lump with multiple openings. What is the clinical diagnosis?

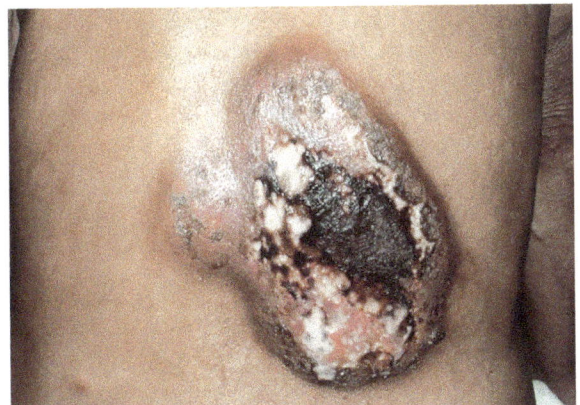

a. Squamous cell carcinoma (SCC)
b. Carbuncle
c. Scrofuloderma

939. This patient complained of enlarged size of nose. What is the clinical diagnosis?

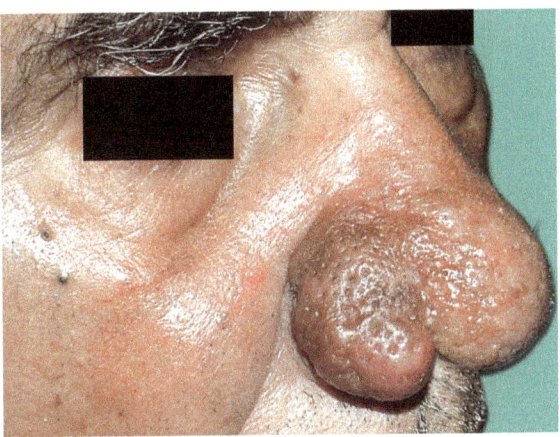

a. Sebaceous hyperplasia
b. Rhinophyma
c. Basal cell carcinoma
d. Squamous cell carcinoma
e. Sebaceous adenoma

940. This patient complained of itching and blistering of both hands for the last one month. What is the clinical diagnosis?

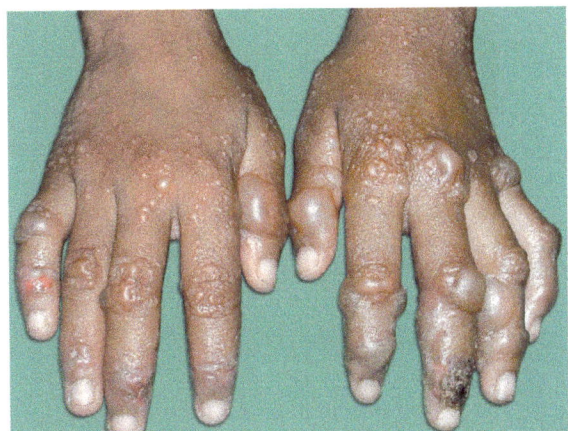

a. Epidermolysis bullosa simplex
b. Pompholyx
c. Id eruption
d. Scabies

941. This patient complained of redness and white scaling of scalp. What is the clinical diagnosis?

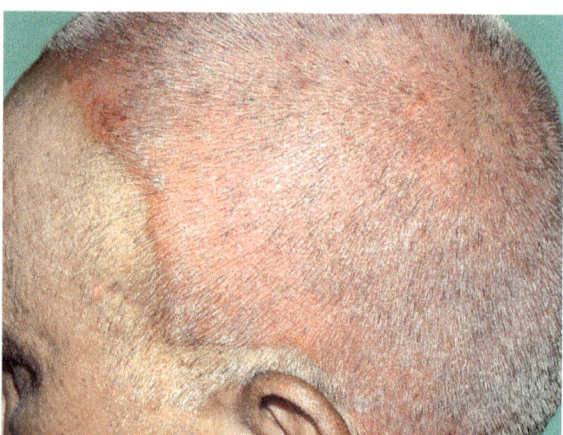

a. Seborrheic capitis
b. Tinea capitis
c. Psoriasis scalp

942. A 30-year-old female complained of itching with hair loss in both axillae for the last 4–5 years. What is the clinical diagnosis?

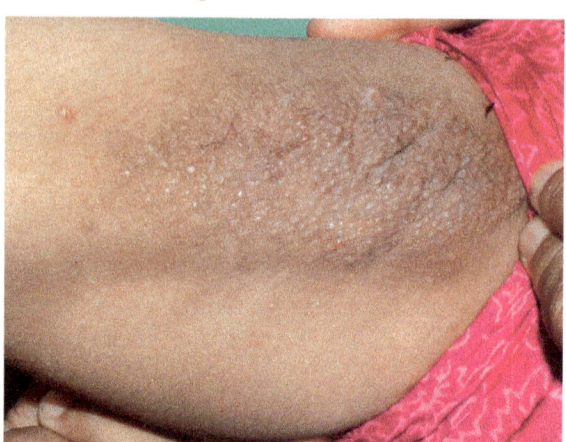

a. Fox-Fordyce disease
b. Pseudoacanthosis nigricans
c. Intertrigo

943. A 4-month-old baby was brought with hair loss in the occipital region. What is the clinical diagnosis?

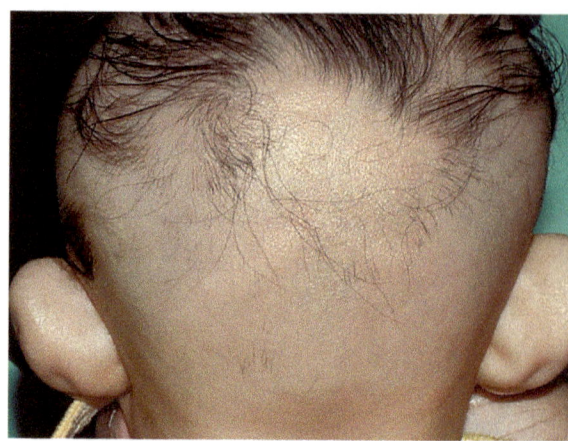

a. Alopecia areata
b. Neonatal occipital alopecia

944. This child was brought with red, painful, and tender swellings on forearm. What is the clinical diagnosis?

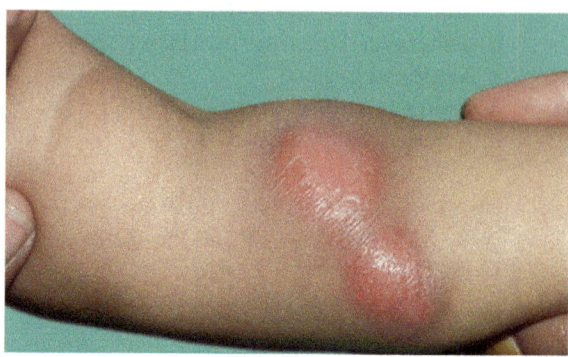

a. Psoriasis
b. Tuberculoid leprosy
c. Abscess
d. Lupus vulgaris

945. A 3-year-old child was brought with two large crusted plaques on shoulder and back for the last seven days. What is the clinical diagnosis?

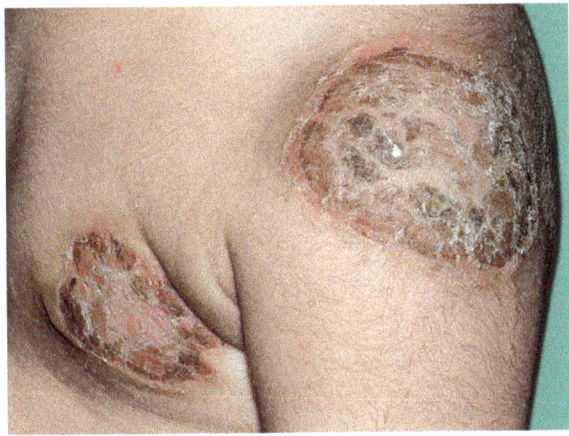

a. Tinea corporis
b. Impetigo contagiosa
c. Psoriasis
d. Discoid eczema

946. She complained of itching and redness under both breasts. What is the clinical diagnosis?

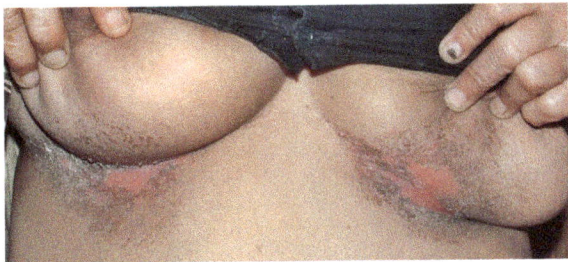

a. Tinea corporis
b. Candidiasis
c. Flexural psoriasis
d. Intertrigo

947. This lady complained eruption of crop of itchy lesions on trunk and extremities for the last seven days. What is the clinical diagnosis?

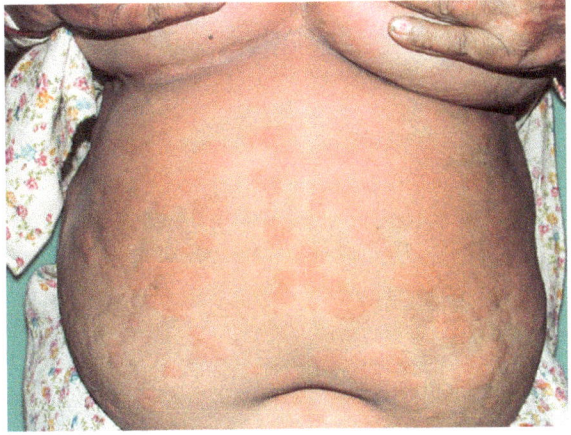

a. Acute urticaria
b. Pityriasis rosea
c. Secondary syphilis
d. Lepromatous leprosy

948. This patient complained of a patch of hair loss. What is the clinical diagnosis?

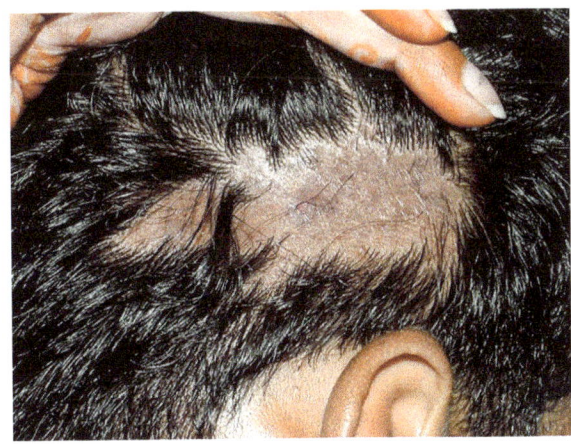

a. Tinea capitis
b. Alopecia areata
c. Trichotillomania
d. Cicatricial alopecia

949. This presented with redness, pain and swelling of foot. What is clinical diagnosis?

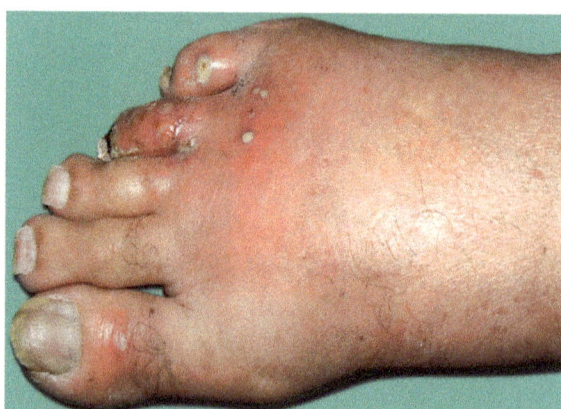

a. Cellulitis foot
b. Erysipelas

950. A 70-year-old male presented with a plaque on his face for the last four years. Margins of the plaque are irregular, slightly raised and thread like. The central part of the lesion is atrophic with crusts at places. What is the clinical diagnosis?

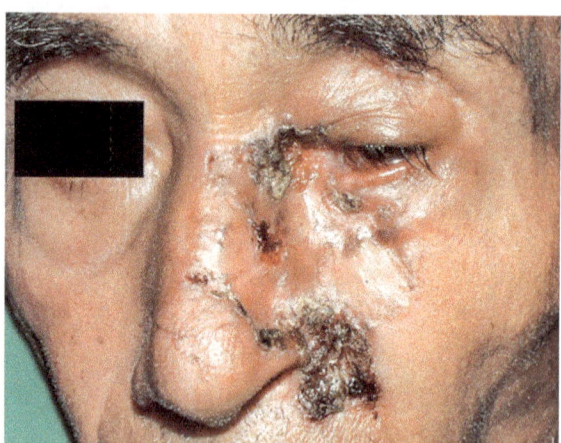

a. Squamous cell carcinoma
b. Basal cell carcinoma

951. This patient developed overnight red patch with burning sensation on *lateral side of his* trunk. What is the clinical diagnosis?

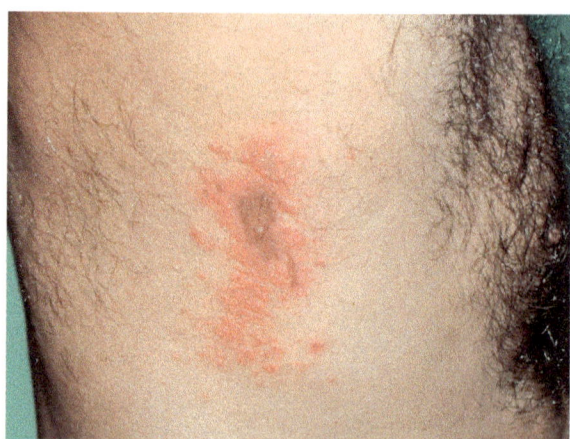

a. Herpes zoster
b. *Paederus dermatitis*

952. This patient complained for itching and redness in groins. What is the clinical diagnosis?

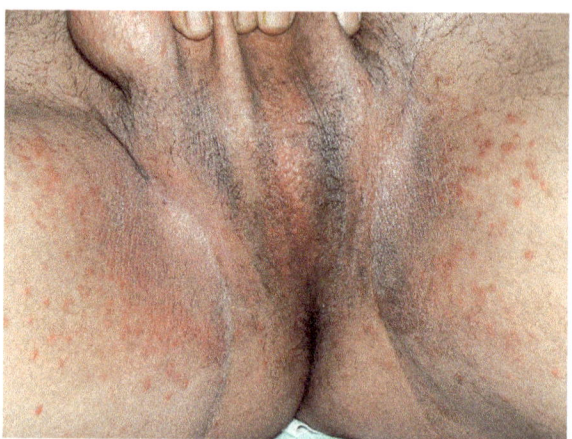

a. Tinea cruris
b. Intertrigo
c. Candidiasis groins
d. Flexural psoriasis

953. This patient complained of red, monomorphic papular lesions on front and back of trunk for the last two months. What is the diagnosis?

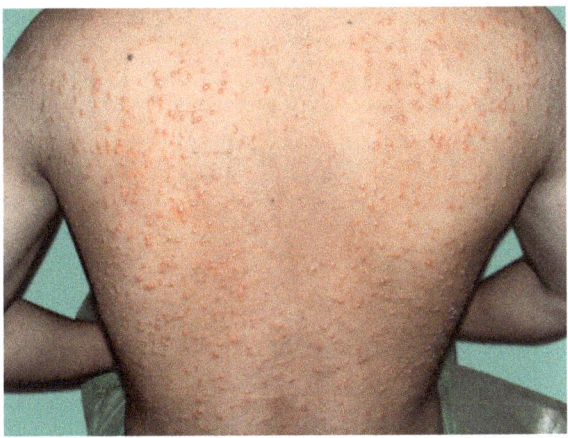

a. Acne vulgaris
b. Chickenpox
c. Acneiform eruption
d. Exanthematous rash

954. This patient complained of scaling and mild itching in this left foot. What is the clinical diagnosis?

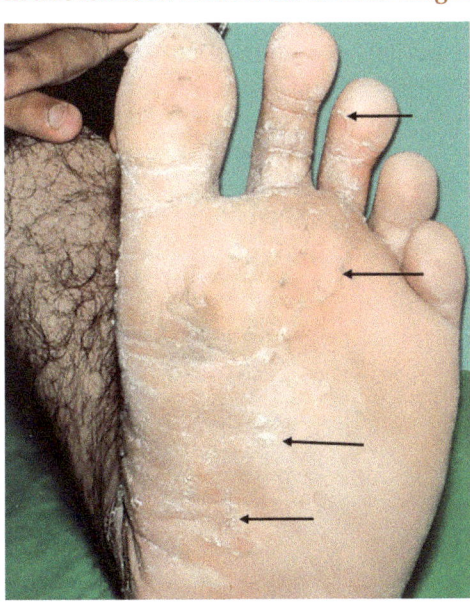

a. Candidiasis sole
b. Hyperkeratotic eczema
c. Keratolysis exfoliativa
d. Tinea pedis

955. She came with genital warts with three months of pregnancy. What is the most appropriate option of treatment for her?

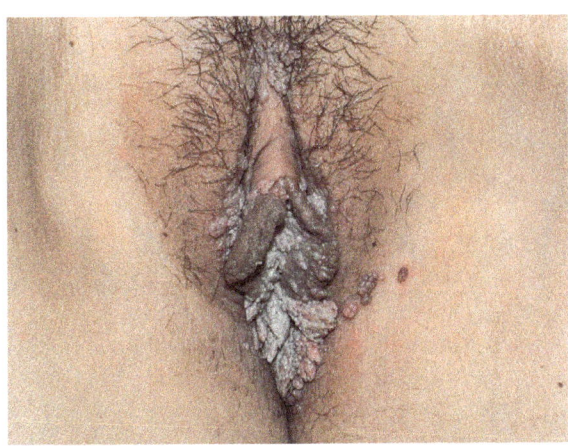

a. Cryotherapy
b. Electrodessication/Lasers
c. Podophyllin application
d. Leave it alone

956. This lady came with swelling of eyelids for the last two days. What is the most probable cause?

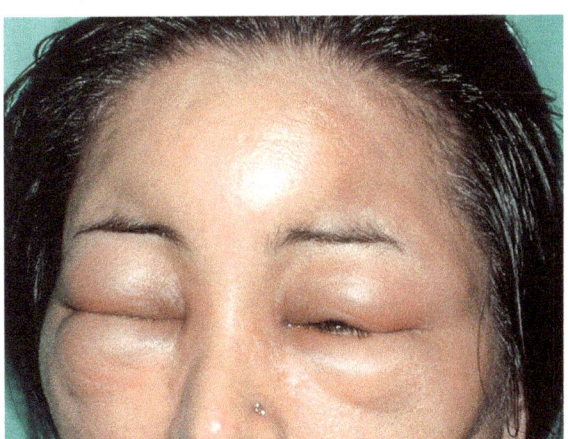

a. Hair dye use
b. Acute urticaria
c. Hypothyroidism
d. Angioedema

957. This patient complained of pigmentation of both legs. What is the most probable cause in this patient?

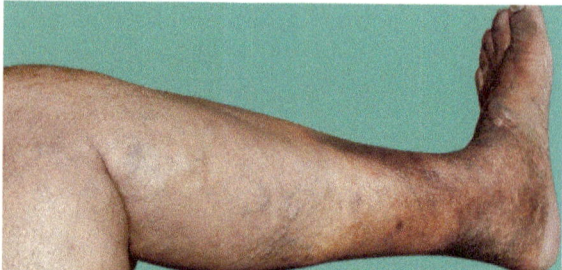

a. Due to topical agents
b. Stasis pigmentation due to varicose veins
c. Due to antihypertensive drugs
d. Schamberg's disease

958. This patient complained of blistering of feet due to mild mechanical trauma. His father and two brothers are also suffering from the same disease. What is the clinical diagnosis?

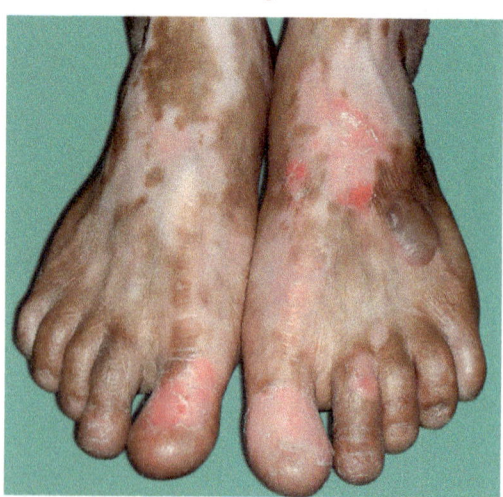

a. Epidermolysis bullosa
b. Porphyria cutanea tarda (PCT)

959. This patient developed a single, painless ulcer two weeks after a sexual contact with a commercial sex worker. Ulcer is red, raised, well-defined. Floor is clean, smooth, brownish red. Base is indurated and can be felt between fingers. Inguinal lymph nodes are enlarged which are discrete, rubbery and painless. What is the clinical diagnosis?

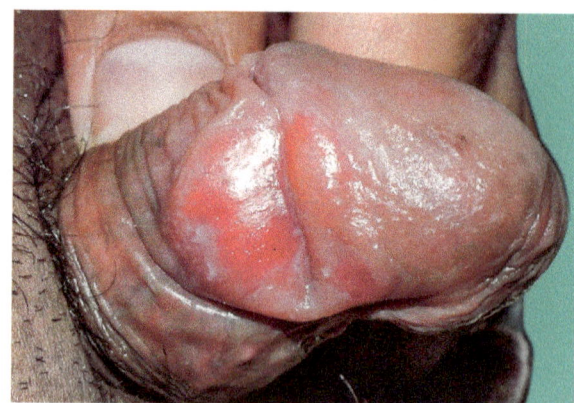

a. Chancroid
b. Syphilitic chancre
c. Donovanosis
d. Herpes genitalis

960. This patient complained of multiple sinuses on both sides of body in the cervical regions, groins and upper thighs for the last one year. What is the closest clinical diagnosis?

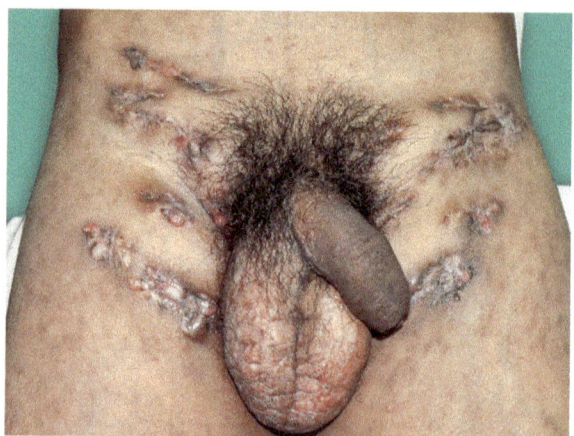

a. Hidradenitis suppurativa
b. Scrofuloderma

961. This patient complained of madarosis and infiltration of ears. He was also having ulcers at tips of his fingers *(MCQ 495)*. What is the clinical diagnosis?

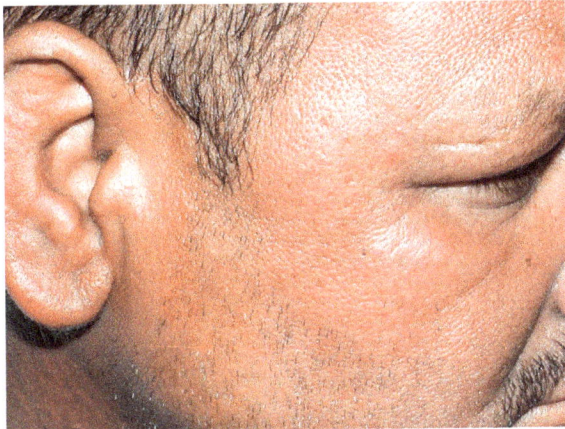

a. Lepromatous leprosy
b. Systemic sclerosis
c. Hypothyroidism (myxedema)
d. Alopecia areata

962. A 33-year-old female complained of hirsutism. She was having 90 kg body weight, oligomenorrhea and acanthosis nigricans in cervical region. What is the closest clinical diagnosis?

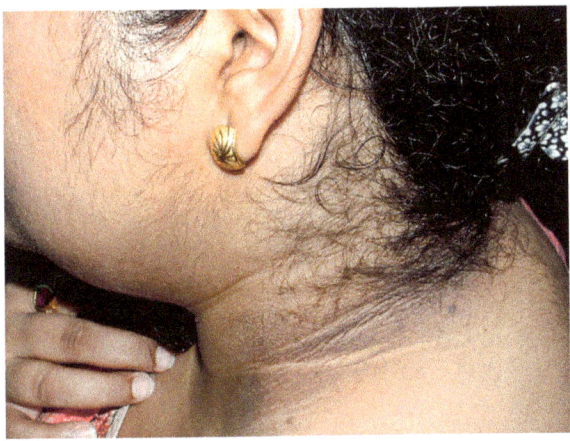

a. Idiopathic hirsutism
b. Non-insulin resistant PCOS
c. Insulin resistant PCOS
d. Androgen producing ovarian tumor

963. This patient had scalp psoriasis. He received systemic steroids that was followed by appearance of multiple small papules with white scaling on his trunk. What is cause and diagnosis?

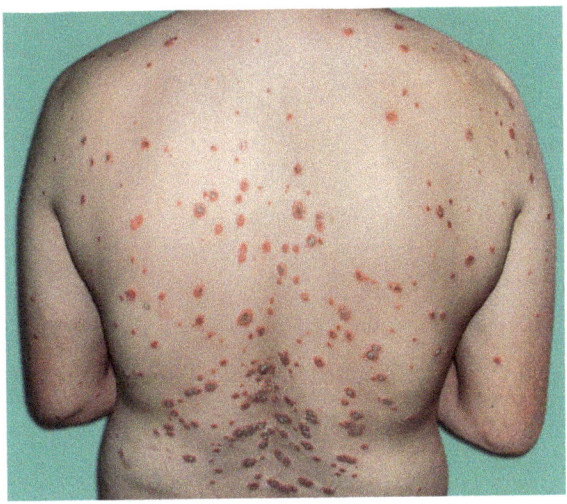

a. Koebner phenomenon
b. Rebound phenomenon
c. FDE due to steroids
d. Steroid induced acne

964. This patient presented with multiple papules on forehead. What is the clinical diagnosis?

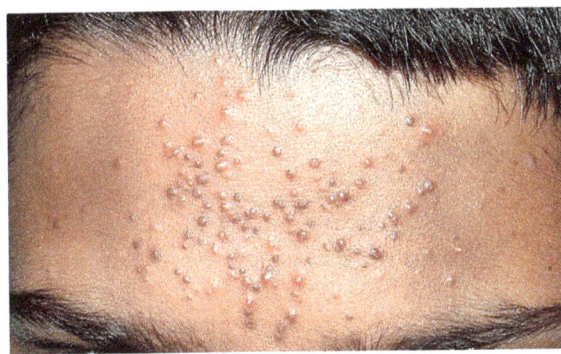

a. Molluscum contagiosum
b. Milia
c. Sand paper comedones
d. Lichen planus
e. Warts

965. A 2-year-old child presented with red plaque on scalp with loss of hair. What is the closest clinical diagnosis?

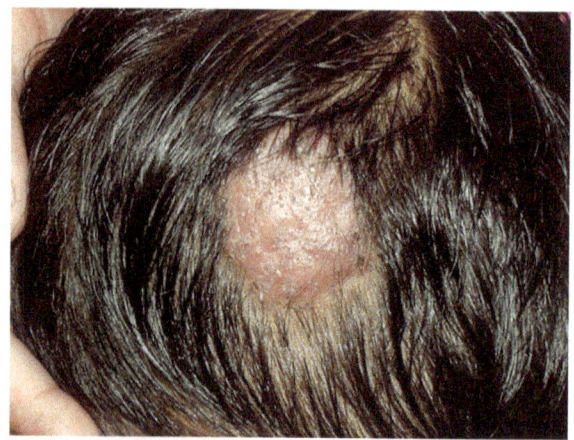

a. Alopecia areata
b. Kerion
c. Trichotillomania

966. A 33-year-old female complained of multiple petechiae and a patch of ecchymosis on her extremities for the last two days. What is closest clinical diagnosis?

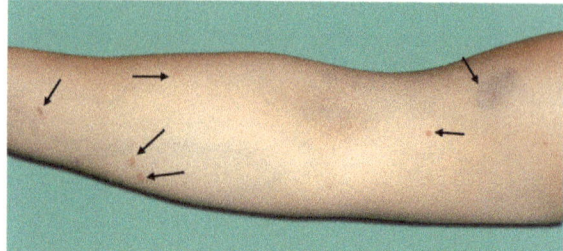

a. Idiopathic thrombocytopenic purpura (ITP)
b. Thrombotic thrombocytopenic purpura. (TPP)
c. Henoch-Schonlein purpura (HSP)
d. Actinic purpura

967. This patient complained of itching and eruption of wheals on stroking with a blunt object. What is the diagnosis of this patient?

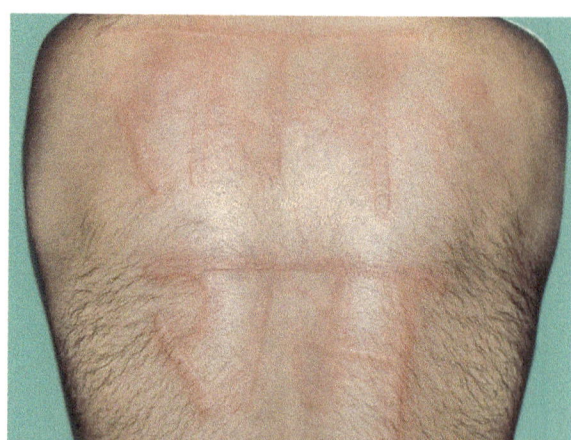

a. White dermatographism
b. Symptomatic dermatographism
c. Darier's sign

968. This patient complained of multiple dark-colored asymptomatic multiple papules on penile shaft. No other parts of body are involved. What is the clinical diagnosis?

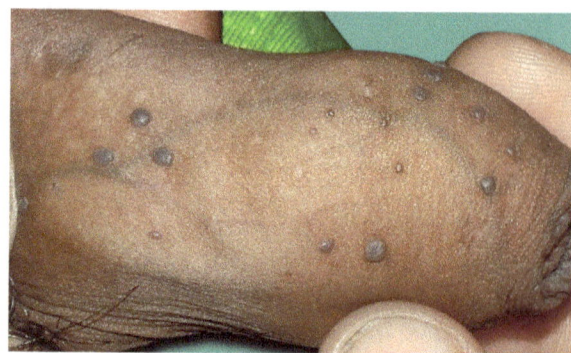

a. Lichen planus
b. Molluscum contagiosum
c. Lichen nitidus
d. Genital warts

969. This patient complained of multiple, itchy dry patches on various parts of body. What is the clinical diagnosis?

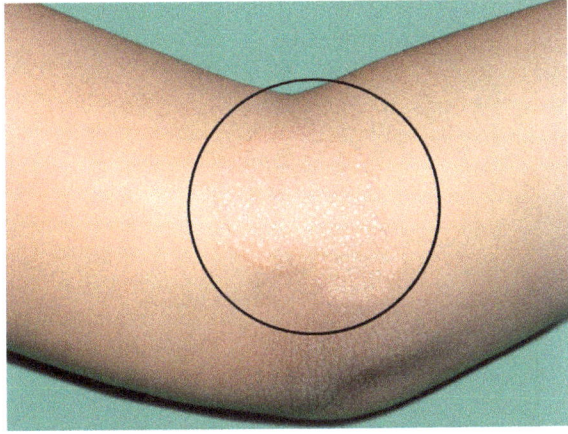

a. Dry discoid eczema
b. Tinea corporis
c. Granuloma annulare
d. Pityriasis alba

970. She complained of itchy red patches on buttocks. What is the clinical diagnosis?

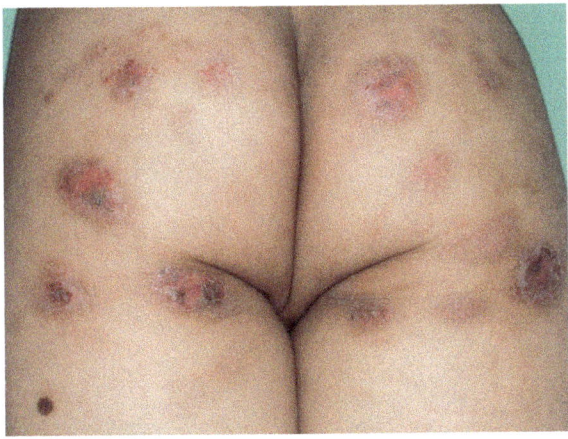

a. Tinea corporis
b. Psoriasis
c. Discoid eczema

971. She complained of painful, tender and red swellings in her axilla for the last 10 days. What is the clinical diagnosis?

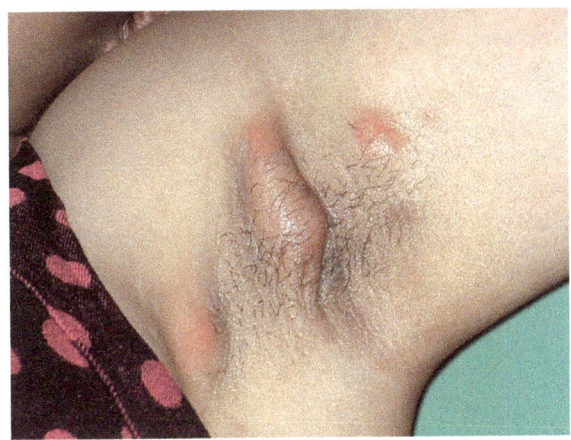

a. Hidradenitis suppurativa
b. Pyogenic abscesses
c. Enlarged lymph nodes

972. This patient presented with multiple red scaly well-defined plaques with little itching. Plaques showed clearing towards center with no loss of sensations. What is the clinical diagnosis?

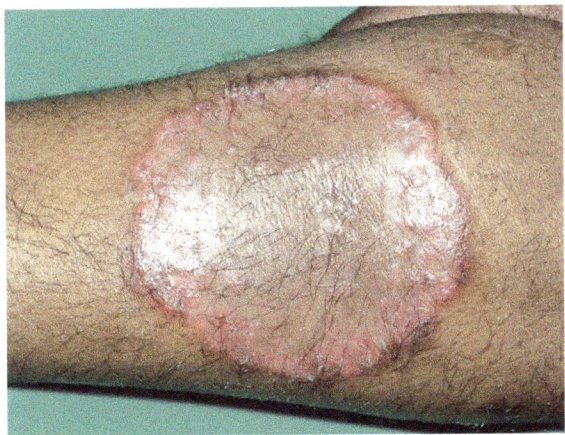

a. Tinea corporis
b. Annular psoriasis
c. Discoid eczema
d. Tuberculoid leprosy
e. Granuloma annulare

973. A 25-year-old male presented with herpes zoster for the last two days. Which one of the following options is most appropriate for this patient?

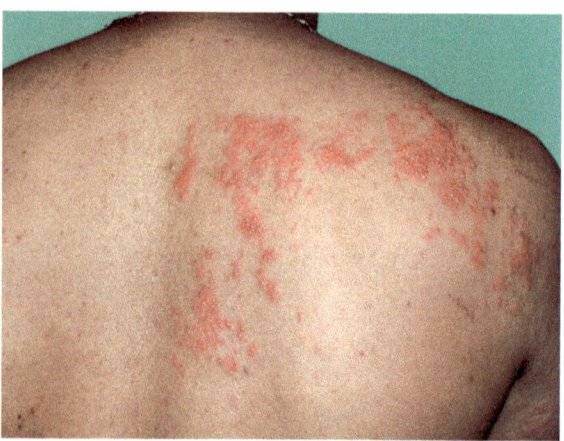

a. Valaciclovir tab + aciclovir cream + analgesics
b. Analgesics + calamine lotion
c. Valaciclovir + analgesics + calamine lotion
d. Analgesics + aciclovir cream

974. She came with itching and redress in groins, perineal region and suprapubic region for the last one week. What is the clinical diagnosis?

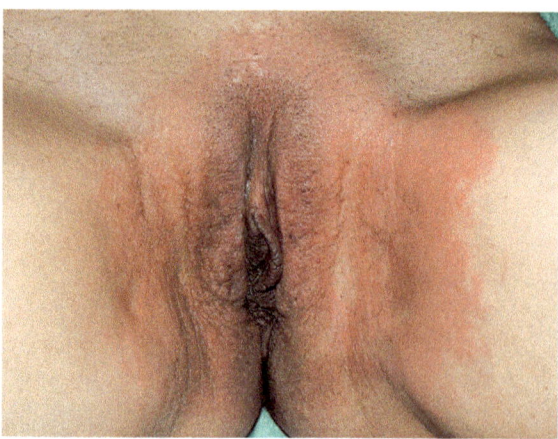

a. Candidiasis
b. Intertrigo
c. Contact irritant dermatitis
d. Tinea cruris

975. This patient presented with reddish hyperkeratotic plaques on trunk and face *(MCQ 26)*. There is no loss of sensations in the plaques. What is the clinical diagnosis?

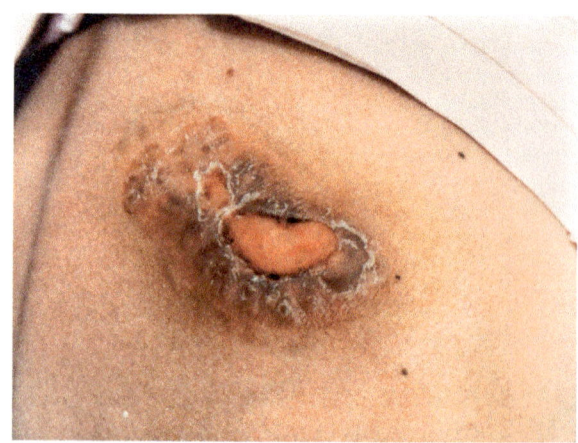

a. Psoriasis
b. Lupus vulgaris
c. Tuberculoid leprosy
d. Chronic cutaneous lupus erythematosus (CCLE)

976. Overnight she developed red patches with pain and burning sensation on the skin of her chest. What is the clinical diagnosis?

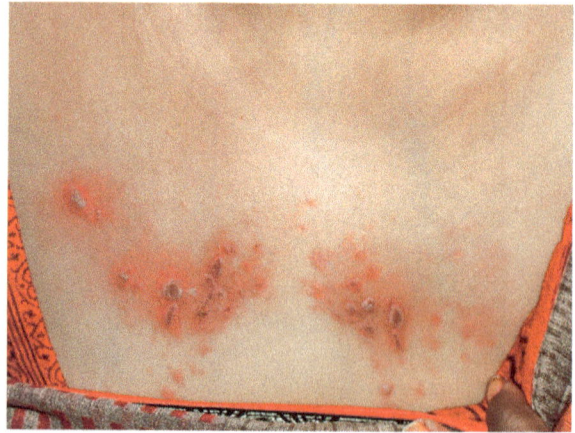

a. *Paederus dermatitis*
b. Herpes zoster
c. Chickenpox

977. Which one of the following drugs in most appropriate for a six months pregnant lady having tinea corporis?

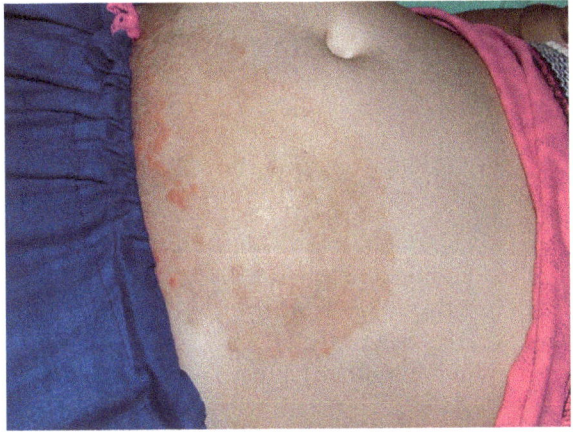

a. Griseofulvin
b. Fluconazole
c. Terbinafine
d. Itraconazole
e. Ketoconazole

978. This child presented with a patch of a hair loss on his scalp. What is the clinical diagnosis?

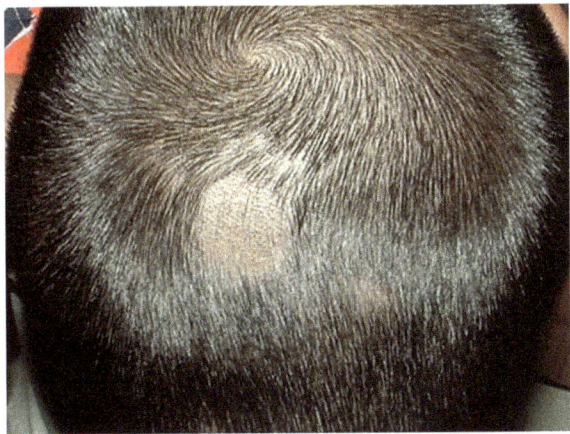

a. Alopecia areata
b. Trichotillomania
c. Tinea capitis

979. This patient complained of erythema and itching on buttocks for the last five days. This is no h/o use of steroids. What is the clinical diagnosis?

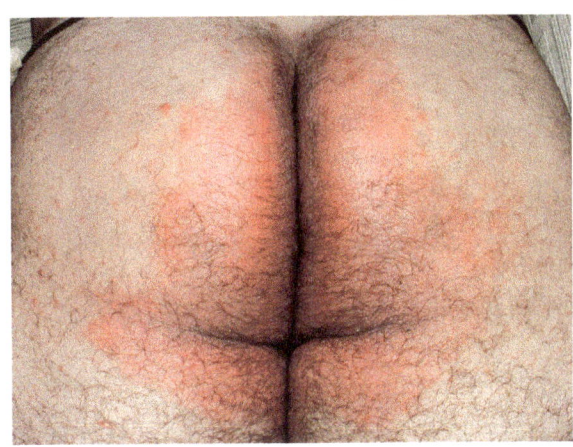

a. Tinea cruris
b. Tinea incognito
c. Contact irritant dermatitis (CID)
d. Candidiasis

980. This patient presented with multiple large itchy plaques on extremities. There is no loss of sensations in the patches. What is the clinical diagnosis?

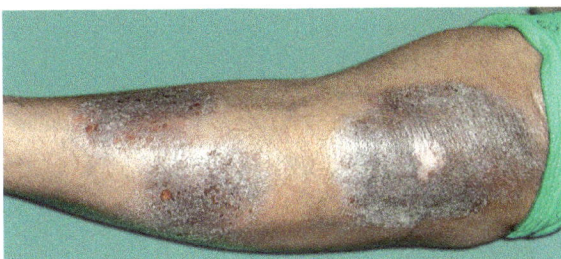

a. Tinea corporis
b. Psoriasis
c. Lichen planus
d. Tuberculoid leprosy
e. Discoid eczema

981. This patient complained of a small patch of hair loss in his moustaches. What is the clinical diagnosis?

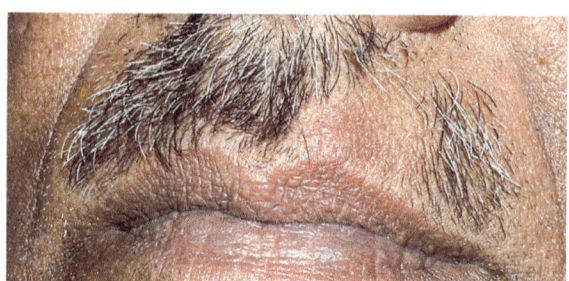

a. Alopecia areata
b. Tinea barbae
c. Trichotillomania

982. A 5-year-old girls presented with a large patch and crop of small macules with fine scaling on trunk and extremities for the last 20 days. It was accompanied by little itching. What is the diagnosis?

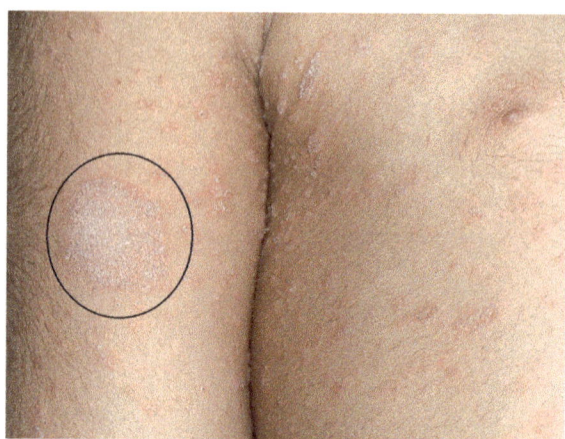

a. Pityriasis versicolor
b. Pityriasis rosea
c. Pityriasis alba

983. This patient presented with multiple various sized asymptomatic ill-defined red plaques on extremities and trunk. There is no loss of sensations in the plaques. What is the clinical diagnosis?

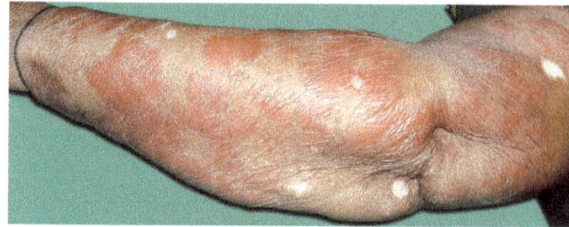

a. Lepromatous leprosy
b. Tuberculoid leprosy
c. Histoid leprosy
d. Indeterminate leprosy

984. This patient is complaining of purple-colored papules on glans and undersurface of prepuce. What is the clinical diagnosis?

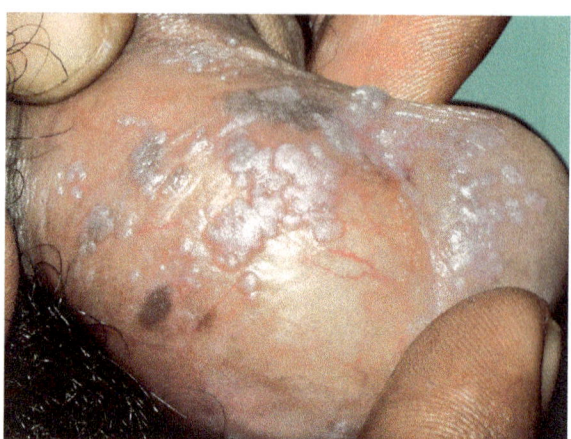

a. Venereal warts
b. Lichen planus
c. Psoriasis

985. A 4-month-old child presented with severely itchy red patches on cheeks. What is the clinical diagnosis?

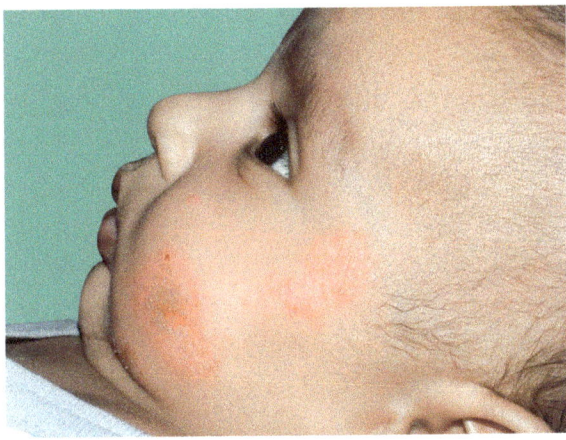

a. Pityriasis alba
b. Discoid eczema
c. Tinea faciei
d. Seborrheic dermatitis

986. A 2-month-old infant was brought with redness of cervical folds and skin behind ears. What is the clinical diagnosis?

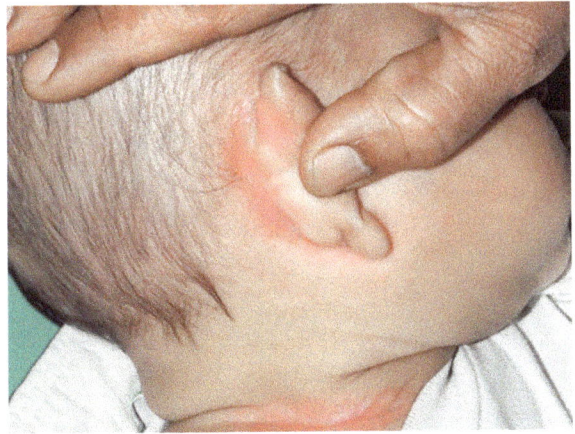

a. Seborrheic dermatitis
b. Infantile atopic dermatitis
c. Candidiasis

987. This patient complained of multiple shiny papular lesions on penile shaft. What is the clinical diagnosis?

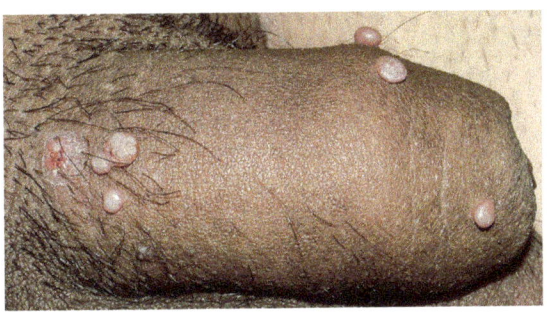

a. Genital warts
b. Molluscum contagiosum
c. Lichen planus

988. She complained of multiple papules on face. What is the clinical diagnosis?

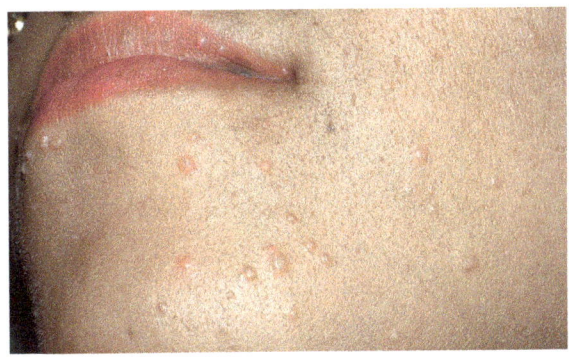

a. Acne vulgaris
b. Milia
c. Molluscum contagiosum
d. Warts

989. This patient complained of itching and scaling of left foot. What is the clinical diagnosis?

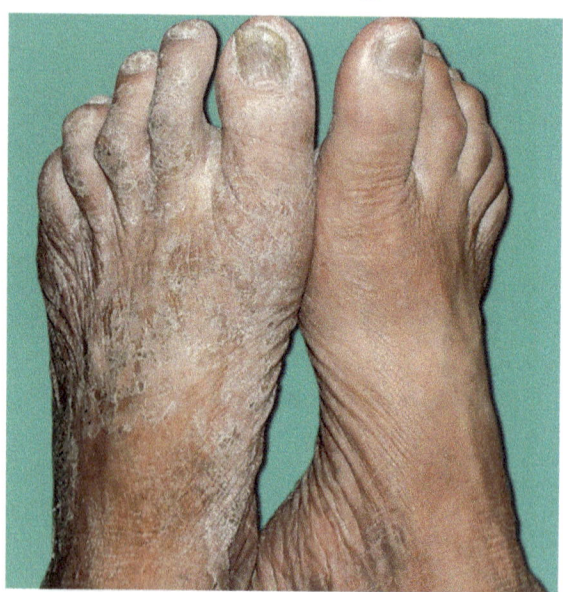

a. Eczema foot
b. Tinea pedis
c. Contact dermatitis to shoes

990. A 10-year-old child presented with a single several centimeters sized hypopigmented macule for the last six years. It is not crossing the midline and is stable. What is the clinical diagnosis?

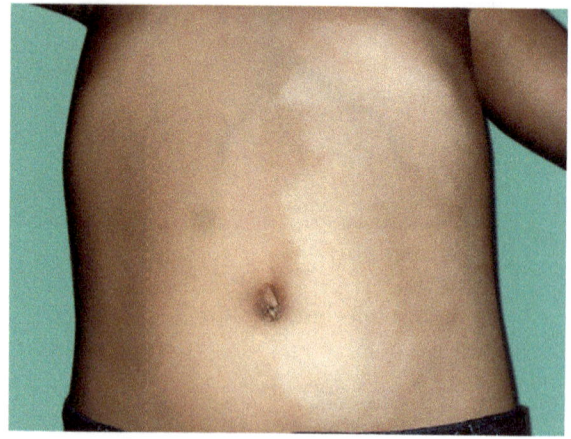

a. Nevus depigmentosus
b. Segmental vitiligo
c. Focal vitiligo

991. This patient presented on lower back with a highly pruritic ill-defined lichenified plaque having increased cutaneous markings. What is the clinical diagnosis?

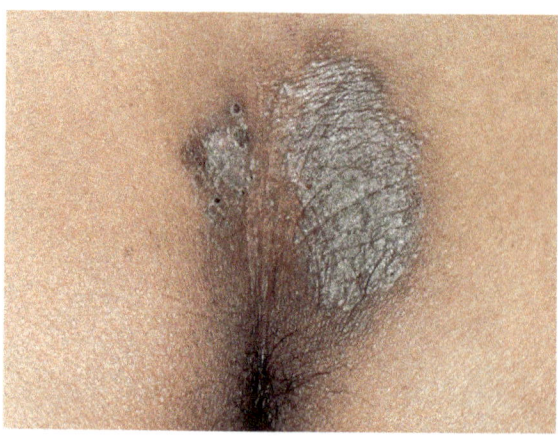

a. Bowen's disease
b. Lichen simplex chronicus
c. Psoriasis

992. This lady complained of itching, fissuring, crusting and pustulation of both lips for the last one month. What is the clinical diagnosis?

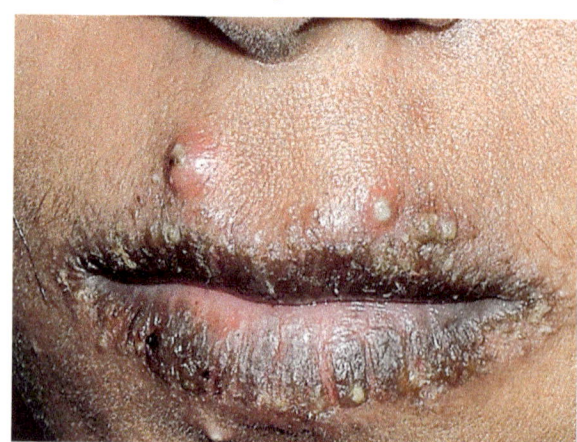

a. Actinic cheilitis
b. Cheilitis due to nutritional deficiencies
c. Cheilitis due to lip-stick

Chapter 4 ✦ MCQs of Dermatology, Venereology and Leprology

993. This patient presented with multiple asymptomatic non itchy yellowish papules on scrotum for the last three years. What is the clinical diagnosis?

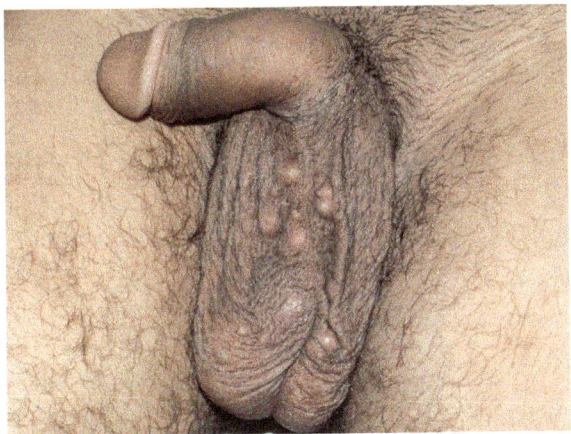

a. Scabies
b. Steatocystoma multiplex
c. Angiokeratomas on scrotum

994. This patient complained of itching redness and scaling at hairline of scalp, eyebrows, moustache and beard region. What is the clinical diagnosis?

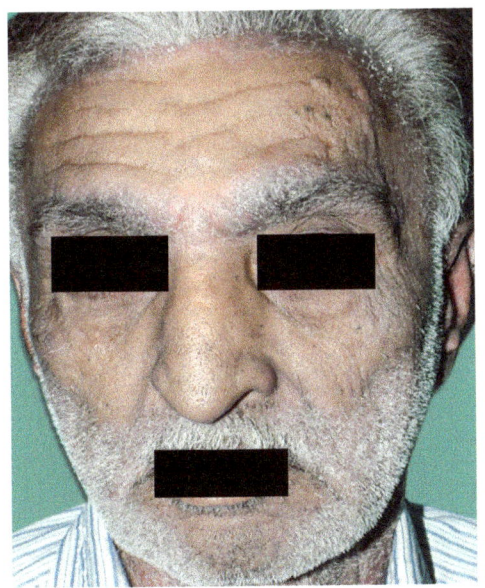

a. Atopic dermatitis
b. Seborrheic dermatitis
c. Psoriasis

995. This patient is complaining of redness, itching, burning and pain sensations of scrotal skin. He is very uncomfortable and cannot sit on chair for prolonged period. What is the clinical diagnosis?

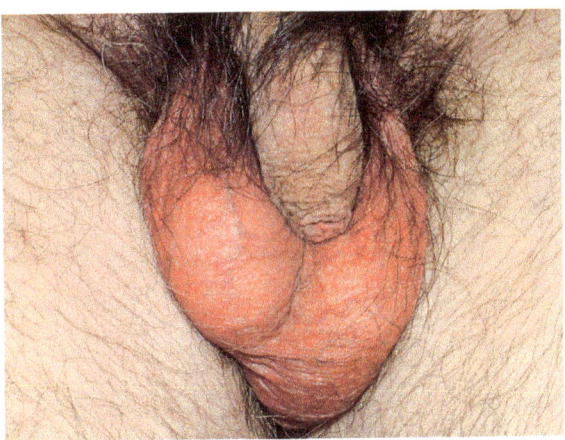

a. Lichen simplex chronicus
b. Red scrotum syndrome
c. Tinea Infection

996. This is a magnified picture of asymptomatic crop of red macules with scaling on the back. Scales are attached peripherally with free edge towards center. Center is giving a wrinkled appearance. What is the clinical diagnosis?

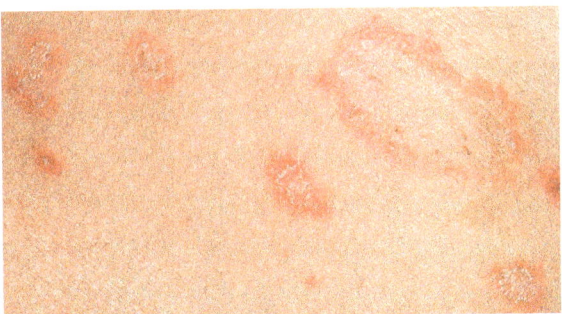

a. Secondary syphilis
b. Pityriasis rosea
c. Psoriasis
d. Exanthematous rash

997. This patient complains of itching on shin for the last 5–6 years. He was having closely set papules on shins. What is the clinical diagnosis?

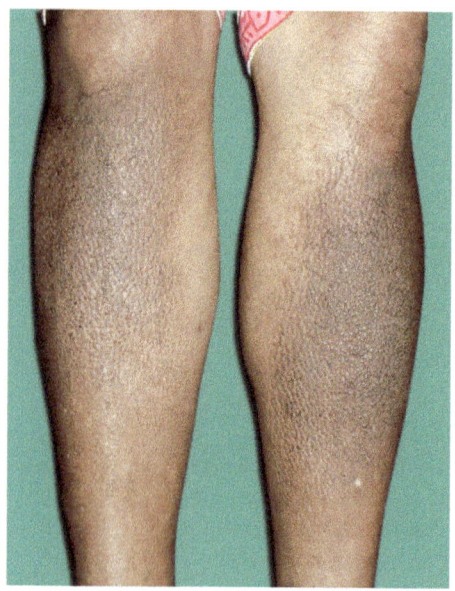

a. Lichen planus
b. Lichen simplex chronicus
c. Lichen amyloidosis

998. This patient complained of bluish discoloration of fingers on exposure to cold. What is the clinical diagnosis?

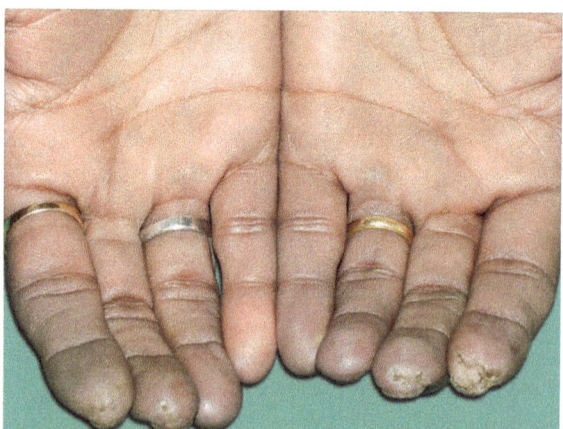

a. Secondary Raynaud's phenomenon.
b. Raynaud's disease
c. Chilblains

999. This patient presented with a chronic non-healing ulcer in the sacral region with watery discharge for the last 10 months. What is the clinical diagnosis?

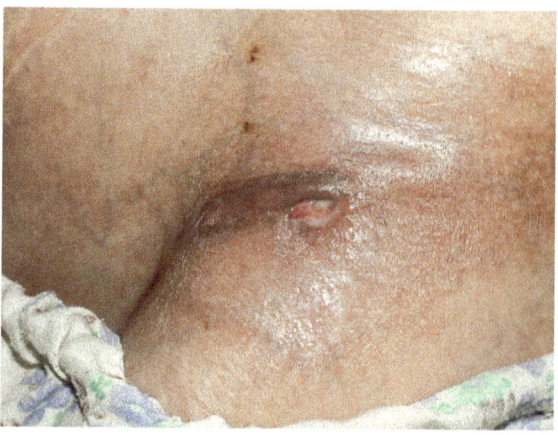

a. Scrofuloderma
b. Pilonidal sinus

1000. A 60-year-old male presented with itching, darkening, thickening of skin of forehead, cheeks and chin for the last many years. Similar changes were also seen on shoulders, extremities and cubital fossae. What is the clinical diagnosis?

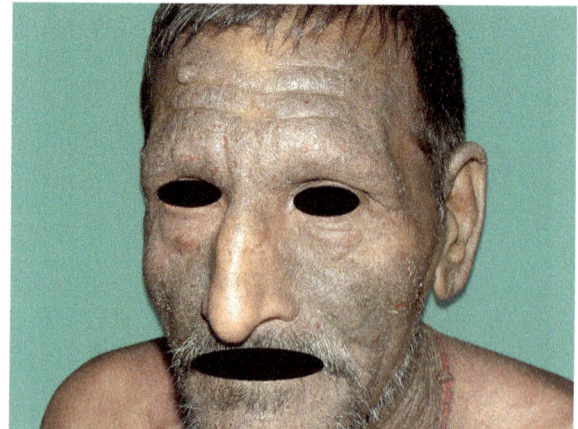

a. Seborrheic dermatitis (SD)
b. Atopic dermatitis (AD)
c. Airborne contact dermatitis (ABCD)
d. Chronic actinic dermatitis (CAD)

Chapter 4 ✦ MCQs of Dermatology, Venereology and Leprology

1001. A newly married girl developed multiple itchy papules on arms and upper chest. What is the clinical diagnosis?

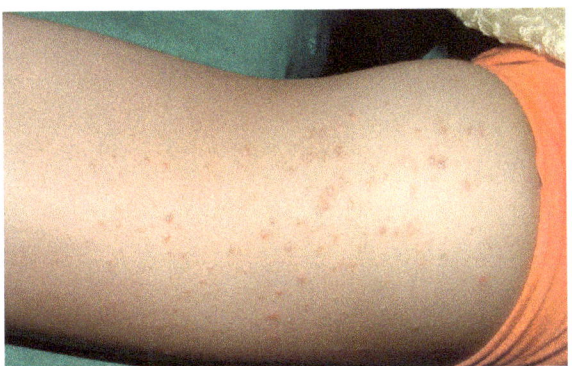

a. Acne vulgaris
b. Acneiform eruption
c. Post-waxing folliculitis

1002. This patient presented with thick hyperkeratotic lesion around nail. What is the clinical diagnosis?

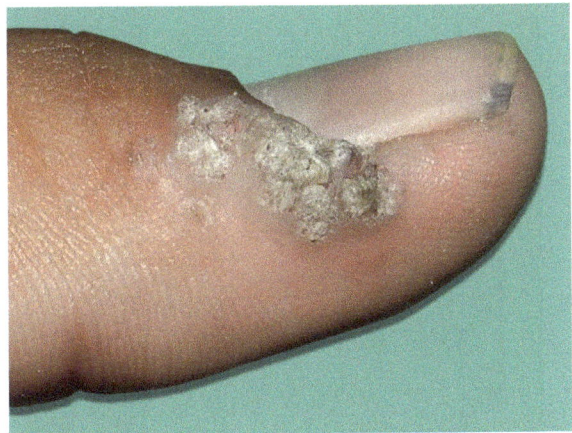

a. Periungual wart
b. Tuberculosis verrucosa cutis
c. Knuckle pad

1003. This patient complained of itching on abdomen. What is the clinical diagnosis?

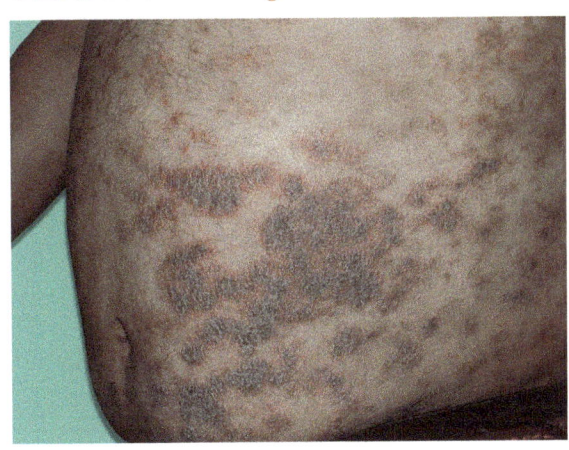

a. Psoriasis
b. Eczema
c. Tinea corporis
d. Lichen planus

1004. This patient complained of itching for the last 1 month. What is the clinical diagnosis?

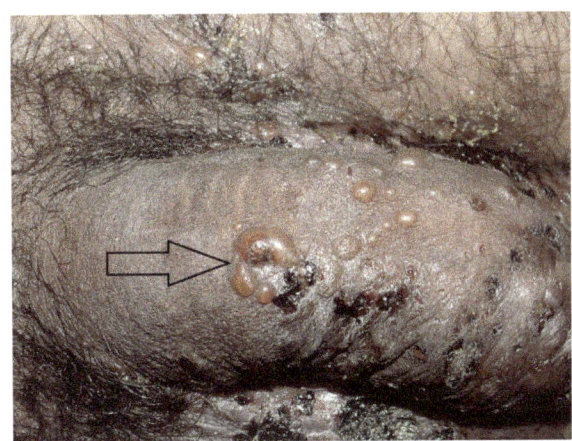

a. Herpes zoster
b. Scabies
c. Linear IgA disease

1005. What is the treatment of choice for this patient having cystic acne?

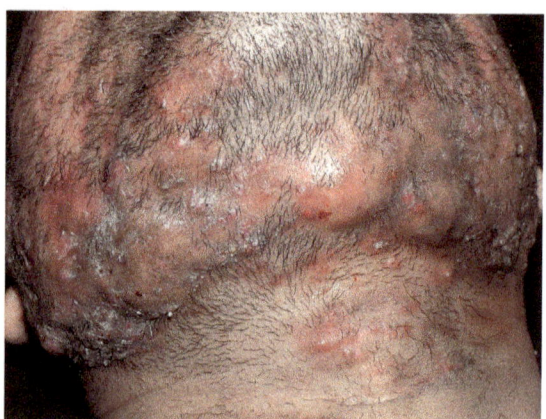

a. Isotretinoin
b. Tetracycline
c. Minocycline
d. Doxycycline

1006. This patient presented with numerous papules having white scaling on the trunk for the last one month. What is the clinical diagnosis?

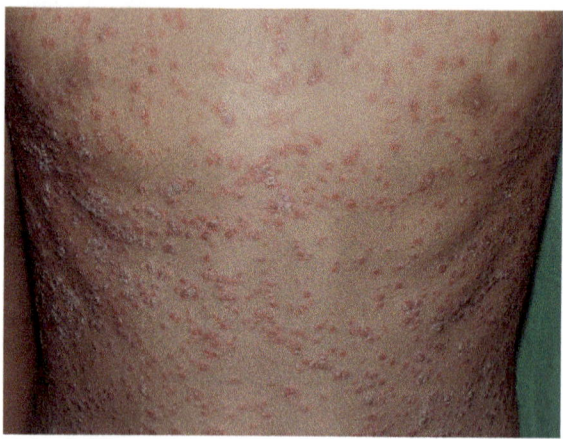

a. Pityriasis rosea
b. Secondary syphilis
c. Exanthematous rash
d. Guttate psoriasis

1007. An adolescent presented with purpuric rash in retiform (net like) pattern on extremities in bilateral symmetrical manner. It was also accompanied by pain abdomen and joint pain. What is the clinical diagnosis?

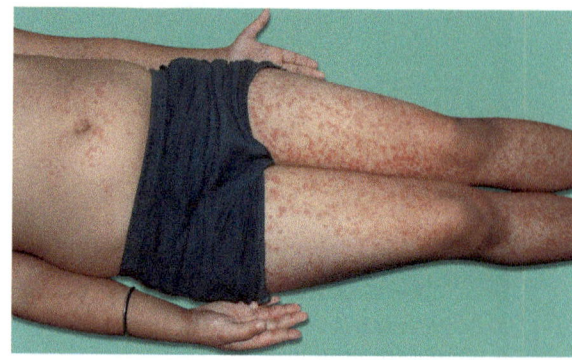

a. Actinic purpura
b. Idiopathic thrombocytopenic purpura (ITP)
c. Henoch-Schonlein purpura
d. Palpable purpura

1008. This patient complained of a recurrent suppurative solitary painless facial papule with crusting for the last six months. It is adherent to the underlying tissues. What is the clinical diagnosis?

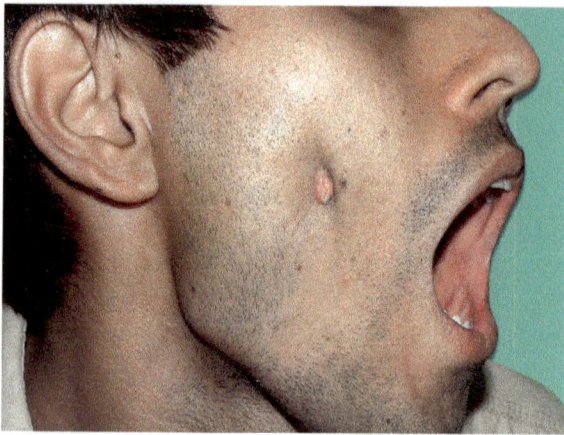

a. Chronic acne cyst
b. Osteomyelitis
c. Cutaneous sinus of dental origin

1009. A 50-year-old patient presented with fleshy irregular growth on glans for the last six months. Inguinal lymph nodes on one side are also enlarged. What is the clinical diagnosis?

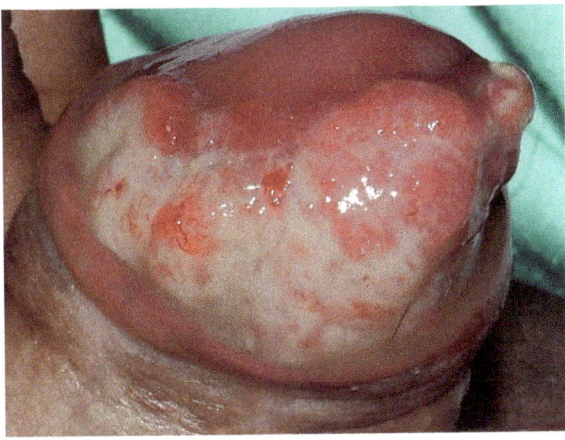

a. Carcinoma penis
b. Genital warts

1010. She presented with a red plaque with slightly raised and thread like margins on her cheek. What is the clinical diagnosis?

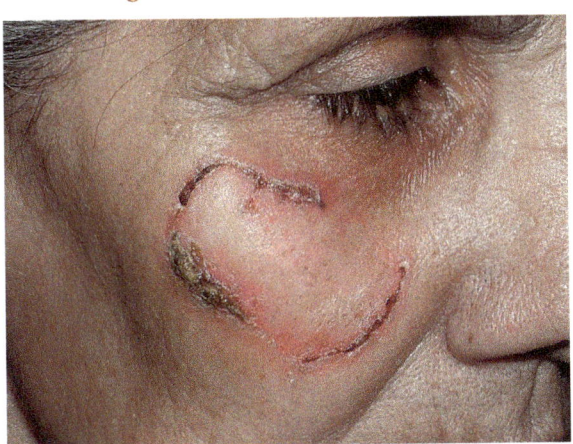

a. Squamous cell carcinoma (SCC)
b. Basal cell carcinoma (BCC)
c. Superficial spreading melanoma (SSM)

1011. A 3-month-old baby was brought with comedones, papules and pustules on cheeks. What is the diagnosis?

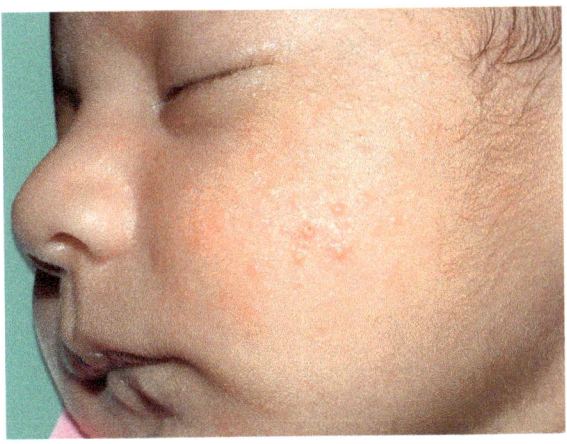

a. Milia neonatorum
b. Erythema toxicum neonatorum
c. Neonatal acne

1012. This patient presented with itching and scaling in the beard region for the last many years. What is the clinical diagnosis?

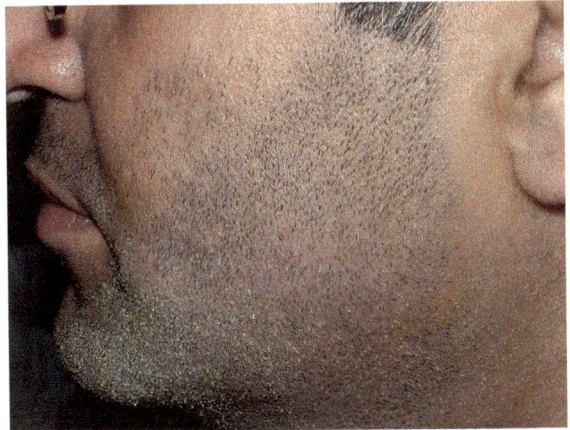

a. Seborrheic dermatitis
b. Atopic dermatitis
c. Tinea faciei

1013. This patient presented with diffuse redness and white scaling of both palms. Dorsal side of hands showed red plaques with white scaling *(next MCQ)*. What is the clinical diagnosis?

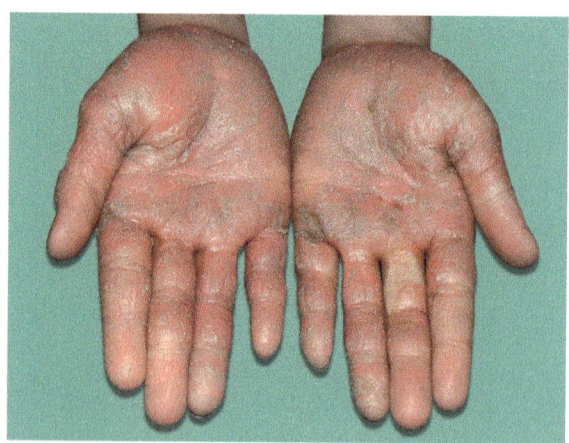

a. Psoriasis
b. Lichen planus
c. Chronic cutaneous lupus erythematosus
d. Hyperkeratotic eczema

1014. This patient presented with red plaques with white scaling. Palms showed diffuse redness, thickening and scaling *(above MCQ)*. What is the clinical diagnosis?

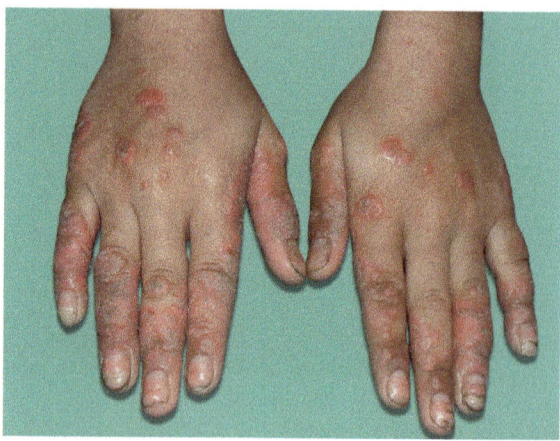

a. Lichen planus
b. Psoriasis
c. Chronic cutaneous lupus erythematosus

1015. This patient developed redness, exfoliation and burning sensation on applications of some cream. Which one of the following creams has she applied?

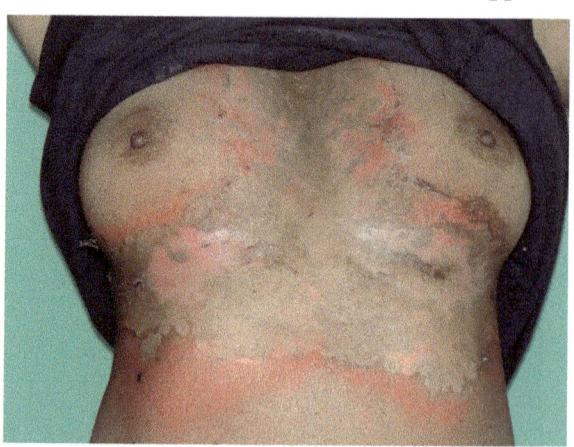

a. Dithranol (Derobin)
b. Podophyllin
c. Corticosteroid cream
d. Acyclovir cream

1016. This patient presented with itchy, violaceous-colored papules on trunk and extremities. What is the clinical diagnosis?

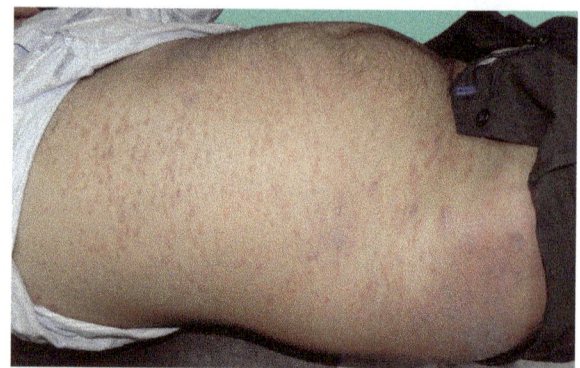

a. Guttate psoriasis
b. Lepromatous leprosy
c. Secondary syphilis
d. Lichen planus
e. Pityriasis rosea

1017. This lady complained of redness, itching and burning sensation on face due to prolonged application of some cream. Which one of the following creams has she applied?

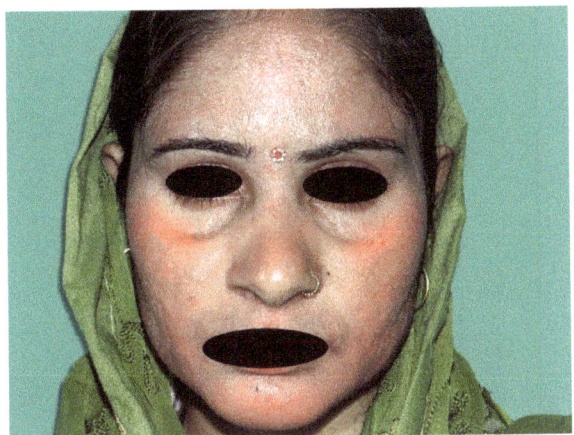

a. Sunscreen lotion
b. Benzoyl peroxide cream
c. Corticosteroid cream
d. Hydroquinone cream

1018. She complained of erythema and itching of face for the last 2–3 years. What is the clinical diagnosis?

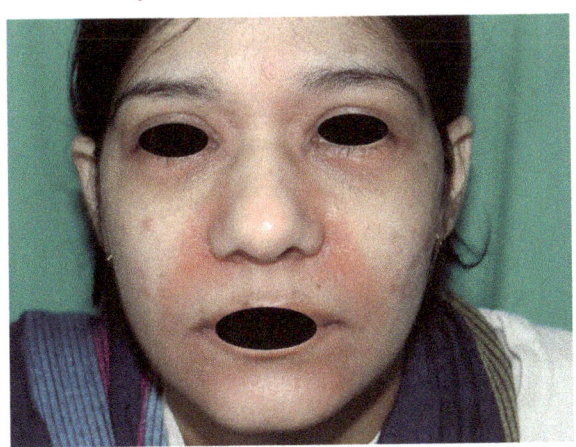

a. Topical steroid damaged face (TSDF)
b. Acne rosacea
c. Butterfly rash
d. Seborrheic dermatitis

1019. This patient applied podophyllin (podowart) incorrectly on genital warts which has led to ulcerations. Which one of the following options is a correct regimen?

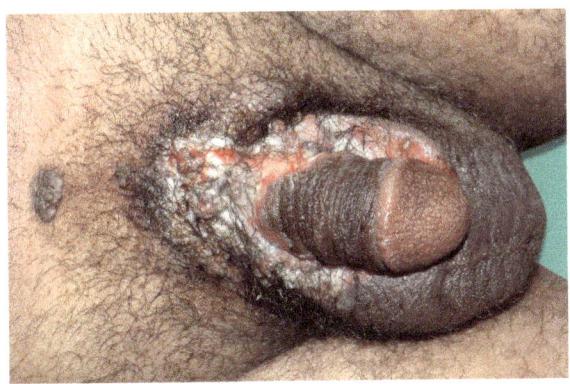

a. Daily application
b. Alternate day application by patient
c. Once in 4–5 days by the dermatologist

1020. A 35-year-old male presented with chronic plantar ulcerations with history of amputation of big toe and adjacent toe. There is a past history of inability to walk long distances. There is no history of loss of sensations. What is the clinical diagnosis?

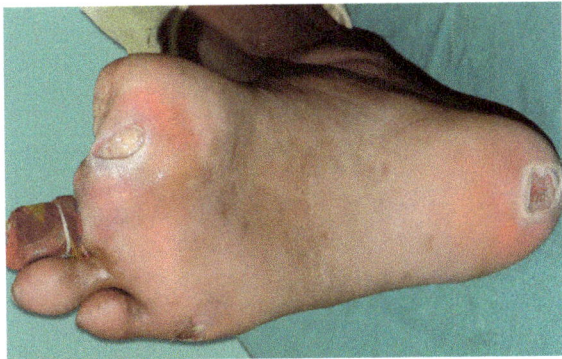

a. Lepromatous leprosy
b. Diabetic trophic ulcerations
c. Buerger's disease
d. Atherosclerotic arterial ulcers

1021. A 15-year-old patient complained of difficulty in walking due to multiple asymptomatic thickenings in soles. What is the clinical diagnosis?

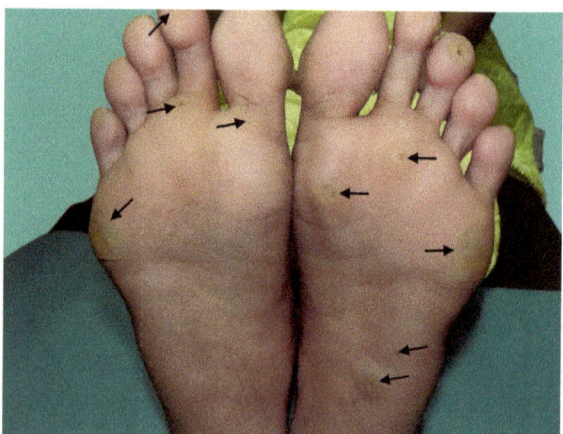

a. Plantar warts
b. Plantar corns
c. Punctate plantar keratoderma

1022. A 35-year-old male patient complained of redness and thickening on nose, cheeks and forehead. Antinuclear antibodies were found to be high. What is the diagnosis?

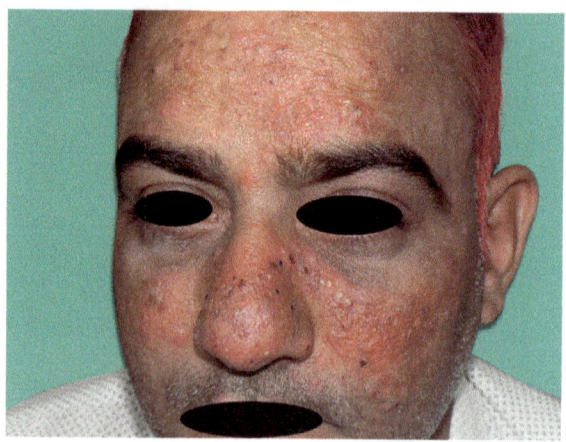

a. Chronic cutaneous lupus erythematosus (CCLE)
b. Systemic lupus erythematosus
c. Acne rosacea
d. Acne vulgaris

1023. A 14-year-old child complained of plantar hyperhidrosis and asymptomatic desquamation of soles for the last two months. What is the clinical diagnosis?

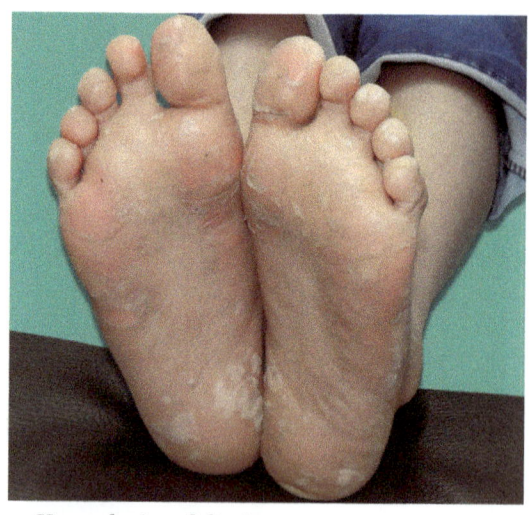

a. Keratolysis exfoliativa
b. Tinea pedis
c. Plantar eczema
d. Plantar psoriasis

1024. This patient complained of redness and white scaling on soles. He also has red plaques studded with white scaling on trunk and scalp. What is the clinical diagnosis?

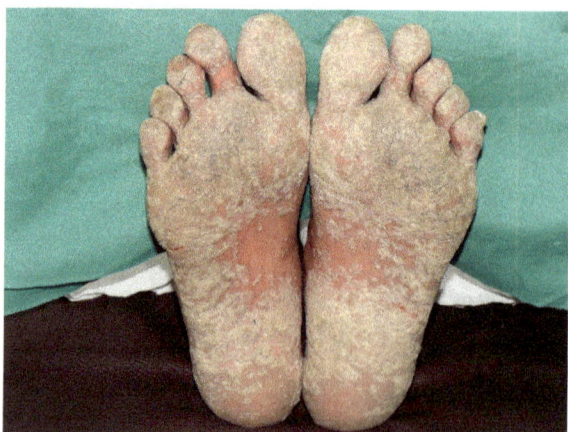

a. Tinea pedis
b. Plantar psoriasis
c. Hyperkeratotic plantar eczema

1025. This patient complained of pigmentation and burning pin pricking sensations on the right side of her back for the last three months. There is a past history of appearance of painful, grouped, small blisters. What is the diagnosis?

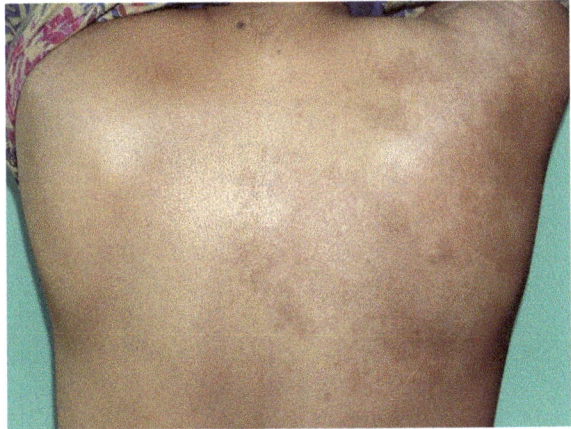

a. Post-herpetic neuralgia (PHN)
b. Notalgia paresthetica

1026. A 35-year-old female presented with papules and pustules on the lower part of cheeks and jawlines. What is the closest clinical diagnosis?

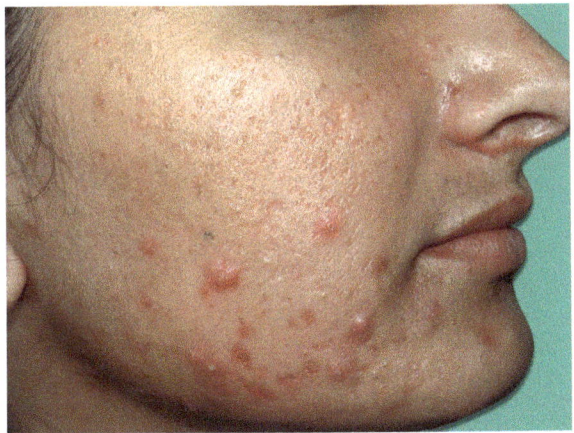

a. Acne vulgaris
b. Acneiform eruption
c. Acne keloidalis
d. Hormonal adult acne

1027. This patient complained of painful white lesion on the inner side of his buccal mucosa for the last two months. What is the clinical diagnosis?

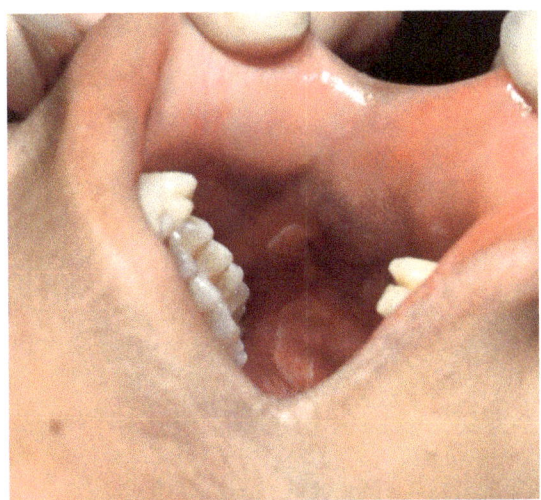

a. Major type oral aphthous ulcer
b. Oral candidiasis
c. Leukoplakia
d. Oral lichen planus

1028. This patient complained of a patch of hyper-pigmentation studded with coarse terminate hairs on his thigh for the last 3–4 years. What is the diagnosis?

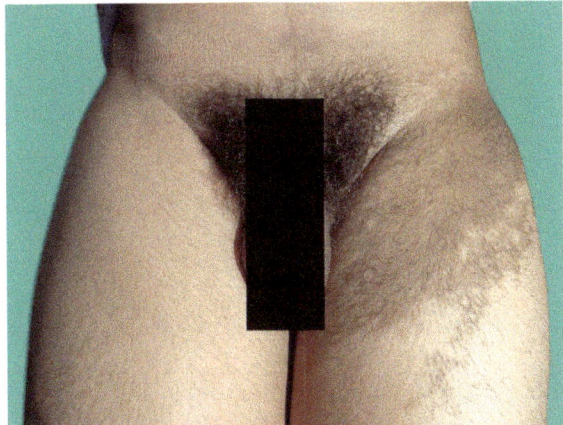

a. Becker's nevus
b. Congenital melanocytic nevus
c. Nevus of Ota

1029. A 40-year-old female complained of excessive loss of scalp hair 3–4 months after Covid infection. What is the clinical diagnosis?

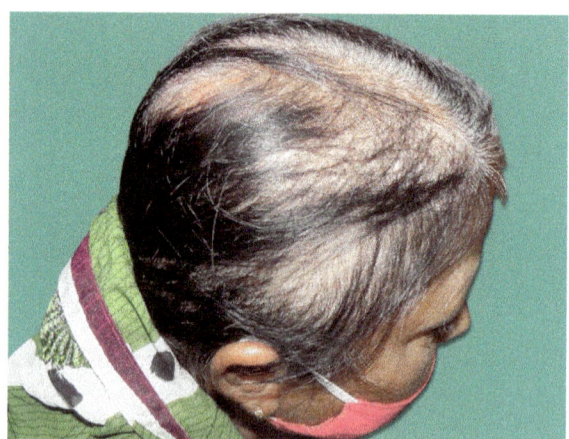

a. Androgenic hair loss
b. Telogen effluvium
c. Alopecia areata
d. Trichotillomania

1030. This patient complained of black-colored patches on his lips for the last two months. What is the clinical diagnosis?

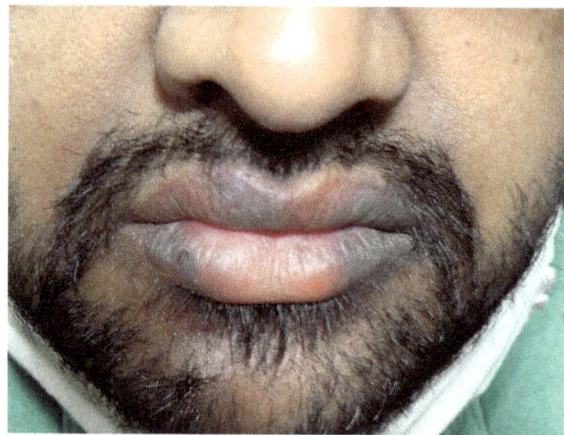

a. Lichen planus lips
b. Fixed drug eruption

1031. This patient complained of painless, firm, subcutaneous multiple nodules on upper extremities for last many years. What is the clinical diagnosis?

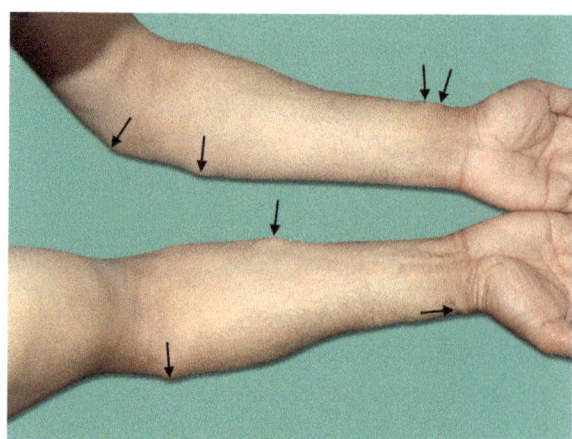

a. Familial multiple lipomatosis
b. Neurofibromatosis type 1

1032. This patient developed striae atrophicans in the groins following continuous application of some cream. Which one of the following creams has he applied?

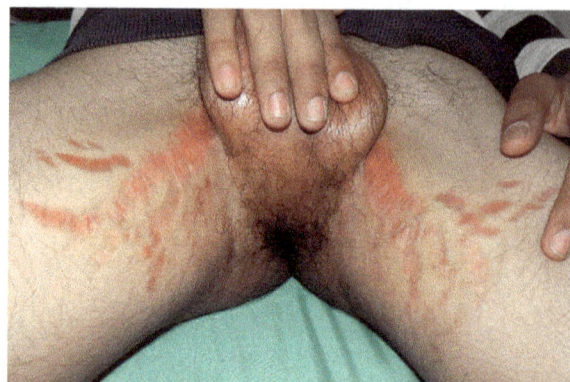

a. Clotrimazole cream
b. Derobin cream
c. Corticosteroid cream
d. Fusidic acid cream

1033. What is the diagnosis of this patient complaining of itching on back and buttocks?

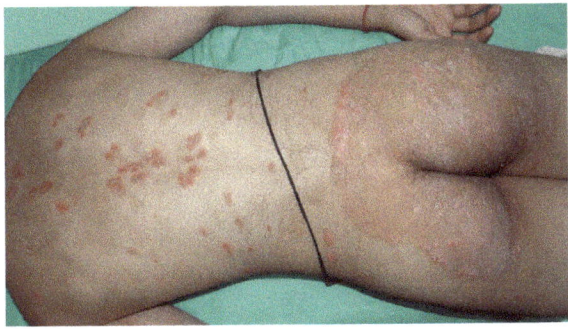

a. Flexural psoriasis
b. Tinea corporis
c. Psoriasis with tinea corporis

1034. This lady complained of multiple small lesions in the genital area, groins and suprapubic region. What is the diagnosis?

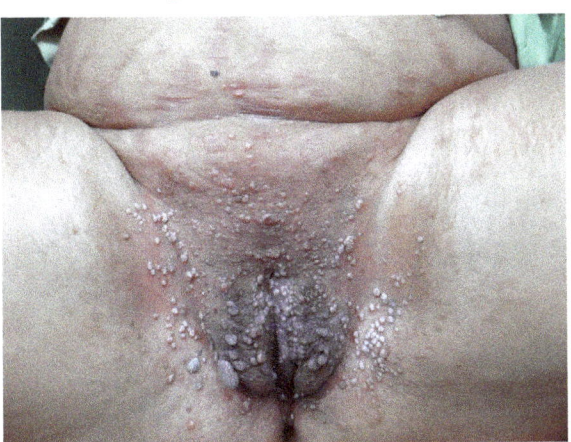

a. Herpes simplex
b. Molluscum contagiosum
c. Genital warts
d. Molluscum contagiosum with genital warts

1035. A 10-month-old female child presented with intensely pruritic red, hyperkeratotic papules in the genital area since birth. What is the clinical diagnosis?

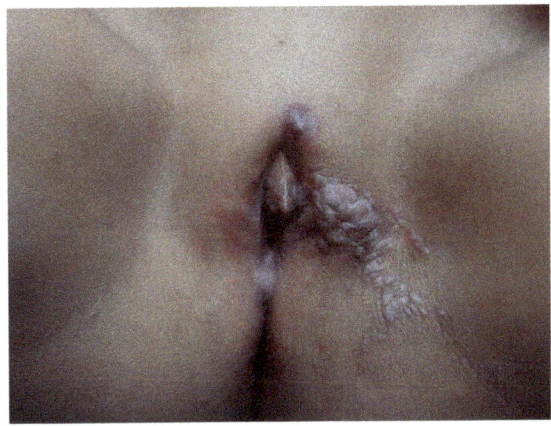

a. Inflammatory linear verrucous epidermal nevus (ILVEN)
b. Genital warts

1036. A 50-year-old patient presented with multiple ulcers on his soles for last three months. He is smoker and is having uncontrolled diabetes. He is also having loss of sensation in his feet and legs. Pulsations of dorsalis pedis artery on the dorsal side of ankle joint can be felt easily. What is the clinical diagnosis?

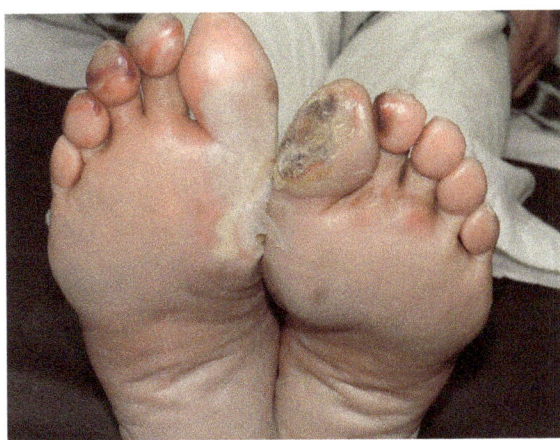

a. Lepromatous leprosy
b. Trophic ulcers due to diabetes
c. Arterial ulcers
d. Buerger's disease

1037. This patient complained of itching and recurrent eruption of papules and pustules on thighs for the last six months. What is the clinical diagnosis?

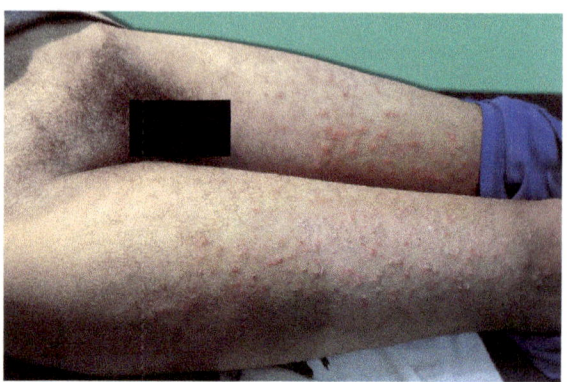

a. Chronic superficial folliculitis
b. Pseudofolliculitis

1038. She complained of itching and redness on her lower eyelids and neighboring areas of cheeks. What is the clinical diagnosis?

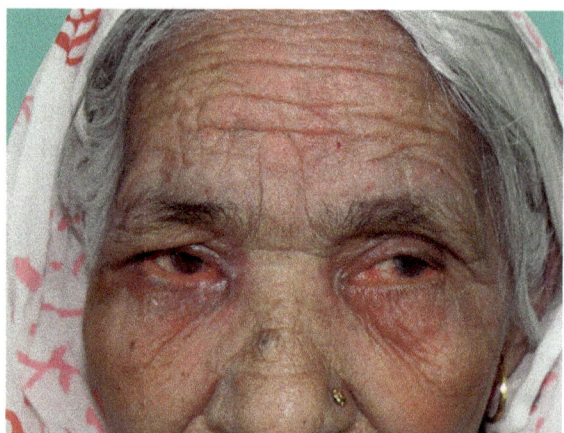

a. Airborne contact dermatitis (A&CD)
b. Allergic contact dermatitis due to eye drops.
c. Chronic actinic dermatitis (CAD)

1039. This patient complained of pruritic, purple-colored papules on lower extremities. What is the clinical diagnosis?

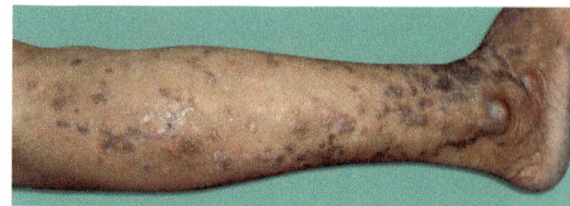

a. Lichen amyloidosis
b. Prurigo nodularis
c. Lichen planus

1040. A 25-year-old male presented with multiple painful ulcers with nonindurated base on his glans and under surface of prepuce five days after exposure with a commercial sex worker. What is the closest clinical diagnosis?

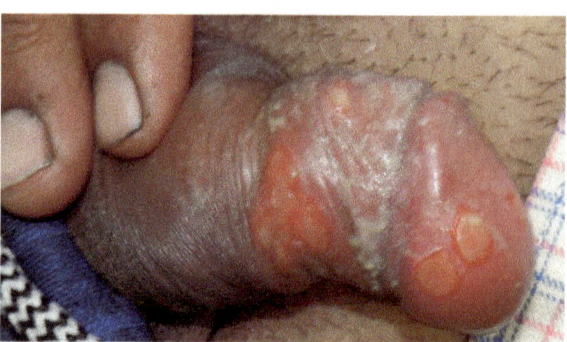

a. Syphilitic ulcer
b. Chancroid
c. Herpes genitalis
d. Lymphogranuloma venereum

1041. This patient complained of desquamation of skin of finger tips without any itching or pain. What is the clinical diagnosis?

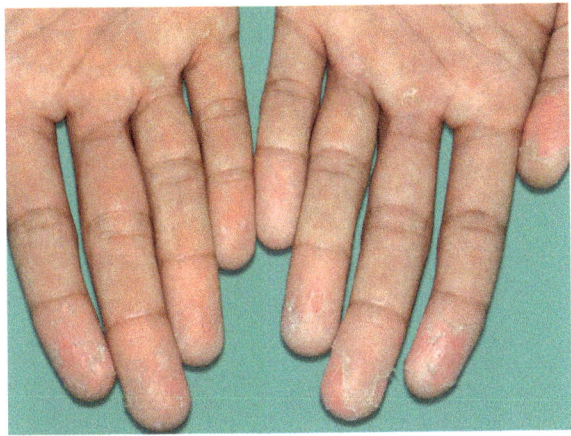

a. Keratolysis exfoliativa
b. Tinea manuum
c. Eczema of finger tips

1042. This patient complained of a red papule on his finger tip with recurrent bleeding for the last two months. What is the clinical diagnosis?

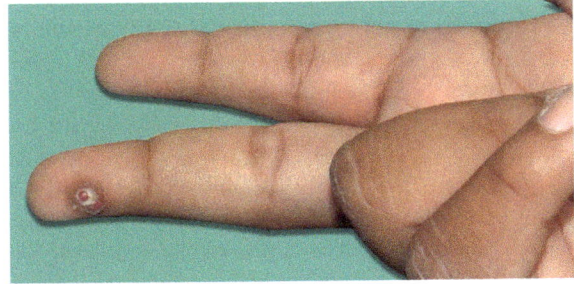

a. Herpetic whitlow
b. Common wart
c. Glomus tumor
d. Pyogenic granuloma

1043. This patient complained of diffuse redness, scaling and itching in the beard region and postauricular region. What is the closest clinical diagnosis?

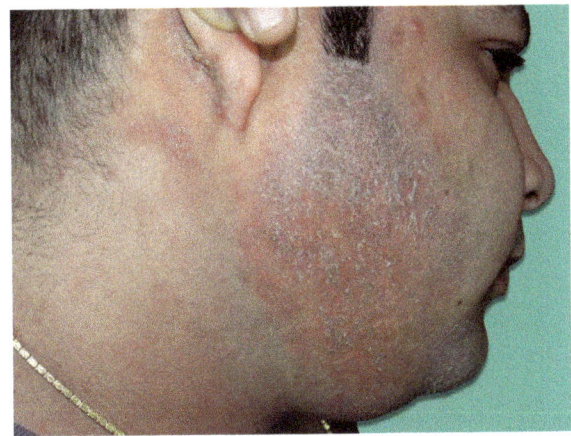

a. Tinea faciei
b. Seborrheic dermatitis
c. Psoriasis

1044. This child came with pain, redness and swelling in the perianal region for the last seven days. What is the clinical diagnosis?

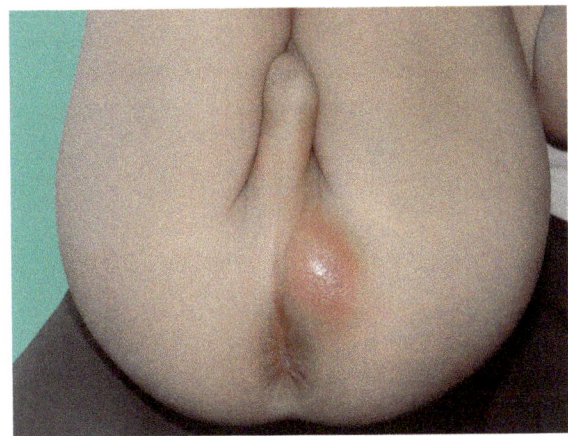

a. Boil
b. Carbuncle
c. Perianal abscess

1045. This patient complained of whiteness inside cheeks and soreness while taking chilly food. What is the clinical diagnosis?

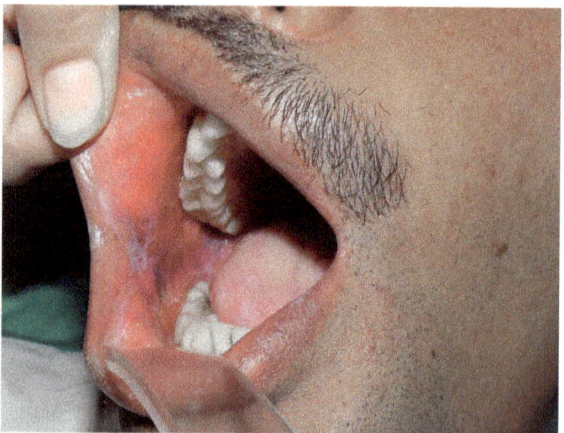

a. Oral lichen planus
b. Oral leukoplakia
c. Oral plaque-like candidiasis

1046. This patient developed following lesions few hours after taking some drug. There is no involvement of mucosae. What is the clinical diagnosis?

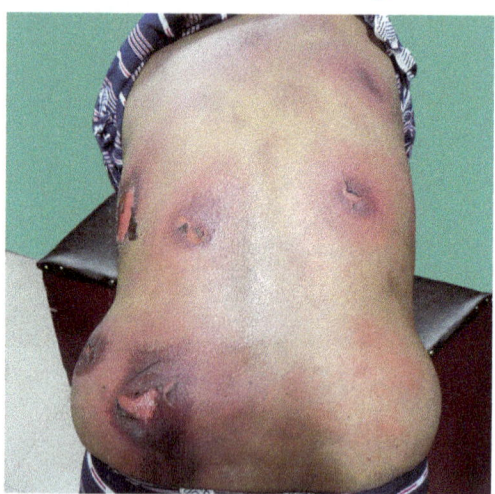

a. Erythema multiforme
b. Fixed drug eruption
c. Stevens-Johnson syndrome
d. Toxic epidermal necrolysis

1047. A 17-year-old patient presented with severe itching on lower extremities for the last one year sparing the other areas. He also complained of night sweats and had lost 25 kg body weight in last one year. X-ray chest showed *(next MCQ)* mediastinal widening. He had no cervical, axillary and inguinal lymphadenopathy. Which one of the following investigations is not required to do?

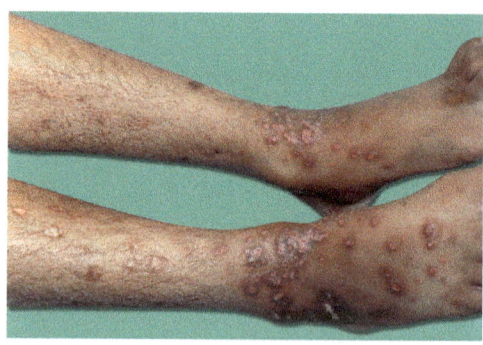

a. Bone marrow examination
b. Mediastinal lymph node biopsy is very important
c. CT-chest
d. USG abdomen for retroperitoneal lymph node
e. Mantoux test

1048. A 17-year-old patient presented with severe itching on lower extremities *(MCQ 1147)* for the last one year sparing the other areas. He also had night sweats and had lost 25 kg body weight in last one year. He had no cervical, axillary and inguinal lymphadenopathy. X-ray chest showed mediastinal widening. Mantoux test is strongly positive. Biopsy of mediastinal lymph nodes showed tubercular granulomas. Which one of the following eruptive tuberculids patient has?

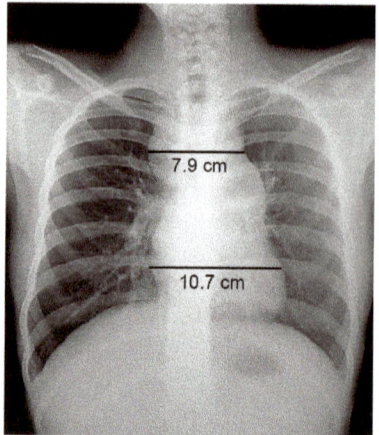

a. Papulonecrotic tuberculids
b. Lichen scrofulosorum
c. Erythema induratum of Bazin

1049. A young male presented with multiple papules for the last six months on scrotal skin with mild itching. What is the clinical diagnosis?

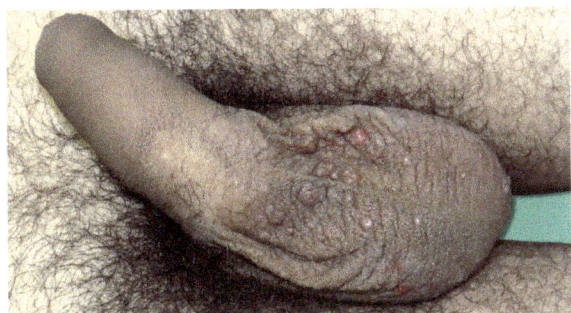

a. Scabies
b. Angiokeratosis
c. Molluscum contagiosum
d. Steacystoma multiplex

1050. Following microphotograph is showing a coronoid lamella as a column of tightly packed parakeratotic keratinocytes within a keratin filled invagination of epidermis. The underlying stratum granulosum is also attenuated. Dermis shows a variable degree of lichenoid lymphocytic infiltrate. What is the closest diagnosis?

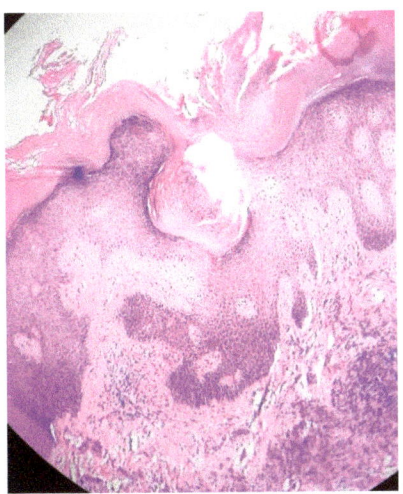

a. Verruca vulgaris
b. Porokeratosis
c. Lichen planus
d. Molluscum contagiosum

1051. She complained of asymptomatic bilateral symmetrical reddish-brown macules on the flexural aspects of forearm and palms, trunk and soles for the last two months. What is the closest clinical diagnosis?

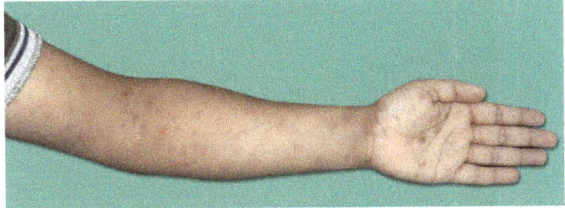

a. Fixed drug eruption
b. Lichen planus
c. Secondary syphilis

1052. A 50-year-old male presented with asymptomatic, multiple, erythematous plaques with no loss of sensation on face and other body parts for the last one year. What is the closest clinical diagnosis?

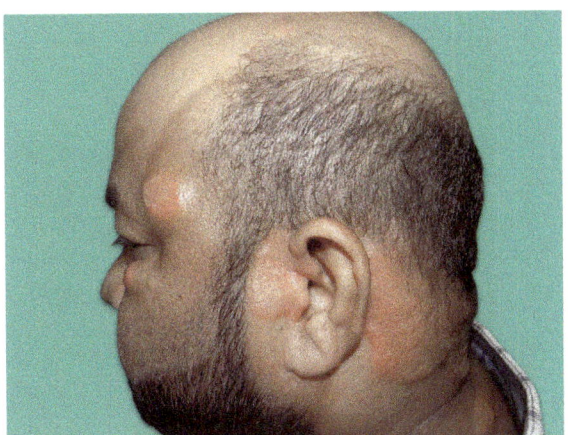

a. Chronic urticaria
b. Lepromatous leprosy
c. Tuberculoid leprosy

1053. This child presented with asymptomatic, multiple, shiny papules on face for the last six months. What is the clinical diagnosis?

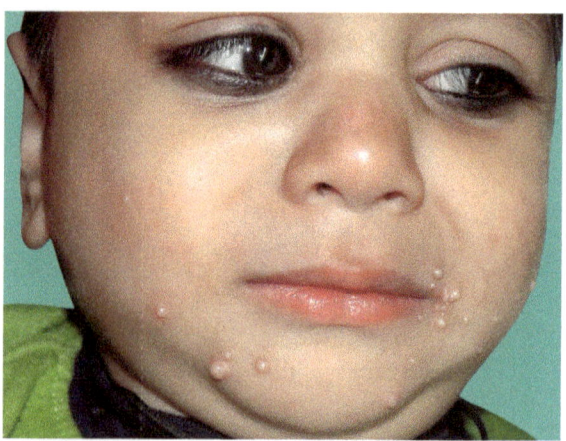

a. Milia
b. Warts
c. Molluscum contagiosum

1054. This child presented with a large and itchy erythematous plaque on the skin of lower abdomen extending up to upper thighs. There is no sensory loss. What is the clinical diagnosis?

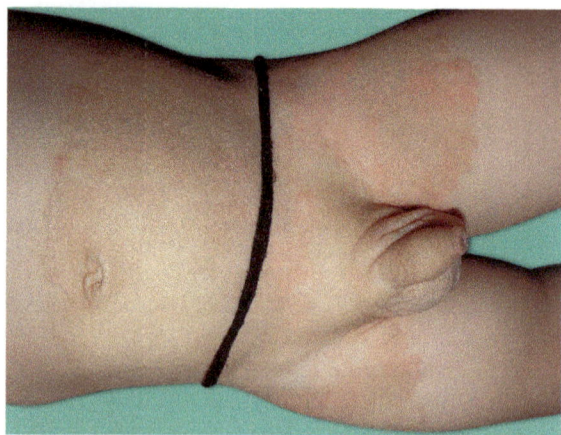

a. Dry eczema
b. Tinea corporis
c. Tuberculoid leprosy

1055. A 26-year-old male patient complained of hair loss for the last one year. What is the closest clinical diagnosis?

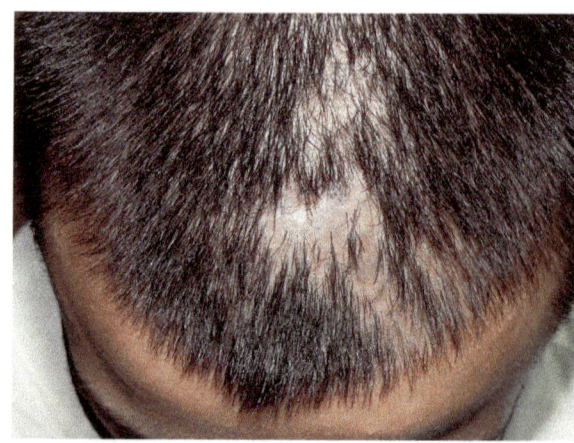

a. Alopecia areata
b. Cicatricial alopecia
c. Trichotillomania
d. Tinea capitis

1056. This patient complained of erosions and fissuring with malodor in groins and axillae *(MCQ 1060)* for the last many years. He is having recurrences and relapses with positive family history. What is the closest clinical diagnosis?

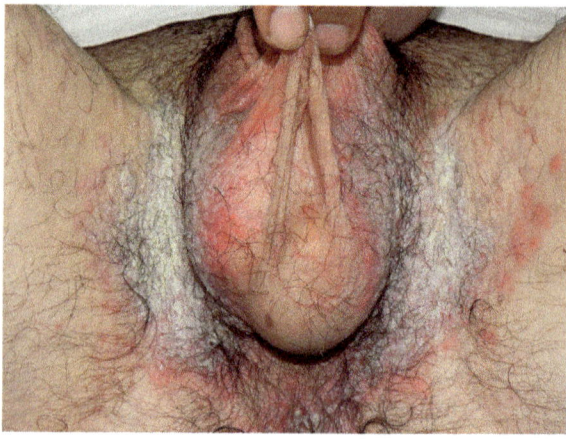

a. Frictional dermatitis
b. Intertrigo
c. Flexural candidiasis
d. Hailey-Hailey disease
e. Seborrheic dermatitis

1057. A 50-year-old male presented with a penile ulcer with unilateral involvement of inguinal lymph nodes for the last one year without remissions and relapses. What is the closest clinical diagnosis?

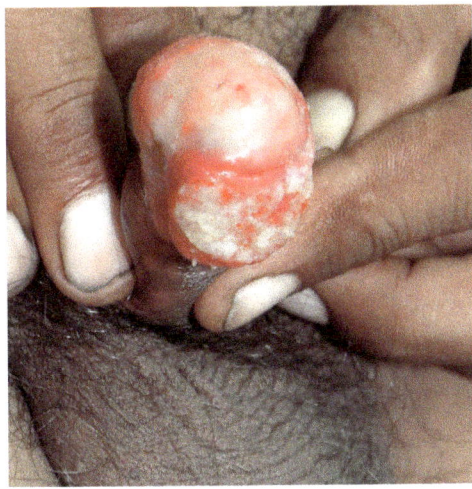

a. Penile carcinoma
b. Syphilitic chancre
c. Chancroid

1058. A 40-year-old presented with extremely itchy small vesicular lesions showing grouping at places on the back for the last few months. He responds excellently to dapsone in every recurrent attack. What is the probable diagnosis?

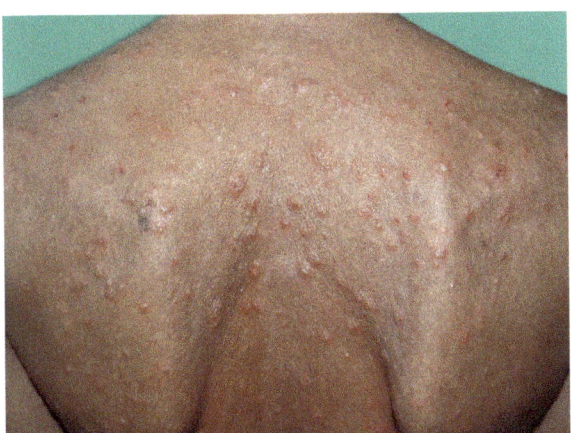

a. Linear IgA dermatosis of adults
b. Dermatitis herpetiformis
c. Erythema elevatum diutinum

1059. This patient complained of mild itching and scaling on both soles for the last one year. His palms are normal. Which one of the following possibilities is a closest clinical diagnosis?

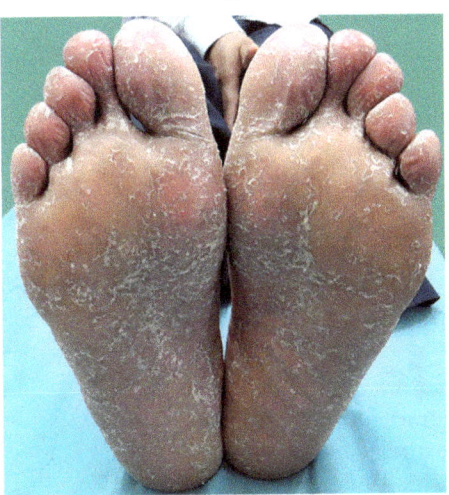

a. Psoriasis
b. Planter keratoderma
c. Tinea pedis
d. Planter eczema

1060. A 20-year-old girl having normal menstrual cycles presented with acne and hirsutism. Which one of the following statements is most appropriate?

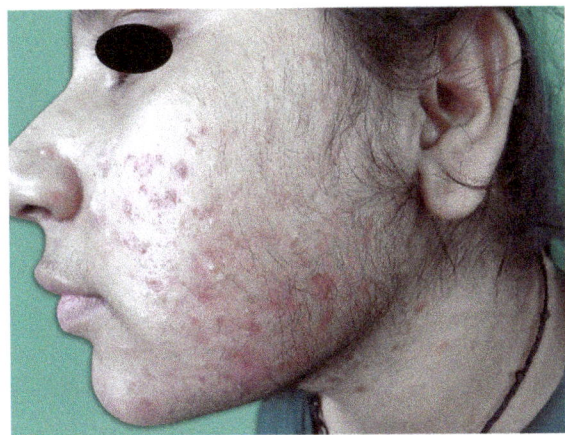

a. She is having acne with idiopathic hirsutism
b. Do USG and hormonal assay
c. Do not bother hirsutism, treat acne

1061. This patient complained of erosions and fissuring with malodor in axillae and groins *(MCQ 1056)* for the last many years. He is having recurrences and relapses with positive family history. What is the closest clinical diagnosis?

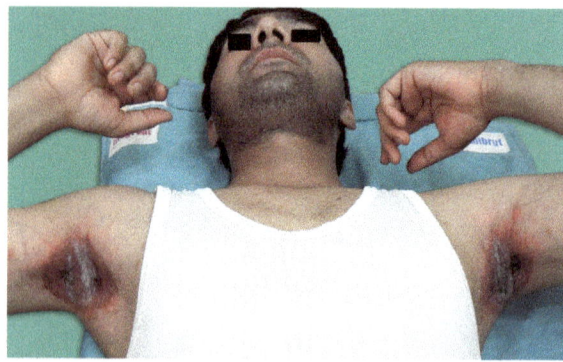

a. Hidradenitis suppurativa
b. Flexural candidiasis
c. Hailey-Hailey disease
d. Seborrheic dermatitis

1062. A 25-year-old man complained of erythema, scaling and mild itching in the nasolabial folds, moustaches, beard regions, scalp, eye brows and eyelashes for the last few years. Which one of the followings is the closest clinical diagnosis?

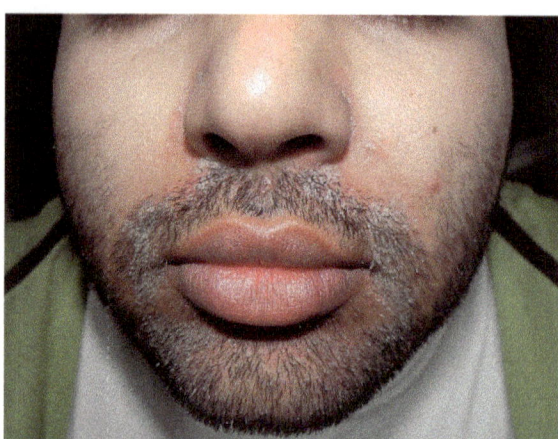

a. Atopic dermatitis
b. Tinea barbae
c. Seborrheic dermatitis
d. Psoriasis

1063. This man presented with dry, red, scaly and well-defined plaques on nose, cheeks and lips for the last five years. Which one of the followings is the closest clinical possibility?

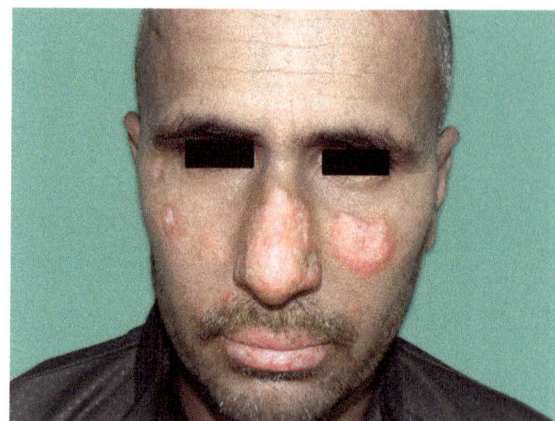

a. Chronic cutaneous lupus erythematosus
b. Systemic lupus erythematosus
c. Psoriasis on face

1064. A 51-year-old male presented with periorbital edema, erythema on forehead, cheeks, temples for the last many years. It is accompanied by difficulty in going upstairs, getting up from chair and combing the hairs. He also has reddish papules on the dorsa of hands *(MCQ 1066)*. What is the closest possibility?

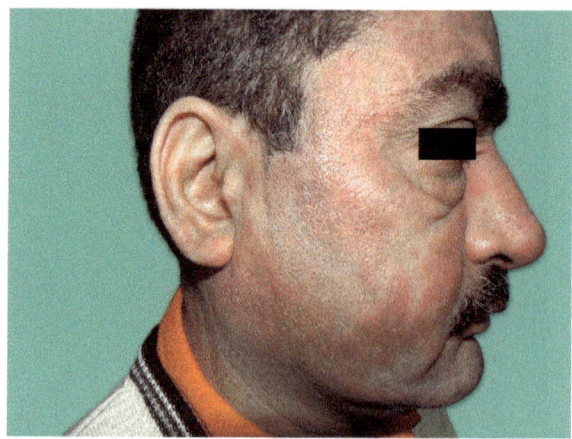

a. Chronic cutaneous lupus erythematosus
b. Systemic lupus erythematosus
c. Psoriasis on face with arthritis
d. Dermatomyositis

1065. This patient presented with red patch with scaling on glans penis for the last one year. What is the clinical diagnosis?

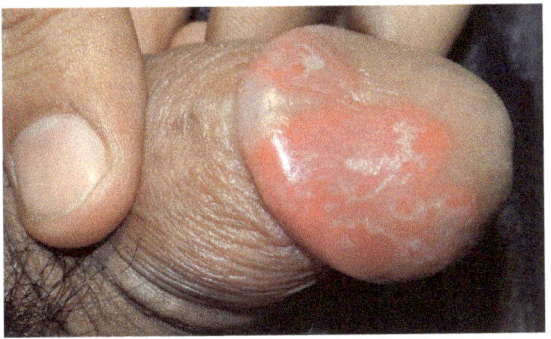

a. Lichen planus
b. Psoriasis
c. Fixed drug eruption
d. Chronic cutaneous lupus erythematosus

1066. A 51-year-old man presented with red violaceous thickening on the dorsa of IP and MP joints. He also had confluent violaceous erythema on forehead and upper cheeks *(MCQ 1064)* along with proximal muscle weakness. What is the closest clinical possibility?

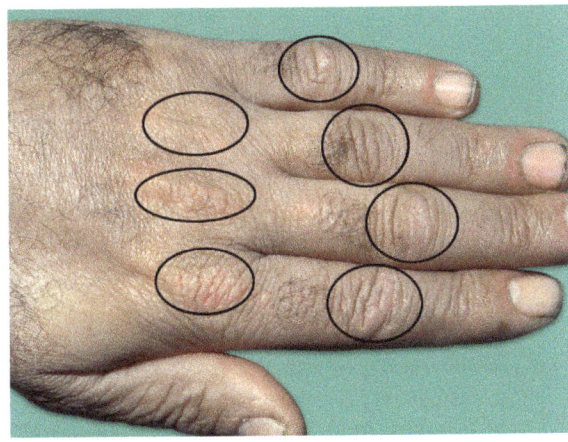

a. Gottron papules
b. Knuckle pads
c. Common warts

1067. A 14-year-old child presented with itching and redness in the groins and axillae for the last one year. What is the clinical diagnosis?

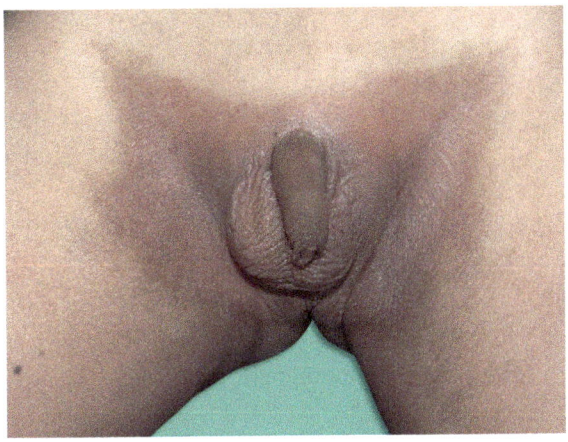

a. Intertrigo
b. Tinea cruris
c. Flexural candidiasis
d. Seborrheic dermatitis

1068. This child presented with inflammatory boggy swelling for the last few months. It is superadded with papules surrounding the hair follicles with easily pluckable hairs. He is not responding to antibiotics. What is the clinical diagnosis?

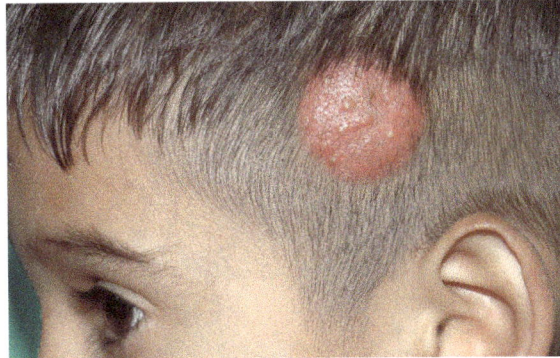

a. Gray patch
b. Kerion
c. Herald patch
d. Abscess

1069. A 55-year-old diabetic patient presented with sudden, painless and nonpruritic large blisters on his feet. What is the clinical diagnosis?

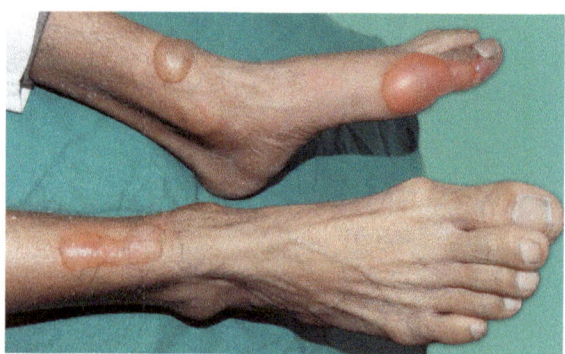

a. Bullous pemphigoid
b. Bullous diabeticorum

1070. Which type of acne scar is it?

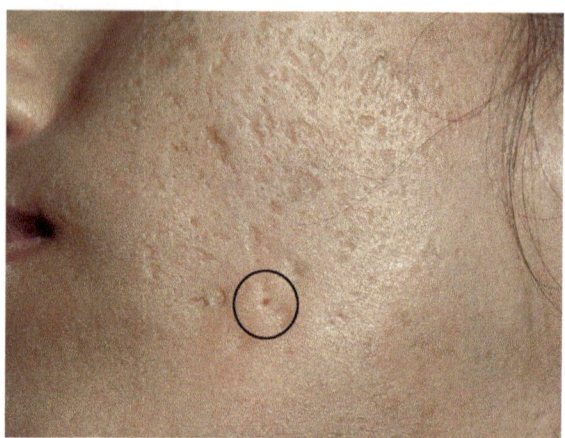

a. Anetoderma
b. Ice pick scar
c. Rolling scar
d. Boxcar scar

1071. A 14-year-old child complained of a patch of hair loss in the frontal region for the last one year. What is the closest clinical diagnosis?

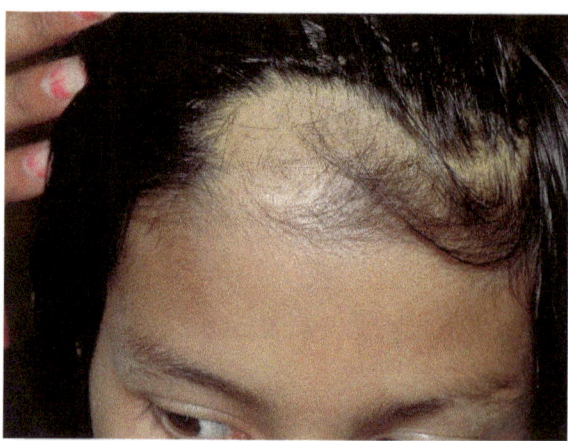

a. Alopecia areata
b. Telogen effluvium
c. Trichotillomania
d. Tinea capitis

1072. A 15-year-old child presented with a red papule on the front of chest for the last six months. At times, it bleeds on slight trauma. What is the closest diagnosis?

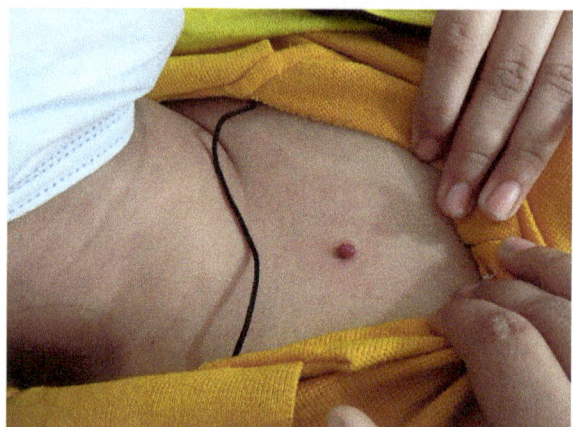

a. Strawberry hemangioma
b. Pyogenic granuloma
c. Cherry angioma

1073. A 50-year-old man presented with itching and redness on face, cubital fossae and popliteal fossae for the last many years. What is the closest clinical diagnosis?

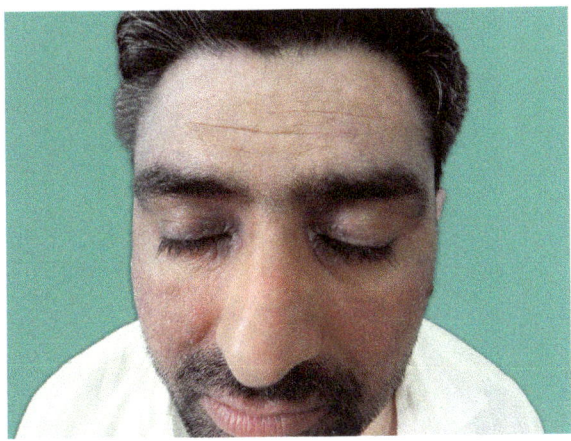

a. Atopic dermatitis
b. Airborne contact dermatitis
c. Seborrheic dermatitis
d. Photosensitive eczema

1074. This patient complained of erythema and itching in the groins and upper part of thighs. What is the clinical diagnosis?

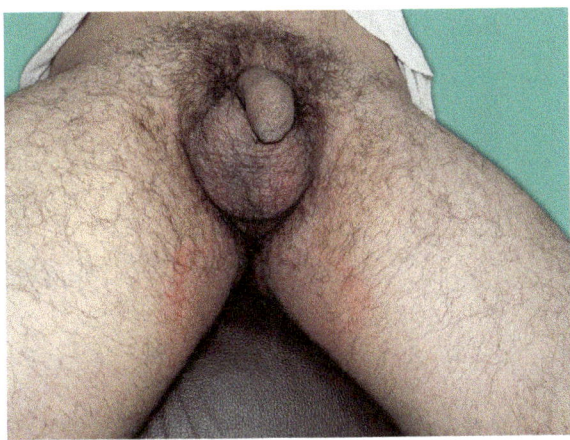

a. Frictional dermatitis
b. Intertrigo
c. Candidal intertrigo
d. Hailey-Hailey disease

1075. This patient presented with macular rash with scaling and mild itching for the last two weeks. What is the clinical diagnosis?

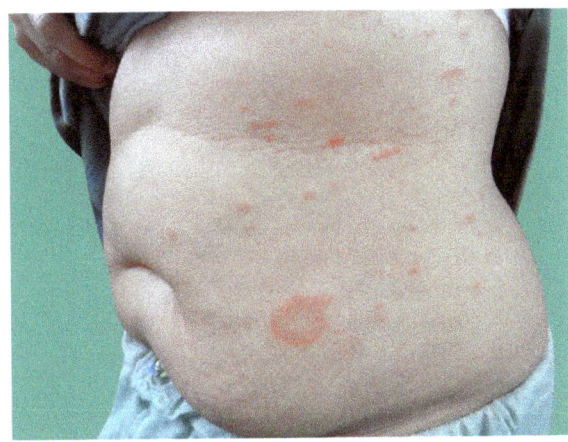

a. Exanthematous rash
b. Pityriasis rosea
c. Secondary syphilis
d. Guttate psoriasis

1076. This man complained of redness and itching on face. There is history of application of some topical cream for the last 2–3 years. Which of the following cream he must have applied?

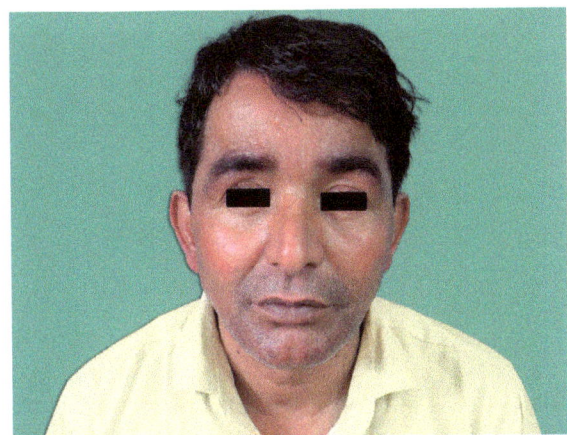

a. Tretinoin cream
b. Salicylic acid cream
c. Derobin cream
d. Steroid cream

1077. What is the name of the deformity of this nail?

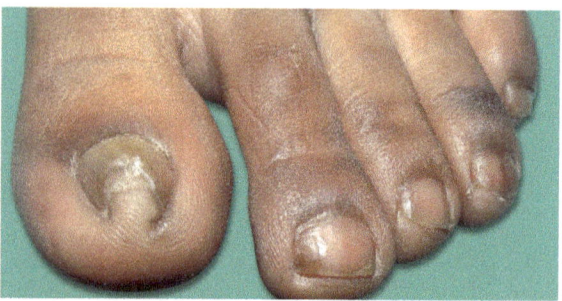

a. Pterygium of nail
b. Pincer nail deformity
c. Koilonychia
d. Clubbing of nail

1078. An 8-year-old child presented with erythema and itching on face, cubital fossae and popliteal fossae for the last many years. What is the closest diagnosis?

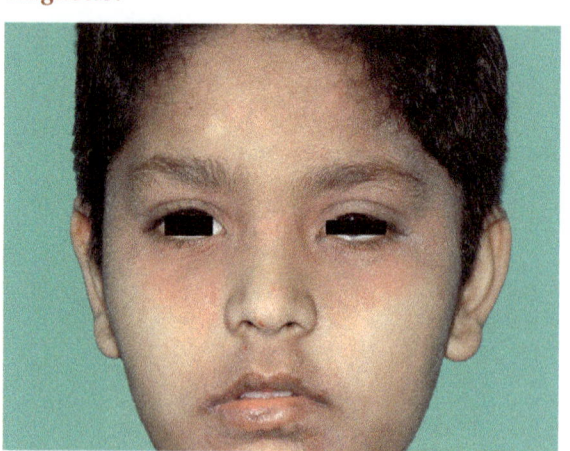

a. Seborrheic dermatitis
b. Chronic urticaria
c. Atopic dermatitis

1079. A 2-year-old child presented with redness and crusting on entire scalp with onset in infancy. What is the clinical diagnosis?

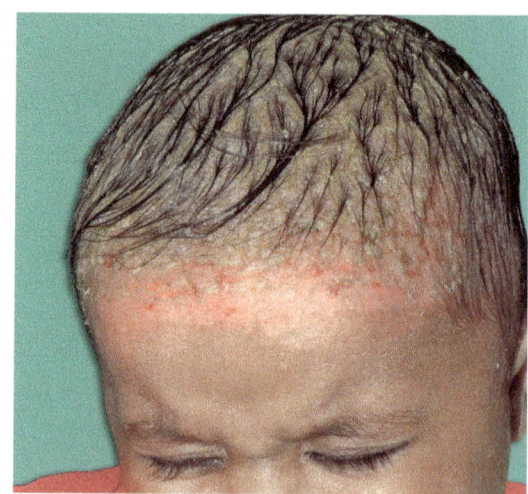

a. Tinea capitis
b. Psoriasis scalp
c. Atopic dermatitis
d. Seborrheic dermatitis

1080. This man presented with a single, skin colored, firm, rapidly enlarging nodule with central keratotic core for the last 2–3 months. What is the closest clinical diagnosis?

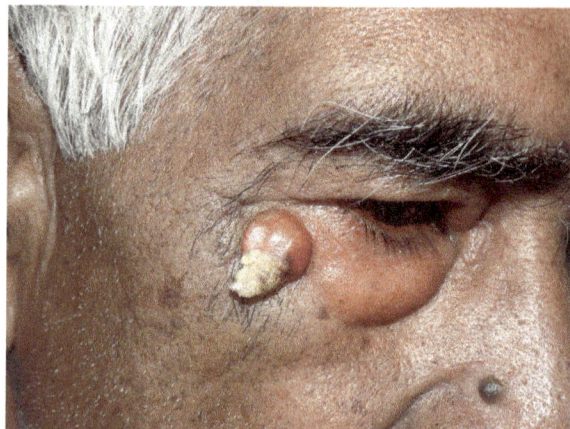

a. Molluscum contagiosum
b. Keratoacanthoma
c. Squamous cell carcinoma
d. Basal cell carcinoma

1081. This patient presented with multiple, shallow, rounded and red patches three months after a sexual contact with a sex worker. What is the closest clinical diagnosis?

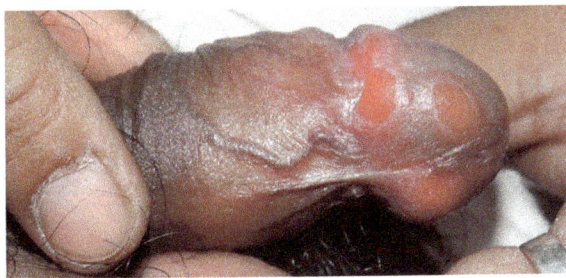

a. Donovanosis
b. Primary syphilis
c. Secondary syphilis
d. Chancroid

1082. This developed these lesions few hours after taking an analgesic. There is no mucosal involvement. What is the clinical diagnosis?

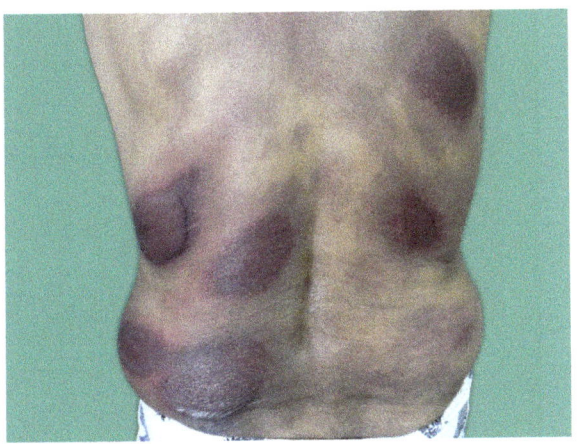

a. Stevens-Johnson Syndrome (SJS)
b. Fixed drug eruption (FDE)
c. Toxic epidermal necrolysis (TEN)
d. Erythema multiforme (EM)

1083. She presented with itchy red macerations in the groins. Involvement is extending beyond the area of contact and has developed irregular fringed margins with satellite vesicles and pustules. What is the clinical diagnosis?

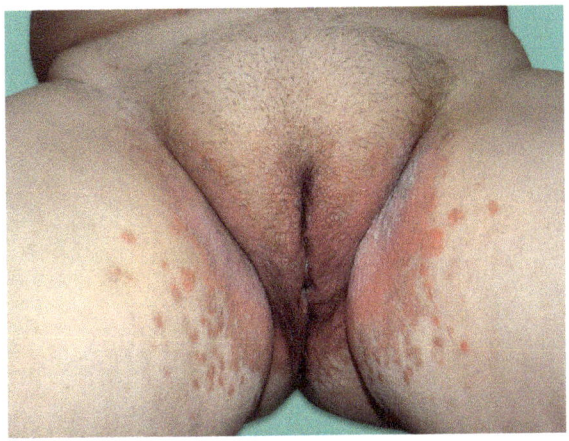

a. Frictional dermatitis
b. Intertrigo
c. Flexural candidiasis
d. Hailey-Hailey disease

1084. A 12-year-old female child presented with multiple, asymptomatic, faintly purplish and circumscribed indurated areas on the extremities for the last two years. The areas are shiny and smooth with absence of hairs. Sensations are intact. What is the clinical diagnosis?

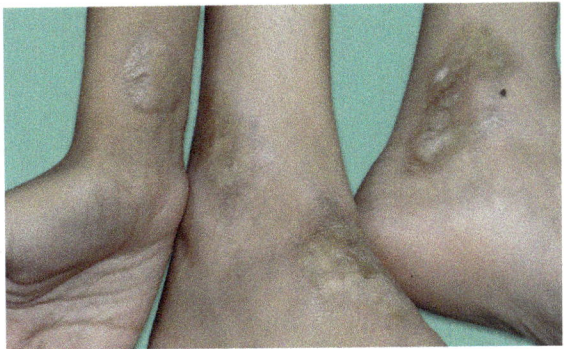

a. Hansens disease
b. Localized morphea
c. Lichen planus
d. Scleredema

1085. This patient presented with single red plaque with loss of sensation and enlargement of great auricular nerve. Which type of leprosy is it?

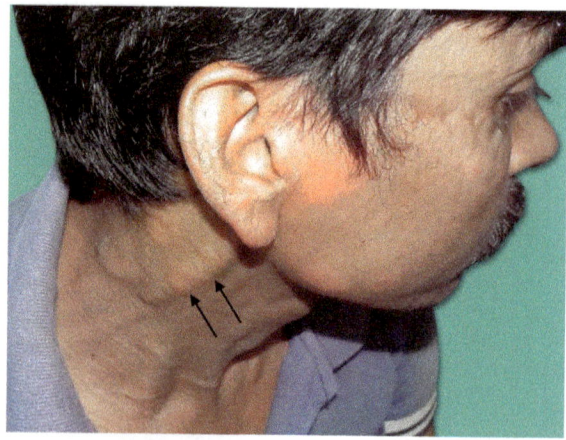

a. Histoid leprosy
b. Multibacillary leprosy
c. Paucibacillary leprosy
d. Indeterminate leprosy

1086. She complained of multiple red plaques with adherent scale on sun exposed parts of face. What is the diagnosis?

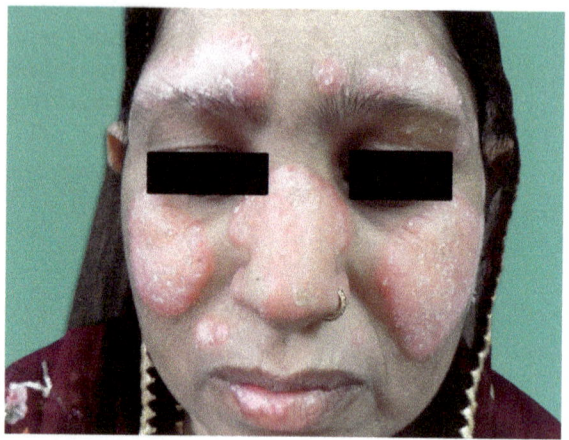

a. Systemic lupus erythematosus
b. Photosensitive eczema
c. Polymorphous light eruption
d. Chronic cutaneous lupus erythematosus

1087. This patient presented with a single red plaque with loss of sensations. What is the clinical diagnosis?

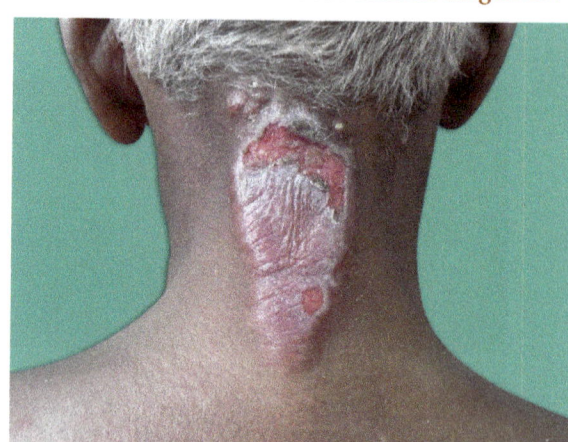

a. Psoriasis
b. Paucibacillary leprosy
c. Chronic cutaneous lupus erythematosus
d. Lupus vulgaris

1088. This patient complained of patchy hair loss. What is the clinical diagnosis?

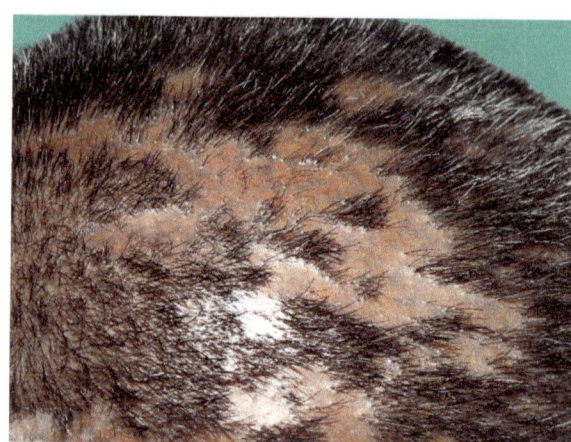

a. Alopecia areata
b. Cicatricial alopecia
c. Non-cicatricial alopecia
d. Pseudopelade of Brocq

1089. This patient developed multiple, painless, fleshy, elevated lesions one month after sexual exposure with a sex worker. What is the closest clinical diagnosis?

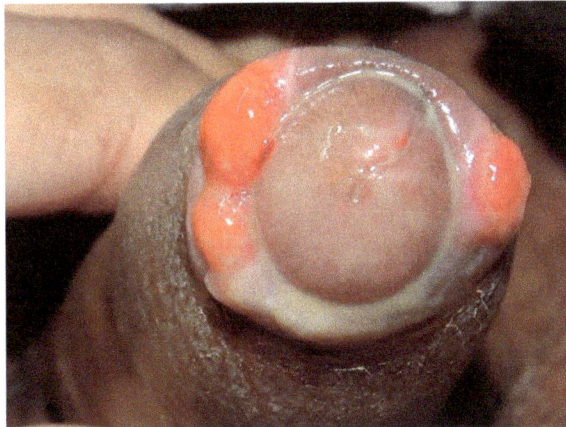

a. Donovanosis
b. Primary syphilis
c. Secondary syphilis
d. Chancroid

1090. This patient presented with a red, single and well-defined plaque with loss of sensations on foot for the last two years. What is the clinical diagnosis?

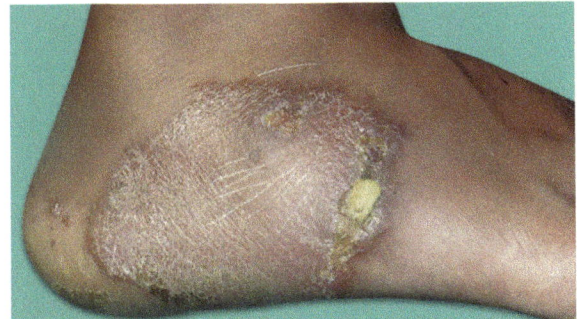

a. Psoriasis
b. Tuberculosis verrucose cutis
c. Paucibacillary leprosy
d. Multibacillary leprosy

1091. This child presented with multiple, thick, dirty brown crusted lesions involving whole back for the last 15 days. Few thin-walled vesicles are also seen. There is no mucosal involvement and no history of prior intake of any drug. What is the clinical diagnosis?

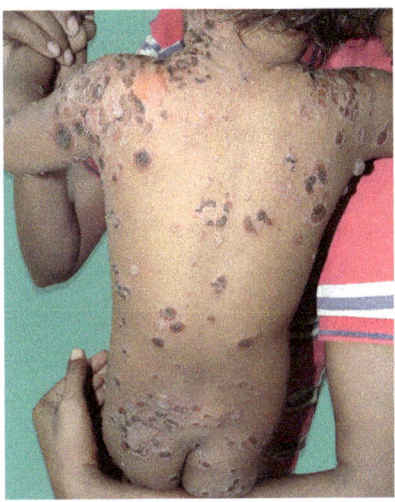

a. Staphylococcal scalded skin syndrome (SSSS)
b. Impetigo contagiosa
c. Pemphigus foliaceous
d. Bullous impetigo

1092. This patient presented with itching, thickening and some redness of palms for the last two years. What is the clinical diagnosis?

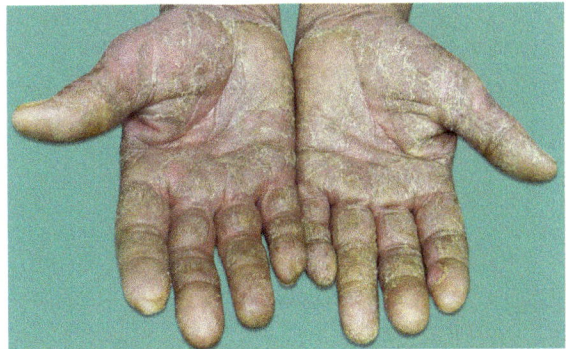

a. Diffuse keratoderma
b. Psoriasis palms
c. Hyperkeratotic eczema

1093. A commercial sex worker developed these flat topped, wet and sessile multiple painless vulval lesions with oozing and macerations for the last 1 month. What is the clinical diagnosis?

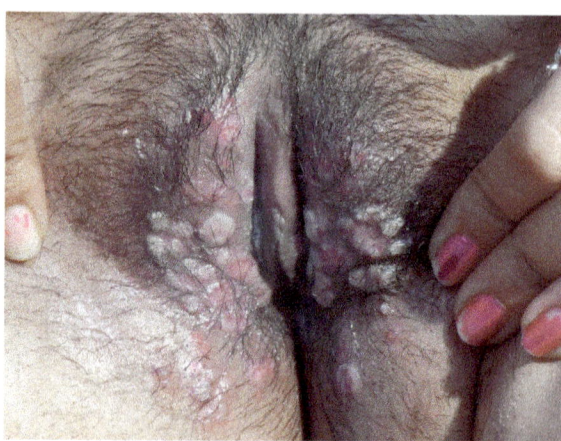

a. Condylomata lata
b. Condyloma accuminata
c. Primary syphilis
d. Chancroid

1094. This patient complained of redness and itching in the groins. What is the closest clinical diagnosis?

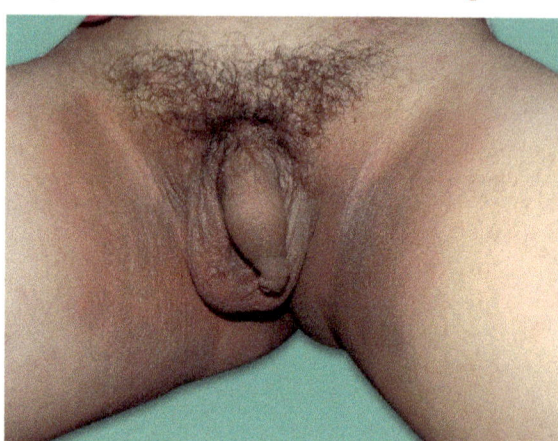

a. Frictional dermatitis
b. Intertrigo
c. Candidal intertrigo
d. Seborrheic dermatitis

1095. A patient was having herpes labialis. One week later, he presented with these lesions on dorsa of hands and forearms. What is clinical diagnosis of this patient?

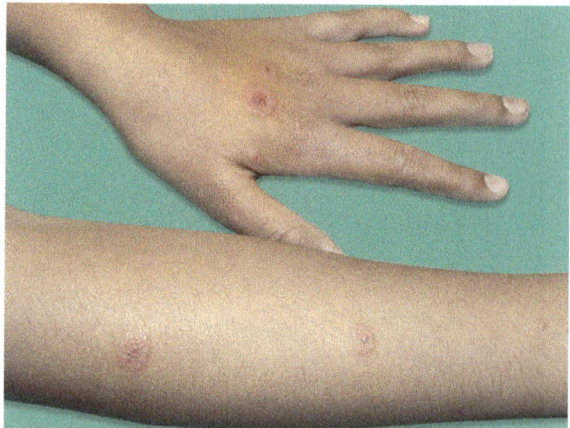

a. Lichen planus
b. Erythema multiforme
c. Chickenpox
d. Impetigo

1096. This patient complained of itching and scaling on the dorsa of both hands with well-defined margins. Palmar surfaces are also involved *(MCQ 1097)*. What is the clinical diagnosis?

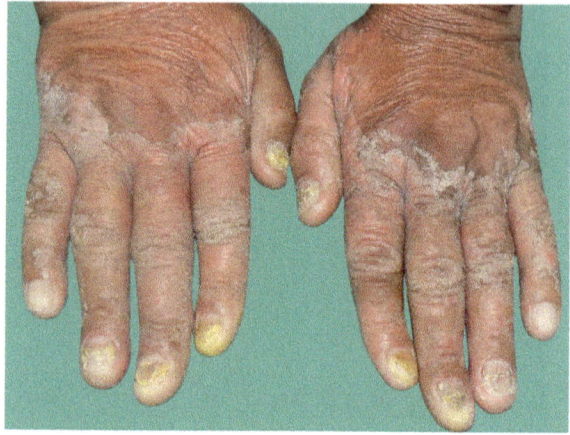

a. Contact dermatitis hands
b. Tinea manuum
c. Candidiasis hands

1097. This patient complained of itching and scaling on both palms. It was extending on to dorsal surfaces also *(MCQ 1096)* with well-defined margins. What is the clinical diagnosis?

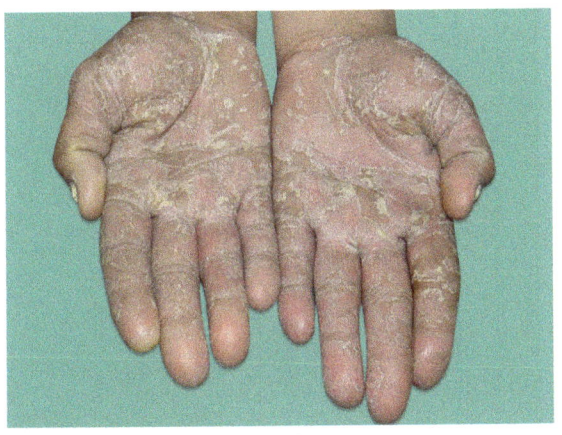

a. Contact dermatitis hands
b. Tinea manuum
c. Candidiasis hands

1098. This patient complained of circular shaped erosions having punched out appearance on both soles. What is the diagnosis?

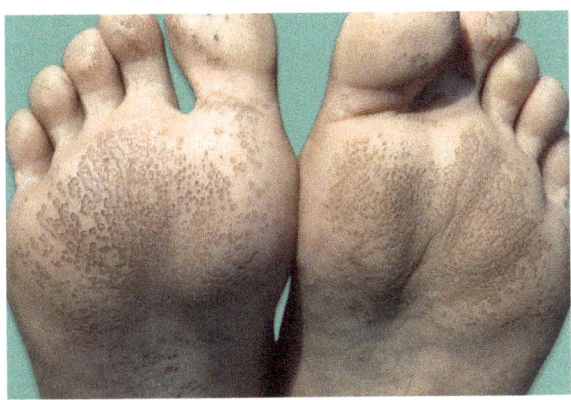

a. Pitted keratolysis
b. Tinea pedis
c. Contact dermatitis

1099. This patient developed a single painless ulcer 20 days after unprotected sexual exposure with a commercial sex worker. What is the clinical diagnosis?

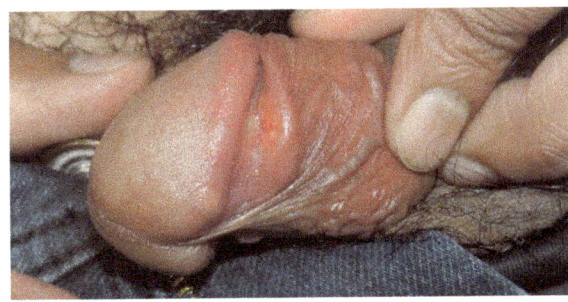

a. Chancroid
b. Donovanosis
c. Primary syphilis
d. Lymphogranuloma venereum

1100. What is the closest diagnosis for the nail involvement for this patient?

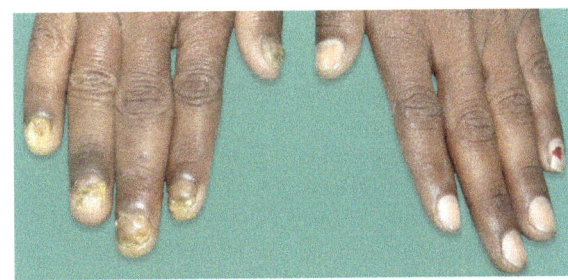

a. Lichen planus
b. Tinea unguium
c. Psoriasis
d. Alopecia areata

1101. A 40-year-old male presented with eruption of painful erythematous nodules on the trunk and extremities with extensive necrosis. On examination, it was found that his ears are swollen and infiltrated. What is the diagnosis?

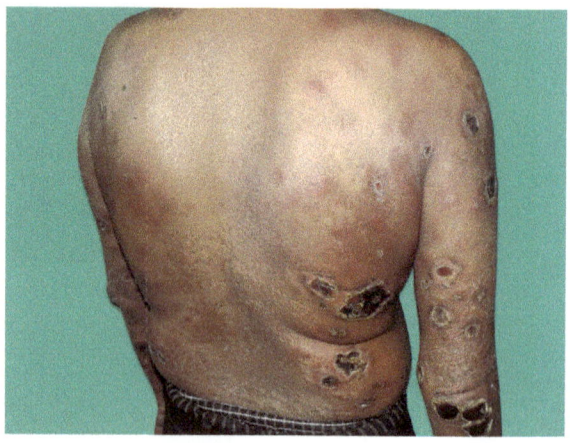

a. Erythema nodosum
b. Erythema nodosum leprosum with necroticans
c. Erythema induratum of Bazin

1102. What is the name of nail dystrophy in the following patient?

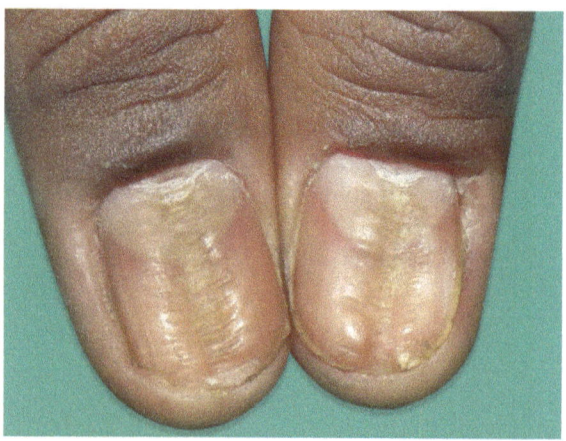

a. Pterygium formation
b. Hellers median nail dystrophy
c. Pincer nail dystrophy

1103. She complained of photosensitivity with hyperpigmentation of sun-exposed areas since infancy. She develops blisters in light exposed skin. There is hypertrichosis in the malar and temple regions. Scarring is there in the ears, nose and fingers. There is brown staining of teeth and reabsorption of terminal phalanges. She is anemic and spleen is enlarged. What is the clinical diagnosis?

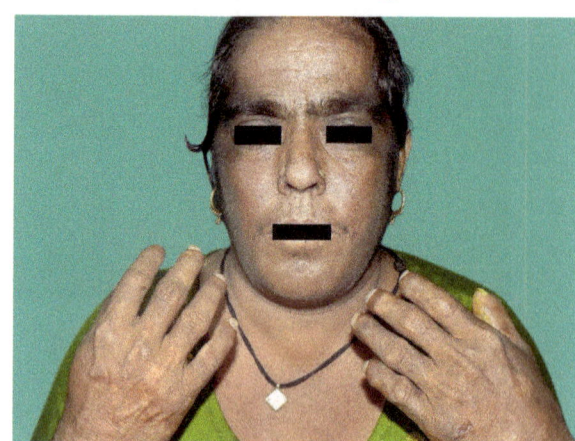

a. Congenital erythropoietic porphyria
b. Porphyria cutanea tarda
c. Systemic sclerosis

1104. This patient presented with mild itching and these lesions for the last six months. What is the diagnosis?

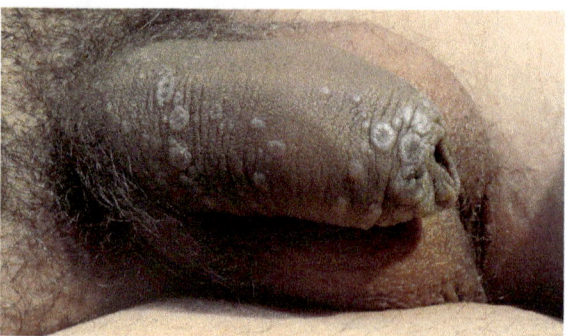

a. Lichen nitidus
b. Scabies
c. Lichen planus
d. Molluscum contagiosum

1105. This patient presented with erythema and itching on buttocks for the last six months. What is the clinical diagnosis?

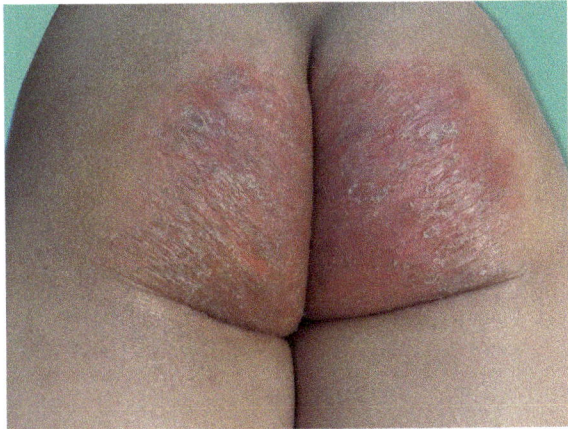

a. Psoriasis
b. Dermatitis
c. Tinea
d. Candidiasis

1106. This lady presented with crusted plaques on buttocks with moderate itching. What is the closest clinical diagnosis?

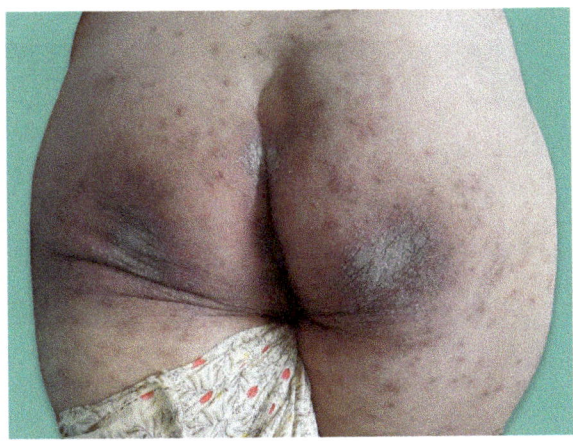

a. Norwegian scabies
b. Dermatitis
c. Tinea
d. Psoriasis

1107. This man presented with multiple patches of alopecia. What is the clinical diagnosis?

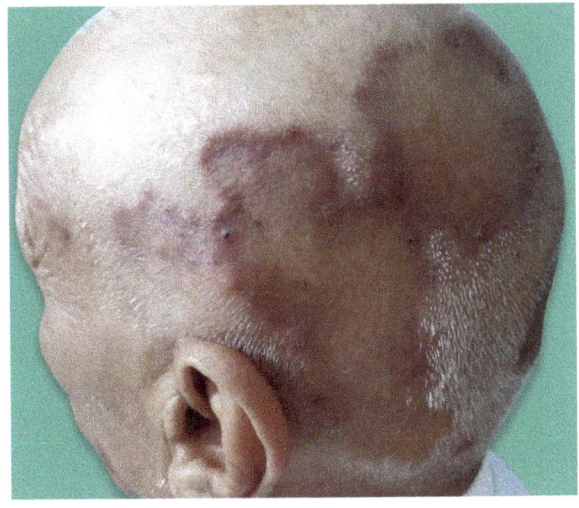

a. Alopecia areata
b. Cicatricial alopecia due to LP or CCLE
c. Pseudopelade of Brocq

1108. A 65-year-old man presented with a single growth on lower lip for the last one year. What is the clinical diagnosis?

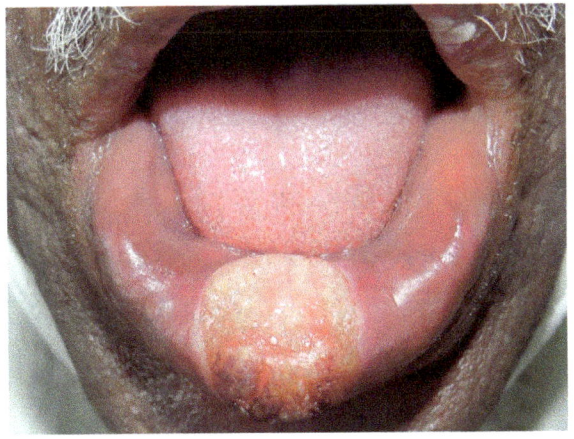

a. Wart on lower lip
b. SCC
c. BCC

1109. A HIV positive patient developed redness and swelling of nostrils that is gradually turning black. What is the clinical diagnosis?

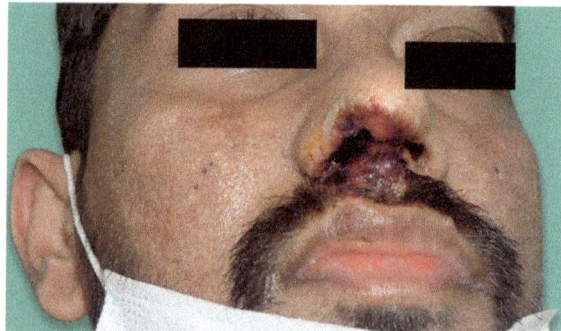

a. Impetigo contagiosa
b. Mucormycosis

1110. A 3-year-old child presented with a longitudinal dark band in the nail plate of his middle finger. What is the clinical diagnosis?

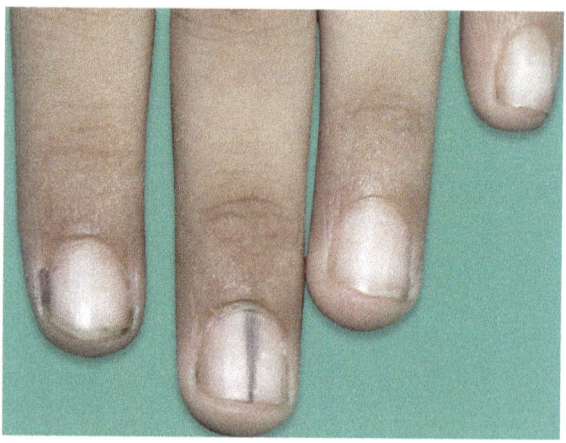

a. Nevus of nail matrix
b. Subungual hematoma
c. Positive Hutchinson's sign (nail unit melanoma)
d. Onychomycotic infection by *Fusarium* species

1111. This lady presented with curdy white soft creamy patches on tongue, inside lips and cheeks for the last few months. These can be wiped off easily with a gauze, leaving behind an area of erythema. What is the diagnosis?

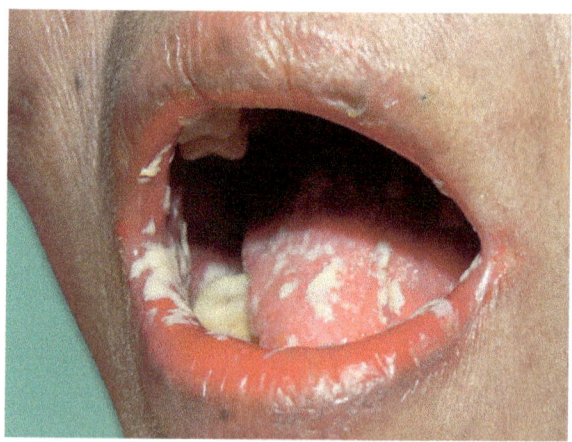

a. Oral thrush
b. Hairy leukoplakia

1112. An unmarried patient presented with these shiny papules and nodules on his penile shaft for the last 5–6 months. There is a history of sexual exposure one year back. What is the diagnosis?

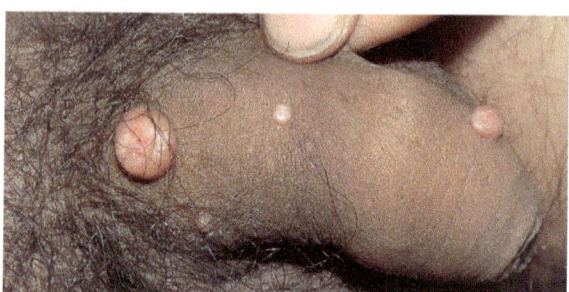

a. Genital warts
b. Molluscum contagiosum

1113. A middle-aged female presented with multiple lesions (Up to 10 mm) predominantly on sun-exposed sites for the last one year. The papules are surrounded by keratotic edge. What is the clinical diagnosis?

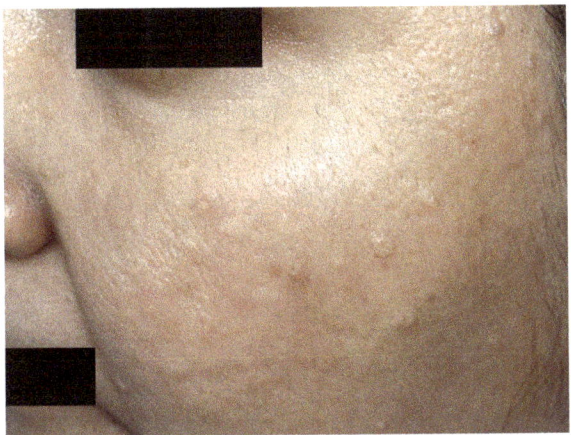

a. Molluscum contagiosum
b. Actinic keratosis
c. Sebaceous hyperplasia
d. Acne vulgaris

1114. This man presented with a single red well-defined plaque with loss of sensations on his face. What is the clinical diagnosis?

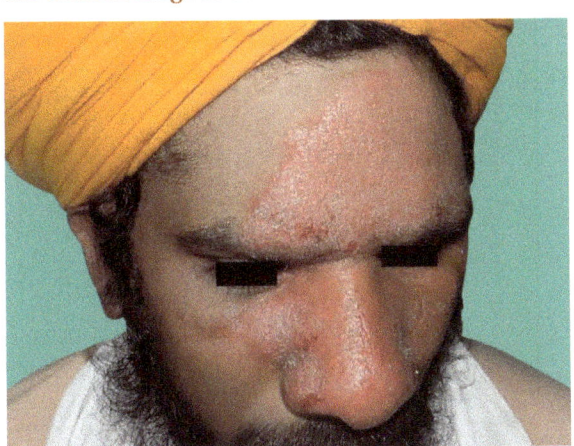

a. Lupus vulgaris
b. Paucibacillary leprosy
c. Lepromatous leprosy
d. Psoriasis

1115. This patient complained of erythema and itching in the groins and suprapubic region. What is the diagnosis?

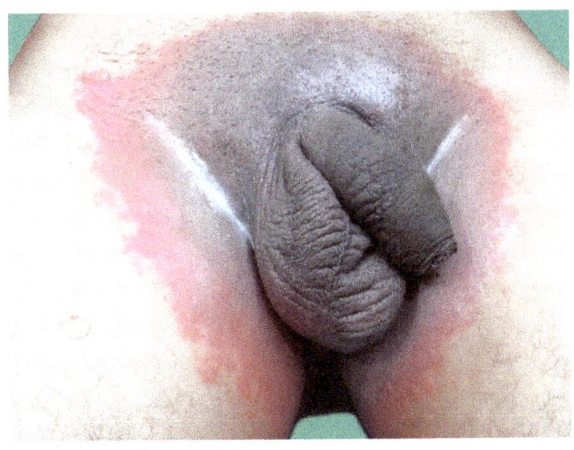

a. Contact dermatitis
b. Tinea dermatitis
c. Candidial intertrigo
d. Hailey-Hailey disease

1116. A 5-month-old female child presented with hyperpigmentation on left side of face since birth. What is the diagnosis?

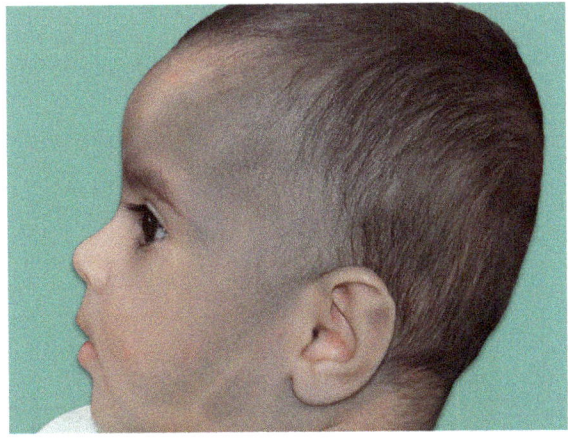

a. Mongolian spots
b. Nevus of Ito
c. Nevus of Ota
d. Becker's nevus

1117. This patient presented with erythema, itching and scaling on the big toe only. Which one of the following is the closest clinical diagnosis?

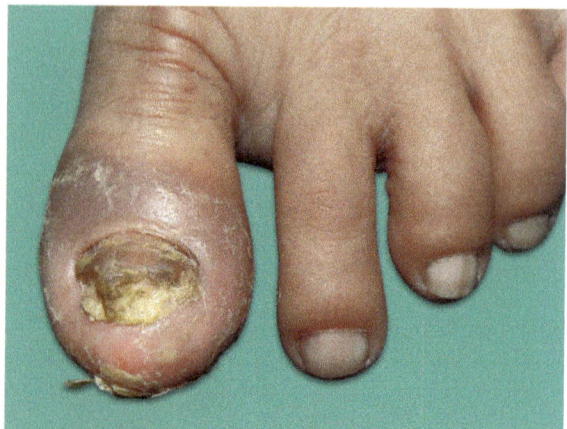

a. Tinea pedis
b. Eczema big toe
c. Acropustulosis

1118. This lady presented with soft, pink, grouped, pedunculated and digitate lesions involving her vulval region for the last one month. What is the diagnosis?

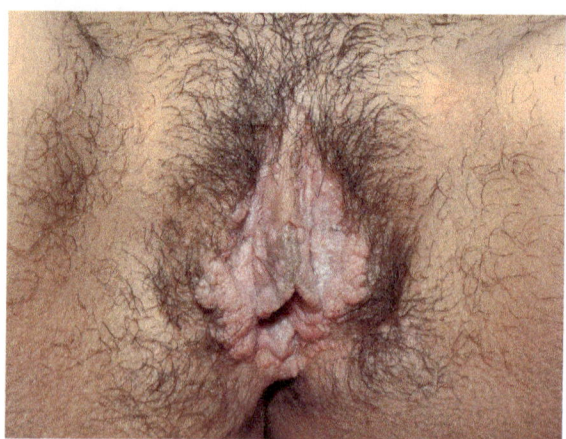

a. Condylomata acuminata
b. Condylomata lata

1119. A 50-year-old male patient presented with uncountable number of digitate warts on both sides of his face, cervical region and chest. There is no history of any immunosuppressive therapy or antineoplastic drugs or HIV infection. Which one of the following treatment options should be opted?

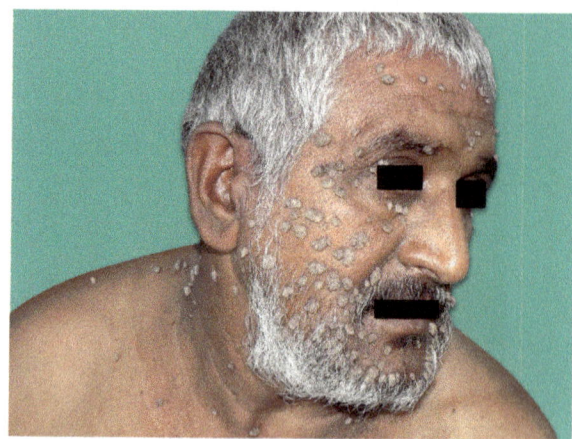

a. Acyclovir orally
b. Podowart topically
c. Immunotherapy
d. Electrodessication
e. Imiquimod cream

1120. An 8-year-old boy complained of loss of eyelashes in both eyes. What is the clinical diagnosis?

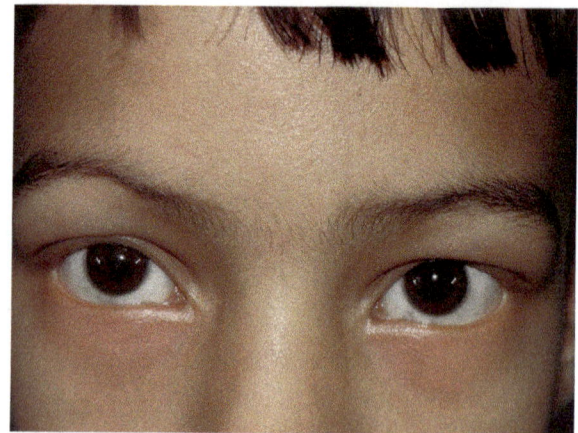

a. Alopecia areata
b. Trichotillomania
c. Tinea infection
d. Seborrheic dermatitis

1121. A 40-year-female complained of following hair loss. What is the closest clinical diagnosis for her?

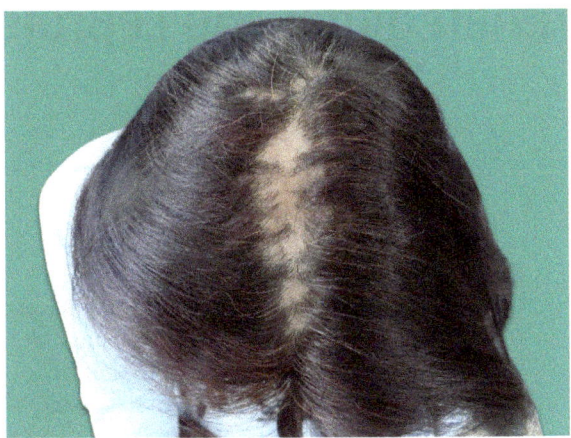

a. Trichotillomania
b. Pseudopelade of Brocq
c. Alopecia areata
d. Christmas tree pattern female androgenic alopecia

1122. A 50-years-old patient developed following nail pigmentation in his thumb only during last one month. Which one of the following options is most appropriate clinical diagnosis?

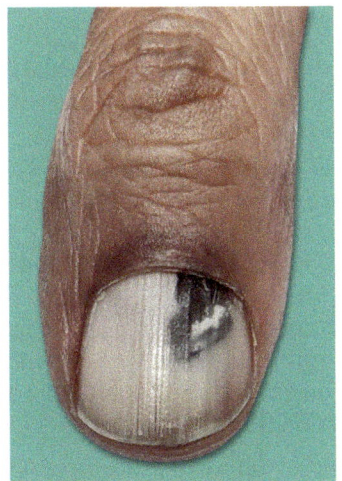

(*Courtesy:* Dr Vijay Shinghal)

a. Nail unit melanoma
b. Subungual hematoma
c. Drug-induced melanonychia
d. Nevus of the nail matrix

1123. This patient developed multiple, smooth, plane topped, 1–5 mm sized, dark colored, asymptomatic papules on the both sides of his cervical regions during past three months of duration. Which one of the following options is the closest clinical diagnosis?

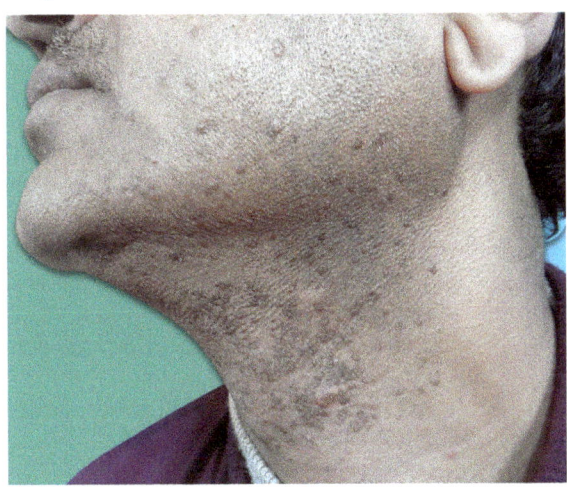

a. Seborrheic keratosis
b. Plane warts
c. Actinic keratosis

Chapter 5: Answers of MCQs in Dermatology, Venereology and Leprology

1. **Ans. b. It is plane warts. Face, dorsa of hands and shins are common sites.**
   - In acne, facial skin is greasy with prominent follicular orifices. There will be white and black comedones.
   - Post chickenpox scars *(MCQ 154)* are depressed ones.
   - In SD nasolabial folds will show redness and yellow greasy scales *(MCQ 171)*.

2. **Ans. b. This patient is having eczema.**
   - It is not tinea manuum because margins are neither well defined nor active. There is a no central clearing also *(MCQ 142)*.
   - Psoriasis plaques typically are raised, well defined and erythematous with silvery white scales *(MCQ 162)*.
   - Lesions in LP are usually purplish papules *(MCQ 21)*.

3. **Ans. d. Almost all patients who are taking isotretinoin have cheilitis. Teratogenicity is another important side effect of isotretinoin.**
   - Azithromycin is safer to use during pregnancy.
   - Tetracycline is not recommended for use during pregnancy and in children below 8 years of age. Milk, iron preparations, antacids and sucralfate reduce its absorption.

4. **Ans. b. Extensive dermatophyte infection needs both topical and systemic antifungal therapy.**
   Topical steroids alone or in combination with antifungal cream should not be used even in the initial period when clinician is sure about fungal infection.

5. **Ans. d. It is topical steroid damaged face (TSDF).**
   Continuous and prolonged use of topical steroid leads to addiction for repeated use and patient presents typically with these features.

6. **Ans. c. It is tuberculoid leprosy which has highest immunity. So, patient has very minimal number (single) of lesions.**
   - In lepromatous leprosy immunity is lowest. So, patient has uncountable skin lesions *(MCQ 155)*.
   - In histoid leprosy also, there will be a crop of asymptomatic glistening papules *(MCQ 47)*.
   - Indeterminate leprosy is an early and transient stage of leprosy. It presents as one or more hypopigmented or slight erythematous ill-defined macules on face of a child.

7. **Ans. d. It is tinea corporis. Central clearing and active margins are its two important features.**
   - Psoriatic plaque typically is erythematous and has silvery white scaling *(MCQ 162)*.
   - Discoid eczema will not have central clearing *(MCQ 194)*.
   - Mother patch of pityriasis rosea has no significant itching. It consists of a dark red peripheral zone and a central wrinkled area *(MCQ 195)*.
   - Intact sensation in a skin patch rules out Hansen's disease *(MCQ 6)*.

8. **Ans. It is a gray patch type of tinea capitis characterized by alopecia with numerous broken hairs and fine scaling.**
   - Alopecia areata presents as totally bald patches of skin having smooth surface with no scaling, inflammation or scarring *(MCQ 156)*.
   - In SD, there will be yellowish greasy scales with no hair loss *(MCQ 153)*.
   - Trichotillomania presents as a patch of hair loss at an easily approachable region of scalp. The bald patch consists of firmly anchored partially broken hairs *(MCQ 167)*.

9. **Ans. c. It is herpes labialis which requires systemic antiviral therapy only for 1 day.**
   Topical antibiotic cream can be advised to prevent secondary infection.

10. **Ans. b. It is tuberculosis verrucosa cutis which is a type of skin tuberculosis associated with high degree of immunity. It is seen at trauma vulnerable sites with characteristic finger like projections.**

- Common warts usually occur as single or grouped, scaly, rough papules or nodules *(MCQ 169)*, not plaques.
- In psoriasis, there will be easily removable silvery white scales.
- LP lesions will be purplish and its hypertrophic variant usually occurs on feet and legs *(MCQ 20)*.

11. **Ans. c. It is kerion which is a type of tinea capitis. Secondary bacterial infection is very common.**
    - Infected sebaceous cyst and abscess will not have hair loss and fluctuation can easily be elicited with fingers.
    - Carbuncle will manifest with discharging pus from multiple follicular openings giving an appearance of a sieve *(MCQ 157)*.

12. **Ans. d. It is chickenpox. Eruption of vesicles surrounded by erythema is a classical presentation.**
    - Measles comprises of maculopapular rash.
    - Acne comprises of papules, pustules, white and black comedones *(MCQ 34)*.
    - Boil is a painful follicular lesion.

13. **Ans. d. All topical steroids cause cutaneous atrophy on prolonged application. Flexures having thin skin are particularly vulnerable.**
    - Dithranol will cause burning and redness *(MCQ 1015)*.
    - Calcipotriol can cause hypercalcemia, if applied for a long period.

14. **Ans. b. This is a typical face of systemic sclerosis patient. Patient usually complains of 'Raynaud's phenomenon.'**
    - SLE manifests as "malar rash" on face *(MCQ 25)*.
    - Scleredema has acute onset with a preceding infectious episode and skin has prominent follicular orifices. Like SS, patient is unable to smile or wrinkle his forehead, but epidermis can be pinched off between thumb and index finger. It is usually not associated with Raynaud' phenomenon also.
    - Generalized morphea do not have these facial features.

15. **Ans. a. Purplish color papules are typical in LP. Genital mucosa is involved in 20–25% of LP patients.**
    - Psoriasis will show red discrete plaques with little scaling *(MCQ 95)*.
    - FDE presents as dusky discoloration and superficial ulceration *(MCQ 160)*.
    - In lichen sclerosus foreskin becomes bluish white that may result in to secondary phimosis *(MCQ 320)*.

16. **Ans. d. It is lichen nitidus which is an uncommon papulosquamous self-limiting disorder. Penile skin is a common site.**
    - Lichen planus lesions have a purplish hue and are itchy *(MCQ 21)*.
    - Papules of scabies will be extremely itchy and are seen on scrotum also *(MCQ 65)*.

17. **Ans. It is PLEVA which is an uncommon papulosquamous disorder characterized by spontaneous resolution.**
    - P. rosea manifests as crop of oval lesions with fine scaling and lesions are seen along the ribs forming "Christmas-tree pattern" *(MCQ 161)*.
    - Pityriasis lichenoides chronica is a chronic disease that comprises of recurrent crops of brown papules with adherent mica like scales.

18. **Ans. b. Herpes zoster ophthalmicus must be treated with antiviral therapy because it is involving a vital organ, i.e., eye.**
    - Antiviral therapy should be started at the earliest preferably within 72 hours of rash onset.
    - Patients older than 50 years of age, ophthalmic zoster, immunocompromised patients, and severe involvement are the indications of antiviral therapy.

19. **Ans. b. Isotretinoin is especially indicated for all types of severe acne, e.g., nodulocystic acne, acne fulminans and acne conglobata.**
    - With isotretinoin complete and long remission is remarkable.
    - It affects all the four pathogenic factors responsible for causation of acne.

20. **Ans. d. Lacy network of white streaks inside cheeks and purplish papules are typical features of LP. Ankle is a typical site for hypertrophic LP.**
    - Common warts have rough hyperkeratotic surface seen on dorsa of hands and feet *(MCQ 169)*.
    - LSC comprises of ill-defined thick plaques seen on shins *(MCQ)*, nape of the neck, vulva *(MCQ 197)* and scrotum *(MCQ 97)*.
    - Prurigo nodularis comprises of extremely itchy discrete papulonodular lesions on extremities *(MCQ 170)*.

21. **Ans. d. These are typical features of cutaneous LP.**
    ❖ Psoriasis will show easily removable silvery white scales *(MCQ 162)*.
    ❖ P. rosea occurs on trunk along the ribs *(MCQ 161)*.
    ❖ Surface of the papules of common warts is rough and hyperkeratotic with no scales *(MCQ 169)*.
    ❖ Parapsoriasis comprises of flat scaly patches that favors non sun-exposed sites.

22. **Ans. b. Asymmetrical nail involvement with subungual hyperkeratosis is typically due to tinea unguium.**
    ❖ Nail psoriasis manifests as yellow discoloration, coarse pitting, subungual hyperkeratosis and onycholysis *(MCQ 88)*.
    ❖ Nail changes in LP shows pterygium formation, longitudinal striations and fissuring and brittleness of nail plate *(MCQ 78)*.
    ❖ In alopecia areata, nail plate shows fine superficial pits *(MCQ 295)* distributed in a geometrical pattern.

23. **Ans. b. Such side effects common with prolonged use of topical steroids.**
    ❖ Corticosteroids stimulate microvascular endothelial cells which lead to occurrence of telangiectasia and abnormal dilatation of capillary vessels.
    ❖ Prolonged use of topical steroids can cause striae atrophicans *(MCQ 13)*.

24. **Ans. a. LP leads to follicular destruction by inflammatory infiltrate and causes atrophic scarring (cicatricial) alopecia of scalp.**
    ❖ Alopecia areata causes non-scarring alopecia characterized by well-defined totally bald patches *(MCQ 156)*.
    ❖ Alopecia due to trichotillomania is also of non-scarring type and is characterized by presence of firmly anchored partially broken hairs in the bald area *(MCQ 167)*.
    ❖ Alopecia due to CCLE show pigmentary changes *(MCQ 76)* and patient will have CCLE lesions on sun exposed areas of face.

25. **Ans. b. Lupus erythematosus is precipitated by sun exposure (photosensitivity) and is typically seen in acute cutaneous lupus erythematosus and in 80% of patients of SLE. Area just below lower eyelids is characteristically spared. SLE is 8 times more commonly seen in females.**
    ❖ Melasma comprises of brownish discoloration with no erythema or edema *(MCQ 182)*.
    ❖ PLE comprises lesions in many morphological forms on sun exposed areas of face namely papules, papulovesicular, EM like lesions *(MCQ 198)*.
    ❖ In SS face gives a characteristic mask like appearance. Forehead skin becomes smooth and shiny with disappearance of lines of expression. Nose becomes small and pinched. Mouth opening gets constricted giving a pursed appearance *(MCQ 14)*.

26. **Ans. d. It is a plaque type lupus vulgaris which is a paucibacillary type of skin tuberculosis with moderate to high degree of immunity.**
    ❖ CCLE depicts red well-defined plaques covered by adherent scales extending in to the orifices of hair follicles. Lesions show erythema and hyper-pigmentation at the periphery *(MCQ 67)*.
    ❖ Such a large lesion is not seen in psoriasis. Psoriatic lesion will comprise of easily removable silvery white scales *(MCQ 162)*. It will not have apple jelly nodules and scarring.
    ❖ Plaque type BCC may demonstrate surface telangiectasia, cystic center and uneven distribution of pigmentation.
    ❖ Sarcoidosis plaques are usually reddish-brown infiltrated plaques that do not have scaling.

27. **Ans. d. It is acneiform eruption, i.e., drug-induced acne. It is commonly seen in patients receiving steroids, antitubercular therapy, antiepileptics, anabolic steroids (protein powder) by athletes. In contrast to acne, it is unusual to find comedones, cysts and scarring.**
    ❖ In acne lesions are pleomorphic and consist of papules, pustules, comedones, cysts and scarring *(MCQ 34)*.
    ❖ Chickenpox presents with a crop of vesicles that are surrounded by irregular area of erythema *(MCQ 12)*.
    ❖ Measles comprises of maculopapular rash.

28. **Ans. a. These are senile comedones.**
    These comedones are not related to acne. Chronic exposure to sun light and smoking are responsible factors.

29. **Ans. c. Well-defined margins and purplish hue are typical features of LP.**
    ❖ Lipstick cheilitis occurs on the vermillion borders of lips varying from a mild redness, scaling and fissuring to edematous crusting *(MCQ 362)*.
    ❖ FDE produces dusky or grayish discoloration *(MCQ 199)*.

- ❖ CCLE on lip manifests as diffuse thickening, redness, ulceration and crusting *(MCQ 201)*.
- ❖ Lip-lick cheilitis is seen as moist fissured eczema involving the perioral region adjoining the vermillion border *(MCQ 93)*.

30. **Ans. b.** Involvement of more than one site by H. Zoster is seen in patients of HIV infection unless proved otherwise. Always rule out HIV infection if H. zoster patient is having:
    - ❖ Recurrence of H. zoster
    - ❖ Simultaneous involvement of two sites
    - ❖ Bilateral involvement
    - ❖ Having tuberculosis along with herpes zoster
    - ❖ In high-risk patients, e.g., truck drivers

31. **Ans. a.** It is pterygium formation which is characteristically seen in LP but is not diagnostic. It results from fusion of proximal nail fold with nail bed and appears as V-shaped fibrotic band of tissue. Longitudinal striations, fissuring and brittleness of nail plate are other commonly seen nail changes in LP *(MCQ 78)*.
    - ❖ Nail psoriasis manifests as yellow discoloration, subungual hyperkeratosis and onycholysis *(MCQ 88)*.
    - ❖ Asymmetrical nail involvement with subungual hyperkeratosis is typically due to tinea unguium *(MCQ 22)*.
    - ❖ In alopecia areata, nail plate shows fine superficial pits *(MCQ 295)* distributed in a geometrical pattern.

32. **Ans. a.** Active border with central clearing is a feature of tinea.
    - ❖ Contact dermatitis due to shoes takes the shape of shoes. It shows hyperkeratosis with no active borders or central clearing *(MCQ 202)*.
    - ❖ It is not eczema as there is no oozing and crusting. Unlike eczema, this patient has well defined active borders with central clearing *(MCQ 213)*.
    - ❖ Candidiasis feet manifests as itchy, moist and red macerations involving interdigital spaces also *(MCQ 210)*.

33. **Ans. c.** Prolonged and high dose of corticosteroids are very well known to cause striae atrophicans.
    - ❖ Phenytoin and antitubercular treatment cause acneiform eruption *(MCQ 43)*.
    - ❖ Anticancer therapy causes anagen alopecia *(MCQ 303)*.

34. **Ans. c.** Face, chest and back are common sites of acne. Acne lesions are pleomorphic that consist of papules, pustules and comedones.

- ❖ DH manifests as extremely itchy urticarial wheals or small vesicles having marked tendency for grouping. Extensors of limbs, trunk, natal cleft and buttocks are common sites *(MCQ 204)*.
- ❖ In drug-induced acne the lesions are monomorphic that comprises of small red papules mainly seen on shoulders, upper arms and trunk *(MCQ 43)*.
- ❖ Chickenpox manifests as crop of vesicles that are surrounded by irregular area of erythema giving a dew drop on rose petal appearance *(MCQ 12)*.

35. **Ans. a.** Use of face wash may cause peeling/burning/dryness/reddening of skin. So, face wash will further aggravate itching and dryness in such patients.

36. **Ans. d.** It is acne keloidalis nuchae which is a variant of acne. It is seen in adults due to chronic folliculitis and is typically seen at this site. It is difficult to treat.
    - ❖ Hypertrophic scar will have a history of injury and surface will be even and smooth *(MCQ 205)*.
    - ❖ SCC may arise from anywhere on the skin and mucous membranes having squamous epithelium. In most cases, it evolves from sun-damaged facial skin in older age. In this patient, age and site do not favor SCC. Lesion is also not soft, friable or verrucous *(MCQ 113)*.
    - ❖ Kerion is a type of tinea capitis that presents as an inflammatory boggy swelling having easily pluckable hairs and pus discharging sinuses *(MCQ 11)*.

37. **Ans. d.** It is 'erythema migrans' which is a hallmark of early cutaneous manifestation of Lyme disease. It is caused by *Borrelia burgdorferi*—a non-venereal spirochete. It is transmitted through the bite of tick Ixodes. In erythema migrans spirochetes are best demonstrated in papillary dermis.
    - ❖ Ring of tinea corporis has well defined active border with central clearing *(MCQ 7)*.
    - ❖ Urticarial wheal lasts for few hours and resolves within 24 hours *(MCQ 206)*.
    - ❖ EM manifests with small target lesions *(MCQ 140)*.

38. **Ans. a.** It is candidal balanoposthitis in a diabetic patient. It is a very common manifestation of diabetes.
    - ❖ Secondary syphilis do not present on glans penis. It can manifests as shallow, round, painless patches edged by dull red areola in oral mucosa. S. syphilis presents as condylomata lata in anal

region and as asymptomatic maculopapular rash on trunk, palms and soles *(MCQ 214)*.
- FDE will cause dusky or grayish colored superficial ulceration *(MCQ 160)*.
- Poor hygiene can cause deposition of smegma *(MCQ 333)* which is a substance made up of oil and dead skin cells which can accumulate under the foreskin in uncircumcised males.

39. **Ans. a. It is pityriasis versicolor which is characterized by asymptomatic, hypopigmented/ discolored macules with fine scaling and presence of satellite lesions at periphery are characteristic.**
    - Macules of vitiligo are usually depigmented, well defined and do not have satellite lesions *(MCQ 181)*.
    - P. rosea presents as crop of discrete oval macules covered by fine scales. Long axes of lesions tend occur parallel to ribs forming a "Christmas tree" pattern *(MCQ 161)*.
    - P. alba presents as invariable sized round or irregular patch of hypopigmentation covered with powdery white scales. Besides face *(MCQ 85)*, arms, shoulders may also have macules of pityriasis alba.

40. **Ans. d. It is tinea imbricata. Concentric rings may also be caused by repeated application of steroid cream. Dermatophyte can be easily demonstrated by KOH smear.**
    - Annular lesions of mid borderline leprosy are infiltrated and asymptomatic lesions *(MCQ 218)*.
    - Granuloma annulare presents as complete or incomplete rings formed by skin colored or violaceous papules. Usually there is no itching, inflammation or scaling *(MCQ 219)*.
    - Discoid eczema presents as disk shaped lesions having well defined edge with no central clearing *(MCQ 194)*.

41. **Ans. c. Lacy network of white streaks with violaceous hue on inner side of cheeks is characteristic of LP.**
    - Leukoplakia is usually unilateral and does not have violaceous hue *(MCQ 230)*.
    - In CCLE, chronic buccal mucosal plaques may resemble leukoplakia. Patient will have red well defined CCLE plaques on sun exposed parts of face with involvement of lower lip *(MCQ 201)*.
    - In P. vulgaris patient will have superficial painful mucosal ulcers with hemorrhagic crusting of lips *(MCQ 184)*.

42. **Ans. c. Bilateral herpes zoster is due to underlying HIV infection unless proved otherwise. Always rule out HIV infection if H. zoster patient is having:**
    - Recurrence of H. zoster
    - Simultaneous involvement of two sites
    - Bilateral involvement
    - Having tuberculosis along with herpes zoster
    - In high-risk patients, e.g., truck derivers

43. **Ans. b. It is drug-induced acne which is commonly seen in patients receiving steroids, antitubercular therapy, antiepileptics, anabolic steroids (protein powder) by athletes. In contrast to acne, it is unusual to find comedones, cysts and scarring.**
    - Antihistamines do not cause drug-induced acne.
    - Anti-tubercular drugs in addition to acneiform eruption also cause lichenoid drug eruption *(MCQ 208)*.
    - Phenytoin in addition to acneiform eruption also causes gum hypertrophy *(MCQ 215)*.

44. **Ans. d. Dusky red discolored lesions are typical of FDE.**
    - SJS and TEN are also caused by drugs, but in addition they also involve 5–10% *(MCQ 81)* and >30% *(MCQ 127)* of body surface respectively.
    - EM can also involve mucosa, but is characterized by presence of target lesions *(MCQ 83)*.

45. **Ans. b. Unilateral involvements usually suggest infective pathology. Hyperkeratosis and scaling are features of dermatophytosis.**
    - Contact dermatitis is usually bilateral.
    - Tubercular involvement is usually verrucous.
    - Palmar psoriasis is usually bilateral and is seen as red plaques with white scaling *(MCQ 231)*.

46. **Ans. d. Acne excoriee patients have psychological illness and they require antidepressants and psychotherapy in addition to anti-acne treatment.**

47. **Ans. c. It is histoid leprosy which is a rare multibacillary type of leprosy. Infiltration of both ears is seen in multibacillary leprosy *(MCQ 101)* unless proved otherwise.**
    - Molluscum contagiosum papules are usually dome-shaped umbilicated papules *(MCQ 209)*.
    - Guttate psoriasis manifests as small sized lesions in rain drop pattern having typical red color and scaling of psoriasis *(MCQ 212)*.
    - Acne on the back presents as pleomorphic lesions that comprises of papules, pustules and comedones *(MCQ 34)*.

48. **Ans. b.** These are milia that are epidermal keratin cysts. They are commonly seen on eye lids and cheeks. They can be squeezed out after disrupting their roof with needle.
    * Acne vulgaris comprises of pleomorphic lesions that comprises of papules, pustules and comedones *(MCQ 216)*.
    * Molluscum contagiosum lesions are shiny, pearly white, dome-shaped and umbilicated papules *(MCQ 224)*.
    * Syringoma is seen as 1–3 mm sized papules in an adult woman. The papules tend to distributed bilaterally symmetrically on cheeks and eyelids.
    * Trichoepithelioma presents as small papules on face around nasolabial folds, chin and forehead *(MCQ 223)*.

49. **Ans. b.** Emollients are quite safe and best for widespread involvement. They normalize hydration of skin and take care dryness, scaling and itching.
    * Use of topical or systemic steroids initially suppresses the disease process. But, later on there is an appearance of a greater number of skin lesions in an aggressive manner than the pretreatment state (**rebound phenomenon: MCQ 316**).
    * Dithranol can be used for few and large plaques without any long-term side effects. Being irritant, its use should be avoided on eyes, genitals and flexures.
    * Calcipotriol is also used for patients having few lesions.

50. **Ans. b.** It is acne rosacea which is seen in middle aged female with involvement of central part of face. The presence of vascular symptoms with absence of comedones suggests the diagnosis of acne rosacea.
    * Acne vulgaris comprises of pleomorphic lesions that comprises of papules, pustules and comedones *(MCQ 216)*.
    * Acute urticaria is not characterized by flushing, but by eruption of wheals *(MCQ 206)*.
    * In drug-induced acne the lesions are monomorphic that comprises of small red papules mainly seen on shoulders, upper arms and trunk *(MCQ 43)*.

51. **Ans. b.** It is squamous hyperkeratotic type of tinea pedis that can easily be proved by KOH smear examination.
    * Keratoderma will manifest as yellowish abnormal thickening of soles *(MCQ 192)*.
    * Candidiasis soles manifests as uniformly red and macerated soles *(MCQ 210)*.
    * Eczema soles manifests as oozing, crusting and cracking *(MCQ 137)*.

52. **Ans. b.** It is scrofuloderma which is an endogenous tuberculosis and results from contiguous spread of infection from underlying tuberculosis focus, e.g., lymph nodes, joints, bone and infected gland.

53. **Ans. a.** It is untreated scrofuloderma involving multiple cervical lymph nodes. Sinuses are having typical bluish margins and correspond to underlying cervical lymph nodes.
    * Predilection sites for hidradenitis suppurativa are axillae, perianal area and groins *(MCQ 111)*.
    * Bacterial sinuses usually do not occur in multiple numbers. Perianal region is a common site for bacterial sinuses *(MCQ 326)*.
    * Sinuses of osteomyelitis are seen over the underlying bone.

54. **Ans. c.** Clofazimine is a red aminophenazone dye which is known to cause red brown cutaneous pigmentation, dryness and ichthyosis *(MCQ 90)*. It usually fades 6–12 months after stopping clofazimine.
    * Rifampicin causes red coloration of urine.
    * Dapsone causes hemolysis and methemoglobinemia that leads to blue coloration of lips.
    * Thalidomide causes teratogenicity.

55. **Ans. c.** It is because of underlying HIV infection unless proved otherwise. Always rule out HIV infection if H. zoster patient is having:
    * Recurrence of H. zoster
    * Simultaneous involvement of two sites
    * Bilateral involvement
    * Having tuberculosis also
    * In high-risk patients, e.g., truck drivers

56. **Ans. b.** It is a classic case of SSSS. Vesicles are filled with sterile clear fluid. It responds nicely to antibiotics. Steroids have no role.
    Absence of mucosal involvement rules out the possibility of pemphigus, SJS and TEN.

57. **Ans. c.** It is lupus vulgaris. Face *(MCQ 26)*, neck, extremities and buttocks are common sites for lupus vulgaris.
    * Leishmaniasis occurs on uncovered parts of body. The face, neck and arms are common sites *(MCQ 237)*.
    * There are no sinuses or granules in favor of mycetoma *(MCQ 272)*.

- Injection abscess will have swelling, redness and tenderness.

58. **Ans. d.** Clinically, it is widening of central parting in a Christmas tree pattern (a common androgenic hair loss in females). TSH and serum ferritin levels should be done.
    - In alopecia areata smooth bald patches are seen *(MCQ 156)*.
    - In trichotillomania, there will be firmly anchored partially broken hairs *(MCQ 167)*.
    - Lupus hairs are coarse, dry, fragile and broken off hairs *(MCQ 89)*.

59. **Ans. c.** It is infantile scabies. Scalp, trunk and soles *(MCQ 74)* are common sites of involvement in infants. If mother is normal, it is difficult to make a diagnosis of infantile scabies. In this case mother is also affected.
    - In SD, soles will not be affected and mother will be normal.
    - Miliaria rubra comprises of uniform red papules with erythema *(MCQ 118)* and mother will be normal.
    - In infantile AD, face is most frequently involved *(MCQ 174)*.

60. **Ans. d.** It is impetigo contagiosa characterized by honey-colored multiple crusted lesions with surrounding erythema. Face is commonly involved in children.
    - IBH manifests as persistent pruritic papules *(MCQ 172)* and secondary infection is uncommon.
    - Chickenpox manifests as vesicles surrounded by erythema *(MCQ 173)*.
    - In pemphigus, usually oral mucosa is involved. Cutaneous erosions are painful and bleed easily *(MCQ 184)*.

61. **Ans. b.** In pediculosis pubis, sharing of bedding and clothing is not the only cause. Close physical contact (usually sexual) is very important. Sexual partner must also be treated.
    It is caused by *Pthirus pubis* which is a dorsiventrally flattened wingless insect having three pairs of legs.

62. **Ans. b.** In scabies papules and pustules have tendency to remain localized to finger web spaces.
    - Pompholyx and id eruption are characterized by vesicles on sides of fingers with normal web spaces *(MCQ 180)*.
    - In candidiasis, there are no vesicles and web spaces will be macerated *(MCQ 183)*.

63. **Ans. c.** It is tuberculous gumma which has resulted from hematogenous dissemination from a distant primary focus. Undermined bluish margins with watery discharge are characteristic features of tubercular ulcer.
    - Lymphangitic form of sporotrichosis occurs on exposed parts, e.g., hands and feet. Its lesions will be in a linear fashion along the lymphatics.
    - Sinuses of osteomyelitis are usually adherent to underlying tissues.
    - Boils present as painful nodules *(MCQ 357)* with pus discharge.

64. **Ans. c.** It is ILVEN which is present since infancy and prefers extremities.
    - Hyperkeratotic eczema will have severe itching and will not be since infancy *(MCQ 2)*.
    - TVC comprises of hyperkeratotic lesion with finger like projections *(MCQ 10)*.
    - LPH comprises of itchy papules and nodules that prefer ankles *(MCQ 20)* and shins.

65. **Ans. c.** Pruritic papules are commonly seen but are not pathognomonic. Burrows are pathognomonic lesions. They are seen as slightly raised and brownish dark tortuous lines 1–10 mm in length on wrists, sides of fingers, web spaces, genitalia *(MCQ 271)* and instep of foot.

66. **Ans. a.** It is not erysipelas. This patient is having cellulitis having indistinct margins due to subcutaneous tissue involvement.
    Erysipelas has distinct margins because infection is superficial and is limited to dermis and upper subcutaneous tissue only *(MCQ 71)*.

67. **Ans. d.** It is crusted or Norwegian scabies. It is usually associated with advanced age, disabled or mentally ill patients. Generalized erythema, scaling, nonpruritic crusts seen on hands, feet and buttocks *(MCQ 647)*. Generalized lymphadenopathy and eosinophilia are common. It is highly infectious and more than a million mites populate the skin. In spite of this fact, pruritus is absent or mild. Patient should be admitted to the hospital and should be kept isolated till the treatment is completed.
    - Psoriasis comprises of red plaques with white scaling *(MCQ 146)*.
    - Tinea corporis presents as red itchy patches with well-defined borders *(MCQ 773)*.
    - Eczema presents as wet, red, ill defined and itchy lesions *(MCQ 970)*.

68. **Ans. d.** She is having CCLE in which plaques have adherent scales that extend in to hair follicles giving a typical "carpet tack" appearance on the undersurface of scales. Involvement of sun exposed area endorses the diagnosis of CCLE.
    - LP is uncommon on face and comprises of purplish lesions *(MCQ 29)*. Psoriatic lesions have easily removable silvery white scales *(MCQ 162)*.
    - *L. vulgaris* manifests as single soft gelatinous plaque with advancing active margin and a trailing scar in the center *(MCQ 26)*.

69. **Ans. d.** It is localized morphea which is characterized usually by shiny and smooth surface with absence of hair. Plaque is usually attached to underlying tissues.
    - Intact sensations rule out the possibility of tuberculoid leprosy in a single plaque *(MCQ 6)*.
    - Hypertrophic scars or keloids are usually red, elevated and are itchy *(MCQ 176)*.
    - Nevus will not be attached to underlying tissues.

70. **Ans. b.** All patients who are older than 50 years should be given systemic antiviral drugs.
    - It should be started within 72 hours of onset of rash. Utility is doubtful if >72 hours have elapsed.
    - Antiviral therapy will limit the extent, duration and severity of pain and rash.
    - It will also minimize the risk of PHN.
    - Topical antiviral cream has no role.
    - Calamine lotion will provide soothing action.

71. **Ans. a.** This is erysipelas which is a superficial bacterial infection. It does not involve the deeper part of dermis and subcutaneous tissue. So, it has sharp well-defined edge to normal tissue.

72. **Ans. a.** It is papular urticaria which is a chronic, self-limiting disorder and takes long time for remission. Papules are persistent that tend to occur in groups and are surrounded by wheal with a central punctum.
    - It is not scabies. Scabies prefers finger webs, wrists, genital and soles.
    - LP papules are purplish in color and prefer peripheral parts *(MCQ 21)* and do not occur at this age.
    - PLC is largely seen in young adults and consists of firm brownish papules with adherent mica like scales.

73. **Ans. a. Permethrin is highly effective. It needs application for 10 minutes only.**

74. **Ans. c.** Scalp, trunk *(MCQ 59)* and soles are common sites of involvement for infantile scabies.
    - Papular urticaria is uncommon in infants and comprises of papules on the exposed peripheral parts *(MCQ 72)*. Mother will be normal.
    - Face *(MCQ 174)* and extensor aspects of limbs are most preferred sites in infantile phase of AD. Mother will be normal.
    - In pyoderma, child will not be irritable. Mother will be normal.

75. **Ans. c. Mechanical removal is uncomfortable and is not recommended.**

76. **Ans. b. It is a cicatricial alopecia due to CCLE.**
    - LP also causes cicatricial alopecia *(MCQ 24)*, but discoid lesions with adherent scaling do not suggest LP.
    - Hair loss in alopecia area is non cicatricial and consists of smooth bald patches *(MCQ 156)*.
    - Hair loss in trichotillomania is also non-cicatricial and consists of firmly anchored partially broken hairs *(MCQ 128)*.

77. **Ans. c. Fexofenadine should be used during renal insufficiency. It is least metabolized in liver and mainly excreted by fecal route. Loratadine should be used in liver insufficiency.**
    Levocetirizine should not be given in patients having renal insufficiency as it is mainly (85%) excreted through kidney.

78. **Ans. c. Pterygium formation is considered as a classical nail change in LP.**
    - Commonly seen psoriatic nail changes are coarse pits *(MCQ 119)*, onycholysis and subungual hyperkeratosis *(MCQ 88)*.
    - In alopecia areata, fine superficial pits are typical *(MCQ 295)* and may have excessive longitudinal ridging *(MCQ 112)*.
    - Tinea unguium usually shows asymmetrical subungual hyperkeratosis *(MCQ 22)*.
    - In Darier's disease, nail plate shows red or white longitudinal streaks which terminate distally in V-shaped notch *(MCQ 178)*.

79. **Ans. d. Epidermolysis bullosa is a heterogenous group of genetically determined skin diseases that manifests at birth or latest during early infancy.**
    - *Pemphigus vulgaris* does not manifest at birth.
    - Early congenital syphilis will manifest with findings in eyes, bones, nails and mucosae.
    - Porphyria does not manifest in neonates. It manifests at later age with fragility and blistering of sun exposed skin.

80. **Ans. b.** Hailey-Hailey disease is also known as familial benign chronic pemphigus that has autosomal dominant inheritance.
    ❖ Tinea cruris manifests with well-defined active margins with no fissuring *(MCQ 4)*.
    ❖ Candidal intertrigo appears as red macerations that extends beyond the area of contact and develops fringed irregular margins with classical satellite vesicles and pustules *(MCQ 253)*.
    ❖ Acantholysis is also seen in PV. But it does not prefer groins only. There will be vesiculobullous lesions at other sites also, e.g., face, trunk, scalp, axillae, etc. Oral mucosa is involved in 50–70% patients of PV *(MCQ 84)*.

81. **Ans. b.** Partial coalescence of lesions, involvement of less than 10% of body surface and more than one mucosa qualify the diagnosis of SJ syndrome.
    ❖ EM major comprises of extensive target lesions with no coalescence. Oral mucosa is involved with blood-stained discharge.
    ❖ In FDE, conjunctiva is not involved. Oral mucosa and glans can be involved simultaneously with no or minimal cutaneous lesions *(MCQ 44)*.
    ❖ In measles, there is conjunctivitis and exanthematous (maculopapular) rash *(MCQ 238)* with no EM like lesions.

82. **Ans. b.** Valaciclovir is a prodrug of acyclovir and 85% of acyclovir is excreted in urine. So, dosage adjustment of valaciclovir is required in patients having renal dysfunction. For patients having creatinine clearance: >50 mL/min—1 g TDS, 30–50 mL/min—1 g BD, 10–29 mL/min—1 g OD and <10 mL/min—500 mg/day.

83. **Ans. b.** Herpes labialis is a known cause of erythema multiforme in which target lesions *(MCQ 140)* are typically seen.
    ❖ In SJS and TEN target lesions can be seen. But, <10% and >30% of body surface area should be involved to qualify the diagnosis of SJS and TEN respectively.
    ❖ More than one mucosa should be involved to make a diagnosis of SJS or TEN.

84. **Ans. d.** It is flexural psoriasis. Pink coloration, scales and well-defined margins are typical features of psoriatic involvement. Axillae, sub mammary folds and umbilicus *(MCQ 245)* are other sites of flexural psoriasis.
    ❖ Tinea cruris will be extremely itchy and margins will be active with central clearing *(MCQ 4)*.
    ❖ In Hailey-Hailey disease, one finds eroded plaques, fissured appearance and moist vegetation. Scaling is not seen *(MCQ 80)*.
    ❖ Candidal intertrigo appears as red macerations extending beyond the area of contact and develops fringed irregular margins with classical satellite vesicles and pustules *(MCQ 253)*.

85. **Ans. b.** Pityriasis alba is a mild eczematous disorder of endogenous type that persists for long periods. Application of emollients is sufficient.
    ❖ Vitiligo patches usually are depigmented and have well defined margins with no scaling *(MCQ 181)*.
    ❖ Nutritional deficiency and worm infestation do not cause such type of hypopigmentation on face.

86. **Ans. b.** ABCD is a typical example of allergic contact dermatitis caused by various types of air borne allergens. It involves upper eyelids and area under the nose and chin, but spares the back of neck.
    ❖ In senile eczema, skin becomes dry, scaly with deep skin markings studded with fine reticulate fissures. It does not cause thickening and lichenification. Forearms, hands and legs *(MCQ 94)* are common sites.
    ❖ Excessive oil application can lead to formation of comedones.
    ❖ Lupus pernio is a specific cutaneous manifestation of sarcoidosis on face. It manifests as asymptomatic infiltrated reddish-brown plaques that tends to involve face in a symmetrical manner. Cheek lesions have prominent telangiectasia.
    ❖ CAD is also known as actinic reticuloid or photosensitivity dermatitis. It is seen as symmetrical, pinkish red, shiny infiltrated plaques mainly on sun exposed sites of face. Lesions show sharp cut off at lines of clothing *(MCQ 196)* with sparing particularly of the depths of skin creases, upper eyelids and skin behind the earlobes.

87. **Ans. d.** It is pityriasis amiantacea which is an uncommon presentation of seborrheic dermatitis.
    ❖ In psoriasis, there, are discrete plaques with silvery white scales *(MCQ 100)*.
    ❖ Tinea capitis presents as patches of baldness having partially broken easily pluckable hair *(MCQ 8)*.
    ❖ CCLE on scalp will manifests as discoid plaques with either adherent scales or cutaneous atrophy *(MCQ 76)*.

88. **Ans. a.** These nail changes are typically seen in psoriasis.

- Tinea unguium usually does not involve all the nails *(MCQ 22)*.
- In alopecia areata, fine superficial pits are typical *(MCQ 295)* and may have excessive longitudinal ridging.
- Pterygium formation, increased longitudinal striations and fissuring in nail plate are common nail changes in LP *(MCQ 78)*.

89. **Ans. c. In SLE hair becomes coarse, dry, fragile and becomes short broken off that are named as 'Lupus hair'.**
    - It is not melasma. Melasma is brownish that chiefly affects upper lip, cheeks, forehead and chin *(MCQ 182)*.
    - Hair loss in LP is of cicatricial type *(MCQ 186)*.
    - Trichotillomania manifests as firmly anchored partially broken hairs in bald area *(MCQ 167)*.

90. **Ans. b. Clofazimine causes brownish red cutaneous pigmentation** *(MCQ 54)*, **dryness and ichthyotic changes.**
    - Dapsone causes hemolysis and methemoglobinemia that result into blue coloration of lips.
    - Rifampicin causes red coloration of urine.
    - Thalidomide causes teratogenicity.

91. **Ans. a. It is angiokeratoma of scrotum. These red papules are ectatic superficial dermal vessels in combination with hyperkeratosis. Patient needs reassurance and is treated symptomatically.**
    - In pediculosis, lice are seen grasping the hairs close to skin surface *(MCQ 61)*.
    - Palpable purpura is either due to vasculitis or vaso-occlusion. It manifests as red papules that does not bleed and is seen on lower extremities *(MCQ 527)* or other dependent areas, e.g., back and gluteal regions.
    - Papules of nodular scabies are not red and do not bleed.

92. **Ans. c. It is steatocystoma multiplex on scrotum. These swellings on scrotum are sebum filled dermal cysts with sebaceous glands in the walls. They can be removed by simple excision or drainage.**
    - Sebaceous cyst has punctum *(MCQ 278)* and do not occur in groups.
    - Nodular scabies manifests as itchy skin-colored papules.
    - Strawberry hemangioma manifests in first month of life as smooth or lobulated scarlet red single tumor *(MCQ 187)* and subsides by the age of 5 years.

93. **Ans. d. It is lip-licking-cheilitis (perioral eczema). It is attributed to the habit of lip licking in children with atopic dermatitis. Application of 1% hydrocortisone ointment is most useful.**
    - Allergic dermatitis due to tooth paste will cause sores in the mouth, swollen gums, an irritated tongue and cheilitis.
    - Iron deficiency and vitamin B-2 (Riboflavin) deficiency will cause persistent dryness and cracking of the lips. Angular cheilitis is the main clinical manifestation of iron deficiency anemia.
    - Dermatitis artefacta is a self-inflicted disorder artificially produced entirely by the action of a fully aware patient in an attempt to gain emotional or psychological benefit. Lesions in dermatitis artefacta invariably appear suddenly overnight and are geometrically shaped or angulated *(MCQ 189)*.

94. **Ans. c. It is asteatotic or senile eczema which is frequently observed in elderly persons during winters. Legs are most commonly involved.**
    - Ichthyosis presents with diffuse and uniform fish like scaling *(MCQ 188)*.
    - Repeated and prolonged heat exposure, e.g., sitting close to fire, use of hot water bottles or heated electric pads causes 'erythema ab igne' that manifests as reticular telangiectatic pigmentation *(MCQ 279)*.

95. **Ans. a. Psoriatic plaques on glans lacks scaling but edges are well defined.**
    - Lichen planus lesions shows violaceous color *(MCQ 15)*.
    - Candidal balanitis presents as soreness, erythema, tiny papules, pustules, superficial erosions and collarette of white scales *(MCQ 38)*.
    - FDE produces dusky discoloration *(MCQ 160)*.

96. **Ans. b. Target lesions are typically seen in erythema multiforme.**
    - SJS and TEN usually involves more than one mucosa and cutaneous lesions are seen on more <10% and >30% of body surface area respectively. Between 10-30% is considered as SJS-TEN overlap. The palmar surface of the hand corresponds to about 0.08% of the body surface area in adults.
    - FDE due to some drug can produce severe oral lesions *(MCQ 44)*. On skin FDE do not exhibit target lesions but can show dusky red macules surrounded by a rim of erythema *(MCQ 191)*.

97. **Ans. c. It is circumscribed neurodermatitis on scrotum. Longstanding itching, repeated scratching and rubbing leads to lichenification which in turn perpetuate itching that completes 'itch scratch cycle'. It is commonly seen on labia majora** *(MCQ 197)*, **scrotum, nape of neck** *(MCQ 263)* **and extremities** *(MCQ 906)*. **Itch scratch cycle should be interrupted by proper counseling, steroid creams and antihistamines.**

   Excessive application of steroid cream never causes lichenification. It causes thinning, atrophy, telangiectasia and hypopigmentation of skin *(MCQ 23)*.

98. **Ans. b. It is port-wine stain or nevus flammeus that presents at birth and manifests unilaterally in the distribution of branches of trigeminal nerve.**
    - While strawberry hemangioma appears in 1st month of life *(MCQ 187)*.
    - Salmon patch tends to disappear by the age of 1 year.
    - Lymphangioma circumscriptum is also noticed at birth, but it presents as discrete or grouped, fluid filled vesicles bulging from skin surface *(MCQ 106)*.

99. **Ans. d. It is a typical case of nevus sebaceous. It can be excised with primary closure with excellent cosmetic results.**
    - In majority of patients BCC occurs after 50 years of age and prefers sun exposed areas of face *(MCQ 193)*.
    - SD manifests as diffuse fine greasy scales on the scalp *(MCQ 138)*.
    - Kerion is one of the types of tinea capitis that manifests as an inflammatory boggy swelling with loss of hairs and discharging sinuses *(MCQ 11)*.
    - Psoriasis on scalp presents as discrete red plaques with silvery white scales *(MCQ 100)*.

100. **Ans. c. Well defined pinkish plaques with silvery white scales are typical of psoriasis.**
     - In SD involvement is usually diffuse with no normal areas of skin in between. Scales are usually fine and greasy *(MCQ 138)*.
     - Tinea capitis is usually not seen at this age. If seen, it will show patches with partial hair loss *(MCQ 8)*.
     - CCLE will manifest with cicatricial alopecia *(MCQ 76)*.

101. **Ans. d. She is a typical case of lepromatous leprosy. Bilateral asymptomatic infiltrated ears in a patient are due to leprosy unless proved otherwise. Absence of remissions and itching are against urticaria.**
     - Myxedema is caused by hypothyroidism that manifests as generalized swelling of face that comprises of thickening of lips, puffiness of eyelids and face *(MCQ 217)*.
     - In PKDL, the rash usually comprises discrete papules on cheeks *(MCQ 361)*, chin, extensors, buttocks and legs. The rash may also comprise of hypopigmented macules at the same sites as those of lepromatous leprosy.
     - Elevated plaques on face with swelling of ear lobules can occur in acute urticaria *(MCQ 194)*. Acute onset, presence of itching and remissions favors the diagnosis of urticaria.

102. **Ans. a. It is pyogenic granuloma which is a misnomer. It is nothing to do with pus. It is a rapidly developed vascular nodule at the site of recent penetrating injury.**
     - Strawberry hemangioma manifests in 1st month of life *(MCQ 187)*.
     - Cherry angiomas are also called as senile angiomas that ate seen mostly on trunk in older individuals *(MCQ 221)*.
     - Boil will present with painful swelling *(MCQ 235)*.

103. **Ans. d. It is Paget's disease of nipple which is an uncommon type of breast carcinoma. It is usually associated with underlying intraductal adenocarcinoma of breast.**
     - Eczema of nipple usually involves both breasts and does not destroy nipple *(MCQ 222)*.
     - Psoriatic plaque will be red color and scaly. It will not destroy nipple.
     - Pyoderma of nipple will have pus, crusting and will not destroy nipple

104. **Ans. b. It is superficial spreading melanoma.**
     - It fulfils all the features that are included in the acronym **ABCDE** (**a**symmetry, irregular/notched **b**order, different **c**olors in lesion, >6 mm **d**iameter, **e**volution, i.e., lesion changes over time) devised for the diagnosis of superficial spreading melanoma.
     - All types of melanocytic nevi have uniform dark or skin colored and are raised above skin surface *(MCQ 120)*.
     - Cafe-au-lait spots are noticed in all patients by the age of 4 years and have uniform color *(MCQ 227)*.

Chapter 5 ✦ Answers of MCQs in Dermatology, Venereology and Leprology

- Bowen's disease is a type of SCC in situ that presents as persistent, red, thin plaque having well defined irregular borders with overlying scale or crust resembling psoriasis *(MCQ 226)*.

105. Ans. c. These are skin tags which may be found associated with insulin resistant diabetes mellitus, pseudoacanthosis nigricans and obesity.
- Mollusca fibrosa are seen on trunk in neurofibromatosis 1 *(MCQ 234)*.
- DPN manifests as small dark brown firm papules commonly on face *(MCQ 228)*.
- Common warts are firm, papules having rough and scaly surface commonly seen on dorsa of hands and fingers *(MCQ 169)*.

106. Ans. b. Axillary folds, shoulders, lower abdominal wall and perineum are common sites for lymphangioma circumscriptum.
- It cannot be herpes zoster as there is no pain or redness and herpes zoster cannot be since childhood.
- Recurrent herpes simplex is seen in the perioral area *(MCQ 9)* and discharge in not expected.
- Vesicles in Hailey-Hailey disease are transient and flaccid. The disease manifests as eroded plaques with fissured appearance in axillae, groins *(MCQ 80)* and neck.

107. Ans. b. Claw hand deformity is due to involvement of ulnar nerve which is one of most commonly involved nerves in Hansen's disease.
- In diabetes sensory neuropathy is prominent and is usually bilateral.
- In carpel tunnel syndrome median nerve is squeezed or compressed as it travels through the wrist that causes pain, numbness, and tingling in the hand and arm.
- The typical symptoms of amyloid neuropathy are due to sensory and autonomic dysfunction. Patients may experience painful paresthesia, numbness and balance difficulties due to sensory dysfunction.

108. Ans. c. It is a mature stage of keratoacanthoma. It will be followed by a resolving stage in which keratin plug is finally shed leaving behind an irregular and puckered scar.
- Short history and absence of rolled out borders do not favor BCC.
- SCC usually arises on sun damaged skin *(MCQ 816)*. While in this patient, facial skin is not showing signs of photo damage, e.g., irregular pigmentation, solar elastosis, telangiectasia and actinic cheilitis.
- Boil does not continue for 2 months.

109. Ans. c. Linear pattern along Blaschko lines since birth is typical for verrucous epidermal nevus.
- TVC, hypertrophic LP and common warts are never present since birth.
- TVC is seen at trauma vulnerable sites *(MCQ 10)*.
- Preferred sites for hypertrophic LP are shins and ankle *(MCQ 20)*.
- Common warts are seen commonly on hands *(MCQ 169)*.

110. Ans. b. Garment or bathing trunk nevus is a congenital melanocytic nevus. Trunk is a common site for this nevus. It is a challenge to treat this nevus which has about 6.3% life time risk of melanoma transformation.
- Spitz and halo nevi are not congenital.
- Spitz nevus is seen in children as acquired, solitary, pink or red, smooth, firm and dome-shaped papule.
- Halo nevus is an acquired melanocytic nevus with a surrounding halo of depigmentation *(MCQ 149)*.
- Junctional nevus is also an acquired melanocytic nevus seen on palms and soles as a macular brown lesion up to 10 cm in size.

111. Ans. It is hidradenitis suppurativa which is a disease of apocrine glands affecting the areas bearing these glands, e.g., axillae, perianal region *(MCQ 343)* and groins *(MCQ 415)*.
- Tubercular adenitis is not characterized by recurrence, sinus tracts and does not occur in perianal region in a widespread manner.
- Fox-Fordyce disease is characterized by intensely itchy, discrete, dome-shaped, pigmented and follicular papules in axillae *(MCQ 232)*.
- Boils are characterized by redness and severe pain not by sinus tracts *(MCQ 971)*.

112. Ans. b. Onychorrhexis and pterygium formation *(MCQ 36)* are characteristic nail changes seen in lichen planus.
- Onycholysis means separation of distal part of nail plate from nail bed *(MCQ 38)*.
- In trachyonychia nail plate becomes rough with accentuated linear striations. When it affects all the nails, it is known as twenty-nail dystrophy.
- Onychomycosis is a fungal infection of the nail *(MCQ 22)*.

113. **Ans. d. It is SCC which can arise anywhere on the skin and mucous membranes having squamous epithelium. Verrucous or cauliflower appearance is very characteristic of SCC.**
    - Nodular melanoma appears as uniformly dark blue or black, dome-shaped lesion *(MCQ 126)*.
    - BCC is particularly seen around eyes, ear and nose *(MCQ 193)*.
    - Lupus vulgaris exhibit active polycyclic outline, central scarring, psoriasiform scaling, erosions and ulcerations *(MCQ 27)*.

114. **Ans. d. It is pyogenic granuloma which is a rapidly developed vascular nodule at the site of a recent penetrating injury.**
    - Strawberry hemangioma develops in first month of life *(MCQ 187)*.
    - Angiokeratoma lesions have hyperkeratotic surface and are multiple *(MCQ 91)*. It is not a site for angiokeratoma.
    - Infected sebaceous cyst will be painful and will not be so red. There will be no history of recurrent bleeding.
    - Cherry angiomas are also known as senile angiomas that are seen in older people as multiple cherry red vascular papules on trunk *(MCQ 221)*.

115. **Ans. d. Infiltration of ear lobules is a characteristic feature of LL. Atrophy of nasal spine in LL causes nasal collapse. Superciliary madarosis is also a feature of LL.**
    - Myxedema is a manifestation of hypothyroidism that manifests as thickening of lips, puffiness of eyelids and face *(MCQ 217)* with no nasal collapse or lobular infiltration.
    - In late syphilis, destruction of nasal cartilage will produce saddle nose deformity with perforation of nose and palate.
    - In traumatic type nasal collapse tip of the nose will also be affected.
    - WG is a lethal necrotizing granulomatous disease of small and medium sized vessels. It involves multiple organs, e.g., upper airways (saddle nose), eyes, kidneys, etc., cutaneous lesions include palpable purpura, tender subcutaneous nodules, infarction of finger tips, gingival hyperplasia, necrotic ulcers of nasal and oral mucosa.
    - In relapsing polychondritis, saddle nose may be due to nasal chondritis. But, auricular chondritis is most typical sign that causes pain, swelling and redness of upper cartilaginous part of pinna sparing the lower non-cartilaginous lobe.

116. **Ans. a. It is SCC usually develops on photo damaged skin at old age.**
    - Granuloma faciale presents as asymptomatic red or violaceous plaques or nodules on nose, preauricular area, ears, cheeks, eyelids and forehead.
    - Lupus vulgaris exhibits psoriasiform scaling, active polycyclic outline with apple jelly nodules *(MCQ 26)*. There may be erosions and ulceration with central scarring, but with no bleeding or pigmentation.
    - This type of leishmaniasis typically presents with painless crateriform (volcanic) ulcer with rolled margin covered with adherent crust *(MCQ 237)*, but with no bleeding. In addition, there are few secondary lesions also.

117. **Ans. d. It is seborrheic keratosis which involves most frequently face and trunk.**
    - The sign of Leser-Trelat comprises of multiple eruptive seborrheic keratosis and is known to be associated with multiple internal malignancies.
    - Skin tags comprises of soft benign pedunculated skin colored or hypopigmented, soft and inelastic papules commonly seen on sides of neck *(MCQ 105)*.
    - Actinic keratosis comprises of macules and papules having rough scaly surface *(MCQ 123)*. Scales are adherent which can be removed with difficulty leaving punctate bleeding.

118. **Ans. c. It is miliaria rubra which is due to blockade of sweat ducts by parakeratotic plugs at intraepidermal level. It is seen in hot and humid conditions on areas of body which are prone to have friction of clothings.**
    - Morbilliform rash is a maculopapular rash in which macules dominate and is caused by drug or viral fever not by hot and humid conditions *(MCQ 238)*.
    - Urticaria is characterized by evanescent, well demarcated, erythematous or pale swellings called wheals *(MCQ 206)*.
    - Erythroderma is characterized by erythema involving whole or nearly whole body with *(MCQ 243)* or without exfoliation *(MCQ 257)*.

119. **Ans. b. These nail changes are seen in psoriasis. Yellow discoloration, subungual hyperkeratosis and onycholysis are other commonly seen nail changes in psoriasis** *(MCQ 38)*.

Chapter 5 ✦ Answers of MCQs in Dermatology, Venereology and Leprology

- ❖ Pterygium *(MCQ 31)* and onychorrhexis *(MCQ 112)* are changes seen in LP.
- ❖ In alopecia areata pitting in fine *(MCQ 295)*.
- ❖ Darier's disease is characterized by red longitudinal streaks which terminates distally in V-shaped notch *(MCQ 178)*.

120. Ans. c. It is compound nevus which shows both junctional activity and nevus cells in dermis. This nevus also contains pigment.
- ❖ Freckles are <3 mm sized light brown macules seen in children that fade with age. Only photoprotection is necessary *(MCQ 240)*.
- ❖ Lentigines are 2-10 mm sized light brown macules seen in middle age and are stable.
- ❖ Intradermal nevus is a non-pigmented nevus containing no melanin *(MCQ 244)*. Nevus cells are present in packets in dermis.

121. Ans. b. It is Lentigo maligna melanoma which is regarded as melanoma is situ. Later it may have vertical growth phase.
- ❖ According to the acronym **ABCDE**, it is having **a**symmetry, poorly defined **b**orders, variation in **c**olor, **d**iameter >6 mm and is showing **e**volution as increase in size.
- ❖ Actinic keratosis manifests as asymptomatic, multiple, 1 mm to 2 cm sized macules or papules with rough scaly surface *(MCQ 123)*.
- ❖ BCC is more common around ears, nose and eyes. It is seen as flesh colored nodule or plaque or non-healing ulcer with rolled border or as patch with thread-like margins *(MCQ 193)*.
- ❖ Acquired melanocytic nevi include compound nevus *(MCQ 120)* which is a dark round raised nodule and intradermal nevus *(MCQ 244)* that is a nonpigmented dome-shaped nodule.

122. Ans. b. It is a large sized infantile hemangioma involving lower eyelid and requires active interventions, e.g., corticosteroids, propranolol, laser, etc. Otherwise, in view of spontaneous regression of small sized infantile hemangiomas *(MCQ 187)*, no active intervention is required in majority of patients.
- ❖ Pyogenic granuloma does not present in first month of life. It consists of a rapidly developed vascular nodule *(MCQ 114)* at the site of a recent penetrating injury. It is unlikely to regress and requires deep excision.
- ❖ Port-wine stain (nevus flammeus) presents at birth as unilateral persistent pink to deep red discoloration in the distribution of sensory branches of trigeminal nerve *(MCQ 98)*.
- ❖ Salmon patch is a blanchable pinkish red macule seen on face and nape of neck that is comprised of fine linear telangiectasia.

123. Ans. d. It is actinic keratosis. Underlying skin is also showing freckles and changes of solar elastosis.
- ❖ Papules of seborrheic keratosis are smooth and do not have scaling.
- ❖ Plane warts are skin colored, smooth, slightly elevated and plane topped papules *(MCQ 1)*.
- ❖ Compound nevi are dark, round or oval papules *(MCQ 120)*. They usually do not occur in multiple numbers at one site. Their surface is not scaly.

124. Ans. c. It is koilonychia.
- ❖ In clubbing, there is a bulbous hypertrophy of terminal phalanx *(MCQ 133)*.
- ❖ Beau' lines refer to transverse grooves in the nail plate parallel to lunula. They reflect some underlying systemic disease for short period, e.g., measles, mumps, etc.
- ❖ In onychogryphosis, nail plate becomes thickened, distorted, opaque, yellowish brown and gives an appearance of oyster shell.

125. Ans. a. It is miliaria profunda which is due to rupture of sweat duct lower down at or below the dermoepidermal junction.
- ❖ *M. crystallina* comprises of tiny thin-walled vesicles not papules. It is due to obstruction of sweat duct at the level of stratum corneum.
- ❖ *M. rubra* manifests as uniformly minute red papules in flexures and areas prone to have friction of clothes *(MCQ 118)*. It is due to blockade of sweat duct at intraepidermal level that leads to leakage of sweat in to epidermis.
- ❖ Milia are thin-walled epidermal keratin cysts seen on cheeks *(MCQ 48)*.

126. Ans. b. It is nodular melanoma which is a second most common subtype of malignant melanoma.
- ❖ A compound nevus is a small dome-shaped pigmented papule raised on epidermal surface *(MCQ 120)*.
- ❖ SCC presents as exophytic tumor having a cauliflower appearance *(MCQ 112)*.
- ❖ BCC has an increased incidence on head and neck. It is seen to have irregular, slightly raised thread-like margins *(MCQ 193)* or non-healing ulcer with rolled border.

127. Ans. c. It is TEN. Involvement of one or more mucosa and >30% of body surface area qualifies the diagnosis of TEN.

- Skin lesions in FDE may or may not accompany mucosal involvement. FDE lesions show characteristic gray color *(MCQ 248)*.
- In SJS <10% body surface is involved *(MCQ 81)*.
- In erythema multiforme target lesions are seen *(MCQ 83)*.

128. Ans. b. It is trichotillomania which is 10 times more often in females than in males. Hair is spared at the nape and at the outer edge of scalp.
- In androgenic alopecia, there is a stepwise miniaturization of hair follicles and terminal hairs are replaced by fine vellus hair. At this age, patient will have widening of central parting in a Christmas tree pattern *(MCQ 190)*.
- In SLE, hair becomes coarse, dry, fragile and becomes short broken off that are named as 'lupus hair' *(MCQ 89)*.
- Alopecia areata shows characteristic "exclamation mark hair" at the periphery of the lesion *(MCQ 156)*.
- Telogen effluvium will have diffuse hair loss *(MCQ 163)*.

129. Ans. b. It is urticarial vasculitis which is characterized by persistence of urticarial wheals for week (>24 hours) and presence of systemic features. It is seen usually 1-3 weeks after parenteral injections, e.g., therapeutic sera, penicillin, radiocontrast media, hepatitis B injections, etc. It usually lasts for 1-4 weeks and runs a benign course.
- Wheals in acute urticaria *(MCQ 206)* disappear within 24 hours to reappear again at another site.
- Morbilliform eruption consists of 2-10 mm sized macules that are confluent at places but without vesiculation or pustulation *(MCQ 238)*.
- EM is characterized by presence of target lesions *(MCQ 83)*.

130. Ans. b. Pruritic, purplish, plain topped papules on peripheral parts are typical features of LP.
- Psoriatic lesions are pink or red and have silvery white scales.
- Prurigo nodularis is uncommonly seen in older adults having atopic dermatitis. It comprises of skin colored extremely itchy, excoriated discrete nodules on arms and legs *(MCQ 170)*.
- TVC is usually a single hyperkeratotic lesion with finger like projections *(MCQ 10)*.

131. Ans. d. It is chickenpox that presents as discrete vesicles with surrounding erythema which gives a typical dewdrop on rose petal appearance.
- Measles has a morbilliform rash *(MCQ 238)*.
- In acne, there are no vesicles.
- Acneiform eruption comprises of acne like lesions *(MCQ 27)* that are induced by certain drugs, e.g., systemic steroids, antiepileptics, antitubercular drugs, etc.

132. Ans. c. It is a manifestation of DM and has no known pathogenesis. Bullae may show intra or subepidermal separations. It runs a benign course.
- In pemphigus vulgaris *(MCQ 184)* and EM *(MCQ 96)* mucosa are usually involved.
- In bullous pemphigoid, bullae are itchy, tense, dome-shaped *(MCQ 285)* and are not localized to legs.

133. Ans. a. It is clubbing which can be associated with carcinoma of lung or other lung diseases.
- Koilonychia refers to concave shape of nail plate both in transverse and longitudinal axes *(MCQ 124)*.
- Subungual hyperkeratosis refers to accumulation of keratinous material under the nail plate. It is typically seen in psoriasis *(MCQ 88)*.
- In onychogryphosis, nail plate becomes thickened, distorted, opaque, yellowish-brown and gives an appearance of oyster shell.

134. Ans. a. It is EM minor in which only target lesions are seen. But mucosal involvement and constitutional symptoms are not there.
- More severe lesions, mucosal involvement and constitutional symptoms are features of EM major *(MCQ 96)*.
- Morbilliform rash is a widespread maculopapular rash that involves mainly trunk *(MCQ 238)*.
- Pityriasis rosea rash comprises of discrete oval macules which are covered by fine scales. Centre of lesions give a wrinkled appearance and prefer trunk along the ribs forming a "Christmas-tree pattern" *(MCQ 161)*.

135. Ans. c. It is prurigo of pregnancy (syn. prurigo gestationis, early onset prurigo). Lesions usually persist through out pregnancy and response to treatment is usually unsatisfactory. But it does not affect fetus and mother.
- PUPPP (late onset prurigo) is seen in first pregnancy in 3rd trimester on abdomen (sparing periumbilical area), thigh, arm and buttocks as urticarial or vesicular or purpuric lesions of same morphological type *(MCQ 259)*.
- Impetigo herpetiformis is an extreme (can cause death) form of pustular psoriasis that presents as

high-grade fever, severe prostration and grouped pin point pustules on fiery red skin. It is also called as generalized pustular psoriasis.
- In pemphigoid gestation is periumbilical vesicles are seen *(MCQ 275)*.
- In prurigo gravidarum (pruritus gravidarum), severe pruritus is localized to palm and soles with no primary skin lesions.

136. Ans. c. It is lichenification which is a feature of chronic eczema due to itching and rubbing.
- Psoriasis is characterized by silvery white scales *(MCQ 146)*.
- Tinea corporis comprises of well-defined light red colored lesions with central clearing *(MCQ 142)*.
- In LP, we find violaceous papules *(MCQ 21)*.

137. Ans. c. It is eczema. Itching, oozing, crusting, fissuring with remissions and relapses are typical features of eczema.
- Tinea on soles is usually of squamous hyperkeratotic type *(MCQ 51)*.
- Keratodermas will show uniform thickening with yellowish discoloration and will show no oozing or crusting *(MCQ 192)*.
- Psoriasis tends to have discrete red plaques with silvery scales with well-defined margins *(MCQ 265)*.

138. Ans. b. It is pityriasis capitis which comprises of fine scaling without redness. It is a manifestation of seborrheic dermatitis on scalp.
- Red coloration of plaque and silvery scales are features of psoriasis *(MCQ 204)*.
- Tinea capitis is predominantly seen between 3–14 years of age and manifests as patches of partial alopecia *(MCQ 8)*.
- Pityriasis alba occurs on face with ill-defined margins *(MCQ 85)*.

139. Ans. a. Presence of Raynaud's phenomenon, facial features and these changes on fingers are typical of systemic sclerosis. Presence of sclerosis proximal to digits is a major criterion for diagnosis of systemic sclerosis.
- SLE manifests as 'malar rash' on face *(MCQ 25)* and does not cause sclerosis of skin.
- Generalized morphea comprises of widespread sclerosis of skin with no systemic disturbances.
- Lichen sclerosus et atrophicus manifests as white sclerotic areas *(MCQ 270)* alone or in combination with involvement of anogenital skin.

140. Ans. c. Target or iris lesions are typically seen in EM.
- In *E. bullosa* simplex blistering is seen on trauma vulnerable sites. Blistering is transient and since childhood *(MCQ 79)*.
- DH is characterized by extremely itchy papules, urticarial wheals and group of small vesicles on back and shoulders *(MCQ 261)*.
- *P. vulgaris* manifests as flaccid blisters, painful cutaneous erosions and hemorrhagic crusting of lips *(MCQ 184)*.

141. Ans. c. It is X-linked recessive ichthyosis which manifests in first week of life and comprise of darker and adherent scales.
- Acquired ichthyosis is seen in later life due to some internal cause or due to some drugs *(MCQ 90)*.
- Ichthyosis vulgaris manifests as white scales sparing diaper area *(MCQ 324)*.
- Malnourishment causes anemia, xerosis and cheilitis.

142. Ans. c. It is tinea corporis having active borders and central clearing.
- Discoid eczema consists of disc or coin shaped lesions composed of dry scaling or microvesicles *(MCQ 194)*.
- Psoriasis manifests as well-defined red plaques studded with silvery white scales *(MCQ 146)*.
- FDE presents as dusky red patches *(MCQ 248)*.

143. Ans. b. Redness of posterior nail fold and loss of cuticle are important features of chronic paronychia.
- Tinea unguium is due to dermatophytes in which there will be no loss of cuticle or redness of posterior nail fold.
- We should never go for nail avulsion except for ingrowing nail.
- Koilonychia is due to iron deficiency *(MCQ 124)*. It should be treated with iron capsules.

144. Ans. b. It is genital warts. VDRL, HIV, HCV and HBsAg must be done in all such patients.
- PPP comprises of 1–3 mm sized flesh colored smooth round papules at the coronal margin *(MCQ 209)*.
- Verrucous SCC manifests as cauliflower like growth *(MCQ 289)*.
- MC comprises of dome-shaped pearly white umbilicated papules *(MCQ 209)*.

145. **Ans. c. 'Exclamation mark' hairs are characteristic of alopecia areata. Loss of eye brows and moustache favors the diagnosis of AA.**
    - Recession of frontal hairline and hair loss at vertex are two main features in male androgenetic alopecia *(MCQ 340)*.
    - Trichotillomania presents as a patch of hair loss at an easily approachable site which is characterized by presence of firmly anchored partially broken hairs in the bald area *(MCQ 128)*.
    - Telogen effluvium is reversible hair loss 3–4 months after some inciting event *(MCQ 163)*.

146. **Ans. b. Reddish pink coloration, silvery white scales and involvement of extensors are typical features of psoriasis.**
    - Guttate psoriasis is characterized by small lesions having rain drop pattern *(MCQ 229)*.
    - Flexural psoriasis occurs in axillae, groins *(MCQ 84)* and under breast *(MCQ 245)*.
    - Annular psoriatic lesions have central clearing *(MCQ 294)*.

147. **Ans. b. Unbearable pain and involvement of single lip suggest the possibility of boil and should be searched.**
    - In angioedema pain is slight and involves both lips *(MCQ 296)*.
    - Granulomatous cheilitis manifests as acute asymmetrical swelling commonly of upper lip. If it is accompanied by fissured tongue and facial paralysis, it called as Melkersson-Rosenthal syndrome.
    - Acute urticaria will also be accompanied by urticarial lesions elsewhere also.

148. **Ans. c. It is senile purpura which is most common type of purpura seen by dermatologists. At old age, skin becomes thin and fragile due to lack of support to cutaneous vessels.**
    - ITP usually causes petechiae *(MCQ 342, 354)*. Majority of patients are children and young adults.
    - HS purpura is mostly seen as crop of small red macules on legs and other dependent areas in a symmetrical manner *(MCQ 332)*. It is seen in children or adolescents.
    - Schamberg's disease (progressive pigmented purpuric dermatosis) is distinct pigmentation seen in dependent part of legs and develops insidiously *(MCQ 365)*.

149. **Ans. c. It is Sutton's nevus which is also called as halo nevus. Excision biopsy is advisable to rule out melanoma.**
    - Nevus of OTA *(MCQ 158)* comprises of facial pigmentation in the region of first two divisions of trigeminal nerve along with pigmentation of cornea, sclera and iris.
    - Intradermal nevus is a acquired melanocytic nevus. It is usually raised, dome-shaped, nonpigmented and are common on face *(MCQ 244)*.
    - Spitz nevus is solitary, pink or red, smooth and dome-shaped. Borders fade in surrounding skin.

150. **Ans. d. Itching, oozing, crusting, recurrence and bilateral involvement are usual features of eczema.**
    - Tinea pedis is usually hyperkeratotic with scaling and does not have oozing or crusting *(MCQ 51)*.
    - Plantar psoriasis presents as well-defined red plaques studded with white scales *(MCQ 265)*.
    - Focal plantar keratoderma comprises of firm to hard thickening of plantar skin at pressure areas *(MCQ 337)*.

151. **Ans. b. These are Mongolian spots which are congenital, benign hyperpigmentations. They fade in early childhood.**
    - Becker's nevus *(MCQ 338)* is usually noticed in adolescence. It is common on shoulder and has terminal hairs.
    - CMN manifests at birth and has terminal hairs *(MCQ 110)*.
    - Nevus of Ito affects acromioclavicular and deltoid regions.

152. **Ans. b. It is due to triamcinolone acetonide injection. It is very common. Effect is also seen along the draining veins.**
    - When depigmentation is idiopathic, it is called vitiligo.
    - Nevus depigmentosus presents at birth *(MCQ 252)*.

153. **Ans. b. Greasy scales, uniform involvement and extension beyond hairline favors seborrheic dermatitis.**
    - Scalp psoriasis comprises of discrete plaques with silvery white scales *(MCQ 100)*.
    - In tinea capitis, there will hair loss *(MCQ 8, 309)* and is uncommon after puberty.
    - Cradle cap manifests during first few weeks of life as adherent greasy scales on scalp *(MCQ 168)*.

154. **Ans. b.** This scarring is caused by chickenpox. So, chickenpox should be treated by systemic antiviral drugs at earliest beyond 13 years of age to avoid scarring which is untreatable.
    - Measles and scarlet fever do not cause vesicular rash.
    - Herpes simplex labialis comprises of groups of small vesicles *(MCQ 9)* and does not cause widespread involvement.

155. **Ans. b.** Asymptomatic bilateral infiltration of ears is always due to lepromatous leprosy (LL) unless proved otherwise. The diagnosis is supported by uncountable lesions on back due to poor immunity in LL.
    - In secondary syphilis lesions are bilateral and symmetrical *(MCQ 293)*, but will not infiltrate ears.
    - In acne there will be papules, pustules and comedones *(MCQ 34)*.
    - In LP there will be itchy violaceous colored papules *(MCQ 339)*.
    - Acneiform eruption comprises of monomorphic papular lesions on trunk and extremities *(MCQ 43)*.

156. **Ans. c.** Total bald patches with 'exclamation mark hairs' at periphery are typically seen in AA.
    - Trichotillomania will show firmly anchored partially broken hairs *(MCQ 167)*.
    - Tinea capitis will not have total baldness. Black dots of broken hairs can be seen in the patch *(MCQ 8)*.
    - In T. effluvium hair loss will be diffuse *(MCQ 163)*. Bald patches are not seen.

157. **Ans. d.** It is carbuncle. Underlying diabetes must be ruled out.
    - Kerion is type of tinea capitis seen on scalp in children *(MCQ 11)*.
    - Furuncle involves a single hair follicle *(MCQ 147)*.
    - Infected sebaceous cyst will be soft and fluctuation can be elicited and will not have multiple follicular openings.

158. **Ans. b.** It is nevus of Ota which is a type of dermal melanocytosis. It is congenital and does not improve with age.
    - Sutton's nevus is a compound nevus surrounded by a halo of depigmentation *(MCQ 149)*.
    - Compound nevus is an acquired melanocytic nevus which is usually dark, round and raised on epidermal surface *(MCQ 120)*.
    - Junctional nevus is seen as brown macule on palms and soles.

159. **Ans. a.** It is a childhood phase of AD in which cubital fossae *(MCQ 207)* popliteal fossae, cervical region, wrists and ankles are characteristically involved.
    - SD has special predilection for scalp, eye brows, eye lashes, nasolabial folds, axillae, inframammary region, umbilicus, groins and natal cleft *(MCQ 171)*.
    - Discoid eczema comprises of disc shaped lesions having well defined edge *(MCQ 194)*.

160. **Ans. d.** Involvement of glans penis is very common due to FDE that may be due to number of drugs. Dusky discoloration is very typical of FDE *(MCQ 248)*. If skin lesions are also present, then it should be differentiated from SJS/EM.
    - LP also involves glans but it does not cause vesiculation *(MCQ 150)*.
    - In SJS and TEN, there is involvement of <10% and >30% of body surface area respectively. There is an involvement of more than one mucosa in TEN and SJS.

161. **Ans. a.** It is pityriasis rosea which is a self-limiting disease and subsides in 6–8 weeks.
    - Psoriatic lesions are reddish and have silvery white scales *(MCQ 162)*.
    - PLEVA lesions are edematous papules with central vesiculation and hemorrhagic necrosis *(MCQ 17)*.
    - Rings of tinea corporis will be large with active borders and central clearing *(MCQ 142)*.

162. **Ans. b.** Well-defined red plaques studded with easily removable silvery white scales are typically seen in psoriasis.
    - Papules of LP are violaceous and are seen on peripheral parts of body with mild scaling *(MCQ 21)*.
    - PLC comprises of firm reddish-brown papules with adherent mica-like scales.
    - Scales of papules/plaques of parapsoriasis are neither silvery white nor easily removable.

163. **Ans. d.** It is telogen effluvium which is caused by typhoid fever in her case. It is a very common inciting etiological factor.
    - In female androgenetic alopecia, common patterns are central parting *(MCQ 190)* and diffuse central thinning with intact frontal hairline *(MCQ 185)*.
    - In alopecia areata, there will be smooth, bald patches *(MCQ 156)*.

- In trichotillomania, there are firmly anchored partially broken hairs *(MCQ 167)* in the bald area.

164. **Ans. b. Retroauricular dermatitis endorses seborrheic dermatitis.**
     - In AD, cubital and popliteal fossae are preferred sites *(MCQ 159)*.
     - In SD preferred sites are scalp, eye brows, eyelashes, nasolabial folds, retroauricular area, flexures, groins, umbilicus and natal cleft.
     - Candidiasis prefers genitals, groins and sub mammary regions *(MCQ 166)*.
     - Psoriasis prefers extensor surfaces.

165. **Ans. a. It is a typical case of chickenpox. In adults, it should be treated with systemic antiviral drugs.**
     - Measles manifests as maculopapular (morbilliform rash) lesions.
     - Acne manifests as papules and pustules *(MCQ 34)*.
     - EM will exhibit target lesions *(MCQ 83)*.

166. **Ans. c. It is intertrigo in which involvement is limited to the contact area of opposing surfaces and has diffuse margins.**
     - Tinea will show well-defined active borders with central clearing *(MCQ 142)*.
     - In flexural psoriasis salmon pink color is retained with well-defined margins *(MCQ 245)*.
     - Candidal intertrigo shows involvement beyond the area of contact and margins are fringed, irregular with satellite vesicles and pustules *(MCQ 179)*.

167. **Ans. c. It is trichotillomania in which patient has compulsive impulse to pull out hair. It manifests at an easily approachable site with characteristic presence of firmly anchored partially broken hairs.**
     - Alopecia areata exhibit smooth bald patches *(MCQ 156)*.
     - Telogen effluvium will have diffuse hair loss *(MCQ 163)*.
     - Androgenic hair loss is not expected at this age.

168. **Ans. b. It is cradle cap which is a common manifestation of infantile SD.**
     - In infantile atopic dermatitis (AD), face is most frequently involved *(MCQ 174)*.
     - Tinea capitis is predominantly seen between 3–14 years and manifests as patches of partial hair loss *(MCQ 8)*.
     - Psoriasis is unusual in infants *(MCQ 204)*. Early peak for age of onset of psoriasis is between 16–22 years.

169. **Ans. a. These are common warts. About 60% of warts disappear spontaneously in 2 years.**
     - LP presents as purplish, plain topped papules with mild scaling *(MCQ 21)*.
     - Psoriasis comprises of red plaques with easily removable silvery white scales *(MCQ 162)*.
     - MC presents as shiny, pearly white, dome-shaped umbilicated papules *(MCQ 209)*.

170. **Ans. c. It is prurigo nodularis. About 65–80% patients are atopic. Emotional stress is also a contributory factor. It runs a protracted course.**
     - Warts also have rough keratotic surface but are skin colored and do not have itching *(MCQ 169)*.
     - LP lesions are violaceous and may be associated with typical LP lesions elsewhere.
     - Central area of plaque of lichen simplex is scaly, thickened, pigmented that merges with normal skin. At periphery, there is indefinite zone of lichenoid papules. Nape of the neck *(MCQ 263)*, ankles *(MCQ 177)* and sides of neck are other sites.

171. **Ans. c. It is SD, showing typically greasy scaling at the sites of seborrheic distribution, e.g., scalp, eye brows, eye lashes, nasolabial folds, inframammary regions, axillae, etc. *(MCQ 175)*.**
     - Manifestations of AD in adult phase are lip-lick cheilitis *(MCQ 93)* and lichenification in the flexures *(MCQ 207)*.
     - In tinea faciei, on careful examination of face will detect a well-defined active border at the periphery of lesion *(MCQ 241)*.
     - ABCD presents as redness, thickening, pigmentation and lichenification on face *(MCQ 86)*.

172. **Ans. a. It is papular urticaria (insect bite hypersensitivity) which is caused by antigen deposited by insect bites that disseminates hematogeneously and lesions often occur far away from the site of bites. It is a type-1 hypersensitivity reaction.**
     - MC comprises of dome-shaped pearly white umbilicated papules *(MCQ 224)*.
     - Scabietic lesions do not occur on face.
     - Impetigo contagiosa comprises of yellowish, thick and dirty brown crusts *(MCQ 60)*.

173. **Ans. c. It is a typical presentation of chickenpox in adults. In adults, it should be treated with antiviral drugs.**
     - Impetigo usually occurs in children with dirty brown thick crusts *(MCQ 60)*.

Chapter 5 ✦ Answers of MCQs in Dermatology, Venereology and Leprology

- *P. vulgaris* comprises of mucosal involvement, flaccid blisters and large painful erosions *(MCQ 184)*.
- Measles consists of red maculopapular rash with no vesicles.

174. **Ans. b. In majority of AD patients, onset in between 3rd and 6th month of age. Face is most frequently involved in infantile phase of AD.**
    - SD favors scalp, eyebrows, eye lashes, nasolabial folds and retroauricular area *(MCQ 171)*.
    - Impetigo contagiosa presents as yellowish, thick and dirty brown crusts *(MCQ 60)*.
    - Measles presents as red maculopapular rash, conjunctivitis, lacrimation and eyes appear red.

175. **Ans. c. It is seborrheic dermatitis. Greasy scales are typical of SD that are typically seen at sites of seborrheic distribution, e.g., scalp, eye brows, eye lashes, nasolabial folds *(MCQ 171)*, axillae, inframammary regions, etc.**
    - Manifestations of AD in adult phase are lip-lick cheilitis *(MCQ 93)* and lichenification in flexures *(MCQ 207)*.
    - Tinea corporis will show well-defined active border and central clearing *(MCQ 142)*.
    - Flexural psoriasis will show salmon pink colored diffuse involvement in axillae, sub mammary regions *(MCQ 245)* and groins *(MCQ 84)* with well-defined borders.

176. **Ans. d. These are keloids. Other sites that show predilection for keloid formation are mandible, shoulders and arm.**
    - Hypertrophic lesions of LP are purplish or reddish brown and are common on ankles *(MCQ 20)* and shins.
    - Hypertrophic scar *(MCQ 205)* usually remains confined to original wound. It is usually asymptomatic and tends to regress with time.
    - CCLE lesions can occur on chest *(MCQ 67)*. They are seen on sun exposed parts as red discoid lesions with hyperpigmented borders and adherent crusts in the center.

177. **Ans. b. Chronic itching and lichenification are features of eczema. Presence of thickening, hyperpigmentation and increased skin markings in combination is described as lichenification.**
    - Psoriatic plaque will be well defined, red and scaly *(MCQ 162)*.
    - LPH also prefers ankle joint but it manifests as thick, elevated, red or purplish papules and nodules *(MCQ 20)*.
    - TVC manifests as asymptomatic well-defined hyperkeratotic plaque with surrounding erythema and finger like projections *(MCQ 10)*.

178. **Ans. c. It is Darier's disease which is an autosomal dominant inherited disease. In addition to these nail changes patient has distinctive persistent multiple firm rough papules *(MCQ 267)*.**
    - LP shows characteristically pterygium formation *(MCQ 31)* and exaggeration of longitudinal lines *(MCQ 78)*.
    - Alopecia areata shows fine superficial pits *(MCQ 295)*.
    - Psoriasis shows yellow discoloration, onycholysis, subungual hyperkeratosis *(MCQ 38)*.

179. **Ans. b. It is flexural candidiasis showing typical features. Underlying diabetes should be ruled out in such patients.**
    - Tinea cruris will show well-defined active margins with clearing towards center *(MCQ 4)*.
    - Flexural psoriasis shows salmon pink color with well-defined margins and white scaling *(MCQ 84)*.
    - Intertrigo is limited to the contact area of opposed surfaces and shows mild erythema and soreness *(MCQ 166)*.

180. **Ans. b. It is ID eruption that refers to small and pruritic vesicles on the sides of fingers in response to an intense inflammatory process elsewhere in the body.**
    - Preferred site for scabies is web spaces, not the sides of fingers. In addition, genitals and buttocks are normal in this patient *(MCQ 62)*.
    - CAD due to cement will present as eczematous papules and plaques *(MCQ 225)*.
    - Pompholyx comprises of various sized vesicles on the sides of fingers, palms and soles *(MCQ 218)*.

181. **Ans. c. It is a segmental vitiligo which is limited to a dermatome. Area supplied by mandibular division of trigeminal nerve is most frequently affected.**
    - N. depigmentosus presents as single circumscribed area of depigmentation with feathered margins *(MCQ 252)*.
    - N. anemicus presents at birth or in infancy as blanchable circumscribed round or oval pale macule surrounded by satellite macules.
    - Focal vitiligo refers to presence of single or few macules in a limited area of body *(MCQ 246)*.

182. **Ans. b.** It is melasma which is predominantly seen in females but is not uncommon in males. It chiefly affects upper lip, cheeks, chin and forehead.
    - SLE has sex predilection for females in the ratio of 8:1. Malar rash consists of erythema and edema which is distributed symmetrically on bridge of nose and malar prominences characteristically sparing nasolabial folds *(MCQ 25)*.
    - Chloasma is a previously used name for melasma, not preferred now.
    - Phototoxic reaction due to systemic or topicals is an abrupt reaction. Melasma develops slowly.

183. **Ans. b.** It is candidal intertrigo for which moisture is an important local pathogenic factor.
    - In scabies, tiny vesicles are seen in the web spaces and on the sides of fingers *(MCQ 62)*.
    - Id eruption refers to small and pruritic vesicles on the sides of fingers *(MCQ 180)* in response to an inflammatory process elsewhere in the body.
    - Tinea manuum often presents as unilateral hyperkeratosis and scaling of palm *(MCQ 45)*

184. **Ans. c.** It is a typical presentation of pemphigus vulgaris.
    - BP comprises of tense dome-shaped blisters in an elderly patient with absence of mucosal involvement and negative Nikolsky's sign *(MCQ 285)*.
    - Linear IgA disease is characterized by tense blisters in clusters as "Cluster of jewels" *(MCQ 266)*.
    - SJS is usually caused by drugs with sudden onset *(MCQ 81)*. It is usually preceded by prodromal symptoms.

185. **Ans. a.** It is androgenic hair loss. Loss of hair from central part of scalp with intact frontal hairline is typical.
    - Absence of firmly anchored partially broken hairs rules out trichotillomania *(MCQ 167)*.
    - Alopecia areata comprises of smooth bald patches *(MCQ 156)*.
    - Telogen effluvium manifests as diffuse hair loss *(MCQ 163)*.

186. **Ans. a.** Lichen planus produces cicatricial type of alopecia.
    - CCLE also produces cicatricial type of hair loss. But unlike LP, it produces depigmentation and hyperpigmentation also *(MCQ 76)*.
    - Trichotillomania produces non-scarring alopecia with the presence of firmly anchored partially broken hairs in the bald area *(MCQ 128)*.

    Hairs are spared at outer edge of scalp and nape of neck *(MCQ 833)*.

187. **Ans. d.** It is strawberry hemangioma (infantile hemangioma) that typically appears in first month of life. In view of spontaneous regression, no active management is required in majority of patients.
    - Pyogenic granuloma is a vascular nodule at the site of recent penetrating injury. It is unlikely to regress and requires excision *(MCQ 114)*.
    - Port-wine stain (nevus flammeus) presents at birth as persistent deep colored macule in the distribution of sensory branches of trigeminal nerve *(MCQ 98)*.
    - Cherry angiomas (senile angiomas) are elevated (1-6 mm) and cherry red colored vascular papules that are seen in old age *(MCQ 221)*.

188. **Ans. b.** It is ichthyosis vulgaris which is a congenital and inherited disease. It is usually persistent and worse in winter.
    - Asteatotic eczema (senile eczema) is frequently observed in elderly persons in winters that superimpose on xerosis *(MCQ 94)*.
    - Clofazimine is an antileprotic drug that causes reddish or brownish black pigmentation of skin and conjunctiva. It may progress to ichthyotic changes *(MCQ 90)* that fades 12 months after stopping the drug.
    - Acquired ichthyosis due to hypothyroidism will not be present since birth and is usually mild.

189. **Ans. c.** It is dermatitis artefacta which refers to self-inflicted lesions by the patient on easily accessible sites of body to seek emotional or psychological benefit. Morphology of these lesions does not fit in to any dermatological disorder.
    - In discoid eczema, lesions are coin shaped *(MCQ 94)* and are itchy.
    - Lupus vulgaris comprises of slowly developing red soft gelatinous plaques *(MCQ 256)*.
    - Psoriasis comprises of red plaques studded with silvery white scales *(MCQ 239)*.
    - Ecthyma is a deeper cutaneous pyogenic infection that comprises of thick adherent crust with underlying shallow and punched out ulcer *(MCQ 299)*.

190. **Ans. d.** Widening of central parting in a Christmas tree pattern is one of the three common patterns of female androgenic hair loss.
    - In telogen effluvium, there will be sudden loss with an etiological factor *(MCQ 163)*.

Chapter 5 ✦ Answers of MCQs in Dermatology, Venereology and Leprology

- There are no firmly anchored partially broken hairs typically seen in trichotillomania *(MCQ 167)*.
- Alopecia areata comprises of smooth bald patches *(MCQ 156)*.

191. Ans. c. It is FDE. Dusky discoloration is typical of FDE *(MCQ 248)*.
- EM major comprises of mucosal lesion with extensive target lesions *(MCQ 96)*.
- In EM minor, there are macules, papules, and target lesions with no mucosal involvement *(MCQ 134)*.
- In SJS at least 2 mucosae are involved with <10% body surface involvement *(MCQ 81)*.

192. Ans. b. It is diffuse plantar keratoderma. Treatment of keratoderma is usually disappointing.
- Eczema presents as oozing, crusting and fissuring *(MCQ 137)*.
- Plantar psoriasis presents as discrete plaques that show pink color and silvery scales *(MCQ 265)*.
- Tinea pedis manifests as hyperkeratosis, scaling with or without erythema *(MCQ 55)*.

193. Ans. c. These are the typical features of BCC. If left untreated, it may cause great destruction to eye and underlying bone.
- SCC in later stages usually become verrucous or gets ulcerated *(MCQ 255)*.
- CCLE lesions are red plaques with regular margins and do not have raised borders *(MCQ 67)*.
- Lupus vulgaris presents with soft gelatinous plaques and does not have raised pigmented thread like margins *(MCQ 26)*.
- MM manifests with pigment dominated nodule, patch or plaque with no thread like margins or central atrophy *(MCQ 121)*.

194. Ans. c. Itching, oozing and crusting are features of eczema.
- Tinea lesions can also be disc shaped. But they will have well-defined active border with central clearing *(MCQ 142)*.
- Psoriatic lesions will have easily removable silvery white scales *(MCQ 162)*.
- LP lesions typically are papules with violaceous color *(MCQ 21)*.

195. Ans. a. It is distinctive pattern of pityriasis rosea. Secondary eruption along the ribs typically forms "Christmas tree" pattern.
- Guttate psoriasis presents as small sized red plaques studded with white scales affecting trunk in a rain drop pattern *(MCQ 229)*.
- Pityriasis versicolor manifests as discolored macules having fine dust like scales *(MCQ 39)*.
- PLEVA presents as crop of polymorphic lesions namely red papules, crusts, vesicles, pustules and erosion *(MCQ 17)*.

196. Ans. b. It is chronic actinic dermatitis (CAD). It is considered as delayed type hypersensitivity (DTH) reaction that occurs after irradiation without any contact of external allergen. It characteristically spares the areas of face not exposed to skin, depth of skin creases and skin behind the earlobes.
- ABCD is characterized by thickening, lichenification and pigmentation because of intractable itching *(MCQ 86)*.
- Lupus pernio is a specific cutaneous manifestation of sarcoidosis. It presents as asymmetrical reddish-brown plaques. Cheek lesions have prominent telangiectasia.
- PMLE is more common in young females that comprises of polymorphic lesions namely papules, papulovesicular, EM like lesions, etc. *(MCQ 198)*.

197. Ans. a. It is lichen simplex chronicus (circumscribed neurodermatitis). Long-standing severe itching leads to lichenification. Other common sites are neck *(MCQ 263)*, **scrotum** *(MCQ 97)*, **extremities** *(MCQ 906)* **and scalp.**
- VVC presents as redness, soreness with scanty, thick curdy white discharge involving vulval skin and adjoining areas *(MCQ 264)*.
- Lichen sclerosus comprises of white well demarcated plaque with waxy or crinkled texture, with purpura and erosions. It often begins first on anterior vulva and periclitorally.
- Herpes simplex presents with grouped vesicles.

198. Ans. b. It is polymorphous light eruption (PMLE). It has onset in hours and resolution in days.
- CAD is a chronic condition seen after 50 years as symmetrical shiny red plaques on face sparing the covered areas *(MCQ 196)*.
- Actinic prurigo is seen as persistent itchy excoriated and crusted papules on face and distal limbs in girls and adult females.
- Hydroa vacciniforme is seen mainly in children as intermittent and symmetrical painful vesicular eruption on exposed area.

- Solar urticaria manifests as intermittent whealing within 5-10 minutes of sun exposure that resolves in 1-2 hours.

199. **Ans. b. Grayish discoloration is typical of FDE.**
    - Lip-lick cheilitis is seen as moist fissured eczema involving the perioral region adjoining the vermillion border *(MCQ 93)*.
    - LP involves only lower lip and has well-defined border *(MCQ 29)*. It may accompany changes inside buccal mucosa.
    - Allergic dermatitis due to tooth paste will cause soreness in the mouth, swollen gums, an irritant tongue and cheilitis.

200. **Ans. c. It is FDE which is supported by sudden appearance of grayish-colored lesion after taking some drug with absence of target lesions. Appearance of lesion only on glans due to offending drug is a minimal reaction in the spectrum (FDE to TEN) of epidermal necrolysis.**
    - LP on glans is a slow and spontaneous development and does not produce bulla *(MCQ 15)*.
    - EM is characterized by target lesions with or without mucosal involvement. *(MCQ 140)*.
    - SJS is characterized by involvement of two mucosa and <10% body surface *(MCQ 81)*.

201. **Ans. c. He is having CCLE. Red plaques with adherent crusts on sun exposed sites of face are typically seen in CCLE.**
    - LP of lip typically has violaceous hue *(MCQ 29)*.
    - Psoriasis usually does not involve face. When involves, it shows red plaques studded with silvery scales *(MCQ 268)*.
    - Lupus vulgaris on face presents as single hyperkeratotic plaque *(MCQ 26)*. It shows scarring in the center and apple jelly nodules at the active edge.

202. **Ans. c. It is allergic contact dermatitis (ACD) due to shoes. ACD is a typical example of delayed type of hypersensitivity in response to variety of exogenous agents. It does not develop on first exposure of allergen.**
    - Candidiasis of feet manifests as red macerations of sole *(MCQ 210)* or between toes.
    - Tinea pedis is usually unilateral and asymmetrical *(MCQ 470)*. Sometimes, it can be bilateral *(MCQ 32)*. But it will show active margins with central clearing.
    - Psoriasis will show red plaques with silvery white scaling.

203. **Ans. c. It is anagen effluvium. The term anagen effluvium is misleading, because in this disorder anagen hairs are not shed. They are broken off within the follicle or at the follicular opening due to systemic anticancer therapy.**
    - Alopecia universalis is a variant of alopecia areata that comprises loss of hair from all parts of body *(MCQ 269)*.
    - Telogen effluvium refers to sudden diffuse hair loss 3-4 months after some inciting event, e.g., typhoid fever, major surgery, abortion, etc. *(MCQ 163)*.
    - Trichotillomania manifests with presence of firmly anchored partially broken hairs in the bald area. Characteristically, hairs at periphery of scalp are spared *(MCQ 128)*.

204. **Ans. a. It is psoriasis scalp. Psoriasis at one year age is unusual. But, red well-defined plaques with silvery white scaling are typical of psoriasis.**
    - Cradle cap manifests in first few months of life as adherent greasy scales with no redness *(MCQ 168)*.
    - Tinea is predominantly seen between 3-14 years and manifests as patches of partial alopecia *(MCQ 8)*.
    - In infantile atopic dermatitis, face is most frequently involved *(MCQ 174)*.

205. **Ans. b. It is hypertrophic scar which is limited to the boundaries of skin injuries and tends to regress with time. It is more responsive to treatment.**
    Keloid extends beyond the boundaries of skin injury. It develops after several months of injury. It is often painful and pruritic. It does not tend to regress with time. It is resistant to treatment with higher rate of recurrence *(MCQ 176)*.

206. **Ans. a. It is acute urticaria that comprises of eruption of itchy wheals. The urticaria with less than 6 weeks is labelled as acute urticaria.**
    - Dermatographism is most common type of physical urticaria. It is seen in 5% of normal persons. When it is accompanied by itching, it is called as symptomatic dermatographism *(MCQ 277)*.
    - Chronic urticaria lasts for >6 weeks.
    - Angioedema is characterized by painful rather than itchy pale or skin-colored subcutaneous swellings affecting face, eyelids and lips *(MCQ 296)*.

Chapter 5 ✦ Answers of MCQs in Dermatology, Venereology and Leprology

207. **Ans. b. It is late childhood AD. Cubital fossae and popliteal fossae are characteristically involved in AD.**
    ❖ Tinea lesions have well defined margins and do not involve in a symmetrical manner *(MCQ 7)*.
    ❖ SD does not prefer cubital or popliteal fossae. It prefers eyelashes, nasolabial folds *(MCQ 171)*.
    ❖ Flexural psoriasis retains the salmon pink color with well-defined margins. It prefers groins *(MCQ 84)*, sub mammary region *(MCQ 245)*.

208. **Ans. b. It is lichenoid eruptions due to ATT. Lichenoid eruptions are extensive and larger than lichen planus. LP consists of small papules with minimal scaling** *(MCQ 21)*.
    ❖ Psoriatic lesion comprises of red plaques with silvery white scaling *(MCQ 162)*.
    ❖ Eczema of hands consists of oozing, crusting, secondary infection, relapses and remissions *(MCQ 220)*.
    ❖ Common warts are seen as discrete papules with rough keratotic surface *(MCQ 169)*.

209. **Ans. c. It is molluscum contagiosum. Central umbilication is a typical feature of MC.**
    ❖ Papules of LP are violaceous that prefers dorsa of hands *(MCQ 21)*.
    ❖ Common warts have rough and hyperkeratotic surface *(MCQ 169)*.
    ❖ Bacterial folliculitis involves the hair follicles *(MCQ 281)*.

210. **Ans. c. It is candidiasis of soles. In such patients diabetes should be ruled out. Repeated washing of feet by psychotic patient can also be responsible.**
    ❖ Tinea pedis is of dry and hyperkeratotic type *(MCQ 51)*.
    ❖ Eczema of soles manifests as itching, oozing crusting with sparing of interdigital spaces *(MCQ 137)*.
    ❖ Pitted keratolysis manifests as circular lesions with punched out appearance *(MCQ 282)*.

211. **Ans. b. It is mid-borderline leprosy. More than three lesions, annular lesions and impairment of sensations are typical features of mid borderline leprosy.**
    ❖ Tuberculoid leprosy (high immunity) manifests as single lesion with loss of sensation *(MCQ 6)*.
    ❖ Indeterminate leprosy manifests as hypopigmented or erythematous macule. Characteristically, margins are not palpable.
    ❖ Lepromatous leprosy (poor immunity) is characterized by uncountable infiltrated lesions *(MCQ 155)*.

212. **Ans. e. It is seborrheic dermatitis. Patches with greasy scales on seborrheic sites are the features of SD.**
    ❖ PF also involves seborrheic sites. But lesions comprise of painful, extensive crusted lesions with surrounding erythema *(MCQ 300)*.
    ❖ Tinea lesions are larger and have active borders with central clearing *(MCQ 142)*.
    ❖ P. rosea comprises of discrete oval lesions covered by fine scales. Lesions are seen parallel to ribs forming a "Christmas tree" pattern *(MCQ 161)*.
    ❖ Pit. versicolor show discolored macules having dust like scales. At center, tend to become confluent. But, at periphery discrete satellite lesions are seen *(MCQ 39)*.

213. **Ans. b. It is eczema of both feet with all typical features.**
    ❖ Tinea pedis of dorsa of feet presents as erythematous plaques with well-defined advancing edge *(MCQ 32)*.
    ❖ Contact dermatitis due to shoes will take the shape of shoes *(MCQ 202)*.
    ❖ Psoriasis of feet shows well defined salmon pink plaques with silvery white scales. Plaques prefer the medial side of foot *(MCQ 292)*.

214. **Ans. b. It is a typical presentation of secondary syphilis as asymptomatic and bilateral symmetrical lesions. Similar lesions on trunk** *(MCQ 293)* **and lower extremities support the diagnosis. VDRL, HIV, HCV and HbsAg must be done in all STD patients.**
    ❖ LP of palm will have itching and violaceous color *(MCQ 231)*. VDRL will be negative.
    ❖ EM lesions usually have pain. Target lesions with central vesicle are typical *(MCQ 83)*. Vesicle is not a feature of secondary syphilis.
    ❖ Psoriasis of palm shows prominent erythema with scaling *(MCQ 233)*.

215. **Ans. c. Gum hypertrophy is typically seen due to phenytoin. Patient additionally has acneiform lesions on trunk** *(MCQ 43)*.
    All the four drugs, i.e., Phenobarbitone, phenytoin, carbamazepine and lamotrigine are considered as high-risk drugs for their association with risk of toxic epidermal necrolysis *(MCQ 127)*.

216. **Ans. d. He is a typical case of acne vulgaris with comedones, papules and pustules.**
    ❖ Acne rosacea is seen middle aged females. It involves central part of face with absence of comedones *(MCQ 50)*.

- Acneiform eruption consists of monomorphic, small, red papules on trunk, arm and shoulders *(MCQ 43)*.
- Milia are 1-2 mm sized uniform dome-shaped white papules on cheeks and eye lids *(MCQ 48)*.

217. Ans. c. She is having typical features of hypothyroidism.
- LL presents with red infiltrated plaques on face. Ear lobes show characteristic infiltration *(MCQ 101)*. Other parts of body also show uncountable red papules and plaques.
- Nephrotic syndrome patient will not have lethargy, constipation. There will be increase in serum triglycerides and decrease in serum proteins.
- In hepatic cirrhosis liver enzymes will be raised.

218. Ans. b. It is pompholyx with typical eruption of deep-seated clear vesicles on the sides of fingers, palms and soles.
- Contact dermatitis manifests as eczema patches, not as vesicles *(MCQ 225)*.
- Id-eruption is an eruption of small vesicles on the sides of fingers in response to an intense inflammatory process elsewhere *(MCQ 180)*.
- Scabies never manifests as such profuse vesicles on the palms. It can present as vesicles in web spaces with secondary infection *(MCQ 62)*.

219. Ans. c. It is granuloma annulare that presents as asymptomatic complete or incomplete rings with no scaling or inflammation.
- Rings of tinea spreads centrifugally very fast with active borders *(MCQ 142)*.
- Intact sensation in the plaques rules out leprosy *(MCQ 211)*.
- Annular psoriasis will show silvery scaling with underlying redness. *(MCQ 294)*.

220. Ans. c. It is eczema hands with typical features, e.g., recurrence, oozing, itching and crusting.
- Tinea manuum is usually unilateral with well-defined advancing border *(MCQ 45)*.
- Psoriatic plaques will maintain red color and silvery scales *(MCQ 239)*.
- Infected scabies shows involvement prominently in the finger web spaces *(MCQ 62)*.

221. Ans. c. These are cherry angiomas (syn. senile angiomas, De Morgan spots). Most patients accept reassurance that no intervention is required.
- Pyogenic granuloma is a vascular nodule *(MCQ 114)* developed at the site of recent penetrating injury. Common sites are upper lip, cheek forehead, etc.
- Strawberry hemangioma appears in first month of life in majority of patients *(MCQ 187)*.
- Angiokeratomas are 1-4 mm sized bright red hyperkeratotic vascular lesions seen on vulva or scrotal skin *(MCQ 91)*.

222. Ans. b. It is eczema of breast with its typical features, e.g., itching, oozing, crusting, ill-defined margins and bilateral involvement.
- Young age of the patient does not favor Paget's disease. Mammary Paget's disease usually presents as unilateral, sharply marginated and crusted plaque, Nipple may or may not be retracted *(MCQ 103)*.
- Pyoderma usually does not have bilateral involvement and has short history.
- Psoriasis will have salmon pink color and silvery white scaling.

223. Ans. b. It is trichoepithelioma which is an uncommon benign tumor arising from hair germ cells. It is usually inherited as autosomal dominant trait. It can be treated by destructive therapies, e.g., cryotherapy, electrodesiccation, etc.
- Syringoma presents as 1-3 mm sized papules seen around cheeks and eyelids in an adult woman. There is a no family history *(MCQ 236)*.
- Acne vulgaris comprises of papules, pustules and comedones on cheeks. *(MCQ 216)*.
- Milia are seen as 1-2 mm sized uniform dome-shaped papules seen on cheeks and eye lids *(MCQ 48)*.

224. Ans. d. It is molluscum contagiosum. It is typically seen as pearly white dome-shaped papules with central umbilication on the face of children.
- Chickenpox manifests as small vesicles surrounded by irregular area of erythema *(MCQ 12)*.
- Milia are 1-3 mm sized papules with no umbilication seen on cheeks and eye lids *(MCQ 48)*.
- Acne vulgaris is seen in older age groups as papules, pustules and comedones *(MCQ 216)*.

225. Ans. e. It is ACD due to potassium dichromate which is one of the ingredients of cement. ACD is a delayed type of hypersensitivity that does not develop on first exposure of allergen.

- ❖ Irritant contact dermatitis develops on single exposure of strong irritant *(MCQ 305)*.
- ❖ Discoid eczema is an endogenous eczema that comprises of coin-shaped lesions *(MCQ 194)*.
- ❖ Pompholyx is also an endogenous eczema that manifests as deep-seated vesicles on palms and soles *(MCQ 218)*.

226. **Ans. d. It is a Bowen's disease that typically presents as single, red, scaly and persistent lesion in an elderly patient not responding to topical steroid creams. It is a premalignant condition.**
   - ❖ Psoriatic lesions are usually multiple and responds to topical steroids *(MCQ 243)*.
   - ❖ SSM does not exhibit scaling and fulfils the features of the acronym ABCDE *(MCQ 121)*.
   - ❖ BCC is commonly seen on head and neck. In untreated patient ulceration is common that shows rolled border *(MCQ 193)*.

227. **Ans. c. It is neurofibromatosis type 1 for which presence of >6 cafe-au-lait spots is one of the important diagnostic criteria.**
   - ❖ SSM is usually single lesion seen in an elderly person as an irregularly shaped macule *(MCQ 121)*.
   - ❖ TSC is a multisystem disorder which usually presents as a diagnostic triad epiloa, i.e., epilepsy, low intelligence and adenoma sebaceum *(MCQ 306)*.
   - ❖ Mongolian spots are bluish black colored-patches of hyperpigmentation seen in lumbosacral region of newborn *(MCQ 151)*.

228. **Ans. d. It is dermatosis papulosa nigra which is a variant of seborrheic keratosis *(MCQ 117)*.**
   - ❖ Milia are small epidermal keratin cysts that present as yellowish 1-2 mm sized papules *(MCQ 48)*.
   - ❖ Senile comedones are seen as open or closed comedones in elderly people in periorbital or malar areas *(MCQ 28)*.
   - ❖ Plane warts on face are skin colored, plain topped multiple lesions *(MCQ 1)*.
   - ❖ Skin tags are 2-5 mm sized soft and inelastic papules commonly seen in obese persons *(MCQ 105)*.

229. **Ans. c. It is guttate psoriasis presenting as rain drop pattern of lesions. It frequently follows Streptococcal infection. It shows a good prognosis.**
   - ❖ Secondary syphilis presents as asymptomatic maculopapular eruption *(MCQ 293)*.
   - ❖ Pityriasis rosea presents as oval-shaped macules on back and front with fine scaling. Macules are present parallel to the ribs forming "Christmas-tree" pattern *(MCQ 161)*.
   - ❖ Discoid eczema constitutes coin-shaped non-scaly lesions *(MCQ 194)*.

230. **Ans. a. It is a non-homogeneous type of OL. There are 30% chances of malignant transformation. Biopsy is mandatory for him.**
   - ❖ Oral LP shows a characteristic lacy network of white streaks with a violaceous hue *(MCQ 41)*.
   - ❖ Oral thrush manifests as creamy white milk curd like patches that can be wiped off with a gauge, leaving area of erythema.
   - ❖ Smoker's keratosis manifests as diffuse whiteness over the palate.

231. **Ans. c. Violaceous color and pruritic papules are typical features of lichen planus.**
   - ❖ CCLE presents as discrete plaques with peripheral hyperpigmentation and central scarring *(MCQ 242)*.
   - ❖ Psoriatic lesions maintain the red color with white scaling *(MCQ 233)*.
   - ❖ Tinea manuum usually shows asymmetrical diffuse hyperkeratosis *(MCQ 45)*.

232. **Ans. d. It is Fox-Fordyce disease which is thought to be due to obstruction of distal part of apocrine sweat ducts as seen in miliaria rubra. It is mainly seen in women. It is not seen before puberty.**
   - ❖ In intertrigo, we do not see papular eruption *(MCQ 166)*.
   - ❖ Chromhidrosis refers to the colored sweat from apocrine glands.
   - ❖ Bromhidrosis is defined as abnormal body odor in axillae due to increased sweating.

233. **Ans. c. It is psoriasis of palms that has maintained its red color and scaling. There are also normal areas of skin in between.**
   - ❖ Tinea manuum usually shows unilateral involvement *(MCQ 45)*.
   - ❖ CCLE of palm will also manifests with red scaly plaques but it has hyperpigmentation at periphery and central scarring *(MCQ 242)*.
   - ❖ Eczema of palms manifests with vesicles, oozing and crusting *(MCQ 250)*.

234. **Ans. c. It is neurofibromatosis type 1. Presence of more than 2 cutaneous neurofibromas and >6 cafe-au-lait spots meet the criteria for the diagnosis of neurofibromatosis type 1.**

- Common warts have rough keratotic surface and are common on hands *(MCQ 169)*.
- Skin tags are seen around the neck in obese individuals *(MCQ 105)*.
- Mongolian spots are bluish black-colored patches seen in lumbosacral region of newborn *(MCQ 151)*. They usually disappear in early childhood.

235. **Ans. b. It is a boil on upper lip. It presents as acute, tender deep seated inflammatory nodule in the hair bearing area of skin.**
    - Pyogenic granuloma presents as vascular nodule at the site of penetrating injury *(MCQ 114)*.
    - Angular cheilitis is type of oral candidiasis. It manifests as redness, fissuring and soreness at angles of mouth *(MCQ 416)*.
    - Herpes simplex labialis is a recurrent HSV infection *(MCQ 9)*. It may precipitate erythema multiforme.

236. **Ans. d. It is syringoma which is a benign tumor showing differentiation towards eccrine sweat glands with characteristic histology. Histology shows tail-like strands of cells on one side that gives a shape of tadpole or comma.**
    - MC presents as discrete, pearly white, dome-shaped and umbilicated papules *(MCQ 224)*.
    - Milia are seen as 1–2 mm sized, uniform, dome-shaped, white and non umbilicated papules on cheeks and eye lids *(MCQ 48)*.
    - Trichoepithelioma presents as 5-8 mm sized skin-colored papules around nose, upper lip and cheek with positive family history *(MCQ 223)*.

237. **Ans. b. It is moist or rural type old world leishmaniasis. Diffuse dermal infiltrate and identification of amastigotes (LD bodies) within the cytoplasm of dermal macrophages is a hallmark of leishmaniasis.**
    - In TVC, there is a granulomatous infiltration consisting of giant cells *(MCQ 10)*.
    - BCC is characterized by presence of palisading arrangement of tumor cells which consist of large dark staining nuclei with scanty cytoplasm *(MCQ 193)*.
    - Sarcoidosis will show noncaseating granulomas.

238. **Ans. a. It is drug-induced morbilliform rash which is a most common type (95%) of drug eruption. In contrast to viral exanthematous eruption, it is not associated with constitutional symptoms or mucosal involvement. It is associated with lymphocytosis.**
    - Erythema multiforme (EM) is characterized by target lesions *(MCQ 83)*.
    - Drug-induced exfoliative dermatitis comprises of redness, scaling and itching *(MCQ 249)*.
    - Drug-induced urticaria will manifests as wheals similar to ordinary urticaria *(MCQ 206)*.

239. **Ans. c. Salmon pink color with silvery white scales and extensor surfaces are typical features of psoriasis.**
    - LP lesions are violaceous papules with little scaling *(MCQ 21)*.
    - Granuloma annulare comprises of complete or incomplete rings formed by small skin colored or violaceous papules *(MCQ 219)*.
    - In LL, lesions are uncountable that are red non scaly papules and plaques *(MCQ 155)*.
    - Lupus vulgaris manifests as reddish-brown and soft gelatinous plaques *(MCQ 256)*.

240. **Ans. b. She is having freckles which are largely genetically determined. They result due to overproduction of melanin in response to stimulation by UV light. They are seen in childhood and fade with age.**
    - Lentigines are 3–10 mm sized that are seen in middle age and are stable.
    - CALMs are 0.5–20 cm sized light brown macules that appear in early childhood *(MCQ 227)*.
    - Nevus of Ota manifests as pigmentation in the distribution of first two division of trigeminal nerve with accompanying pigmentation of sclera also *(MCQ 158)*.

241. **Ans. c. It is tinea faciei with typical inflamed and well-defined border.**
    - Pityriasis versicolor is characterized by discolored or hypopigmented skin lesions studded with dust like scales *(MCQ 39)*. Face is not a common site for pityriasis versicolor.
    - PLE comprises of eruption of papules, vesicles and redness within few hours of sunlight exposure *(MCQ 198)*.

242. **Ans. b. It is chronic cutaneous lupus erythematosus (CCLE) of palms. Lesions are showing adherent scales, hyperpigmentation at the periphery and central scarring.**
    - Psoriasis of palms will maintain its red color and white scaling *(MCQ 233)*.
    - Tinea manuum usually shows unilateral involvement *(MCQ 45)*.
    - Eczema of palms manifests as vesicles, oozing and crusting *(MCQ 250)*.

243. **Ans. a. It is erythroderma due to psoriasis.** Erythema, itching, scaling and involvement of whole or nearly whole body qualify the term erythroderma. Red or Salmon pink color, silvery white scales and areas of normal skin in between favor the underlying cause as psoriasis.
    - In seborrheic dermatitis, there are no skip areas and scales are greasy rather than white *(MCQ 257)*.
    - DHS comprises of exfoliative rash, fever, lymphadenopathy, eosinophilia and internal organ involvement *(MCQ 249)*.
    - Patch stage of MF presents as multiple red or violet red patches of variable sizes that favors non exposed parts of body *(MCQ 254)*.

244. **Ans. c. It is intradermal melanocytic nevus that may also show overlying telangiectatic vessels and one or two coarse terminal hairs.**
    - Cellular nevus (mole) is a broad term that includes three most common types of acquired melanocytic nevi, i.e., junctional, compound, intradermal.
    - Compound nevus is usually dark, round or oval and raised on epidermal surface *(MCQ 120)*.
    - Junctional nevi are often seen on palms and soles as brown macules up to 10 cm in size that tends to be uniform and regular.

245. **Ans. c. It is flexural psoriasis.** Salmon pink color, well-defined margins and white scaling are typical features of psoriasis. Groins *(MCQ 84)*, axillae, sub mammary region, umbilicus are common sites for flexural psoriasis.
    - Flexural candidiasis presents as red maceration in body folds and shows fringed irregular margins with classical satellite vesicles and pustules at the periphery *(MCQ 253)*.
    - SD manifests as greasy scales, ill-defined margins, involvement of other site of seborrheic distribution *(MCQ 175)*.
    - Tinea corporis will have well-defined active borders with central clearing *(MCQ 142)*.

246. **Ans. a. It is focal vitiligo that refers to the presence of single or few macules in a limited area of body.**
    - Segmental vitiligo is limited to a dermatome. Mandibular region is a common site *(MCQ 181)*.
    - N. depigmentosus is a congenital nonprogressive disorder that presents as single circumscribed area of depigmentation with feathered margins and do not cross the midline *(MCQ 252)*.
    - N. anemicus presents at birth or in infancy as blanchable circumscribed round or oval pale macule surrounded by satellite macules.

247. **Ans. a. These are Beau's lines.** It reflects temporary interference in nail formation due to some systemic disease, e.g., measles, mumps, etc.
    - Koilonychia refers to the concave shape of nail plate both in transverse and longitudinal axes. Most commonly, it is associated with iron deficiency anemia *(MCQ 124)*.
    - In onychogryphosis, nail plate becomes thickened, distorted, opaque, yellowish brown and gives an appearance of oyster shell.
    - In clubbing, there is a bulbous hypertrophy of terminal phalanx *(MCQ 133)*.

248. **Ans. c. It is fixed drug eruptions in which eruption characteristically recurs at the same site on subsequent administration of drug.**
    - EM manifest with characteristic target lesion *(MCQ 83)*.
    - Pemphigus manifests with involvement of oral mucosa and vesicles on various parts of body *(MCQ 184)*.
    - Exanthematous eruption consists of maculopapular rash on trunk and extremities *(MCQ 238)*.

249. **Ans. d. It is drug hypersensitivity syndrome (DHS)** which comprises of triad of fever, skin rash and internal organ involvement. It is also known as drug rash with eosinophilia (>1,500/mm^3) and systemic symptoms (DRESS). It is a serious condition and is usually managed with oral corticosteroid therapy.
    - Morbilliform rash comprises of 2–10 mm sized red macules which may get confluent at places *(MCQ 238)*. It is not associated with fever, lymphadenopathy or internal organ involvement.
    - Pemphigus foliaceous comprises of transient flaccid blisters and crusting at seborrheic sites *(MCQ 300)*.
    - Drug-induced ichthyosis is seen as dry fish like in later part of life *(MCQ 90)*, not since birth.

250. **Ans. d. It is eczema of palms characterized by itching, vesicles and crusting.**
    - Psoriasis presents as red plaque with white scaling *(MCQ 233)*.
    - Tinea manuum manifests as asymmetric diffuse hyperkeratosis *(MCQ 45)*.
    - LP of palm presents as discrete papules with violaceous hue *(MCQ 231)*.

251. **Ans. b.** Leukoplakia refers to a white lesion of oral mucosa that cannot be rubbed off or attributed to any known cause, e.g., tobacco, candidiasis, dermatological disorder, etc. It is a non-homogeneous type of oral leukoplakia at ventrolateral aspect of tongue that is one of the high-risk sites. Soft palate and floor of the mouth are other high-risk sites. Biopsy must be done to see for any dysplasia.
    - Oral LP shows a characteristic lacy network of white streaks with a violaceous hue *(MCQ 41)*.
    - Hairy leukoplakia is also seen on lateral side of tongue as vertical white ridges giving a hairy appearance. It is seen in AIDS patients.
    - Smoker's keratosis manifests as diffuse whiteness over palate.

252. **Ans. d.** It is nevus depigmentosus which is a congenital non-progressive depigmentary disorder. Its margins are feathered and do not cross the midline.
    - Nevus anemicus also presents at birth but as a blanchable circumscribed round or pale macule surrounded by satellite macules.
    - Focal vitiligo refers to a single or few macules in a limited area of body and appears later in life *(MCQ 246)*.
    - Segmental vitiligo is limited to a dermatome. Mandibular region is a common site *(MCQ 181)*.

253. **Ans. a.** It is flexural candidiasis under breast. Groins is another common site *(MCQ 179)*.
    - SD will manifest with greasy scales with involvement of other sites of seborrheic distribution also *(MCQ 175)*.
    - Tinea corporis will have well-defined active borders with central clearing *(MCQ 142)*.
    - Flexural psoriasis in sub mammary folds will have salmon pink color, well-defined margins and white scaling *(MCQ 245)*.

254. **Ans. b.** It is a patch stage mycosis fungoides (MF). MF is rare disease and is one of the types of cutaneous T-cell lymphomas. These patches favor the non-sun exposed parts of body.
    - Psoriasis plaques have silvery white scaling and favor extensors *(MCQ 146)*.
    - Drug-induced morbilliform rash comprises of macules and maculopapular rash on trunk and extremities *(MCQ 238)*.
    - Urticarial vasculitis lesions are *(MCQ 129)* tender or painful, lasts for few days and are associated with systemic features, e.g., fever, arthropathy, lymphadenopathy, etc.

255. **Ans. b.** It is squamous cell carcinoma (SCC) of lower lip. It is having highest rate of metastasis. About half of the patients already have metastasis at the time of diagnosis.
    - Basal cell carcinoma (BCC) usually presents as nonhealing ulcer with rolled border. It is particularly seen around eyes, nose or ear *(MCQ 193)*.
    - Malignant melanoma usually does not present with exophytic or cauliflower appearance. It usually has some black pigmentation *(MCQs 121, 126)*.
    - Orificial tuberculosis is seen in patients of advanced internal tuberculosis. It presents as small red nodule which breakdown to form typical tubercular ulcer.

256. **Ans. c.** It is lupus vulgaris manifesting with multiple lesions. Limited involvement to one extremity is an important clue that indicates an infected disorder. Apply jelly nodules are typically seen in lupus vulgaris. This type of skin tuberculosis is characterized by psoriasiform lesions *(MCQ 26)*.
    - Psoriasis, hyperkeratotic eczema and LP usually do not limit their involvement to one part of body.
    - LPH is characterized by purplish papulonodular lesions that are usually seen on shins and ankle joint *(MCQ 20)*.
    - Multiple lesions in Hansen's disease will also be seen on other areas of body. When limited to one part, then it will have impaired sensation *(MCQ 211)*.

257. **Ans. b.** It is non-psoriatic erythroderma. It has a long list of etiological factors. It is to be treated by systemic and topical steroids. All possible investigations should be done to find out the cause.
    - Exanthematous eruption is a sudden eruption due to some drug. It comprises of maculopapular rash on trunk and extremities *(MCQ 238)*.
    - Psoriatic erythroderma will manifest with red color and white scaling. We may find areas of normal uninvolved skin in between *(MCQ 243)*. Patient may give past history of psoriatic lesions. It is treated by methotrexate.
    - Term exfoliative dermatitis is used for patients of erythroderma when exfoliation is more prominent than redness.

258. **Ans. a.** It is pincer nail dystrophy. Pinching of nail bed by the over curved nail plate resembles the shape of tool pincer. It may be inherited or acquired in later life due to some systemic disease.

- Pterygium is characteristically seen in LP *(MCQ 31)*.
- Subungual hyperkeratosis refers to accumulation of keratinous material under nail plate *(MCQ 88)*. It is seen typically in psoriasis.
- In onychogryphosis, nail plate gets thickened, distorted, opaque, yellowish brown and gives an appearance of oyster shell.

259. Ans. b. It is toxemic rash of pregnancy (syn. pruritic urticarical papules and plaques of pregnancy, i.e., PUPPP and late onset prurigo). It does not pose risk to fetus and recovers after delivery.
- Prurigo of pregnancy is characterized by excoriated papules on extensor surfaces of extremities in 2nd trimester of pregnancy *(MCQ 135)*
- Impetigo herpetiformis is generalized pustular psoriasis during pregnancy that is characterized by high grade fever and severe prostration. It is a serious condition *(MCQ 260)*.
- Pemphigoid gestationis is least common vesiculobullous eruption seen in majority of patients during 2nd or 3rd trimester of pregnancy *(MCQ 275)*.
- Prurigo gravidarum (syn. cholestasis of pregnancy, pruritus gravidarum) is typically seen during 3rd trimester. It causes severe pruritus which is generalized or localized to palms and soles. It poses fetal risks.
- Chickenpox will present as vesicles surrounded by irregular area of erythema giving a dew drop on rose petal appearance *(MCQ 274)*.

260. Ans. b. She has developed generalized pustular psoriasis (GPP). It is an emergency. High dose of acitretin (1 mg/kg/day) is the treatment of choice and will control it rapidly. Ciclosporin and methotrexate are also effective drugs.
- Psoriasis with secondary infection will not produce high-grade fever or severe prostration.
- Psoriatic erythroderma is characterized by red plaques and silvery scaling *(MCQ 243)*.
- Acropustulosis is a type of localized pustular psoriasis which involves tips of fingers and toes *(MCQ 376)*.

261. Ans. c. This is a typical case of DH that responds dramatically to dapsone without any systemic steroid.
- In PF, itching is not a prominent feature. There is diffuse involvement on chest, upper back *(MCQ 300)* and lesions do not have the tendency of grouping.
- PV is characterized by flaccid bullae and painful erosions that are often large, bleed easily and have tendency to spread peripherally. Oral mucosa is involved in 70% of patients *(MCQ 184)*.
- In SD, interscapular region is a site of predilection that will have greasy scales *(MCQ 212)*.

262. Ans. a. It is bullous impetigo in which split of epidermis is just below the *S. granulosum*, so bullae are flaccid. It is caused by *S. aureus*, so fluid is turbid that form dark crusts. Pathology is not generalized. So, Nikolsky sign is negative.
- In BP, bullae are subepidermal. So, they are tense, dome-shaped and last longer. Contents are not turbid *(MCQ 285)*.
- PV is characterized by flaccid bullae, large painful erosions that have tendency to spread peripherally. Oral mucosa is involved in 70% of patients *(MCQ 184)*.
- Ecthyma is characterized by thick adherent crusts that can be removed with difficulty *(MCQ 299)*.

263. Ans. b. He is having circumscribed neurodermatitis in cervical region. Long-standing severe itching has led to lichenification. Other common sites are vulva *(MCQ 197)*, scrotum *(MCQ 97)*, extremities and scalp.
- Benign acquired AN is seen in obese patients in cervical region *(MCQ 273)*, axillae, groins and natal cleft. These patients do not have itching.
- CAD spares the area not exposed to sun, e.g., retroauricular area, depth of skin creases *(MCQ 298)*. In addition, CAD will involve the face also which is not involved in this patient.
- ABCD will involve the area exposed to air allergens, e.g., face *(MCQ 86)* cervical region and extremities.

264. Ans. b. It is a typical presentation of VVC in a diabetic female. Similar presentation is also seen in males *(MCQ 38)*.
- LSC of vulva presents as thickening, pigmentation and increased skin markings of vulval skin *(MCQ 197)*.
- Lichen sclerosus comprises of white demarcated plaque with waxy or crinkled texture with purpura and erosions.
- Vagina is resistant to gonococci. Sites of gonococcal infection are cervix and urethra. Vaginal discharge is not appreciable unless there is severe cervicitis or associated trichomonas infection.

265. **Ans. c. It is plantar psoriasis.**
    - Tinea pedis does not present as thick plaques, but as superficial hyperkeratosis with white scales *(MCQ 51)*.
    - Plantar keratoderma presents as yellowish thickening with no scales *(MCQ 192)*.
    - Eczema of soles presents as itching, oozing, crusting and fissuring *(MCQ 137)*.

266. **Ans. c. This child is having CBDC which is also called as linear IgA dermatosis of childhood. It responds dramatically to dapsone without any systemic steroid.**
    - P. vulgaris is characterized by mucosal involvement, flaccid blisters and painful cutaneous erosions *(MCQ 184)*.
    - BP comprises of tense dome-shaped blisters (with no clustering) in an elderly patient with no mucosal involvement *(MCQ 285)*.
    - DH comprises of extremely itchy wheals or small vesicles (seldom found intact) on shoulders *(MCQ 261)*, extensors, buttocks and natal cleft.

267. **Ans. b. This man is having Darier's disease which is an autosomal dominant condition having characteristic histopathology** *(MCQ 785)*.
    - Seborrheic dermatitis involves mainly seborrheic sites and comprises of fine greasy scales *(MCQ 175)*.
    - Ichthyosis vulgaris comprises of white fish likes scales *(MCQ 188)*.
    - Pseudoacanthosis nigricans comprises of darkening, thickening of skin of cervical region axillae and groins, giving a velvety appearance. It is seen in obese individuals *(MCQ 273)*.

268. **Ans. b. This man is having psoriasis. Involvement of face is uncommon in psoriasis, but red plaques with silvery white scaling and involvement of extensors are typical features of psoriasis.**
    - In SD scales are greasy that are seen in nasolabial folds and eyelashes *(MCQ 171)*.
    - CCLE lesions show predilection for sun exposed area on face *(MCQ 201)* and scales are adherent in CCLE.
    - When tinea involves whole face, patient will complain of erythema burning and scaling. Careful examination will always be able to detect a well-defined active border *(MCQ 241)*.
    - In topical steroid damaged face, patient will present as burning, redness, papules and pustules with no well-defined border *(MCQ 5)*.

269. **Ans. c. It is alopecia universalis which is a variant of alopecia areata. In addition to scalp, hairs of all other body parts are also lost. They respond to systemic steroids.**
    - Ophiasis is also a variant of alopecia areata *(MCQ 297)*. This term is used when there is hair loss at the periphery of the scalp.
    - In anagen effluvium also, there is hair loss at all body sites. Hairs are broken off due to anticancer chemotherapy *(MCQ 203)*.
    - Telogen effluvium refers to sudden and diffuse loss of scalp hair 3–4 months after an inciting event *(MCQ 163)*, e.g., after typhoid fever, major surgery, abortion, etc.

270. **Ans. b. It is lichen sclerosus et atrophicus which is a connective tissue disease. The term "white spot disease" is also used for lesions on trunk and limbs.**
    - Vitiligo is an idiopathic hypomelanotic disorder due to the absence of melanocytes in vitiligo macules *(MCQ 181)*.
    - Lichen planus presents as violaceous pruritic papules on peripheral parts of body *(MCQ 21)*.
    - Morphea appears as faintly purplish circumscribed indurated area on skin *(MCQ 69)*.

271. **Ans. d. All are true.**
    Pruritic papular lesions on genitals and in finger webs are commonest scabietic lesions. But they are not pathognomonic. The burrows are pathognomonic of scabies.

272. **Ans. b. It is mycetoma foot which is a type of deep fungal infection. It is characterized by chronic painless and firm swelling of trauma vulnerable part of body, e.g., foot, hand and gluteal region (rare). Swelling is studded with sinuses with discharge of colored granules.**
    - Tinea pedis is a superficial fungal infection characterized by scaling *(MCQ 32, 51)*.
    - Scrofuloderma is endogenous tuberculosis that results from underlying tuberculous focus. It is characterized by ulcer having thin bluish margins with watery discharge *(MCQ 53, 52)*.
    - Osteomyelitis comprises of sinuses adherent to underlying bone with no swelling of the part.

273. **Ans. b. It is pseudoacanthosis nigricans seen as a result of obesity. Insulin resistance is commonly seen in these patients. This type of acanthosis nigricans is also common in females having PCOS** *(MCQ 315)*.
    - CAD is characterized by itching. CAD spares the area not exposed to sun, depth of skin creases and skin behind ear lobes *(MCQ 298)*.

- LSC is characterized by severe itching. It is also characterized by skin thickening which also involves skin creases that leads to increased skin markings *(MCQ 263)*. Involvement is irrespective of sun exposure.
- In malignancy associated AN, and pigmentation is not limited to the hyperkeratotic areas. Palms will show thickening. Nails become brittle and hairs may shed.

274. Ans. b. It is chickenpox during pregnancy with typical vesicular eruption on erythematous base. During 3rd trimester, it should be treated with antiviral therapy.
- In toxemic rash of pregnancy, involvement is diffuse and comprises of papules or vesicles which are surrounded by erythema. Spontaneous recovery is characteristic *(MCQ 259)*.
- Prurigo of pregnancy comprises of excoriated papules on extensor surfaces in 2nd trimester *(MCQ 135)*.
- In pemphigoid gestationis, tense vesicles are seen around umbilicus *(MCQ 275)*.
- Prurigo gravidarum comprises of severe pruritus which is generalized or localized to palms and soles with no primary skin lesions. Serum levels of bile acids, SGOT and SGPT should be checked.

275. Ans. d. It is pemphigoid gestationis. In majority of patients, it manifests in 2nd or 3rd trimester of pregnancy and poses risk to fetus. There is increased risk of recurrence in subsequent pregnancies.
- Bullous pemphigoid bullae are usually seen after 60 years *(MCQ 285)* that may contain hemorrhagic fluid.
- PV is characterized by flaccid bullae, painful erosions and mucosal involvement in 70% of patients *(MCQ 184)*.
- In bullous impetigo, split is below stratum granulosum. Bullae are thick walled flaccid with turbid contents. They rupture less rapidly and form dark yellow crusts *(MCQ 262)*.

276. Ans. b. It is neonatal occipital alopecia which is a non-scarring physiological self-limiting alopecia seen in occipital region of 2–5 months old babies. Area is not totally bald and boundaries are not well defined.
- Alopecia areata comprises of totally bald, smooth and well-defined patches *(MCQ 156)*.
- Ophiasis is a variant of alopecia areata and refers to loss of hairs in periphery of scalp *(MCQ 297)*.
- Pseudopelade of Brocq is an uncommon idiopathic, chronic, asymptomatic, non-inflammatory, slowly progressive and patchy cicatricial alopecia. It is more common in females after the age of 40 years with female: male ratio 3:1 *(MCQ 284)*.

277. Ans. b. Dermatographism is seen in 5% of the normal individuals. This response is called as triple response of Lewis. When it is accompanied by itching, it is called as symptomatic dermatographism.
- Black dermatographism refers to black discoloration on stroking with soft metals.
- White dermatographism is seen in atopic patients. It is due to capillary vasoconstriction on light stroking.
- Darier's sign is seen in mastocytosis. It is elicited by stroking of reddish-brown cutaneous lesions of mastocytosis.

278. Ans. c. It is a typical sebaceous cyst having punctum. Punctum represents the pilosebaceous unit.
- Patient with acne cyst will have papules, pustules and comedones also *(MCQ 19)*.
- A dermoid cyst is present at birth. It contains structures such as hair, fluid, teeth, etc. It grows slowly and is not tender unless ruptured. They usually occur on the face, in the skull, lower back, inside ovaries, etc.
- Boil is an acute painful deep-seated inflammatory nodule around a hair follicle *(MCQ 147)*.

279. Ans. b. It is erythema ab igne. It is due to repeated or prolonged exposure to infrared radiation, e.g., sitting close to the fire, use of hot water bottles, heated pads for chronic backache, etc.
- Senile purpura presents as geometric-shaped dark purplish patches on forearm and dorsa of hands *(MCQ 148)*.
- Asteatotic eczema (senile eczema) is seen in elderly persons as dry scaly skin with prominent and deep skin markings *(MCQ 94)*.
- Ichthyosis refers to dry, rough skin having diffuse and uniform fish like scales. It involves almost whole skin *(MCQ 188)*.

280. Ans. b. It is smegma which is an accumulation of sebum combined with desquamated dead cells. It is benign and should be washed off twice a week.
- Venereal warts (condylomata acuminata) present as soft pink filiform or digitate lesions *(MCQ 283)*.
- Candidal balanoposthitis presents as superficial erosions and collarette of white scales *(MCQ 38)*.

- Verrucous carcinoma presents as slow growing exophytic tumor with cauliflower like appearance in older patient *(MCQ 289)*.

281. **Ans. d. It is superficial folliculitis which is a follicular infection confined to the follicular osteum.**
    - Pseudofolliculitis results from penetration of sharp tips of shaved hair to the neighboring skin. It is seen in males having curly hairs *(MCQ 291)*.
    - CSF comprises of profuse eruption of follicular pustules on legs. It is chronic and recalcitrant to treat *(MCQ 286)*.
    - Boils are deep-seated painful inflammatory nodules *(MCQ 147)*.

282. **Ans. d. It is pitted keratolysis which is caused by digestion of keratin by keratinophilic *Corynebacterium*.**
    - Candidiasis manifests as redness, maceration and soreness *(MCQ 210)*.
    - Tinea pedis manifest as dryness and hyperkeratosis *(MCQ 51)*.
    - Eczema manifests as oozing, crusting *(MCQ 137)*.

283. **Ans. b. It is condylomata acuminata which is also called as genital warts. It is STD and fresh warts can be treated with podophyllin.**
    - Smegma is a benign deposit with cheese like appearance with off white color *(MCQ 280)*.
    - Condylomata lata is a manifestation of secondary syphilis. It manifests as soft, sessile, flat-topped papules. Anal region and groins *(MCQ 287)* are common sites.
    - Pearly penile papules is a physiological condition which is seen as 1–3 mm sized, flesh colored, smooth and round papules in a row or rings around coronal margin *(MCQ 290)*.

284. **Ans. d. It is pseudopelade of Brocq. It is an uncommon idiopathic, chronic, asymptomatic, non-inflammatory, slowly progressive and patchy cicatricial alopecia. It is more common in females after the age of 40 years with female: male ratio 3:1.**
    - Trichotillomania is characterized by presence of firmly anchored partially broken hairs in the bald area *(MCQ 167)*.
    - Alopecia areata is a non-scaring and reversible hair loss that comprises of smooth bald patches. Skin looks normal with no scarring, atrophy or inflammation *(MCQ 156)*.
    - Folliculitis decalvans is characterized by redness and swelling and pustules around the hair follicle (folliculitis) that leads to destruction of the follicle and consequent permanent hair loss.

285. **Ans. a. It is bullous pemphigoid which is seen at older age. Being subepidermal, bullous pemphigoid bullae are tense. Mucosa is less frequently involved in BP.**
    - In PV, vesicles are due to suprabasal cleft. So, vesicles are flaccid and rupture easily and mucosa is involved in 70% of patients *(MCQ 184)*.
    - In PF, vesicles are subcorneal, transient and may not be obvious. Oral lesions are usually not found *(MCQ 300)*.
    - In EM target lesions are found *(MCQ 83)*.
    - DH presents as pruritic small vesicles having tendency of grouping. Common sites are buttocks, natal cleft and shoulders *(MCQ 261)*.

286. **Ans. d. It is chronic superficial folliculitis in which involvement is limited to osteum. It is often chronic and recalcitrant to treat.**
    - Pseudofolliculitis comprises of papules and pustules on shaved skin due to penetration of sharp tips of shaved hairs to the neighboring skin *(MCQ 291)*.
    - Boil present as deep-seated inflammatory nodule around hair follicle *(MCQ 147)*.
    - Impetigo contagiosa comprises of dried, thick, dirty brown (honey colored) crusts *(MCQ 147)*.

287. **Ans. b. It is condylomata lata in the groin which is a manifestation of secondary syphilis and is highly infectious. It is more common in anogenital region.**
    - Condylomata acuminata (genital warts) is characterized by filiform or digitate lesions. It is more common on glans *(MCQ 283)* and anal region.
    - Intertrigo shows erythema and soreness limited to the opposing surfaces and has ill-defined margins *(MCQ 166)*.
    - T. cruris shows red plaques with well-defined margins extending to the adjacent part of thigh *(MCQ 4)*.

288. **Ans. c. It is linear IgA dermatosis in adult. Being subepidermal blistering, vesicles are tense. Vesicles typically tend to occur in clusters to form "collarette of blisters".**
    - *Paederus dermatitis* can cause blistering *(MCQ 386)*. It is neither widespread nor lasts for one month.
    - In PF, cleavage being superficial, blisters are flaccid that rupture easily and are not obvious *(MCQ 300)*.

❖ BP presents as tense, dome-shaped blisters in an elderly patient *(MCQ 285)*.

289. **Ans. c. It is verrucous SCC which has good prognosis. But, in the presence of involvement of inguinal l. nodes, prognosis is poor.**
    ❖ Condylomata acuminata (genital warts) shows filiform or digitate lesions. It is very common on glans *(MCQ 283)* and anal region.
    ❖ Smegma is cheese like physiological subpreputial deposit *(MCQ 280)*.
    ❖ Lichen planus on glans manifests as violaceous plaques *(MCQ 15)* that are never hyperkeratotic.

290. **Ans. b. It is pearly penile papules which is a physiological condition. These are angiofibromas. Patient takes it as penile warts. Reassurance is usually sufficient to anxious patients.**
    ❖ Condylomata acuminata (genital warts) presents as asymmetrical filiform or digitate lesions not limited to coronal sulcus *(MCQ 283)*.
    ❖ Condylomata lata (secondary syphilis) presents as soft, flat topped, sessile papules in anal region or groins *(MCQ 287)*.
    ❖ Lichen planus shows violaceous papules *(MCQ 15)*.

291. **Ans. b. It is pseudofolliculitis barbae which is due to mechanical reason. It is seen in males who have curly hairs. Penetration of sharp tips of shaved hairs to the neighboring skin is responsible for this disorder.**
    ❖ In CSF, involvement is confined to follicular osteum. It is mainly seen on lower extremities as profuse tiny follicular pustules *(MCQ 286)*.
    ❖ Acne vulgaris manifest as comedones involving mainly face *(MCQ 216)*.
    ❖ Boils present as painful papules or nodules *(MCQ 147)*.

292. **Ans. a. It is psoriasis of foot showing red color, white scaling and well-defined margin. Typical psoriatic nail changes also support the diagnosis of psoriasis.**
    ❖ Eczema plaques are not red. They are oozy with crusting with no definite margins *(MCQ 213)*.
    ❖ LP on feet presents as hyperkeratotic, violaceous papules around ankle *(MCQ 130)*.
    ❖ LL also manifests with numerous lesions. But lesions do not have scaling, but are red, glistening and infiltrated lesions *(MCQ 155)*.

293. **Ans. b. He is a typical patient of secondary syphilis presenting with asymptomatic bilateral symmetrical papulosquamous (non-vesicular) lesions. Involvement of palms and soles is classic. VDRL, HIV, HCV and HbsAg must be done in all STD patients.**
    ❖ Guttate psoriasis is usually seen in children as small sized red papules with white scaling *(MCQ 229)*. VDRL will be negative.
    ❖ LP lesions usually are not profuse. They are violaceous *(MCQ 339)* and pruritic.
    ❖ P. rosea lesions are usually macules with fine scaling *(MCQ 161)*. Papules are not found. Palms and Soles are not involved in PR.

294. **Ans. c. He is having annular psoriasis which is a rare presentation of psoriasis showing central clearing in the plaques. But red color and silvery scaling are still present.**
    ❖ Rings of granuloma annulare are usually incomplete with no scaling, inflammation or itching *(MCQ 219)*.
    ❖ Intact sensation in the plaque rules out leprosy *(MCQ 211)*.
    ❖ Tinea circinata presents as circular, pruritic, sharply marginated lesions with raised edges *(MCQ 142)*.

295. **Ans. d. Fine superficial pits are typically seen in alopecia areata. It is supported by the presence of alopecia areata patches on the scalp.**
    ❖ In psoriasis, pits on nail plates are coarse *(MCQ 119)*. Other psoriatic nail changes are also not there, e.g., yellow discoloration, subungual hyperkeratosis, etc.
    ❖ Darier's disease manifests as red longitudinal streaks *(MCQ 178)* that terminates distally in V-shaped notch.
    ❖ In tinea unguium, nail plate becomes rough and thickened with subungual hyperkeratosis. Involvement is asymmetrical *(MCQ 22)*.

296. **Ans. c. This child is suffering from ordinary angioedema. If, it involves tongue and larynx, it can cause breathing difficulties. Itching is not a prominent feature because edema occurs in deeper areas where sensory endings are few.**
    ❖ Urticarial swelling of lips and eyelids will not last more than 1–2 days.
    ❖ Swelling in myxedema is not acute and is not so severe *(MCQ 217)* and involves the other parts of the body also. It is not accompanied by itching
    ❖ Hereditary angioedema is an autosomal dominant condition that does not have urticarial

lesions but is often accompanied by GIT and urinary symptoms.

297. **Ans. b. It is ophiasis which is an uncommon variant of alopecia areata. It is recalcitrant to treat.**
    - Trichotillomania is characterized by presence of firmly anchored partially broken hairs in the bald area *(MCQ 167)*.
    - Pseudopelade of Brocq comprises of irregular slightly depressed area of scarring alopecia on vertex *(MCQ 284)*.
    - Anagen effluvium refers to breakage of hairs within the follicle or at the level of scalp due to anticancer chemotherapy *(MCQ 203)*.

298. **Ans. c. It is chronic actinic dermatitis that predominantly affects photo-exposed sites. It occurs in response to irradiation without any contact of external allergen. In this patient, it characteristically spares the depth of skin creases. At other sites, it shows clear margins from covered areas** *(MCQ 196)*.
    - Benign acquired AN is seen in obese patients involving cervical region *(MCQ 273)*, axillae and groins. It does not have itching.
    - LSC shows diffuse margins, does not spare the depth of creases *(MCQ 263)*.
    - ABCD involves the exposed areas of body *(MCQ 86)*. It involves upper eyelids and area under the nose and chin, but spares the back of neck.

299. **Ans. b. It is ecthyma which is a deep pyogenic infection. It heals with scarring in few weeks.**
    - Infected discoid eczema will be larger disc or coin-shaped itchy lesions *(MCQ 194)*.
    - Tuberculous gumma is an endogenous skin tuberculosis that presents as ulcers having watery discharge and bluish margins *(MCQ 63)*.
    - Pyoderma gangrenosum presents as painful ulcer surrounded by zone of erythema *(MCQ 367)* and base is covered with pus. It is usually associated with underlying systemic disease.

300. **Ans. b. It is pemphigus foliaceous which is involving the seborrheic sites. Only crusted and scaly lesions with surrounding erythema are seen. Vesicles are thin walled and transient because acantholysis is subcorneal. Oral mucosa is usually not involved.**
    - In PV, cleft in suprabasal. So, vesicles stay longer and are usually seen as flaccid blisters. Oral lesions are seen in 70% of patients. *(MCQ 184)*
    - In BP vesicles and bullae are subepidermal, tense and dome-shaped *(MCQ 285)*.
    - In linear IgA dermatosis, lesions are subepidermal and are seen in clusters as "cluster of jewels" or "collarette of blisters" *(MCQ 288)*.

301. **Ans. b. He is having neurofibromatosis type 1. The presence of 2 or more of any neurofibromas is one of its diagnostic criteria.**
    - Bilateral vestibular schwannomas and meningeal or glial tumors are essential features of neurofibromatosis type 2.
    - TSC comprises of a triad (epiloia) of epilepsy, low intelligence and adenoma sebaceum *(MCQ 306)*.
    - Common warts have rough hyperkeratotic surface and are common on hands *(MCQ 169)*.

302. **Ans. a. He is having pseudoacanthosis nigricans. It is due to insulin resistance and these patients are prone to suffer from diabetes mellitus.**
    - Darier's disease comprises of multiple, firm gray colored papules on seborrheic areas of trunk and extremities *(MCQ 267)*.
    - PCOS is a disease of females. It comprises of menstrual irregularities, polycystic ovaries and hormonal changes.
    - Seborrheic dermatitis comprises of greasy scales at seborrheic sites *(MCQ 175)*.

303. **Ans. b. Androgen secreting tumor has caused these virilizing (formation of male secondary sex characteristics) features. Ultrasound and CT abdomen should be done to rule out adrenal tumor.**
    - PCOS does not have sudden onset. Clitoromegaly is not its feature. It comprises of menstrual irregularity, hormonal changes and increased size of ovaries
    - Cushing syndrome is due to systemic steroids and manifests as moon face *(MCQ 307)*.
    - During menopause, less estrogen may cause the vulva and vaginal mucosa to become thinner, drier, and less elastic or flexible.

304. **Ans. a. This child has developed Stevens-Johnson syndrome (SJS). The diagnosis is favored by partial coalescence of lesions, involving <10% of body surface and involvement of 2 mucosae.**
    - In EM major, one mucosa can be involved; involvement of skin is not also extensive *(MCQ 83)*.
    - In FDE, lesions are usually dusky red macules. Large number of skin lesions and conjunctival involvement are not features of FDE *(MCQ 248)*.
    - In TEN, area involvement is >30% *(MCQ 127)*.

Chapter 5 ✦ Answers of MCQs in Dermatology, Venereology and Leprology

305. **Ans. c.** It is acute irritant contact dermatitis (ICD) to the cream applied. ICD is a non-immunological inflammatory response to first exposure to strong irritant.
    ❖ ACD is a delayed type hypersensitivity that does not develop on first exposure to allergens *(MCQ 301)*.
    ❖ FDE appears few hours after oral administration of drug as red or dusky red macules *(MCQ 248)*.
    ❖ Pompholyx is an endogenous eczema that manifests as deep-seated vesicles on palms and soles *(MCQ 218)*.

306. **Ans. a.** It is tuberous sclerosis complex (TSC) which is an autosomal dominant inherited disease with multisystem involvement.
    ❖ Neurofibromatosis type 1 comprises cutaneous neurofibromas *(MCQ 301)*.
    ❖ Plane warts are slightly elevated, smooth and plane topped lesions *(MCQ 1)*.
    ❖ Acne presents as papules, pustules in adolescent age *(MCQ 216)*.

307. **Ans. b.** It is Cushing syndrome that occurs when body is exposed to high levels of the cortisol hormone for a long time. It is also called as hypercortisolism which is caused by the use of high dose of corticosteroid medication. Forehead is non androgen dependent area. Hair growth at this site is due to raised cortisol levels.
    ❖ Hair growth in PCOS is seen in androgen dependent area, i.e., beard region and these patients do not have moon-shaped face *(MCQ 315)*.
    ❖ Androgen secreting tumor presents with hirsutism, virilizing features, e.g., *(MCQ 321)* clitoromegaly, deepening of voice, male pattern baldness and menstrual irregularities. They do not have moon face.
    ❖ Hypothyroidism presents as thickening of lips puffing of face and eyelids *(MCQ 217)*.

308. **Ans. b.** It is Koebner phenomenon which is also called as isomorphic phenomenon. It is also seen in patients of lichen planus *(MCQ 346)* and warts *(MCQ 389)*.
    ❖ Rebound phenomenon refers to appearance of a greater number of lesions in an aggressive manner than the pretreatment state *(MCQ 316)*.
    ❖ Auspitz's sign refers to the appearance of pinpoint bleeding spots on scraping a cutaneous lesion. It can be demonstrated in psoriatic lesions *(MCQ 316)*.
    ❖ Grattage test refers to demonstration of easy removal of silvery white scales from psoriatic plaque with the edge of a glass slide *(MCQ 322)*.

309. **Ans. b.** It is tinea favosa which is an uncommon type of tinea capitis and is characterized by cup-shaped crusts. Crusts are composed of fungal elements. It may show cicatricial alopecia.
    ❖ Scalp psoriasis shows discrete plaques with white scales and with no hair loss *(MCQ 314)*.
    ❖ SLE scalp consists of broken off hairs and non-cicatricial hair loss *(MCQ 89)*.
    ❖ Pityriasis amiantacea consists of large and dry, micaceous scales which get separated from scalp but remain entangled in hair *(MCQ 87)*.

310. **Ans. d.** Distal interphalangeal joint is typically involved in psoriasis. Arthritis is seen in only less than 10% of psoriasis patients.
    ❖ Involvement of proximal interphalangeal (PIP) and metacarpophalangeal (MCP) joints is most frequent in rheumatoid arthritis *(MCQ 313)*.

311. **Ans. b.** He is having anhidrotic ectodermal dysplasia which is a rare X-linked recessive genetic disease. Hypotrichosis, hypodontia and partial or complete absence of sweat glands are its characteristic features.
    ❖ Hypothyroid patient will have puffiness on face. He will feel cool and will show loss of hair from outer 1/3 of eye brows. They will not have hypodontia *(MCQ 217)*.
    ❖ In androgenic alopecia, patient will not lose hair from eyebrows, eyelashes or beard region *(MCQ 415)*.
    ❖ Alopecia universalis patients will not have heat intolerance or hypodontia *(MCQ 269)*.

312. **Ans. c.** It is neurofibromatosis type 1. The presence of ≥6 cafe-au-lait spots is an important criterion for the diagnosis for this disorder.
    ❖ Mongolian spots are bluish-colored patches in lumbosacral region in a newborn *(MCQ 151)*.
    ❖ TVC comprises of epilepsy, low intelligence and adenoma sebaceum *(MCQ 306)*.
    ❖ One to five cafe-au-lait spots can be seen in 10% of normal population.

313. **Ans. a.** Ulnar deviation of fingers is a typical deformity of rheumatoid arthritis.
    ❖ In psoriasis, distal interphalangeal joint is typically involved *(MCQ 310)*.
    ❖ In osteoarthritis, weight bearing joints (knees, hips, lumbosacral) are predominantly involved.

314. **Ans. b.** It is scalp psoriasis with typical discrete plaques studded with silvery white scales.
    - Tinea capitis is characterized by hair loss *(MCQ 309)*.
    - Pityriasis amiantacea consists of large, dry, micaceous scales which get separated from scalp but remain entangled in hairs *(MCQ 87)*.
    - Seborrheic capitis is characterized by fine greasy scales *(MCQ 153)*.

315. **Ans. c.** She is having polycystic ovarian syndrome (PCOS) with typical presentation. She is having insulin resistance also as indicated by presence of obesity and acanthosis nigricans. Diagnosis is confirmed by hormonal changes and ovarian size >10 cc on ultrasonography.
    - Idiopathic hirsutism consists of normal menses, normal hormonal levels and normal sized ovaries *(MCQ 328)*.
    - Androgen secreting tumor is characterized by hirsutism and virilizing features *(MCQ 321)*.
    - Cushing syndrome consists of moon face, hirsutism on non-androgen dependent sites *(MCQ 307)*.

316. **Ans. d.** It is rebound phenomenon due to systemic steroids. So, systemic steroid should not be given to psoriatic patients. Topical steroids should also be avoided except at certain sites, e.g., scalp, axillae, etc.
    - Koebner phenomenon refers to development of pathologic lesions in traumatized uninvolved skin *(MCQ 308)*.
    - Isomorphic phenomenon is another name of Koebner phenomenon.
    - Auspitz's sign is an appearance of pinpoint bleeding spots on scrapping with a glass slide of a psoriatic lesion *(MCQ 329)*.

317. **Ans. c** It is periungual fibroma which is seen in the patient of tuberous sclerosis complex (TVC). These periungual fibromas are also called as Konen's tumors. TVC comprises a triad (epiloia) of epilepsy, low intelligence and adenoma sebaceum *(MCQ 306)*.
    - Periungual warts are rough and hyperkeratotic papules *(MCQ 325)*.
    - Skin tags are soft and pedunculated papules commonly seen on the sides of neck in obese individuals *(MCQ 105)*.
    - Cutaneous horns are hard reddish-brown horn like growths *(MCQ 345)*.

318. **Ans. c.** It is Darier's disease which is an autosomal dominant condition having characteristic histopathology.
    - In pseudoacanthosis nigricans, there is a darkening and thickening of cervical and axillary skin giving a velvety appearance *(MCQ 273)*.
    - S. dermatitis is characterized by fine greasy scales in seborrheic sites *(MCQ 175)*.
    - Ichthyosis vulgaris shows white fine fish like scales sparing diaper area *(MCQ 188)*.

319. **Ans. b.** She is having Down syndrome (mongolism) which is a congenital anomaly due to trisomy of chromosome 21. Its incidence increases with maternal age.
    - Isotretinoin can cause skeletal and cardiovascular abnormalities.
    - Thalidomide can cause phocomelia, if taken during 1st trimester.
    - Systemic steroids can cause cleft palate, harelip, cardiac septal defect if taken during the 2nd trimester.

320. **Ans. c.** It is balanitis xerotica obliterans (BXO) which is seen in lichen sclerosus et atrophicus. In later stage, it may result in to acquired phimosis.
    - Vitiligo will not cause soreness or phimotic changes *(MCQ 412)*.
    - Candidiasis will not cause white discoloration of prepuce *(MCQ 38)*.
    - Smegma comprises of deposition of off white and cheesy material under the foreskin *(MCQ 333)*.

321. **Ans. c.** She is having androgen secreting tumor. This patient has high testosterone levels which has caused virilizing features (male sex characters), i.e., hirsutism and clitoromegaly. Ultrasound and CT abdomen should be done to rule out adrenal tumor.
    - Idiopathic hirsutism is seen in young females having normal menses, normal hormonal level and normal size of ovaries *(MCQ 328)*.
    - PCOS comprises of menstrual irregularities, hormonal abnormalities and increased size (>10 cc) of ovaries *(MCQ 315)*.
    - Cushing syndrome is seen in patients who are on long term high dose of systemic steroids. These patients have moon face, hypertrichosis on non-androgen dependent sites, e.g., forehead *(MCQ 307)*.

Chapter 5 ✦ Answers of MCQs in Dermatology, Venereology and Leprology

322. **Ans. a. It is grattage test which is elicited on psoriatic cutaneous plaques.**
    - Koebner phenomenon refers to the development of pathological lesions in traumatized uninvolved skin *(MCQ 308)*.
    - Auspitz's sign is an extension of grattage test. On further scrapping, it demonstrates the appearance of pinpoint bleeding spots. This test has diagnostic value for psoriasis *(MCQ 329)*.
    - Rebound phenomenon refers to the appearance of new psoriatic lesions in uninvolved skin in an aggressive manner *(MCQ 316)*. It happens in patients of psoriasis during steroid therapy or after its withdrawal.

323. **Ans. a. This patient is having anhidrotic ectodermal dysplasia which is a rare X-linked genetic disease. It is characterized by hypodontia, hypotrichosis *(MCQ 311)* and partial or complete absence of sweat glands.**
    - Hypothyroidism never causes hypodontia.
    - Hutchinson's teeth are most common stigmata of congenital syphilis. Hypodontia is not a feature of congenital syphilis. Sides of incisors converge towards cutting edge and take the shape of a screw driver.

324. **Ans. b. This child is having ichthyosis vulgaris in which diaper area is characteristically spared. It is an autosomal dominant condition and is seen in both sexes.**
    - XLRI manifests in 1st week of life and comprises of dark colored scales and spares cubital *(MCQ 335)* and popliteal folds.
    - Acquired ichthyosis is seen in later life due to some internal cause or due to some drug *(MCQ 90)*.
    - Atopic dermatitis causes dryness and itching. It does not cause ichthyotic changes.

325. **Ans. b. It is periungual wart which is seen in children who habitually suck their fingers.**
    - Periungual fibroma is a manifestation of TVC seen as firm, reddish and smooth growth *(MCQ 317)*.
    - Cutaneous horn is a hard, reddish brown horn like growth *(MCQ 345)*.
    - A corn is a sharply circumscribed and usually a painful callosity over a bony prominence *(MCQ 350)* due to sustained friction or pressure.

326. **Ans. c. It is a perianal sinus which is a very common condition. It requires surgical excision.**
    - Boil is painful and does not have recurrent discharge. Duration will be small *(MCQ 147)*.
    - Skin tag will not have discharge and is pedunculated *(MCQ 331)*.
    - Sinuses in hidradenitis suppurativa are multiple and are accompanied by scarring *(MCQ 343)*.

327. **Ans. a. It is typical aphthous ulcer having yellowish pseudomembrane and erythematous margin. It is painful and recurrent.**
    - Behcet's disease in a rare multisystem disease characterized by oral and genital ulcers and iridocyclitis.
    - Mucous patches of secondary syphilis are shallow, round and painless lesions edged by dull red areola.
    - P. vulgaris ulcers are painful and are usually accompanied by hemorrhagic crusting of lips *(MCQ 344)*.

328. **Ans. b. She is having idiopathic hirsutism. It is seen in young females with/without family history.**
    - PCOS comprises of menstrual irregularities, hormonal abnormalities, increased size of ovaries, acanthosis nigricans and hirsutism *(MCQ 315)*.
    - Hypertrichosis refers to presence of localized or generalized excess of hair irrespective of androgen excess *(MCQ 334)*.
    - Steroid induced hirsutism will be accompanied by moon face, striae *(MCQ 307)*.

329. **Ans. b. It is Auspitz's sign which has a diagnostic value in making a clinical diagnosis of psoriasis.**
    - Grattage test refers to demonstration of easy removal of silvery white scales from a cutaneous lesion *(MCQ 322)*. It is seen in psoriasis.
    - Koebner phenomenon refers to development of pathologic lesions in traumatized uninvolved skin. It is seen in psoriasis *(MCQ 308)*, lichen planus *(MCQ 346)*, cutaneous warts *(MCQ 389)*.
    - Rebound phenomenon refers to appearance of a greater number of skin lesions in an aggressive manner than the pretreatment state. It is due to use of systemic steroids in patients of psoriasis *(MCQ 316)*.

330. **Ans. c. He is having Down syndrome (mongolism) which is a congenital anomaly due to trisomy of chromosome 21. Its incidence increases with maternal age.**
    - Systemic steroids can cause cleft palate, hare lip and cardiac septal defects if given during second trimester.

- Isotretinoin can cause skeletal and cardiovascular abnormalities.
- Thalidomide can cause phocomelia if taken during first trimester.

331. **Ans. d. It is a large skin tag. Commonly affected sites for skin tags are cervical region** *(MCQ 105),* **axillae and groins.**
    - Cutaneous horn is a horn like hard growth *(MCQ 345).*
    - Molluscum contagiosum papules are usually smaller, multiple dome-shaped, pearly white and umbilicated *(MCQ 209).*
    - Venereal warts are firm, hyperkeratotic and multiple *(MCQ 398).*

332. **Ans. b. It is Henoch-Schonlein purpura (HS purpura) which is mostly seen in children on legs and other dependent area in a symmetrical manner.**
    - CML can present as large ecchymotic patches due to platelet dysfunction *(MCQ 390).*
    - ITP usually causes petechiae (MCQ 342, 354). Majority of patients are children and adolescents.
    - Senile purpura is seen at old age as geometric-shaped dark purplish patches *(MCQ 148).*

333. **Ans. d. It is smegma which is composed of sebum and desquamated dead cells. It is completely benign and patient is advised to wash it at least twice a week.**
    - In LP, there are no deposits. LP comprises of violaceous papules *(MCQ 15).*
    - In BXO, patient will complain of whiteness of foreskin and difficulty in retraction of foreskin *(MCQ 320).*
    - In candidiasis, patient will complain of soreness, erythema and white scales. Blood sugar level is found to be high *(MCQ 38).*

334. **Ans. d. It is hypertrichosis which refers to the presence of localized or generalized excess of hair irrespective of androgen responsive areas. This is usually since birth or childhood. Underlying spina bifida should be ruled out.**
    - Idiopathic hirsutism refers to growth of facial hair without any detectable abnormality *(MCQ 328).*
    - Androgenic secreting tumor will present with sudden hirsutism and virilizing features (MCQs 303, 321).
    - Steroid induced hypertrichosis will be accompanied by moon face, striae and other side effects of systemic steroids *(MCQ 307).*

335. **Ans. a. This boy is having X-linked recessive ichthyosis (XLRI) that affects only males and does not improve with age.**
    - Ichthyosis vulgaris manifests between 3-12 months of age. Scales are white and spares diaper area *(MCQ 324).*
    - Acquired ichthyosis appears later in life. It can be due to some internal cause or due to some drug *(MCQ 90).*
    - Atopic dermatitis causes dryness and itching. It does not cause ichthyotic changes.

336. **Ans. c. It is drug-induced morbilliform (exanthematous) rash which is due to drug. It should be differentiated from that due to viral infection. Drug-induced rash is usually seen in adults, does not involve mucous membrane, has no constitutional symptoms and is associated with eosinophilia.**
    - Erythroderma (exfoliative dermatitis) comprises of redness and scaling *(MCQ 249).*
    - Urticaria comprises of itchy wheals which appear and disappear *(MCQ 206).*
    - EM comprises of target shaped lesions *(MCQ 83).*

337. **Ans. c. It is focal plantar keratoderma. Keratoderma comprises of abnormal thickening of palms and soles.**
    - T. pedis is characterized by hyperkeratosis and scaling *(MCQ 51).*
    - Plantar psoriasis plaques are red with scales *(MCQ 265).*
    - Eczema of soles is characterized by itching oozing, crusting and recurrence *(MCQ 150).*

338. **Ans. c. It is Becker's nevus (pigmented hairy epidermal nevus) which is usually first noticed during adolescence.**
    - Nevus of Ota is usually congenital and comprises of grayish hyperpigmentation on one side of face in the distribution of first two divisions of trigeminal nerve *(MCQ 158).*
    - Nevus of Ito is a variant of nevus of Ota. It affects acromioclavicular and deltoid regions.
    - CMN is a pigmented hairy nevus since birth *(MCQ 341).*

339. **Ans. d. It is lichen planus. Violaceous color of papules, itching and mucosal involvement are typical features of LP.**
    - Secondary syphilis manifests as asymptomatic, bilateral symmetrical papules on trunk and extremities *(MCQ 293).*

Chapter 5 ✦ Answers of MCQs in Dermatology, Venereology and Leprology

- In LL, lesions will be asymptomatic and reddish *(MCQ 155)*. These patients usually have swelling and infiltration of ears *(MCQ 101)*.
- Acne comprises of papules, pustules and comedones *(MCQ 34)*.
- Acneiform eruption consists of monomorphic, small, red papules on trunk and extremities *(MCQ 43)*.

340. Ans. d. This is typical androgenetic alopecia.
- Trichotillomania in adults is most common in females (7:1). It is characterized by the presence of firmly anchored partially broken hair and a peripheral rim of intact hairs *(MCQ 128)*.
- T. effluvium causes a diffuse hair loss *(MCQ 163)* due to some inciting cause.
- A. areata causes patchy hair loss which are smooth *(MCQ 156)* with complete hair loss *(MCQ 269)*.

341. Ans. a. It is congenital melanocytic nevus (CMN). Cosmetic concern and its malignant potential are two main reasons for which it should be excised, if possible.
- Becker's nevus is acquired epidermal pigmented hairy nevus that manifests during adolescence *(MCQ 338)*.
- Nevus of Ota is grayish pigmentation on one side of face in the distribution of first two divisions of trigeminal nerve *(MCQ 158)*.

342. Ans. d. She is having idiopathic thrombocytopenic purpura (ITP). Thrombocytopenia causes petechiae when platelet count is <50,000/cc.
- HS purpura is mostly seen in children on legs and other dependent areas in a symmetrical manner *(MCQ 332)*.
- CML can manifests as large ecchymotic patches due to platelet dysfunction *(MCQ 390)*. The count of platelet maybe normal.
- Senile purpura is seen at older age as geometric-shaped dark purplish patches *(MCQ 148)*.

343. Ans. c. It is hidradenitis suppurativa. Involvement is limited to sites of apocrine glands, i.e., perianal region, axillae *(MCQ 111)*. Abscesses, sinuses and scarring are characteristic.
- Bacterial sinuses are usually one or two *(MCQ 326)*.
- Multiple sinuses in scrofuloderma are seen over the underlying lymph nodes *(MCQ 53)*.
- Boils will be painful, large and not limited to site of apocrine glands. They will be found elsewhere also.

344. Ans. c. She is having pemphigus vulgaris which is an autoimmune disease. Hemorrhagic crusting of lips and flaccid blisters are typical features.
- DH is characterized by extremely pruritic papules, group of small vesicles on extensors, back *(MCQ 261)* and natal cleft.
- Pemphigoid comprises of tense bullae with no mucosal involvement *(MCQ 285)*.
- Secondary syphilis is characterized by shallow, dull red and painless mucous patches with asymptomatic papulosquamous eruption on trunk *(MCQ 293)* and extremities.

345. Ans. c. It is a cutaneous horn which is a morphological diagnosis. It can be caused by variety of disorders. Excision biopsy is treatment of choice.
- Periungual fibroma is a manifestation of tuberous sclerosis complex and is seen on nail fold *(MCQ 317)*.
- Periungual warts are hyperkeratotic plaques on nail folds *(MCQs 325, 364)*.
- Skin tags are 2–5 mm sized soft papules on the sides of neck in obese persons *(MCQ 105)*.

346. Ans. b. It is Koebner phenomenon which is also known as 'isomorphic phenomenon'. It refers to the development of pathologic lesions in the traumatized 'uninvolved skin' of persons having certain cutaneous diseases, e.g., psoriasis *(MCQ 308)*, warts *(MCQ 346)*, lichen planus, etc.
- Rebound phenomenon refers to appearance of a greater number of psoriatic lesions in an aggressive manner than the pretreatment state *(MCQ 316)*. It is seen in patients of psoriasis receiving systemic steroids.
- Grattage test is demonstrated in psoriasis as easy removal of silvery scales with the edge of a glass slide *(MCQ 322)*.
- Auspitz's sign is also demonstrated in psoriasis as an extension of grattage test. On further scrapping, pin point bleeding spots are visible in psoriatic lesion *(MCQ 329)*.

347. Ans. c. These are hyphae of dermatophytes. Branching septate hyphae is a typical feature of dermatophytes.
- Coarse and short filaments together with groups of spherical thick-walled spores give a 'spaghetti and meatballs' appearance *(MCQ 363)*.

- Candida shows pseudomycelia with cluster of budding grapes like yeast cells *(MCQ 644)*.
- Chromoblastomycosis shows sclerotic thick-walled cells singly or in clusters.

348. Ans. c. It is Milker's nodule which is caused by Paravaccinia virus from the infected cow teats. Initially, it presents as a slightly painful papule. Later, dark color crust forms on depressed centre of nodules.
- Boils are very painful, deep seated inflammatory nodules around hair follicles *(MCQ 147)*.
- *M. contagiosum* usually are not so large, uncommon on hands and do not have dark central crust. They have central umbilications *(MCQ 224)*.
- Warts usually do not get infected. They present as rough hyperkeratotic papules *(MCQ 169)*.

349. Ans. d. It is X-linked recessive ichthyosis (XLRI). It is characterized by dark colored scales sparing the cubital and popliteal folds. It is only seen in males.
- Ichthyosis vulgaris manifests between 3–12 months of life. Scales are white and spares diaper area *(MCQ 324)*.
- Acquired ichthyosis is seen in later life due to some internal cause or due to some drug *(MCQ 90)*.
- Atopic dermatitis does not cause ichthyotic changes. In later stage, it can cause lichenification *(MCQ 177)*.

350. Ans. b. It is a corn. A corn (type of callosity) is a sharply circumscribed and usually a painful callosity over a bony prominence.
- A callus (type of callosity) is an evenly thickened broader area of hyperkeratosis. It is usually noticed under the heads of metatarsals *(MCQ 369)*.
- Warts are usually multiple and are not found on bony prominences *(MCQ 364)*.
- Knuckle pads are idiopathic fibromatosis seen on dorsal side of interphalangeal joints *(MCQ 355)*.

351. Ans. c. It shows Gram negative diplococci inside neutrophils. It makes presumptive diagnosis of gonorrhea by finding Gram negative reniform diplococci inside the neutrophils in pus smear examination.
- Demonstration of acantholytic cells in Tzanck smear makes the diagnosis of pemphigus vulgaris *(MCQ 373)*.
- Presence of LD bodies (amastigotes) inside the histiocytes is seen in leishmaniasis *(MCQ 368)*.
- Acid fast bacilli in slit smear examination are seen in leprosy *(MCQ 388)*.

352. Ans. a. Induration 15 mm X 15 mm in tuberculin test cannot be interpreted as doubtful because induration 10–12 mm is taken as positive. Between 5–10 mm is regarded as doubtful.
- Positive response indicates previous exposure to *T. bacilli*.
- It also suggests partial immunity against new tuberculosis infection.

353. Ans. c. It is alarming, HIV infection must be ruled out. Recurrence of herpes zoster or bilateral herpes zoster *(MCQ 42)* or simultaneous herpes zoster at two sites *(MCQ 30)* are due to underlying HIV infection unless proved otherwise.
- In addition, there is high probability of HIV infection in patients having disseminated herpes zoster.
- HIV testing should also be done in high-risk herpes zoster patients, e.g., truck driver, patient having tuberculosis of lungs, etc.

354. Ans. b. She is having idiopathic thrombocytopenic purpura (ITP). Thrombocytopenia usually causes petechiae when platelet count falls below <50,000/cc.
- Senile purpura is seen at older age as geometric-shaped dark purplish patches *(MCQ 148)*.
- HS purpura is mostly seen in children on legs and other dependent areas in a symmetrical manner *(MCQ 332)*.
- CML shows large ecchymotic patches due to platelet dysfunction *(MCQ 390)*. Count of platelet may be normal.

355. Ans. d. These are knuckle pads. It is a misnomer, because this uncommon idiopathic fibromatosis is seen on the interphalangeal joints not on knuckles. Treatment is unsatisfactory.
- Common warts are rough hyperkeratotic papules *(MCQ 169)*.
- Callus is an evenly thickened broader area of hyperkeratosis usually noticed under the heads of metatarsals *(MCQ 369)*.
- Corn is sharply circumscribed and is usually a painful callosity over a bony prominence *(MCQ 350)*.
- Gottron papules are seen in dermatomyositis as red and violaceous papules on the dorsa of IP and MP joints *(MCQ 1066)*.

356. **Ans. d. It is molluscum contagiosum. Dome-shaped, pearly white papules with central umbilication are its typical features.**
    - Acne vulgaris comprises of papules, pustules and comedones *(MCQ 34)*.
    - Acneiform eruption comprises of monomorphic, small red papules on trunk and shoulders *(MCQ 43)*.
    - Acne conglobata is severe nodular form of acne. It comprises of nodules, abscesses and scars.

357. **Ans. b. It is furuncle or boil. It is defined as deep folliculitis and perifolliculitis. It presents as acute painful, necrotic and deep-seated inflammatory nodule around a hair follicle.**
    - Angioedema refers to acute subcutaneous uniform swelling of lips, eyelids *(MCQ 296)*. When it involves tongue, it can cause breathing difficulty.
    - Granulomatous cheilitis can also manifest as swelling of upper lip. It usually presents as chronic and symmetrical swelling of lips *(MCQ 366)*. If it is accompanied by fissured tongue and facial paralysis, it is called Melkersson-Rosenthal syndrome.

358. **Ans. b. It is pityriasis capitis in which involvement is confined to scalp. It is a manifestation of seborrheic dermatitis.**
    - PV is characterized by hypopigmented or discolored macules on trunk, arms and cervical region *(MCQ 39, 421)*.
    - P. alba is characterized by ill-defined hypopigmented patch on face *(MCQ 85)*.
    - P. rosea comprises of discrete oval lesions forming 'Christmas tree' pattern on trunk *(MCQ 161)*. Lesions are covered by fine scales.

359. **Ans. b. It is adult phase atopic dermatitis. Manifestations of adult phase of AD are similar to those of late childhood phase. It characteristically involves flexures of knees and elbows, cervical region and face.**
    - ABCD does not involve flexures. It involves uncovered parts. Face is predominantly involved *(MCQ 86)*.
    - SD involves the nasolabial folds, axillae, groins, inframammary regions and other seborrheic sites *(MCQ 171)*.
    - Darier's disease manifests as firm, gray, rough and firm papules at seborrheic sites *(MCQ 267)*.

360. **Ans. c. It is infected dermatitis. Here microorganism or their byproducts play a causative role in this type of eczema. Dermatitis has developed around the pus discharging ear canal. Eczematization around infected wound due to roadside injury is also common** *(MCQ 498)*.
    - Impetigo contagiosa presents as yellowish thick dirty brown crusts *(MCQ 60)*.
    - Scrofuloderma is a type of endogenous skin tuberculosis that presents as a sinus *(MCQ 52)* having thin bluish margins with watery discharge.
    - Ecthyma is deep pyogenic infection that presents as thick adherent crust *(MCQ 299)*.

361. **Ans. b. It is post-kala-azar dermal leishmaniasis (PKDL). PKDL is a complication of visceral leishmaniasis. Cutaneous manifestations in PKDL include hypopigmented macules, papules, nodules and plaques and erythema on face. In PKDL, dermal macrophages are laden with amastigotes (LD bodies). Diagnosis is proved by biopsy and finding antibodies to RK 39.**
    - In MC, papules will be pearly white and umbilicated *(MCQ 224)*.
    - Intradermal nevi are seen in older patients and may show overlying telangiectatic vessels or one or two coarse terminal hairs *(MCQ 244)*.
    - Trichoepithelioma papules are usually small multiple and are seen particularly around nose and upper lip *(MCQ 223)*.

362. **Ans. b. It is a contact allergic dermatitis due to lipstick. Ricinoleic acid has been identified as a common cause in lip cosmetics.**
    - CID develops on first exposure *(MCQ 305)*. While sensitization is prerequisite for clinical manifestation of CAD.
    - Lip-lick cheilitis is attributed to the habit of lip licking and involves the perioral region adjoining the vermillion border *(MCQ 93)*.
    - FDE has acute onset and is characterized by dusky color *(MCQ 199)*.

363. **Ans. d. It is pityriasis versicolor. It is showing coarse and short filaments together with groups of spherical thick-walled spores giving a 'spaghetti and meatballs' appearance.**
    - Branching septate hyphae is a typical feature of dermatophytes *(MCQ 347)*.
    - Candida shows pseudomycelia with clusters of budding grapes like yeast cells *(MCQ 644)*.
    - Chromoblastomycosis shows sclerotic thick-walled cells singly or in groups.

364. **Ans. a. It is periungual wart.**
    - TVC presents as hyperkeratotic plaque surrounded by erythema. Margins usually show finger like projections *(MCQ 10)*.
    - Periungual fibroma is a manifestation of tuberous sclerosis complex. It presents as smooth, firm and reddish excrescence on the nail fold *(MCQ 317)*.
    - Corn is a sharply circumscribed and usually painful callosity over a bony prominence *(MCQ 350)*.

365. **Ans. b. It is Schamberg's disease which presents as distinct pigmentation of dependent parts of legs due to extravasation of RBC and deposition of hemosiderin. Margins are indistinct.**
    - Senile purpura is seen at old age as geometric-shaped dark purplish patches *(MCQ 148)*.
    - LPP is a characterized by dark brown macules on sun exposed areas and flexural folds.
    - CML may present with large ecchymotic patches due to platelet dysfunction *(MCQ 390)*.

366. **Ans. a. He is having granulomatous cheilitis which is a rare idiopathic inflammatory disorder that usually affects young adults. When it is accompanied by facial paralysis and fissured tongue, then this clinical triad is named as Melkersson-Rosenthal syndrome.**
    - Angular cheilitis presents as erythema and maceration at angles of mouth. It is predisposed by ill-fitting dentures, oral candidiasis, nutritional deficiency, diabetes and HIV infection.
    - Cheilitis glandularis is a painless enlargement of lower lip in an elderly patient. It results from inflammation of minor salivary gland ducts.
    - Actinic cheilitis is a premalignant condition. It presents as ill-defined white, atrophic and scaly plaque on lower lip.

367. **Ans. c. It is pyoderma gangrenosum which is a rare idiopathic disorder of neutrophilic infiltration having common association with underlying systemic disease. It requires high dose of systemic steroids as first line treatment.**
    - Ecthyma is a deeper pyogenic infection having indurated base and margin *(MCQ 299)*.
    - Tuberculous chancre will be painless and will have watery discharge *(MCQ 382)*.
    - Boil presents as painful deep-seated inflammatory nodule *(MCQ 357)*.

368. **Ans. b. The presence of numerous amastigotes inside the histiocytes (called as LD bodies) and outside the histiocytes confirm the diagnosis of leishmaniasis.**
    - Acantholytic cells in Tzanck smear are seen in pemphigus vulgaris *(MCQ 373)*.
    - Gram negative diplococci are seen in pus smear in gonorrhea patient *(MCQ 351)*.
    - AFB in slit skin smear are seen in leprosy *(MCQ 388)*.

369. **Ans. c. It is a callus (syn. tylomata) which is evenly thickened broader area of hyperkeratosis usually noticed under the heads of metatarsals. It develops at the site of recurrent friction. Callus principally develops on feet, soles or palms.**
    - In fact, callus is term used to describe a bigger lesion. Besides friction, callus can also be seen due to palmoplantar keratoderma.
    - Corn is a type of callus. It generally occurs on lateral side of toes as thick localized area having conical or circular shape *(MCQ 369)*.
    - Plantar warts present as firm painful lesions which are seen as black dots *(MCQ 410)*. They are more painful when squeezed side to side.
    - Keratoderma is a disease which manifest as callus in response to repeated shear or friction *(MCQ 337)*.

370. **Ans. a. It is incontinentia pigmenti which is a rare X-linked dominant disease and is seen mainly in females. This congenital widespread linear pigmentation is along the lines of Blaschko. It is lethal for males in the embryonic stage.**
    - Dyskeratosis congenita is a degenerative skin disease. It comprises of reticulate pigmentation, leukoplakia patch in mouth, nail atrophy and bone marrow failure.
    - Peutz-Jeghers syndrome presents as pigmented macules in oral mucosa and perioral lentiginosis around nose and mouth. It might be associated with GIT polyp or malignancy of any other organ.
    - CALMs are light brown macules. These are considered as markers of many disorders. CALMs are seen in 90% patients of neurofibromatosis type 1 *(MCQ 227)*.

371. **Ans. b. It is lichen amyloidosis which is a localized cutaneous amyloidosis. It is diagnosed by demonstration of amyloid material in the papillary dermis sparing blood vessels and adnexal structures.**
    - Lichen planus is characterized by violaceous pruritic papules *(MCQ 381)*.

Chapter 5 ✦ Answers of MCQs in Dermatology, Venereology and Leprology

- Prurigo nodularis comprises of 1–2 cm sized extremely itchy cutaneous nodules on lower extremities *(MCQ 170)*.
- Darier's disease comprises of multiple rough, firm, gray colored papules at seborrheic sites *(MCQ 267)*.

372. Ans. d. It is superficial palmoplantar warts (mosaic warts). Hyperhidrosis is a predisposing factor. It is often painless and tends to be persistent.
- LP of palms will show papules with violaceous color *(MCQ 231)*.
- In pompholyx, on puncturing with a needle fluid will come out from deep seated vesicles *(MCQ 218)*.
- Corns are seen on pressure points and skin markings continue over the corn surface.
- Deep palmoplantar warts are deep seated and do not coalesce *(MCQ 310)*.

373. Ans. b. It is showing acantholytic cells in Tzanck smear. These are large round cells having large dark staining nucleus, perinuclear halo and a peripheral rim of condensed cytoplasm. The presence of acantholytic cells in smears made from vesicles or bullae confirms pemphigus.
- LD bodies are seen in leishmaniasis *(MCQ 368)*.
- Gram negative diplococci inside neutrophils are seen in pus smear made in gonorrhea *(MCQ 351)*.
- AFBs in slit skin smear are seen in Hansen's disease *(MCQ 388)*.

374. Ans. d. Strong reaction (>20 mm × 20 mm) does not indicate protection. A large necrotic response or blister formation suggests either susceptibility or presence of active disease. A small necrotic response indicates protection.
- A large necrotic response or blister formation suggests either susceptibility or presence of active disease.
- Small necrotic response indicates protection.

375. Ans. b. It is molluscum contagiosum with typical dome-shaped and pearly white papules with central umbilications.
- Milker's nodule is mainly seen on uncovered parts, e.g., face *(MCQ 385)* and hands *(MCQ 348)*. It shows a dark-colored crust on the depressed centre of nodules.
- Common warts are seen on exposed part of body as hyperkeratotic papules *(MCQ 169)*.
- Acne conglobata is severe nodular form of acne comprising of nodules, abscesses, scars and comedones.

376. Ans. a. It is acropustulosis which is a localized type of pustular psoriasis involving distal parts of big toes and adjoining toes. Treatment is disappointing.
- Keratoderma blennorrhagica is a cutaneous manifestation of Reiter's disease on the soles. It manifests as papule, nodule or horny excrescences.
- Eczema is characterized by oozing and crusting *(MCQ 213)*.
- Tinea pedis shows patches with well-defined borders *(MCQ 32)*.

377. Ans. b. It is a cutaneous manifestation of hepatitis B infection. Urticaria, lichen planus like lesions and erythema nodosum are some other manifestations of hepatitis B infection.
- Papular urticaria is seen in children on exposed parts and do not involve trunk *(MCQ 72)*.
- Pityriasis rosea is seen as a crop of discrete oval shaped lesions covered by fine scales. Lesions are distributed symmetrically on trunk in "Christmas tree pattern" *(MCQ 161)*.
- Gianotti-Crosti syndrome (infantile papular acrodermatitis) is seen between 6 months and 12 years. It presents as multiple red brown 1–10 mm sized papules (may coalesce in to plaque) and papulovesicles. The lesions are flat topped or dome-shaped and distributed often asymmetrically on cheeks, extensors of extremities, and the buttocks. Generalized lymphadenopathy is common. It is self-limiting and lasts for 5 days–12 months.

378. Ans. d. It is diabetic dermopathy (syn. diabetic shin spots). Its pathogenesis is not understood.
- Granuloma annulare is also seen in diabetics as asymptomatic incomplete rings of small smooth skin colored or reddish papules *(MCQ 219)*.
- Lichen amyloidosis is seen as discrete highly pruritic papules on shins *(MCQ 371)*.
- Diabetic rubeosis is seen as rose reddening of face, hands and feet in long standing diabetes patients.

379. Ans. b. It is lymphocytoma cutis which is a pseudolymphoma which means lymphocytic infiltration without malignant transformation.
- Mycetoma is a deep fungal infection which is characterized by swelling with discharging granules *(MCQ 272)*.
- Mycosis fungoides is a cutaneous-T-cell lymphoma in which T-cells colonize the

epidermis (epidermotropism) to form clusters *(MCQ 408)*.
- ❖ Actinic reticuloid also shows dermal lymphocytic infiltration but it manifests on sun exposed areas *(MCQ 298)*.

380. **Ans. b. He is having urethritis with frank pus discharge. It can be due to gonococcal or non-gonococcal organisms or both. So, it is best called as urethral syndrome and he should always be given treatment for both.**
    - ❖ Balanoposthitis patient will have white discharge from undersurface of prepuce not from urethral opening *(MCQ 38)*.
    - ❖ Reiter's disease comprises of a triad of non-gonococcal urethritis, polyarthritis and conjunctivitis or iritis.
    - ❖ Smegma is a cheesy deposit under the prepuce. It is composed of sebum and desquamated cells *(MCQ 280)*.

381. **Ans. b. It is lichen planus having all typical features.**
    - ❖ Lichen amyloidosis comprises of highly pruritic, closely set skin-colored papules *(MCQ 317)*.
    - ❖ Psoriasis comprises of red plaques with white scaling *(MCQ 239)*.
    - ❖ Prurigo nodularis comprises of 1-2 cm sized highly pruritic nodules on shins *(MCQ 170)*.

382. **Ans. a. It is a typical tuberculous chancre at trauma vulnerable site. Smear for AFB should be made from the discharge.**
    - ❖ *P. gangrenosum* presents as a painful ulcer with surrounding erythema *(MCQ 367)*.
    - ❖ Perianal sinus presents as small opening having recurrent pus discharge *(MCQ 326)*.
    - ❖ Carbuncle presents as multiple openings from a painful dome-shaped lump and gives an appearance of sieve *(MCQ 157)*.

383. **Ans. c. It is hyperkeratotic palmar eczema having typical features of eczema.**
    - ❖ Psoriasis is characterized typically by red color and normal areas of skin in between *(MCQ 233)*.
    - ❖ DLE lesions are disc shaped and are surrounded by rim of hyperpigmentation *(MCQ 242)*.
    - ❖ LP lesions are small papules showing violaceous color *(MCQ 231)*.
    - ❖ Palmoplantar keratoderma is characterized by asymptomatic, yellowish uniform thickening *(MCQ 486)*.

384. **Ans. d. It is a black dot type of tinea capitis showing black dots due to broken hairs at the surface of scalp.**
    - ❖ Alopecia areata comprises of variable sized well defined totally bald patches *(MCQ 145)*.
    - ❖ Trichotillomania shows the presence of firmly anchored partially broken hairs. It is seen on easily accessible sites *(MCQ 167)*.
    - ❖ Pseudopelade of Brocq is an idiopathic cicatricial (scarring) alopecia seen in females *(MCQ 284)*.

385. **Ans. d. It is Milker's nodule which is caused by Paravaccinia virus from the infected cow teats. Initially, there is formation of slightly tender papule. Later, dark colored crust forms on depressed centre.**
    - ❖ Molluscum contagiosum usually do not get infected and comprises of pearly white, dome-shaped and umbilicated papules *(MCQ 224)*.
    - ❖ Impetigo contagiosa comprises of honey-colored crusted lesions *(MCQ 60)*.
    - ❖ Chickenpox comprises of vesicular lesions surrounded by an irregular area of erythema *(MCQ 173)*. Lesions do not persist for one month. It affects face, trunk and extremities.

386. **Ans. d. It is *Paederus dermatitis* (syn. dermatitis linearis or blister beetle dermatitis). It is a peculiar irritant dermatitis provoked by coelomic fluid released by an insect of genus Pederus. It does not bite or sting. The symptoms are due to vesicant action of pederin.**
    - ❖ Erythema multiforme (EM) comprises of typical target lesion which consists of central zone of erythema or purpura, middle zone of edema and a peripheral zone of well-defined erythema *(MCQ 140)*.
    - ❖ Fixed drug eruption (FDE) manifests as dusky red macules which occasionally evolve into bulla *(MCQ 200)*.
    - ❖ Bullous impetigo comprises of thick-walled small bullae. Initially, its contents are clear, later it becomes turbid *(MCQ 262)*.

387. **Ans. b. It is sycosis barbae which is a subacute or chronic deep folliculitis that commonly involves the beard region. It presents as edematous papule or pustule with hair in the centre.**
    - ❖ In CSF, involvement is confined to the osteum. It comprises of profuse eruption of follicular pustules on lower extremities *(MCQ 286)*.
    - ❖ Boils comprises deep folliculitis and perifolliculitis. They present as acute deep-seated red and tender nodules *(MCQ 357)*.
    - ❖ Pseudofolliculitis barbae is caused by penetration of sharp tips of shaved hairs and comprises of papules and pustules on shaved skin *(MCQ 291)*.

Chapter 5 ✦ Answers of MCQs in Dermatology, Venereology and Leprology 353

388. **Ans. c. Red structures are lepra bacilli. Demonstration of lepra bacilli in slit skin smear or skin biopsy is considered as one of the three cardinal features for the diagnosis of leprosy.**
    - Gram negative diplococci are seen in pus smear examination in gonorrhea patient *(MCQ 35)*.
    - Acantholytic cells in Tzanck smear are seen in pemphigus patient *(MCQ 373)*.
    - LD bodies inside the histiocytes are seen in leishmaniasis *(MCQ 368)*.

389. **Ans. d. It is Koebner phenomenon shown by facial plane warts. It is also known as 'isomorphic phenomenon'. It refers to the development of pathologic lesions in the traumatized 'uninvolved skin' of person having certain cutaneous diseases, e.g., psoriasis** *(MCQ 308)*, **lichen planus** *(MCQ 346)*, **warts, etc.**
    - Grattage test is demonstrated in psoriasis as easy removal of silvery scales with the edge of a glass slide *(MCQ 322)*.
    - Auspitz's sign is also demonstrated for psoriasis. On further removal of scales by glass slide, pinpoint bleeding spots are visible *(MCQ 329)*.
    - Rebound phenomenon refers to appearance of a greater number of psoriatic lesions in an aggressive manner than the pretreatment state *(MCQ 316)*. It seen in patients of psoriasis receiving systemic steroids.

390. **Ans. c. It is due to chronic myelocytic leukemia (CML) in this patient. Large ecchymotic patches in a young patient are usually due to platelet dysfunction. Platelet count may be normal. But platelets are abnormal and not functioning properly. Thrombocytopenia usually causes petechiae when count is <50,000/mcL** *(MCQs 342, 354)*.
    - ITP usually causes petechiae *(MCQs 342, 354)*. Majority of patients are children and adolescents.
    - Senile purpura is seen at older age. Skin shows senile changes. It becomes thin, fragile, inelastic and skin markings become prominent *(MCQ 148)*.
    - HS purpura is mostly seen in children on legs and other dependent areas in a symmetrical manner *(MCQ 332)*.

391. **Ans. c. It is erythrokeratoderma variabilis (syn. erythrokeratoderma congenitals progressiva symmetrica, erythrokeratoderma figurate variabilis) with all the typical clinical features. It is a rare autosomal condition that usually presents at birth or below 1 year of age. This disorder of cornification is associated with noninflammatory erythema. Lesions are bizarrely shaped, polycyclic and can occur at any site.**
    - Seborrheic dermatitis presents with greasy scales and ill-defined margins *(MCQ 175)*.
    - Tinea incognito does not last so long and is not asymptomatic *(MCQ 451)*.
    - Flexural psoriasis manifests with salmon pink color and white scales *(MCQs 84, 245)*.

392. **Ans. c These are common warts on face with typical rough and hyperkeratotic surface of papules.**
    - Adenoma sebaceum presents as red brown, telangiectatic, discrete and firm papules *(MCQ 306)*. It is seen in tuberous sclerosis complex.
    - Molluscum contagiosum comprises of pearly white dome-shaped umbilicated papules *(MCQ 224)*.
    - Impetigo contagiosa comprises of multiple honey-colored crusted lesions *(MCQ 60)*.

393. **Ans. c. It is candidiasis both feet. It may be caused if feet remain wet for longer time, e.g., frequent washing of feet due to some psychotic reason.**
    - Tinea pedis comprises of hyperkeratosis and white scaling *(MCQ 51)*.
    - Pitted keratolysis presents as circular, superficial erosions on soles *(MCQ 282)*.
    - Contact dermatitis to shoes will affect the dorsa of feet and will take the shape of shoes *(MCQ 202)*.

394. **Ans. b. It is a dry type housewife contact dermatitis. Initially, it affects thumb, index finger and middle finger. Then, it involves the entire palms. Moist type primarily affects dorsa of the hands** *(MCQ 413)*.
    - Tinea manuum affects asymmetrically and manifests as scaling *(MCQ 45)*.
    - Lichen planus manifests as papules with violaceous coloration *(MCQ 231)*.
    - Allergic dermatitis in mason affects the dorsa of hands and fingers *(MCQ 225)*.

395. **Ans. b. It is allergic contact dermatitis due to hair dye. Para-phenylenediamine (PPD) is the causative ingredient. Initial application has sensitized her. Sensitization is a prerequisite for allergic dermatitis.**
    - Acute irritant dermatitis develops due to irritants and sensitization is not a prerequisite. It does not develop again if applied in appropriate amount *(MCQ 305)*.

- Angioedema refers to dermal or subcutaneous swelling that commonly involves lips, eyelids and genitalia *(MCQ 296)*. In most of the patients, it is idiopathic.

396. **Ans. b.** It is endothrix type of hair involvement by the dermatophyte. It is showing huge number of small sized spores inside the hair shaft replacing the intrapilary keratin, but leaving the cortex intact. Branching hyphae are also visible outside the follicle.
     - Candida in KOH smear appears as pseudomycelia in clusters of grape-like yeast cells *(MCQ 644)*, filament like elongated cells showing end to end connection (pseudohyphae) and septate hyphae.
     - Coarse and short filaments together with group of spherical thick-walled spores give a 'spaghetti and meatballs' appearance *(MCQ 363)*.
     - Presence of Sarcoptes scabiei can be confirmed if mite, eggs *(MCQ 651)* or short legs with bristles are detected.

397. **Ans. a.** It is superficial palmoplantar warts (mosaic warts). Hyperhidrosis is a predisposing factor. It is often painless and tends to be persistent.
     - LP papules will show violaceous coloration *(MCQ 231)*.
     - Pompholyx comprises of deep-seated vesicles *(MCQ 218)*. On puncturing with a needle, fluid will come out.
     - Corns are seen at pressure points *(MCQ 359)*. Skin markings will continue over corn surface.
     - Deep palmoplantar warts are deep and do not get coalesce *(MCQ 410)*.

398. **Ans. a.** It is condylomata acuminata which is also called as venereal warts. Usually, venereal warts on this area are soft and pink. In this patient, dark color is because of long untreated duration.
     - SCC is usually a single, exophytic, cauliflower like growth *(MCQ 289)*.
     - Seborrheic keratosis also comprises of pigmented papules, but these are seen on face, extremities and upper trunk *(MCQ 117)* in elderly persons.
     - Condylomata lata is a manifestation of secondary syphilis. It comprises of flesh-colored flat-topped papules with oozing and macerations. Common sites are anal region and groins *(MCQ 287)*.

399. **Ans. d.** It is idiopathic thrombocytopenic purpura (ITP). Most of ITP patients are children or adolescence. ITP usually presents as crop of petechiae or small sized few ecchymotic patches. Large sized multiple ecchymotic patches are due to platelet dysfunction *(MCQ 390)*.
     - HS purpura presents as retiform crop of small purpuric lesions on legs and dependent area in a symmetrical manner *(MCQ 332)*.
     - CML presents in adult or middle aged as large ecchymotic patches *(MCQ 390)*.
     - Actinic purpura is a synonym of senile purpura that presents in older people as geometric-shaped dark and purplish patches *(MCQ 148)*.

400. **Ans. b.** It is tinea faciei. Many times, typical lesions of tinea on face are not found because of certain reasons, e.g., absence of scaling, steroid application, exacerbation by sunlight giving an impression of photo dermatosis. Careful examination and KOH smear *(MCQ 347)* will make correct diagnosis.
     - It is difficult to differentiate from steroid dermatitis *(MCQ 5)* if patient has applied topical steroid. KOH smear will show absence of dermatophytes.
     - ABCD presents as chronic intractable itching, redness, scaling, pigmentation, thickening and lichenification *(MCQ 86)*.
     - PLE manifests within few hours of sun exposure and comprises of many morphological forms of lesions, e.g., papules, vesicles, etc. *(MCQ 198)*.

401. **Ans. a.** It is a manifestation of adult phase atopic dermatitis. The presentation is similar to that of late childhood phase of AD. It characteristically involves flexures of knees and elbows, cervical region and face.
     - SD involves nasolabial folds, axillae, groins, inframammary regions and other seborrheic sites *(MCQ 171)*.
     - Intertrigo comprises of diffuse macerated erythema involving the opposing surfaces of body folds, e.g., groins *(MCQ 166)* in obese persons. Face will be normal.
     - ABCD will involve the exposed parts of body. Face is characteristically involved *(MCQ 86)*.

402. **Ans. c.** She is having xeroderma pigmentosum which is an autosomal recessive disease. Both sexes are affected equally. There is a lack of ability to repair UV radiation damaged DNA.
     - Freckles are light brown macules of <3 mm size. They are seen in sunlight exposed skin in fair skin individuals *(MCQ 240)*.
     - RTS comprises of sparse hairs on scalp and eyebrows, short stature, abnormalities of teeth and nail.

- Actinic keratosis develops at older age. It comprises of 1–2 cm sized macules and rough hyperkeratotic papules. Papules have adherent scales which can be removed with difficulty *(MCQ 123)*.

403. **Ans. b. She is having pemphigus foliaceous (PF). Blister formation is at granular cell layer. So, vesicles are flaccid and transient.**
     - In PV, acantholysis is at supra basal level. So, blisters last longer than PF. Oral mucosa is involved in 70% of patients *(MCQ 184)*.
     - In BP, blistering is subepidermal. So, blisters last still longer. Oral mucosa is usually not involved *(MCQ 285)*.
     - In linear IgA dermatosis blistering is subepidermal. Blisters may occur in clusters or try to form collarette, i.e., new lesions form around the previous lesion *(MCQ 288)*.

404. **Ans. c. He is a typical patient of actinic lichen planus.**
     - DLE comprises of red, well defined plaques with adherent scales *(MCQ 67)*.
     - Actinic keratosis presents as 1 mm to 2 cm sized macules and papules having scales which can be removed with difficulty. It is seen in older patients *(MCQ 123)*.
     - XP manifests in childhood as relentless progression of freckling, dryness and dark rough keratotic papules *(MCQ 402)*.

405. **Ans. b. It is neonatal acne that manifests between 3 months to 24 months. It is thought to be due to transplacental stimulation of adrenal glands. It is managed by topical benzoyl peroxide.**
     - ETN presents as blotchy erythematous macules. The macules have 1–3 mm sized vesicle or a pustule in the center *(MCQ 432)*.
     - Milia presents as 1–3 mm sized white papules on cheeks and chin *(MCQ 497)*.
     - Sebaceous gland hyperplasia presents as tiny <1 mm sized yellow papules on nose, cheeks and chin. These sites have highest density of sebaceous glands.

406. **Ans. b. These are Fordyce spots which are visible sebaceous glands. They can appear on penile skin, labia, lips. On the foreskin they are called as Tyson's gland and on areola as Montgomery's tubercles.**
     - Lichen nitidus presents as asymptomatic, shiny, flat topped discrete, pinpoint to pinhead sized papules on shaft of penis *(MCQ 16)*, forearms, buttocks, chest, etc.
     - Syringoma presents as 1–3 mm sized papules commonly in females on face *(MCQ 236)*, cheeks and neck.
     - Molluscum contagiosum presents as pearly white, dome-shaped umbilicated papules in scattered manner *(MCQ 531)*.

407. **Ans. b. It is larva migrans. Lesions creep or migrate due to moving parasite in the skin. It is caused by hookworm.**
     - Granuloma annulare comprises of complete or incomplete rings of skin or red-colored papules *(MCQ 219)*.
     - Tinea corporis will present as itchy plaques with well defined borders and central clearing *(MCQ 40)*.

408. **Ans. c. It is a tumor stage of mycosis fungoides. It is cutaneous T-cell lymphoma (CTCL). Histopathology is showing epidermotropism by T-cells which is diagnostic of CTCL. Electron beam therapy is treatment of choice for tumor stage.**
     - Psoriasis does not form tumor. Psoriatic plaques will have silvery scaling *(MCQ 162)*.
     - Lupus vulgaris also will not form tumor. It manifests as soft gelatinous plaque with scarring in the centre. Usually, plaques are not multiple *(MCQ 26)*.
     - SCC usually forms a single exophytic tumor with cauliflower like appearance *(MCQ 113)*.

409. **Ans. a. He is having chilblains (syn. perniosis, erythema pernio). It is due to persistent constriction of larger arterioles with dilatation of superficial vessels. It is caused by exposure to cold.**
     - Raynaud's phenomenon is an episodic attack of well demarcated blanching or blue coloration of digits on exposure to cold. In chronic cases nail may become brittle or deformed. Finger tips may show scars *(MCQ 496)*.
     - Urticaria presents as wheals which do not last for >24 hours. Erythema of urticaria will not be limited to distal part of extremities. It will be found on other parts also *(MCQ 501)*.
     - Contact dermatitis on hands will show oozing and crusting *(MCQ 413)*.

410. **Ans. b. Deep warts are sharply defined and deep seated. On pairing with scalpel, surrounding collar becomes evident. On further paring, multiple small bleeding points are seen.**
     - Corns are seen at pressure points. Skin markings will continue over corn surface.

- Pitted keratolysis is seen as circular, punched out and superficial erosions on soles *(MCQ 282)*.
- Superficial palmoplantar warts are seen as superficial hyperkeratoses which coalesce at places *(MCQs 372, 397)*.

411. Ans. d. It is tinea faciei. Always have a high index of suspicion of tinea faciei whenever patient complains of redness and itching on face. Search for border of tinea and do KOH smear *(MCQ 347)* examination.
- PLE manifests within few hours of sun exposure. It comprises of eruption of many morphological forms of lesions, e.g., papules, vesicles, etc. *(MCQ 198)*
- Topical steroid damaged face (TSDF) is characterised by erythema, papules, and pustules *(MCQ 5)*.
- ABCD presents as chronic intractable itching, redness, scaling, pigmentation, thickening and lichenification *(MCQ 86)*.

412. Ans. a. He is having vitiligo on glans. It is a uniformly depigmented macule with no change in texture and is well defined.
- Lichen planus will show violaceous color and lacy network *(MCQ 15)*.
- Lichen sclerosus et atrophicus will show bluish white coloration of foreskin which can progress to phimosis *(MCQ 320)*.
- Leukoplakia is a precancerous condition which is common inside the mouth *(MCQ 230)*. It is uncommon on glans.

413. Ans. a. This is a moist type housewife's contact dermatitis. It is of allergic type and is seen on the dorsa of hands. Dry type of house wife contact dermatitis is of irritant type and seen on palmar aspect extending to dorsal aspects of thumbs, index and middle fingers *(MCQ 513)*.
- Discoid eczema will present as disc or coin shaped lesions *(MCQ 194)*.
- Pompholyx comprises of deep-seated vesicular lesions *(MCQ 218)*.
- Infected dermatitis is an eczematisation around infected wound *(MCQ 489)* or other infective focus *(MCQ 360)*.

414. Ans. c. It is miliaria crystallina. Obstruction of sweat duct is at the level of stratum corneum and vesicle formed is sub corneal. It is seen in febrile patients having profuse sweating.
- In miliaria rubra, blockade is at intraepidermal level. It manifests as uniformly minute red papules *(MCQ 477)*.
- In miliaria profunda, duct ruptures below dermo epidermal junction. It manifests as 1–3 mm sized, firm papules on trunk and extremities *(MCQ 125)*.
- SSSS presents as widespread erythema and blistering in response to toxin meditated pathogenesis *(MCQ 56)*.

415. Ans. b. It is hidradenitis suppurativa in the groins. It shows autosomal dominant inheritance and is considered to be due to occlusion and dilatation of ducts of apocrine glands. It is seen in areas having apocrine glands, e.g., axillae *(MCQ 111)*, perianal region *(MCQ 343)* and groins. It is characterized by small tender abscesses, scarring, sinus tracts with seropurulent discharge.
- Scrofuloderma sinus usually has bluish thin margins and watery discharge *(MCQ 52)*.
- Fox-Fordyce disease is a chronic, itchy papular eruption in the region bearing apocrine glands *(MCQ 232)*.
- Intertrigo refers to erythema and soreness in opposing surfaces of body folds. Sinus is not its feature *(MCQ 166)*.

416. Ans. d. It is angular cheilitis. It is predisposed by oral candidiasis, ill fitting denture, nutritional deficiency, diabetes and HIV infection.
- Cheilitis glandularis results from inflammation of minor salivary gland ducts. It presents as painless enlargement of lower lip in an elderly patient.
- Granulomatous cheilitis is a rare idiopathic disease which presents as chronic swelling of upper lip *(MCQ 366)*. When it is accompanied by facial paralysis and fissured tongue, it is named as Melkerson-Rosenthal syndrome.
- Actinic cheilitis is a premalignant condition that presents as ill defined white, atrophic and scaly plaque on lower lip *(MCQ 529)*.

417. Ans. c. It is lupus miliaris disseminatus faciei (LMDF). Because of granulomatous pathology, it was thought to be tubercular, but evidences didn't support. It responds to tetracyclines, isotretinoin and dapsone.
- Acne vulgaris comprises of papules, comedones and pustules *(MCQ 216)*.
- Acneiform eruption is common on trunk and shoulders *(MCQs 27, 43)*.
- Eruption of perioral dermatitis is prominent in nasolabial and perioral area *(MCQ 503)* sparing the lip margins.

- Acne rosacea is common in middle aged females. Lesions are common in central part of face *(MCQs 50, 853)*. Persistent facial erythema is a common feature.

418. **Ans. a.** It is diascopy. The pressure of glass slide will empty the blood from superficial vessels. If skin redness is due to blood within the vessels (erythema), it will blanch on pressure. If redness is due to extravasated blood into skin (petechiae or purpura), it will not blanch on pressure. It is used in patients of purpura, nevus anemicus and granulomatous diseases for detection of apple jelly nodules.
    - Dermatoscopy is skin surface microscopy with the handheld instrument called dermatoscope which is equipped with a light source and magnifying capability. It differentiates between melanocytic and non-melanocytic lesions.
    - Grattage test is simple bedside test used to diagnose a psoriatic plaque. Easy removal of white scales with the edge of glass slide favours psoriasis *(MCQ 232)*.

419. **Ans. b.** It is collodion baby which is a characteristic entity where child is born with an extra shining membrane named collodion. About 90% of collodion babies will develop autosomal recessive ichthyosis of severe type. Collodion babies require good nursing care in high humidity atmosphere with monitoring of body temperature. Prevention of infection is of utmost importance.
    - Harlequin ichthyosis may have similar facial appearance, but it will have fusion of fingers and toes. Ears will be bound down to scalp.
    - In restrictive dermopathy, skin is thin and transparent making the underlying blood vessels prominent.

420. **Ans. b.** It is filiform warts. They can be also be found on nostrils *(MCQ 430)*, angle of mouth *(MCQ 440)*, cervical region *(MCQ 450)*.
    - Milia are 1-2 mm sized, uniform dome-shaped, non umbilicated white papules *(MCQ 48)*.
    - Skin tags are soft, round and inelastic papules commonly seen on the sides of neck *(MCQ 105)*.
    - Molluscum contagiosum are small pearly white dome-shaped umbilicated papules *(MCQ 224)*.

421. **Ans. d.** In PV lesions can be hypopigmented *(MCQ 39)* or discolored. Trunk, neck and arms are common sites of involvement.
    - P. capitis is a manifestation of seborrheic dermatitis as white scales. Involvement is confined to scalp *(MCQ 358)*.
    - P. alba presents as ill-defined hypopigmented patches on face covered with fine white scales *(MCQ 85)*.
    - P. rosea presents as a crop of discrete macules oval in shape in a 'Christmas tree' pattern on trunk *(MCQ 161)*. Lesions are covered by white scales.

422. **Ans. d.** He is having Buerger's disease (thromboangiitis obliterans). It is seen in smokers only. Feet are more common to be involved *(MCQ 478)*. Upper extremities are involved only in 1/3 of patients.
    - Chilblains presents as erythema, burning and itching of fingers and toes on exposure to cold in severe winter *(MCQ 409)*.
    - Digital necrosis due to metoprolol: If a non smoker patient is taking metoprolol, then metoprolol should be considered as an etiological factor *(MCQ 487)*.
    - Raynaud's phenomenon is seen as episodic attacks of sequential and well demarcated changes in distal parts on exposure to cold, i.e., pallor, cyanosis and redness. It is seen bilaterally in all fingers and is common *(MCQ 496)* in patients of connective tissue disorders.

423. **Ans. b.** It is hyperkeratotic type of tinea pedis. It is showing white scaling with well-defined borders and is involving single foot.
    - Candidiasis usually involves both feet *(MCQ 393)* and show itchy red macerations.
    - Pitted keratolysis presents as superficial circular shaped erosion on soles *(MCQ 282)*.
    - Keratolysis exfoliativa is an asymptomatic desquamation of palms *(MCQ 452)* and occasionally the soles. It is self limiting, harmless and only requires emollients.

424. **Ans. a.** It is diaper dermatitis or diaper rash. It is characteristically sparing the skin inside the folds. It develops because of prolonged wetness, infrequent change of diapers, prolonged contact of urine, feces. It is an example of irritant contact dermatitis and involvement is confined to area covered by diapers. Bacteria and Candida are common causes of diaper rash.
    - Intertrigo is a dermatitis inside the skin folds *(MCQ 166)*.
    - Tinea cruris presents with well defined border with some clearing towards centre *(MCQ 4)*.
    - Flexural psoriasis presents as red colored plaques and scaling in body folds *(MCQs 84, 245)*.

425. **Ans. a.** It is pyogenic granuloma. It is a misnomer because it is nothing to do with pus. It is rapidly developed vascular nodule at the site of recent penetrating injury. It is composed of lobular proliferation of small vessels.
    - Cherry angiomas (senile angiomas) are most common vascular anomaly seen on trunk after the age of 70 years *(MCQ 221)*.
    - Strawberry hemangioma appears in first month of life as smooth, scarlet red single tumor *(MCQ 187)*.
    - Lymphangioma circumscriptum is noticed during childhood as discrete or grouped fluid filled vesicles bulging from the skin. Patient complains of blood-stained lymph from the vesicles *(MCQ 106)*.

426. **Ans. b.** She is having hyperthyroidism with exophthalmos. If she has thyroid dermopathy, then this triad is called as Graves' disease.
    - Orbital tumor will cause exophthalmos in one eye.
    - Hypothyroidism will not present with exophthalmos. It presents as puffiness of lids, lips. Loss of outer one-third of eyebrows may be there *(MCQ 217)*.
    - Goiter refers to swelling of thyroid gland due to iodine deficiency.

427. **Ans. c.** It is soft corn with a rubbery texture. It is a painful lesion that occurs between toes. Soft corns develop from ill-fitting shoes that cause friction.
    - Plantar warts are usually multiple. On paring, it shows multiple bleeding points *(MCQ 410)*.
    - A corn is a small lesion of thickened skin with central core *(MCQ 350)*.
    - Callus is a painless thickening of outermost layer of skin due to repeated friction. It can develop on hands or feet *(MCQ 369)*.

428. **Ans. c.** It is alopecia areata which is a chronic inflammatory disease involving the hair follicles. Scalp *(MCQ 156)* and beard *(MCQ 488)* are commonly involved sites.
    - Hypothyroidism and lepromatous leprosy can show the hair loss from eyebrows, but from outer one third *(MCQ 495)*.
    - Trichotillomania shows the presence of firmly anchored partially broken hairs *(MCQ 128)* from an easily accessible site of scalp. Eyebrow is least common site.

429. **Ans. c.** It is squamous cell carcinoma. It is exophytic ulcer with raised and thick borders. Ulceration is a common feature of SCC.
    - BCC is particularly common around eye, ear or nose *(MCQ 193)*.
    - Ulcerative lupus vulgaris will have trailing scar in center and apple Jelly nodules at the advancing margin.
    - Malignant melanoma does not present with a big ulcer. It will have black pigmentation also. It presents as papules or nodules *(MCQ 126)*.

430. **Ans. d.** It is digitate warts in the nostril.
    - Molluscum contagiosum are pearly white, dome-shaped umbilicated papules (MCQ).
    - Filiform warts are small (1–2 mm) and elongated. They are seen at angle of mouth *(MCQ 440)*, eye lids *(MCQ 420)*, cervical region *(MCQ 450)*.
    - Skin tags are soft, inelastic, round papules commonly seen on the sides of the neck in obese individuals *(MCQ 105)*.

431. **Ans. c.** It is tinea barbae which is also called as tinea sycosis or barber's itch. It includes the involvement of beard and/or moustache areas with involvement of coarse terminal hairs. We should have high index of suspicion especially when patient is not responding to antibiotics. KOH smear will clinch the diagnosis.
    - Boil will present as tender swelling of upper lip *(MCQ 357)*.
    - CSF presents as profuse eruption of follicular eruption on lower extremities *(MCQ 286)*.
    - Sycosis barbae is a subacute or chronic deep bacterial infection of hair follicles of beard region or upper lip. It presents as red papule with hair in the center *(MCQ 387)*.

432. **Ans. b.** It is erythema toxicum neonatorum. It is seen in 70% of term neonates within 2–10 days of life. The vesicle reveals numerous eosinophils.
    - Neonatal acne manifests as white or black comedones, papules and pustules on cheeks *(MCQ 405)*.
    - Milia are seen as 1–3 mm sized papules on cheeks, chin *(MCQ 497)*.
    - TNPM manifests as tiny brown macules, papules, vesicles in the mandibular area and forehead. The papules lack surrounding erythema.

433. **Ans. b.** He is a typical case of lepromatous leprosy having gloves and stockings type of anesthesia. Ulcers at fingertips are due to loss of sensations.

Infiltration of ear lobules is always due to LL unless proved otherwise. Loss of outer 1/3 eyebrows is common in LL.
- Myxedema is a characteristic feature of hypothyroidism and may have loss of outer 1/3 of eyebrows. But it will not have loss of sensation or ear lobule infiltration *(MCQ 217)*.
- Alopecia areata can have loss of hair of eyebrows *(MCQ 428)* but not especially from the outer one third.
- Systemic sclerosis presents as mask like face *(MCQ 14)*. Calcinosis cutis of tip of finger is a common feature *(MCQ 496)*.

434. Ans. c. It is discoid eczema which is typically showing symmetrical involvement with scaling and crusting.
- Dermatitis artefacta lesions are linear or bizarre shaped and appears in very short period *(MCQ 494)*.
- Psoriatic plaques are red with silvery white scaling *(MCQ 146)*.
- Tinea corporis will show well-defined border with central clearing *(MCQ 142)*. Oozing and crusting are not features of tinea.

435. Ans. d. It is herpes zoster with pain and typical grouped vesicles with unilateral involvement.
- *Paederus dermatitis* manifests on uncovered parts *(MCQ 444)*.
- Scabies manifests as extremely itchy papules not vesicles *(MCQ 65)*.
- Herpes genitalis presents as group of small vesicles *(MCQ 445)*.

436. Ans. c. It is oral candidiasis (oral thrush). It can be caused by underlying diabetes, anemia, leukaemia, HIV infection, immunosuppressant drugs, corticosteroids, etc.
- Oral leukoplakia refers to white lesions of oral mucosa that cannot be rubbed off *(MCQs 230, 251)*.
- Oral lichen planus presents as lacy network of white streaks *(MCQ 41)*.
- Smoker's keratosis is caused by chronic irritation due to use of the tobacco in various forms. It manifests as diffuse whiteness over of the palate with dark brown staining of teeth.

437. Ans. b. It is lichen planus soles. Pruritic, papular, purplish lesions on peripheral parts are its typical features.
- Psoriasis comprises of red plaques with scaling *(MCQ 858)*.
- Eczema is characterized by oozing, crusting and fissuring *(MCQ 137)*.
- CCLE presents as red plaques with adherent scales *(MCQ 242)* with borders of hyperpigmentation.

438. Ans. b. It is mid-borderline leprosy. Impaired sensations and 4–6 skin lesions together qualify the diagnosis of mid borderline Leprosy.
- Tuberculoid leprosy (high immunity) comprises of single plaque with loss of sensations *(MCQ 6)*.
- Lepromatous leprosy (least immunity) comprises of numerous uncountable skin lesions *(MCQ 155)*.
- Indeterminate leprosy refers to early transitory stage of leprosy whose immunological status yet not been determined. It presents as hypopigmented or slight red ill-defined patch. Sensations may not be impaired. If edges are palpable, then it is no longer indeterminate type.

439. Ans. b. It is a typical patient of acquired perforating dermatosis. It is due to transepidermal extrusion of dermal material commonly associated with diabetes and chronic renal failure. Umbilication is due to central hyper keratotic crust.
- Molluscum contagiosum presents as pearly white, dome-shaped umbilicated papules *(MCQ 224)*.
- Prurigo nodularis presents as a highly pruritic nodular lesions *(MCQ 170)*.
- Lichen planus presents as purplish papules *(MCQ 381)*.

440. Ans. a. It is filiform wart which can also be seen on eye lids *(MCQ 420)*, in nostrils *(MCQ 430)*, cervical region *(MCQ 450)*.
- Skin tags are soft, round, smooth surfaced, inelastic papules commonly seen on the sides of neck in obese persons *(MCQ 105)*.
- Plane warts are smooth, only slightly elevated, rounded or polygonal lesions in large number *(MCQ 389)*.
- Molluscum contagiosum comprises of pearly white, dome-shaped umbilicated papules *(MCQ 224)*.

441. Ans. a. It is 'black dot type' of tinea capitis showing group of black dots due to broken hairs at surface of scalp.
- Alopecia areata comprises of variable sized, well-defined, totally bald patch *(MCQ 145)*.
- Trichotillomania shows the presence of firmly anchored partially broken hairs. It is seen on the easily accessible sites *(MCQ 167)*.

- Cicatricial alopecia is also called scarring alopecia. It is irreversible hair loss because damaged hair follicles are replaced by fibrous tissue, e.g., pseudopelade of Brocq *(MCQ 284)*.

442. **Ans. c. It is fixed drug eruption. Dusky red macules or vesicles are typical of FDE.**
     - Erythema multiforme minor comprises of macules, papules and target lesions *(MCQ 134)*.
     - In erythema multiforme major, mucosal involvement is prominent in addition to target lesions *(MCQ 96)*.
     - SJS comprises of involvement of 2 or more mucosae with <10% cutaneous involvement *(MCQ 81)*.

443. **Ans. b. It is a segmental necrotizing granulomatous neuritis which is a rare pure neuritic leprosy. High resolution ultrasonography will assess the thickness and morphological alteration in the nerve. Thickening of peripheral cutaneous nerve is one of the cardinal features for the diagnosis of leprosy. Involvement of one nerve and more than one nerve are considered as paucibacillary and multibacillary leprosy respectively for the treatment point of view.**
     - To qualify the diagnosis of tuberculoid leprosy, at least one cutaneous plaque should be there *(MCQ 6)*.
     - Amyloid neuropathy typically presents as distal sensory symptoms, e.g., numbness and paraesthesia.

444. **Ans. b. It is *Paederus dermatitis* (syn. dermatitis linearis, blister beetle dermatitis). It is the peculiar irritant dermatitis provoked by an insect of genus Pederus. Coelomic fluid released by this insect has a potent vesicant action which produces the skin lesion. Lesion is characteristically linear and has a grayish white slough in the center.**
     - Herpes zoster presents as grouped vesicles on erythematous base *(MCQ 70)*.
     - Dermatitis artefacta lesions are seen on easily approachable sites *(MCQs 189, 494, 500)* as bizarre shaped lesions.

445. **Ans. b. It is primary genital herpes characterized by tiny grouped vesicular lesions with an incubation period of 2-5 days. They may soon break down to leave behind multiple small painful superficial erosions *(MCQ 471)*.**
     - Herpes zoster comprises of grouped vesicular lesions in a dermatome and is preceded by pain *(MCQ 435)* not by sexual exposure.
     - Syphilitic chancre comprises of painless ulcer with indurated base *(MCQ 453)*.
     - Chancroid ulcers are painful and multiple ulcers *(MCQ 489)*.
     - Lymphogranuloma venereum presents as inconspicuous single painless papule or ulcer which usually go unnoticed. It does not present as vesicle.

446. **Ans. c. It is xanthelasma palpebrarum. It is most common xanthoma that manifests on medial aspects of upper eyelids. It is triggered by hyperlipidaemia, hypothyroidism and diabetes.**
     - Necrobiotic xanthogranuloma is a rare multisystem histiocytic disorder that presents as asymptomatic indurated yellowish plaque in periorbital region. Majority of patients are associated with monoclonal gammopathy.
     - Sarcoidosis can involve any part of eye. Eyelid involvement is rare.
     - Systemic amyloidosis may manifest as petechiae and purpura on eye lids, chest, beard region and cheeks. When amyloid papule or plaques is pinched or rubbed, hemorrhage occurs, it is described as 'pinch purpura'.

447. **Ans. a. It is cutis verticis gyrata which is a folded hyperplasia of scalp. It is one of the cutaneous manifestations of acromegaly which is due to over production of growth hormone.**
     - Primary hypertrophic osteoarthropathy (HO) is a rare hereditary disorder that comprises of digital clubbing, pachydermia (thickening of skin of face and\or scalp), periostosis (swelling of periarticular tissue) hyperhidrosis.
     - Secondary type of HO results from cardio-pulmonary, hepatic disease and certain malignancies. It develops in men (65-75 years). Bone changes are rapid and painful. Skin changes may be mild or absent.

448. **Ans. b. It is acrodermatitis enteropathica which is a rare autosomal recessive metabolic disorder seen in young children who have lower zinc absorption than adults. It is seen typically after weaning. Top feeds have lower zinc bioavailability than breast milk. These children respond dramatically to oral supplementation of zinc in the dose of 2 mg/kg/day.**
     - Babies with biotin deficiency will have ataxia, conjunctivitis, lethargy, vomiting, diarrhea, periods of unconsciousness, seizures, hair loss.

- Seborrheic dermatitis comprises of yellow greasy scales favoring scalp *(MCQ 466)*, flexures and diaper area.
- In AD, face is most commonly *(MCQ 174)* involved. Involvement of extensors of limbs is also common.

449. Ans. a. She is having submucosal fibrosis. It is a chronic, irreversible debilitating condition associated with areca nut chewers. Areca nut is a chief component of betel quid. In late stage, these patients may have leukoplakia which is precancerous.
- Smoking also causes brown staining of teeth, but do not cause fibrosis.
- Smoker's keratosis manifests as diffuse whiteness over palate.
- Scleroderma patient presents as thin lips and radiating furrows giving a "fish mouth" or "purse string" appearance to oral aperture *(MCQ 454)*.

450. Ans. c. In the presence of such a huge number of filiform warts, underlying any immunodeficiency should be looked for, e.g., HIV infection, leukemia, etc.
- M. contagiosum can be in multiple numbers, but they are pearly white, umbilicated papules *(MCQ 224)*.
- Skin tags are seen on sides of neck *(MCQ 105)* as soft, inelastic papules.
- Plane warts are also seen in multiple, but they are plane toped, round or polygonal flat lesions *(MCQ 389)*.

451. Ans. d. It is tinea incognito which refers to those patients in which tinea infection becomes unrecognizable due to modification by topical or systemic steroids. When pustular lesions are not responding to various courses of antibiotics, then we must do KOH smear examination.
- CSF is a profuse eruption of follicular pustules on lower extremities *(MCQ 286)*. It is often chronic and resistant to treat.
- Infected scabies will definitely involve the genitals in such a severe case. But it is spared in this patient.
- Typical tinea corporis is characterized by ring shaped lesions with well-defined borders *(MCQ 40)*.

452. Ans. a. It is keratolysis exfoliativa. It is commonly associated with hyperhidrosis. It is self limiting, harmless and only requires emollients.

- Candidiasis will involve the interdigital spaces and presents as maceration *(MCQ 183)*.
- Eczema comprises of itching, oozing and crusting *(MCQ 383)*.
- Tinea manuum is usually asymmetrical *(MCQ 45)* and involve one palm.

453. Ans. b. It is typical syphilitic chancre which is characteristically painless with indurated base. Its incubation period is 9-90 days. VDRL, HIV, HBsAg and HCV must be done in all STD patients.
- Chancroid is characterized by multiple painful ulcers with non-indurated base with an incubation period of 3-10 days *(MCQ 489)*.
- Lymphogranuloma venereum presents as a small painless inconspicuous papule or ulcer which often go unnoticed (incubation period 3-30 days).
- Granuloma venereum (donovanosis) ulcers are painless, elevated, velvety and granulomatous which bleed easily (incubation period 1-5 weeks).

454. Ans. b. She is having systemic sclerosis manifesting with typical facial features. Presence of Raynaud's phenomenon with these facial features confirms systemic sclerosis.
- Submucosal fibrosis comprises of progressive inability to open mouth *(MCQ 449)*. It is caused by habit of betel quid chewing.
- SLE on face presents as malar rash on cheeks and short, broken hair on scalp *(MCQ 89)*.

455. Ans. b. It is lip and tip vitiligo (syn. acrofacial vitiligo). It refers to involvement of finger tips and perioral region. It is least responsive to the medical treatment due to absence of hair.
- Leukoderma is commonly used term by laymen. It implies acquired depigmentation of skin irrespective of etiology, e.g., vitiligo, depigmentation after using bindi *(MCQ 474)*, etc.
- Generalized vitiligo (vitiligo vulgaris) is common type of vitiligo. It comprises widespread involvement in a symmetrical manner *(MCQ 511)*.
- Universal vitiligo refers to involvement of >90% of body surface *(MCQ 638)*.

456. Ans. b. It is pompholyx manifesting as vesicles on the sides of fingers.
- Herpetic whitlow is an infection of herpes simplex virus. It presents as painful single or

group of vesicles on the nail fold close to nail affecting typically fingers or thumb
- Id eruption is a pompholyx like vesicles on the sides of fingers *(MCQ 180)*. It is an auto-eczematisation in response to distant fungal or bacterial infection.
- Infected scabies involves finger webs rather than sides of fingers *(MCQ 62)*. Moreover, it will accompany genital involvement.

457. **Ans. b. It is a condylomata lata which is a manifestation of secondary syphilis. It manifests at mucocutaneous junctions, e.g., vulva, anal region, in the groins** *(MCQ 287)*, **etc. It is highly infectious. VDRL, HIV, HCV and HBsAg must be done in all STD patients.**
    - Condylomata acuminata is caused by HPV virus. It presents as soft, pink and digitate lesions *(MCQ 496)*.
    - Chancroid presents as multiple painful ulcers *(MCQ 489)*.
    - Herpes infection presents as grouped vesicular lesions *(MCQs 445, 471, 512)*.

458. **Ans. b. It is acute paronychia presenting as severe pain and tenderness. It is evident by presence of localized pus which usually points close to the nail. It needs immediate drainage.**
    - Glomus tumour is a nail bed vascular tumour that presents as spontaneous pain in relation to nail bed. A bluish or small red patch can be seen under the nail plate.
    - Chronic paronychia presents as redness of posterior nail fold with loss of cuticle. Nail plate shows discoloration and formation of irregular transverse ridges *(MCQ 481)*.
    - Herpetic whitlow is a herpetic paronychia caused by primary inoculation of herpes virus. It presents as very painful single or a group of vesicles on the nail fold close to nail.

459. **Ans. d. Recurrence of herpes zoster is rare and is always alarming. Always rule out underlying HIV infection and lymphoreticular disorders if patient is having one of the following presentations.**
    - Recurrence of herpes zoster *(MCQ 353)*
    - Simultaneous involvement of two sites *(MCQ 30)*
    - Bilateral involvement *(MCQ 42)*
    - Disseminated herpes zoster *(MCQ 879)*

460. **Ans. c. It is tinea unguium. Infective pathology usually affects asymmetrically.**
    - Nail changes in LP includes pterygium formation *(MCQ 31)*, longitudinal striations *(MCQ 112)*.
    - Typical psoriatic nail changes are yellow discoloration, subungual hyperkeratosis *(MCQ 38)* and coarse pitting of nail plate *(MCQ 119)*.
    - In Darier's disease, red longitudinal band and V-shaped notch at the free margin of nail is characteristic *(MCQ 178)*.

461. **Ans. d. He is having tuberculoid leprosy which has highest immunity. So, lesions are very small in number and are well defined with loss of sensations.**
    - Indeterminate leprosy refers to early transitory stage of leprosy whose immunological status not yet determined. It presents as an ill-defined macule.
    - Histoid leprosy is a multibacillary leprosy which presents as crop of asymptomatic, smooth glistening, firm and non-tender papules *(MCQ 47)*.
    - Lepromatous leprosy has least immunity. So, it presents with huge number of small lesions *(MCQ 155)*. Infiltration of ears is very common feature *(MCQ 101)*.

462. **Ans. c. It is ingrown toe nail in which edge of nail plate has grown into lateral nail fold. Big toe is mostly likely to be affected. Partial or complete avulsion of nail plate is usually required.**
    - Chronic paronychia is characterized by loss of cuticle, redness of posterior nail fold and dystrophy of nail plate *(MCQ 481)*.
    - Tinea unguium is characterized by thickening and roughening of nail plate with subungual hyperkeratosis *(MCQ 22)*.
    - Acute paronychia is associated with severe pain with or without localization of pus. Nail plate has not grown in to nail fold and full nail plate will be visible *(MCQ 458)*.

463. **Ans. b. These are black comedones (black heads) which are commonly seen in acne. These are not unique for acne because they can be seen in other disorders also, e.g., senile comedones** *(MCQ 28)*.
    - White comedones are slightly elevated papules which are also seen in acne *(MCQ 415)*.
    - Milia are 1–2 mm sized uniform dome-shaped white papules with non-umbilicated top. These are commonly located on cheeks and eye lids *(MCQ 48)*.
    - DPN is a variant of seborrheic keratosis. It presents as small dark brown papules *(MCQ 228)*. They do not have any keratotic impaction in the center.

464. **Ans. b.** The closest clinical diagnosis is superficial spreading melanoma. It is having all the features of the acronym ABCDE devised for its diagnosis. Melanoma is highly malignant. In this patient, it is difficult to excise and manage it.
    ❖ Extramammary Paget's disease (EMPD) affects the apocrine bearing sites, e.g., vulva, perianal region, scrotum and penis. Though vulva is most common to be affected. But it presents as moist, well defined, red and scaly patch.
    ❖ SCC presents as exophytic cauliflower like or as nodule or red erosive plaque *(MCQ 113)*.
    ❖ BCC and SCC are seen in sun exposed areas. BCC is common around the ear, eye and nose *(MCQ 193)*.

465. **Ans. b.** It is pyogenic granuloma which is a rapidly developed vascular nodule at the site of recent penetrating injury. Finger, forehead, cheeks and upper lip are the common sites.
    ❖ Single wart usually cannot be so large. Warts are usually multiple *(MCQ 392)*.
    ❖ Strawberry hemangioma appears in first month of life as scarlet red single tumor *(MCQ 189)*.
    ❖ Keratoacanthoma is seen in middle aged person on sun exposed sites *(MCQ 108)*.

466. **Ans. a.** It is infantile seborrheic dermatitis which usually manifests by the 3 months of age. It spontaneously disappears by the age of 8 months. Fine, white greasy scales are typical.
    ❖ Atopic dermatitis usually manifests after 3 months of age. Face is commonly involved *(MCQ 174)*.
    ❖ Tinea capitis is not common at this age. It presents as patchy hair loss *(MCQ 8)*.
    ❖ Cradle cap is a common clinical form of infantile seborrheic dermatitis. It manifests as adherent greasy scales on scalp *(MCQ 168)*.

467. **Ans. b.** It is malar rash (butterfly rash) which is considered as a specific lesion of SLE (seen in 80% of patients). It spares the involvement of nasolabial folds.
    ❖ In dermatomyositis, it does not spare the nasolabial folds and one third of patients have Gottron's papules over knuckles.
    ❖ PLE manifests within few hours of sun exposure with many morphological lesions, namely papules, vesicles, EM like lesions on sun exposed areas of face *(MCQ 198)*.
    ❖ Melasma is dark skin coloration on sun exposed areas on face. It is symmetrically distributed on cheeks having irregular borders. Erythema is not its feature *(MCQ 23)*.

468. **Ans. a.** It is a typical case of alopecia areata with a well defined, smooth, totally bald patch.
    ❖ Tinea barbae will present as patch with raised red inflamed border.
    ❖ Alopecia totalis is a variant of alopecia areata. It refers to loss of all scalp hairs.
    ❖ Ophiasis refers to loss of hair in a band like pattern along the margins of scalp *(MCQ 297)*. It is seen in children and is recalcitrant to treat.

469. **Ans. a.** It is condylomata acuminata which is caused by HPV. Its incubation period is 3 weeks to 8 months. HPV-16 and HPV-18 types are high risk types which are present in majority of cervical carcinomas. VDRL, HIV, HCV and HBsAg should be done in all patients of STDs.
    ❖ Condylomata lata is a manifestation of secondary syphilis. It manifests as soft, flat, painless papules with oozing and maceration *(MCQ 457)*.
    ❖ Molluscum contagiosum presents as shiny, dome-shaped, discrete and umbilicated papules *(MCQ 510)*.
    ❖ Angiokeratoma of vulva presents as multiple, smooth surfaced vascular papules, which bleeds if traumatized *(MCQ 542)*.

470. **Ans. a.** It is tinea pedis. Well defined margins and unilateral involvement are good points in favor of tinea.
    ❖ Eczema is characterized by itching, oozing, crusting and recurrence *(MCQ 213)* and is usually bilateral.
    ❖ ACD will take the shape of shoes in both feet *(MCQ 202)*.
    ❖ Candidiasis is usually limited to soles *(MCQ 210)* or between toes *(MCQ 393)*.

471. **Ans. a.** It is primary genital herpes. Grouped tiny vesicles or superficial grouped erosions within an incubation period of 2–5 days is typical. VDRL, HIV, HBsAg and HCV should be done in all STD patients.
    ❖ H. zoster is characterized by many groups of tiny vesicles in a dermatome. It is preceded by pain not by sexual exposure *(MCQ 435)*.
    ❖ Chancroid is characterized by multiple, painful ulcers *(MCQ 489)*.
    ❖ Syphilitic chancre is characteristically a painless ulcer with an indurated base *(MCQ 453)*.

472. **Ans. c.** These are typical kissing lesions of *Paederus dermatitis*. The coelomic fluid released by the insect has touched the opposing surfaces of

popliteal fossa and has caused the mirror imaged lesions.
- ❖ Atopic dermatitis in popliteal fossae will involve the whole depth of popliteal *(MCQ 159)* fossae on both sides.
- ❖ Discoid eczema will manifest with discoid lesions with oozing and crusting on other body parts also, e.g., trunk and extremities.

473. **Ans. b. He is having acromegaly which is caused by excess of growth hormone. Prognathism, cutis verticis gyrata and acral hypertrophy are typical features of acromegaly.**
- ❖ Hypothyroid patient can present as acral hypertrophy. But, prognathism is not its feature. Face shows puffiness of lips, eyelids and cheeks *(MCQ 217)*.
- ❖ Cutis verticis gyrata alone can be an idiopathic finding. But, in combination with prognathism and acral hypertrophy it cannot be without cause.

474. **Ans. b. It is leukoderma due to bindi. Leukoderma is an acquired depigmentation due to some known cause. It is due to p-tertiary butylphenol (PTBP) which is an ingredient in adhesives used in sticker types of bindis. This chemical is a known melanotoxic agent.**
- ❖ It cannot be called as bindi vitiligo as the term vitiligo is used for an idiopathic acquired depigmentation.
- ❖ Focal vitiligo refers to single or two vitiligo macules in a limited area of body *(MCQ 246)*.
- ❖ Segmental vitiligo is limited to dermatome. Distribution of mandibular division of trigeminal nerve is most frequently affected area *(MCQ 181)*.

475. **Ans. b. These are white comedones (closed comedones) which are seen in acne patients. They form when dead skin cells and bacteria plug hair follicle.**
- ❖ Open comedones are slightly raised lesions with dark-colored keratotic follicular impaction in the center *(MCQ 463)*.
- ❖ Milia are 1–2 mm sized, uniform dome-shaped white papules with non-umbilicated top. These are commonly locally located on cheeks and eyelids *(MCQ 48)*.
- ❖ Syringoma presents as 1–3 mm size skin-colored papules in women affecting chiefly face *(MCQ 236)*.

476. **Ans. d. She is having borderline lepromatous leprosy which has very low immunity. So, she has >8 lesions but still countable.**
- ❖ Lichen planus comprises of violaceous and itchy papular lesions *(MCQ 21)*.
- ❖ Psoriasis comprises of red papules with white scaling *(MCQ 162)*.
- ❖ Discoid eczema comprises of itchy, coin shaped and wet lesions *(MCQ 194)*.

477. **Ans. c. It is miliaria rubra (heat rash) which is also common in infants. It is caused by obstruction of sweat gland ducts at the deeper level. It usually occurs on covered parts of skin.**
- ❖ TNPM papules and pustules have no surrounding erythema. They rupture easily leaving collarette of scales and pigmented macules.
- ❖ ETN presents as red macules with tiny papule or vesicle in the center. It is common on face *(MCQ 432)*.
- ❖ Scabies can present as papules and pustules which are not closely placed *(MCQ 59)*. It will accompany the involvement of soles *(MCQ 74)*.

478. **Ans. a. He is having Buerger's disease with typical h/o intermittent claudication (pain in legs). This disease is only seen in smokers.**
- ❖ Hypertensive ulcer is extremely painful, but with no history of intermittent claudication. It prefers the region just above the ankle in posterolateral aspect.
- ❖ Venous ulcer is seen on medial lower aspect on leg (gaiter area). Ulcer is shallow and have flat margins *(MCQ 532)*. Pain improves on leg elevation and rest.
- ❖ Arterial ulcer is seen on the toes as sharply defined punched out ulcers *(MCQ 514)*.

479. **Ans. a. She is having borderline lepromatous leprosy which has very low immunity. So, lesions are multiple (>8), but still countable.**
- ❖ Psoriasis comprises of red plaques studded with white scales *(MCQ 162)*.
- ❖ Eczema comprises of itching, lichenification and ill-defined margins *(MCQ 213)*.
- ❖ Lupus vulgaris comprises of usually single psoriasiform plaque with active margin at periphery and trailing scar in the center *(MCQ 256)*. If multiple, involvement will be asymmetrical *(MCQ 256)*.

480. **Ans. d. Asymmetrical involvement of nails suggests infective pathology. Well defined border of patch is typical of tinea.**
- ❖ Psoriasis will involve nails of both hands and is characterized by yellow coloration, subungual hyperkeratosis *(MCQ 88)*.
- ❖ Eczema of hands manifest as oozing, crusting and usually do not involve nails *(MCQ 220)*.

481. **Ans. a. It is chronic paronychia. Involvement of index and middle fingers, loss of cuticle, redness and swelling of nail folds are typical features. Dystrophy of nail plate is due to chronic inflammation of posterior nail fold.**
    - Tinea unguium presents as rough and thick nail plate with subungual hyperkeratosis. Involvement is asymmetrical and may be associated with tinea manuum *(MCQ 480)*.
    - Acute paronychia presents as painful swelling of nail fold with/without localized pus *(MCQ 458)*.
    - Nail psoriasis presents as yellowish discoloration, coarse pitting and subungual hyperkeratosis *(MCQ 119)*.

482. **Ans. c. It is psoriasis with typical red color and silvery white scaling.**
    - Lichen planus presents with purplish papular lesions *(MCQ 381)*.
    - Discoid eczema presents as itchy lesions with oozing and crusting *(MCQ 434)*.
    - Pityriasis rosea presents as crop of oval scaly lesions on trunk along the ribs forming a 'Christmas tree pattern' *(MCQ 161)*.

483. **Ans. a. It is Hailey-Hailey disease which is also known as chronic benign familial pemphigus. It is an autosomal dominant disease. There is formation of transient flaccid vesicles which have a tendency to spread peripherally. Fissured appearance is highly characteristic. Groins** *(MCQ 80)* **and axillae are most commonly involved.**
    - Intertrigo refers to mild redness, soreness, maceration with no sharply define margins. It is seen on the opposing surfaces of body folds in obese individuals *(MCQ 166)*.
    - Candidal intertrigo manifests as red maceration in body folds extending beyond the area of contact. It shows irregular fringed margins with satellite vesicles and pustules *(MCQ 253)*. Flexural psoriasis manifests as red color with white scales in flexural sites, e.g., groins *(MCQ 84)*.

484. **Ans. a. Large hands in this patient are as a part of general somatic hypertrophy due to excessive production of growth hormone (GH). GH also produces prognathism and cutis verticis gyrata.**
    - Acropachy refers to the dermopathy associated with Graves' disease. It is soft tissue swelling of hands along with clubbing of fingers. Metacarpal bones may show periostitis.
    - Insulin resistance can produce large hands. These patients will also have acanthosis nigricans.
    - Pachydermoperiostosis comprises of pachyderma (thick facial Skin), periostosis (periosteal new bone formation) hyperhidrosis and acropachia (digital clubbing).

485. **Ans. d. It is seborrheic capitis. Fine white scaling involving entire scalp is a classical presentation.**
    - Tinea capitis presents as patchy hair loss and scaling *(MCQ 8)*.
    - Psoriasis is characterized by patchy involvement with normal skin in between *(MCQ 314)*. Patches are red and studded with white scales.
    - AD typically involves face in almost all patients *(MCQ 174)*. Involvement of flexures of knees and elbows *(MCQs 159, 207)* is also very common.

486. **Ans. d. It is a typical case of plantar keratoderma.**
    - Psoriasis is characterized by reddish pink color and areas of normal skin in between *(MCQ 233)*.
    - Hyperkeratotic eczema is characterized by itching, thickening, fissuring *(MCQ 383)*.
    - DLE lesions are discrete and surrounded by a rim of hyperpigmentation *(MCQ 242)*.

487. **Ans. d. It is digital necrosis due to metoprolol. Beta-blockers inhibit vasodilatation and decreases peripheral blood flow. Characteristically, hands and feet of these patients are cold and do not respond to analgesics. These patients should be put on other antihypertensive drugs.**
    - FDE appears half an hour to 8 hours after administration of drug as dusky red macules *(MCQ 191)*.
    - Raynaud's phenomenon manifests as sequential color change (pallor, cyanosis and erythema) and usually affects more than one fingers. It is usually associated with the connective tissue diseases *(MCQ 496)*.
    - Buerger's disease manifests as gangrene and intermittent claudication in young male smokers *(MCQ 422)*.

488. **Ans. c. It is tuberculoid leprosy having very high immunity. So, number of patches is very few. Any cutaneous patch with loss of sensation is a cardinal feature for the diagnosis of leprosy.**
    - LL has lowest immunity. So, it comprises of numerous uncountable skin lesions *(MCQ 155)*.
    - Indeterminate leprosy refers to early transient stage whose immune status is yet to be determined. It presents as red or hypopigmented ill defined macule.

❖ Mid-borderline leprosy has its place in the mid of the two poles of leprosy and comprises of 4–8 lesions. Annular lesions are characteristic of this type *(MCQ 211)*.

489. **Ans. b. He is having chancroid (soft sore). Multiple, painful and non-indurated ulcers with an incubation of 3–10 days is typical of chancroid. VDRL, HIV, HBsAg and HCV should be done in all STD patients.**
   ❖ Syphilitic chancre is typically a painless with an indurated base *(MCQ 453)*.
   ❖ Lymphogranuloma venereum presents as small painless inconspicuous papule or ulcer that usually go unnoticed.
   ❖ Granuloma venereum ulcers are painless, elevated, granulomatous and bleeds easily.

490. **Ans. a. It is candidiasis. Long time exposure to water, predisposes to candidiasis. Interdigital web spaces between fingers and toes *(MCQ 393)* are commonly involved.**
   ❖ T. manuum manifests as asymmetrical involvement *(MCQ 45)*.
   ❖ Irritant or allergic contact dermatitis will show involvement of whole hand.
   ❖ Dry type housewife's dermatitis commonly involves dorsa of thumb, index finger and middle finger or entire palm *(MCQ 394)*.

491. **Ans. a. It is lichen planus of tongue with typical violaceous color of patches.**
   ❖ Scrotal tongue is a fissured tongue and is seen in 10% of normal individuals *(MCQ 530)*.
   ❖ Geographic tongue (benign migratory glossitis) is seen in 3% of general population. It is seen as bald red areas of varying sizes that are surrounded by white border *(MCQ 635)*. It is seen in Reiter's syndrome, diabetes, atopic dermatitis, etc.
   ❖ Oral leukoplakia is usually single and white plaque. OL on ventrolateral aspect of tongue is a high-risk site for SCC *(MCQ 251)*.

492. **Ans. a. It is subungual melanoma (advanced stage) that arises from tissues of nail bed. It needs early detection. A large pigmented lesion, irregular colors, broad band of pigmentation, ill defined edges, nail dystrophy and Hutchinson's sign (pigmentation of proximal nail fold) are the features which suggest a strong possibility of malignant melanoma. A positive history of injury does not rule out the possibility of melanoma.**
   ❖ Subungual hemorrhage may occur in adjacent nails also. Usually, subungual hematoma has a sharply demarcated curved proximal limit.
   ❖ Tinea unguium does not have swelling or black pigmentation and usually affects multiple nails *(MCQ 22)*.
   ❖ Glomus tumor is a rare benign tumor of glomus body, a thermoregulatory structure. It presents as triad of symptoms, i.e., pain, pinpoint tenderness and hypersensitivity to cold. The diagnosis is often difficult because it is small and situated deep in finger tip. Radiologically, it appears as mild indentation to scalloping of phalangeal cortex. It can present as bluish or small red patch under the nail plate.

493. **Ans. c. It is CCLE lower lip. The plaque is typically surrounded by a rim of hyperpigmentation. Brim of the nose and lower lip are commonly involved sun exposed sites.**
   ❖ Cheilitis simplex (common cheilitis, chapped lips) presents as cracking, fissuring and desquamation of lower lip. Frequent lip licking promotes it.
   ❖ Actinic cheilitis is caused by long-term sun exposure. It presents as very chapped lips *(MCQ 529)*. Later on, it may become white and scaly. If left untreated, it may cause SCC.
   ❖ Lichen planus of lip give a violaceous color *(MCQ 29)*.

494. **Ans. c. It is dermatitis artefacta which is a self-inflicted artificially produced cutaneous disease entirely by the action of a fully aware patient in an attempt to assume a patient's role. Patient intention is to seek emotional or psychological benefit.**
   ❖ Eczema shins is characterized by oozing and crusting *(MCQ 434)*.
   ❖ Diabetic dermopathy presents as brown scar like atrophic macules on shins *(MCQ 378)*.
   ❖ Pretibial myxedema presents as waxy looking indurated nonpitting nodules or plaques on anterolateral aspects of both legs. It is a manifestation of hyperthyroidism.

495. **Ans. d. He is a typical case of lepromatous leprosy having gloves and stockings type of anesthesia of hands and feet. Infiltration of both ear lobules is always due to lepromatous leprosy unless proved otherwise.**
   ❖ Urticarial swelling of ear lobules *(MCQ 194)* will be acute and will not last more than one day. It will be accompanied by wheals and itching on other body parts also.

- Myxedema patient can have loss of outer one third of eyebrow. But it presents characteristically with puffiness of face, eyelids and lips *(MCQ 217)*. There will be no loss of sensations of hands.
- In systemic sclerosis, calcinosis cutis at the tips of finger may give an impression of ulceration *(MCQ 496)*. But the patient will have mask like face *(MCQ 14)* with history of Raynaud's phenomenon.

496. Ans. b. It is Raynaud's phenomenon which is typically seen in patients of systemic sclerosis usually as the earliest and presenting feature.
- Chilblains presents as redness, swelling, itching and burning of fingers and toes on exposure to cold *(MCQ 409)*.
- Buerger's disease is an inflammation of smaller and medium sized arteries. It is seen in young smokers and manifests as intermittent claudication, ulcer and gangrene in distal part of extremities *(MCQ 478)*.
- DVT is noticed 7-10th day after major surgery. Patient complains of pain and swelling in the calf or in whole limb with swelling and dusky coloration. D-dimer test is highly sensitive, but is less specific for DVT.

497. Ans. b. It is milia neonatorum which is one of the most common transient skin conditions seen in the neonates. They are benign epidermal keratin cysts seen in nearly half of full-term neonates. It resolves spontaneously within few weeks of life.
- Sebaceous gland hyperplasia is seen as <1 mm sized yellow papules on nose, cheeks and chin where sebaceous gland density is highest.
- Neonatal acne is seen as tiny white or black, comedones on cheeks *(MCQ 405)*.
- TNPM is less common. It presents as tiny pustules and dark macules in mandibular area and forehead.

498. Ans. b. It is infected dermatitis. Here microorganisms or their by-products play a causative role in dermatitis. In this patient, it has developed around an infected wound. Infected dermatitis around a pus discharging ear canal is also a good example *(MCQ 360)*.
- Madura foot is deep fungal infection. It is characterized by chronic swelling of foot with sinuses having seropurulent discharge containing granules *(MCQ 272)*.
- Scrofuloderma is an endogenous skin tuberculosis. It is characterized by sinus with thin bluish margin and thin watery discharge *(MCQ 52)*.
- Impetigo contagiosa is seen in children with skin lesions having thick and dirty brown crusts *(MCQ 60)*.

499. Ans. c. Involvement of flexures behind knees and elbows is classically seen in childhood phase of AD.
- SD involves the seborrheic sites, e.g., scalp *(MCQ 485)*, nasolabial folds, axillae, groins, etc.
- Intertrigo comprises of diffuse macerated erythema involving opposing surfaces of body folds in obese persons *(MCQ 166)*.
- T. corporis comprises of patches with well defined active borders *(MCQ 142)*.

500. Ans. c. She is having dermatitis artefacta. These are inflicted by herself in an attempt to assume a patient role. She needs psychological treatment from psychiatrist. Left hand is easy approachable for her right hand. Lesions are not fitting into any other dermatological condition.
- Lichen planus comprises of violaceous, pruritic papular lesions *(MCQ 29)*.
- Discoid eczema lesions will be oozy, discoid or coin shaped *(MCQ 194)*.
- Housewife contact dermatitis of wet type will show eczema on dorsa of both hands *(MCQ 413)*.

501. Ans. a. It is widespread or extensive urticaria. Urticaria is characterized by wheals that disappear within 24 hours and reappear at other sites.
- Exanthematous rash (morbilliform rash) is maculopapular rash that usually develop 1-2 weeks after the initiation of drug therapy *(MCQ 238)*. Wheals are not its feature.
- Erythroderma comprises of redness, itching and scaling *(MCQ 257)*.
- Patch stage of mycosis fungoides presents as multiple red or violet red patches that favor non-sun exposed parts of body *(MCQ 254)*.

502. Ans. b. It is en coup de sabre which is a linear type of localized morphea. It gives a resemblance to sabre cut. So, it is named so. Morphea refers to sclerosis of skin without systemic involvement.
- Lichen sclerosus et atrophicus presents as small asymptomatic Ivory white round macules or papules on trunk especially around umbilicus *(MCQ 270)*.
- Scleredema presents as non-pitting, symmetrical, cutaneous induration with no sharp demarcation between involved and uninvolved skin. Epidermis can be pinched off between thumb and index finger indicating that epidermis is normal.

- Dermatomyositis characteristic lesion comprises of confluent macular violaceous erythema on eyelids, cheeks, temples and forehead.

503. **Ans. b. It is perioral dermatitis. Application of potent topical steroid cream around mouth is a common etiological factor.**
     - Gram-negative folliculitis usually occurs in patients with existing acne. It presents as superficial follicular pustules with surrounding redness.
     - LMDF presents as papules with no pustules or comedones *(MCQ 417)*.
     - Acne rosacea lesions are seen in middle-aged female in central part of face with persistent facial erythema *(MCQ 50)*.
     - Lip-lick cheilitis is a moist fissured eczema adjoining the vermilion border *(MCQ 93)*. It is attributed to the habit of lip-licking.

504. **Ans. b. It is eczema shins having itching, oozing and crusting.**
     - Psoriasis comprises of red plaques studded with white scales *(MCQ 162)*.
     - Lichen planus presents as purplish papular lesions *(MCQ 381)*.
     - Diabetic dermopathy presents as brown scar like atrophic macules on shins *(MCQ 378)*.

505. **Ans. b. She is having borderline lepromatous leprosy which has very low immunity. So, number of skin lesions is multiple, i.e., >8. Still, it is countable.**
     - Lupus vulgaris presents as single or multiple psoriasiform plaques with active border at the periphery and trailing scar in the center *(MCQ 26)*.
     - Sarcoidosis presents as reddish-brown papules or nodules. Apple jelly nodules can be seen on diascopy.
     - Actinic lichen planus presents as well-defined annular lesions having deep hyperpigmented center and violaceous thread like peripheral rim *(MCQ 404)*.

506. **Ans. a. This child is having epidermolysis bullosa simplex having an autosomal dominant inheritance. Cleavage being intraepidermal, scarring is absent.**
     - Chronic benign familial pemphigus (Hailey-Hailey disease) is also an autosomal dominant condition. It usually manifests in third or fourth decade as transient flaccid vesicles in groins or axillae and gives a typical fissured appearance *(MCQs 80, 483)*.
     - EB acquisita is seen in adults. Cleavage is subepidermal and blisters heal with scarring.
     - Fragility and blistering of sun exposed skin is a common feature of all cutaneous porphyrias.

507. **Ans. b. It is dry discoid eczema which is common in atopic individuals.**
     - Pityriasis rosea comprises of oval scaly lesions distributed along the ribs on trunk forming a 'Christmas-tree' pattern' *(MCQ 161)*.
     - Parapsoriasis comprises of red plaques that favor non-sun exposed sites, e.g., trunk, etc.
     - In senile eczema (asteatotic eczema) skin becomes dry, scaly with prominent and deep skin markings *(MCQ 94)*.

508. **Ans. c. These are rolling scars which are broad depressions with sloping edge to give a saucer shape.**
     - Macular scars are flat scars at skin level and seen primarily as discoloration of skin *(MCQ 543)*.
     - Anetoderma refers to flat thin atrophic scars due to loss of elastic tissue *(MCQ 565)*.
     - Boxcar scars are wider scars, round or oval in shape with vertical walls. They are found in areas like lower cheeks and jaw where skin is relatively thick *(MCQ 520)*.

509. **Ans. b. It is tinea incognito which refers to modified tinea infection which is not recognizable due to lack of typical clinical features. Picture is modified due to topical or systemic steroids. Branching septate hyphae in KOH smear are typically due to dermatophytes** *(MCQ 347)*.
     - Tinea corporis comprises of typical erythematous ring shaped or other shaped lesions with well defined active borders *(MCQ 142)*.
     - Pityriasis versicolor is common on back and shoulders and presents as hypopigmentation *(MCQ 39)*. KOH smear will show short filaments with group of spherical thick-walled spores *(MCQ 363)*.
     - Candidiasis presents as itchy red macerations in body folds. It develops fringed irregular margins with classical satellite vesicles and pustules *(MCQ 253)*. KOH smear will show pseudohyphae and spores appearing as bunch of grapes *(MCQ 644)*.

510. **Ans. b. It is molluscum contagiosum in the perineal region which is transmitted most likely by sexual contact.**
     - Genital warts have rough hyperkeratotic surface *(MCQ 562)*.
     - Skin tags at this site are usually not multiple *(MCQ 331)* and have narrow pedicle.
     - Scabies comprises of itchy small papules.

511. **Ans. c.** It is vitiligo vulgaris (syn. generalized vitiligo) which is most common type having widespread involvement in a symmetrical manner.
    - Leukoderma refers to acquired pigmentation due to some known cause *(MCQ 474)*.
    - Universal vitiligo refers to involvement of more than 90% of body surface *(MCQ 638)*.
    - Segmental vitiligo involves a dermatome. Area supplied by mandibular division of trigeminal nerve is most frequently affected *(MCQ 181)*.

512. **Ans. c.** It is recurrent herpes genitalis. It is difficult to prevent recurrence after the resolution of primary genital herpes. The virus persists in the roots of sacral plexus. Stress and fatigue can precipitate recurrence. Recurrent attacks are usually less severe. VDRL, HIV, HBsAg and HCV should be done in all STD patients.
    - Fixed drug eruption manifests as dusky red color *(MCQ 160)* and does not present as group of vesicles.
    - Candidal balanoposthitis presents as little soreness, erythema and collarette of white scales *(MCQ 38)*.
    - Lymphogranuloma venereum presents as small painless inconspicuous papule or ulcer which often go unnoticed. It does not have a recurrent presentation.

513. **Ans. a.** It is a dry type of housewife dermatitis. It affects palmar aspects of hands *(MCQ 394)* and extends to the dorsal side of thumb, index finger and middle finger.
    - Discoid eczema presents as disc or coin shaped lesions *(MCQ 194)*.
    - Tinea manuum usually has asymmetrical involvement and show well defined advancing border *(MCQ 480)*.
    - Infective dermatitis is an eczematization around an infected wound or an infected focus *(MCQ 360)*.

514. **Ans. d.** It is arterial ulcer. It is usually seen after the age of 45 and patient may not be smoker. He may complain of intermittent claudication. Pedal pulse may be absent or feeble.
    - Tuberculous ulcer has thin, bluish undermined margins with watery discharge *(MCQ 382)*.
    - Hypertensive ulcer is seen on posterolateral aspect of leg just above ankle. They are painful and have some relief with dependency.
    - Venous ulcer is seen in gaiter area with hyperpigmentation and varicose veins *(MCQ 532)*.

515. **Ans. d.** She is having tuberculoid leprosy. This type has highest immunity. So, has least number of skin lesions. Loss of sensations in skin lesions is a cardinal feature of leprosy.
    - Indeterminate leprosy refers to early and transient stage of leprosy. It presents as red or hypopigmented macule. When edges are palpable, it is no longer indeterminate leprosy.
    - Lupus vulgaris is a skin tuberculosis having moderate to high immunity. It presents as red soft gelatinous plaques. But it will not have loss of sensations *(MCQ 26)*.
    - Lepromatous leprosy has lowest immunity and will present with uncountable number of skin lesions *(MCQ 155)*.

516. **Ans. d.** It is superficial spreading melanoma fulfilling all the features according to the acronym ABCDE for the clinical diagnosis of melanoma.
    - Mongolian spots are bluish or slate brown-colored patches in the lumbosacral region of new born *(MCQ 151)*.
    - Bowen's disease presents as persistent red scaly or crusted plaque *(MCQ 226)*.
    - Extramammary Paget's disease presents as red, moist, persistent scaly eczematous patch in the region of vulva, groins, axillae and perineum.

517. **Ans. a.** It is butterfly rash due to SLE which is 8 times more common in females. It is characteristically sparing the nasolabial folds. Investigations should be done to find antinuclear, anti-DNA and anti-Smith antibodies.
    - Rash due to dermatomyositis will not spare nasolabial folds.
    - Melasma is a dark brown pigmentation with irregular borders. Redness is not a feature. Hair will be normal *(MCQ 598)*.
    - Nevus of Ota is usually unilateral. Rarely, it can be bilateral. It presents at birth as bluish gray coloration in the area supplied by first two divisions of trigeminal nerve. Cornea, sclera, Iris are also involved *(MCQ 158)*.

518. **Ans. a.** It is umbilical granuloma. It forms due to delayed separation of umbilical cord remnant and low-grade infection. Later, a salmon pink friable mass persists which is termed as umbilical granuloma. It is an overgrowth of granulomatous tissue that persists after separation of umbilical cord.
    - Umbilical hernia presents as small bulge near umbilicus. It becomes larger when the baby cries or coughs.

- Vitellointestinal duct forms a connection between umbilicus and ileum. It may remain patent and get prolapsed. These patients will present with intestinal obstruction or intussusceptions, etc.
- Umbilical polyp is rare congenital lesion resulting from persistence of omphalomesenteric duct.

519. **Ans. b. It is chronic paronychia which has caused dystrophy of nail plate. It is characterized by red glistening inflamed posterior nail folds.**
    - In tinea unguium, posterior nail fold will be normal. Nail plate becomes rough thickened with subungual hyperkeratosis. Involvement will be asymmetrical *(MCQ 22)*.
    - In LP, nails show increased longitudinal ridges *(MCQ 112)*. Pterygium formation is typical *(MCQ 31)*.
    - In psoriasis, nails show yellowish discoloration, subungual hyperkeratosis and onycholysis *(MCQ 88)*.

520. **Ans. b. These are boxcar scars which are wider than ice pick scars. They can be found in areas like lower cheeks and Jaw where skin is relatively thick.**
    - Anetoderma refers to flat thin macular atrophic scars due to loss of elastic tissue *(MCQ 565)*.
    - Macular scars are flat scars at skin level and seen primary as discoloration of skin *(MCQ 543)*
    - Hypertrophic scars are seen as pink raised and firm lesions due to excessive collagen deposition *(MCQ 533)*.

521. **Ans. c. It is por-twine-stain (nevus flammeus). It presents at birth as unilateral persistent pink, several centimetre sized macule in the distribution of sensory branch of trigeminal nerve. It usually persists throughout life.**
    - Strawberry hemangioma presents as round or oval smooth scarlet red single tumor. It is not present at birth but appears in first month of life *(MCQ 187)*.
    - Salmon patch presents as blanchable dull pinkish irregular macule on the nape of the neck, forehead, nose, etc. Lesion tends to disappear by the age of 1–2 years.
    - Cherry angioma is a most common vascular anomaly. It is seen as 1–6 mm sized cherry red colored firm papules after the age of 70 years *(MCQ 221)*.

522. **Ans. b. It is pityriasis versicolor with typical discrete satellite lesions at the margin. KOH smear is showing typical 'spaghetti and meat balls' appearance** *(MCQ 363)*.
    - Tinea corporis will have well defined margins. KOH will show branching septate hyphae *(MCQ 347)*.
    - Candidiasis clinically presents in body folds as soreness and wet maceration *(MCQ 253)*. KOH smear will show pseudohyphae and spores with bunch of grapes like appearance *(MCQ 644)*.
    - Pityriasis alba presents as irregular patch of hypopigmentation covered with powdery white scales. Face is common site *(MCQ 85)*. KOH will be negative.

523. **Ans. a. It is a typical presentation of superficial basal cell carcinoma presenting as well demarcated eczema like plaque, with thread like margin. The area near the eye, ear and nose are common sites.**
    - SCC usually arises on photo damaged skin *(MCQ 816)* and usually has a verrucous appearance or is an ulcerated one *(MCQs 255, 113)*.
    - Malignant melanoma usually has a black component and may abide by the features of acronym ABCDE *(MCQ 121)*.
    - Actinic keratosis comprises of multiple 1 mm to 2 cm sized macules having rough scaly surface. Lesions have adherent scale which can be removed with difficulty *(MCQ 123)*.

524. **Ans. b. It is *Paederus dermatitis* presenting typically as red patch having white necrotic slough in the center.**
    - Herpes zoster is usually preceded by pain. Rash comprises of group of vesicles on erythematous base *(MCQ 70)*.
    - Petechiae or purpura do not follow a linear pattern. Patches will not have a central slough *(MCQ 354)*.
    - Palpable purpura comprises of visible non-blanching hemorrhages. They are 1 mm to several centimetres sized raised lesions *(MCQ 527)*. They can be touched or felt on palpation. It is a kind of vasculitis secondary to some underlying serious disease. It is seen on lower extremities or dependent parts of body.

525. **Ans. b. It is lepromatous leprosy with scrofuloderma. Chronic infiltration of ears is always due to lepromatous leprosy unless proved otherwise. Sinuses with watery discharge over the underlying lymph nodes are due to scrofuloderma which is an endogenous type of tuberculosis. Both these diseases are of multibacillary type and are seen in a patient having very low immunity. It is rare to see tuberculosis and leprosy simultaneously in a patient.**
    - Urticaria can also present with swelling of ear lobules *(MCQs 194, 683)*. But it will have itching with remissions and relapses.

- Hidradenitis suppurativa is a disease of the areas of skin bearing apocrine glands characterized by abscesses, scarring and sinuses. It is seen in axillae *(MCQ 111)*, perianal region *(MCQ 343)* and groins *(MCQ 415)*.

526. **Ans. a. These are common warts having rough scaly surface and are in group. It is involving an isolated site.**
     - LPH presents as thick elevated, hyperkeratotic purplish plaque. Common sites are shin and ankle joint *(MCQ 20)*.
     - TVC presents as single plaque and margins may show finger like projections *(MCQ 10)*.
     - Keloids are often painful and non-scaly with firm to hard consistency. Common sites are chest *(MCQ 176)* upper back, shoulder, etc.

527. **Ans. b. It is palpable purpura which is due to small vessel cutaneous vasculitis. In majority of patients, it is idiopathic. In others, it can be due to some secondary cause. When purpuric lesions are palpable, they are called signature lesions or palpable purpura.**
     - HSP presents as purpuric lesions on the extensors of limbs and buttocks in a symmetrical manner *(MCQ 322)*.
     - ITP presents as petechiae when platelet count falls below 50,000 per mcL *(MCQ 354)*.
     - TTP presents with fever, hemolytic anemia and neurological symptoms. LDH level is increased.

528. **Ans. b. It is SCC sole. Exophytic and cauliflower appearance is typical of SCC.**
     - TVC is a type of skin tuberculosis having high immunity which presents as a dry and warty plaque. Bleeding and ulceration are not the features of TVC *(MCQ 620)*.
     - BCC presents in the area around eye, ear, and nose *(MCQ 198)*.
     - Madura foot is a deep mycosis which presents as painless, non-pitting swelling of foot. It is studded with multiple nodules and sinuses which discharge colored granules *(MCQ 272)*.

529. **Ans. b. It is actinic cheilitis which is caused by chronic ultraviolet exposure typically affecting lower lip obliterating vermilion border. It is a precancerous condition.**
     - Lichen planus shows violaceous coloration *(MCQ 29)*.
     - CCLE will show red plaque with peripheral border of hyperpigmentation *(MCQ 493)*.

530. **Ans. a. It is scrotal tongue (synonyms; furrowed tongue, plicated tongue, grooved tongue). It is usually present since birth but may not be noticed until gets older. If patient is also having granulomatous cheilitis and facial nerve palsy, then this triad is called 'Melkersson-Rosenthal syndrome'.**
     Geographic tongue (benign migratory glossitis) is seen in 3% of general population. It is seen as bald areas of varying sizes that are surrounded by white border *(MCQ 635)*. It is also seen in Reiter's disease, diabetes, atopic dermatitis, etc.

531. **Ans. d. He is having molluscum contagiosum with typical umbilicated papules.**
     - PPP consists of 1-3 mm sized flesh-colored papules in a row around coronal margin *(MCQ 290)*.
     - Scabies cannot be asymptomatic *(MCQ 291)*.
     - Fordyce spots are 1-3 mm sized uniform papules on penile skin *(MCQ 407)*.
     - Lichen nitidus presents as asymptomatic shiny, flat topped, discrete and pinpoint to pinhead sized papules on the shaft of penis *(MCQ 16)*.

532. **Ans. a. It is typical varicose ulcer in the medial lower aspect of leg (gaiter area) showing hyperpigmentation and varicose veins.**
     - Hypertensive ulcers are seen on posterolateral aspect of lower part of leg just above ankle. They are very painful and get some relief with dependency.
     - Arterial ulcer is seen on the toes as sharply defined punched out ulcer *(MCQ 514)*.
     - Tuberculous ulcers have thin bluish margin with watery discharge *(MCQ 382)*.

533. **Ans. a. The hypertrophic acne scars are seen as pink raised and firm lesions which are due to deposition of excessive collagen deposition.**
     - Anetoderma refers to flat thin macular atrophic scar due to loss of elastic tissue *(MCQ 565)*.
     - Boxcar scars are wider than ice pick scars. They are round or oval in shape with vertical walls. They are found in areas like lower cheeks and jaw where skin is relatively thick *(MCQ 520)*.
     - Macular scars are flat scars at skin level and are seen primarily as discoloration of skin *(MCQ 543)*.

534. **Ans. a. It is a plaque type lupus vulgaris presenting with a slowly evolving lesion having advancing polycyclic active margin. Buttock is one of the common sites for involvement. It shows a strongly positive tuberculin test.**
     - Psoriasis prefers extensor surfaces and manifests with silvery white scaling *(MCQ 162)*.

- Plaque of chronic cutaneous lupus erythematosus prefers sun exposed sites *(MCQ 201)* and comprises of plaques with depigmented atrophic center and hyperpigmented border.
- Leishmaniasis is seen at bite prone sites. It has tendency for ulceration and crusting *(MCQ 237)*.

535. **Ans. a. It is a Becker's nevus (pigmented hairy epidermal nevus). It is usually first noticed during adolescence in the region of shoulder, chest and scapular region *(MCQ 338)*. It is thought to be androgen dependent and is usually unilateral.**
    - Localized hypertrichosis is irrespective of androgen dependent area and can be congenital *(MCQ 334)*.
    - Nevus of Ota manifests as hyperpigmentation on one side of face in the distribution of the first two divisions of trigeminal nerve *(MCQ 158)*.

536. **Ans. b. It is paraphimosis in which foreskin get trapped behind the glans penis and cannot be easily reduced back to its normal flaccid position covering the glans. It requires reduction at the earliest.**
    - Phimosis is a condition in which penile foreskin is too tight to be pulled back to reveal glans. It may cause difficulty in micturition.
    - Balanoposthitis is an inflammation of prepuce and glans.

537. **Ans. b. It is X-linked recessive ichthyosis which is rare and affects only males. Onset in 1st week of life, dark polygonal scales, sparing of cubital fossae in a male child are its typical features.**
    - Ichthyosis vulgaris manifests between 3–12 months of age. Scales are white or light colored. It spares characteristically diaper area *(MCQ 141)*.
    - Asteatotic eczema is seen in elders. Skin becomes dry scaly with deep skin markings with fine reticulate superficial fissures *(MCQ 94)*.
    - Atopic dermatitis patient has severe itching. Whole body skin becomes dry. Face is a commonest to be involved *(MCQ 174)*.

538. **Ans. b. This absorption of phalanges along with sclerosis of skin is due to systemic sclerosis. Phalangeal absorption is commonly associated with calcinosis.**
    - In lepromatous leprosy, distal phalanges may show absorption, but metacarpal and carpal bones remain unchanged *(MCQ 550)*.
    - In psoriatic arthritis, absorption of distal phalanx, increased joint space and sharp margins of bony surfaces, ulnar deviation of fingers are typical changes *(MCQ 310)*.
    - Hyperparathyroidism classically affects radial aspects of proximal and middle phalanges of 2nd and 3rd fingers.

539. **Ans. a. It is addisonian pigmentation which is caused by stimulant effect of ACTH on melanocytes. It causes pigmentation of sun exposed sites, scars and palmar creases. Pigmentation of oral mucous membrane is invariable.**
    - Peutz-Jeghers syndrome is characterized by pigmented macules in oral mucous membrane. In addition, there is a perioral lentiginosis around nose and mouth.
    - In Cushing's syndrome, body is making too much cortisol from adrenals or any tumor other than pituitary gland. It is called Cushing's disease, when too much cortisol is produced from primary pituitary pathology in which there is continuous secretion of ACTH and MSH. The patient will have symptoms associated with elevated level of serum corticosteroids, e.g., weight gain, diabetes, hypertension, osteoporosis, moon facies, etc.
    - Various drugs can induce mucocutaneous pigmentation in different patterns, e.g., tetracyclines, antimalarials, phenothiazines, OCPs, cytotoxic drugs, etc. Hydroxychloroquine typically triggers pigmentation of palatal mucosa.

540. **Ans. b. This gangrene is due atherosclerotic peripheral vascular disease. Diabetes, hypertension and atherosclerotic changes in an old patient are predisposing factors. Patient may or may not be a smoker.**
    - Buerger's disease is a peripheral vascular disease in a young smoker *(MCQs 422, 478)*.
    - Metoprolol is a beta blocker which can cause gangrene of mild degree in peripheral parts *(MCQ 487)*.
    - Vasopressors used in shock, sometime can cause symmetrical peripheral gangrenous changes.

541. **Ans. a. It is due to acute urticaria. Lips and eyelids are commonly involved. Subsidence within 24 hours is enough to make diagnosis of urticaria. Urticarial lesions on other parts of body may not be there.**
    - Itching is not a feature of angioedema because it involves deeper layer of skin. It is rather painful. It may involve eyes, lips *(MCQ 296)*, larynx and tongue and may cause breathing difficulty.
    - Cheilitis glandularis presents as painless enlargement of lower lip in an elderly person. It is due to inflammation of minor salivary gland ducts.

- Granulomatous cheilitis manifests as acute symmetric swelling of upper lip without any itching. Later on, scaling, fissuring and erosions may develop.

542. **Ans. b. It is genitogluteal porokeratosis. The peripheral threadlike raised border is typical. Histopathological examination *(MCQ 1049)* typically shows coronoid lamella as a column of tightly packed parakeratotic keratinocytes within a keratin filled invagination of epidermis.**
    - Genital warts are non-itchy pedunculated, filiform or digitate lesions. The lesions may fuse to form cauliflower masses *(MCQ 935)*.
    - Condylomata lata presents as flat-topped papules with oozing and macerations *(MCQ 457)*.
    - Molluscum contagiosum presents as discrete, dome-shaped, shiny and umbilicated papules *(MCQ 510)*.

543. **Ans. a. These are macular scars which are flat scars at skin level and seen primarily as discoloration of skin.**
    - Hypertrophic scars are seen as pink, raised and firm lesions due to excessive collagen deposition *(MCQ 533)*.
    - Anetoderma refers to flat, thin, macular atrophic scars due to loss of elastic tissue *(MCQ 565)*.
    - Boxcar scars are wider than Ice pick scars. They are round or oval in shape with vertical walls. They are found in the area of lower cheeks and jaw *(MCQ 520)*.

544. **Ans. b. It is a typical case of acute hemorrhagic edema of infancy (AHEI). It is rare small vessel vasculitis which is seen under the age of two years. It is characterized by cocade (rosette) pattern purpuric targetoid lesions predominantly on cheeks, ears and extremities. Mucosa and trunk are spared with no systemic or visceral involvement. Spontaneous recovery occurs within few weeks.**
    - HSP presents as purpuric lesions on extensors of limbs and buttocks *(MCQ 354)* in a symmetrical manner.
    - Term palpable purpura is used when purpuric lesions are palpable and can be felt upon palpation. It is common on limbs *(MCQ 527)*.
    - ITP presents as petechiae when platelet count falls below 50,000 mcL *(MCQ 354)*.

545. **Ans. b. These atrophic changes on glans and under surface of prepuce are due to prolonged self application of steroid cream by the patient. Topical steroids are known to cause atrophy *(MCQs 13, 23)*.**
    - FDE is an acute presentation that comprises of dusky red coloration *(MCQ 160)*.
    - Candidal balanoposthitis is characterized by redness and white flakes *(MCQ 38)*.
    - Secondary syphilis mucous patches are shallow rounded, painless and edged by dull red areola. It also presents as condylomata lata in the anal and groin regions *(MCQ 287)*.

546. **Ans. c. It is oral submucosal fibrosis due to betel quid chewing. It is a chronic irreversible condition caused by areca nut which is a component of betel quid. In later stages, patient may have leukoplakia which is precancerous.**
    - Scleroderma patient presents as thin lips and perioral radiating furrows giving a "fish mouth" or "purse string" appearance to oral opening *(MCQ 454)*.
    - Smoker's melanosis causes brown to black pigmentation of oral tissues, i.e., gums, palate, cheeks, larynx, etc. Lower labial gingiva is typically involved. It does not cause difficulty in opening of mouth.

547. **Ans. a. It is herpes zoster with typical morphology of lesions. There is history of chickenpox in mother during 6th month of pregnancy.**
    - Chickenpox is characterized by discrete vesicular lesions with surrounding erythema on trunk and extremities *(MCQ 12)*.
    - *Paederus dermatitis* comprises of overnight eruption of red and edematous rash usually of linear type. Characteristically, there is a grayish white necrotic slough in the center of the rash *(MCQ 144)*.
    - Lymphangioma circumscriptum is noticed at birth or in the childhood as grouped vesicles with watery or blood-stained discharge from vesicles *(MCQ 106)*.

548. **Ans. b. It is a gluteal abscess which requires incision and drainage.**
    - Sebaceous cyst is generally seen in young and middle-aged persons. It is rare in children. It is not painful unless infected. It is seen as elastic dome-shaped swelling with the punctum *(MCQ 278)*.
    - Strawberry hemangioma presents as sharply circumscribed painless scarlet red single tumor. It appears in first month of life *(MCQ 187)*.
    - Cellulitis presents as painful red indurated plaque with indistinct margin *(MCQ 66)*.

549. **Ans. a.** It is idiopathic thrombocytopenic purpura which is commonly seen in children. Thrombocytopenia <50,000/mcL usually causes petechiae. Spontaneous remission is expected in the most of the children.
    - Henoch-Schonlein purpura is also common in children. But it is seen as net like pattern of purpuric lesions on extensors of lower limbs, buttocks in a symmetrical manner *(MCQ 332)*.
    - Dermatitis artefacta is a self-inflicted condition by the patient. The lesions suddenly appear overnight in the geometric shapes or angulated *(MCQ 494)*. They are not of purpuric type.
    - TTP presents with the fever, hemolytic anemia and neurological symptoms.

550. **Ans. a.** This deformity is due to lepromatous leprosy in which metacarpal and carpal bones remain unchanged. It is accompanied by loss of sensations.
    - In systemic sclerosis, it is accompanied by tight bound skin and Raynaud's phenomenon *(MCQ 538)*.
    - Hyperthyroidism classically affects radial aspects of proximal and middle phalanges of 2nd and 3rd fingers.
    - Psoriatic arthritis shows typically resorption of distal phalanx, increased joint space, sharp margins of bony surfaces and ulnar deviation of fingers.

551. **Ans. b.** It is an addisonian pigmentation which is caused by stimulant effect of ACTH on the melanocytes. Intraoral pigmentation is considered as initial sign. It causes pigmentation of sun exposed sites, palmar creases and oral mucous membrane.
    - Peutz-Jeghers syndrome comprises of pigmented macules in oral mucosa. In addition, there is perioral lentiginosis around nose and mouth.
    - Cushing's disease is caused by continuous secretion of ACTH and MSH by pituitary pathology. The patient will have symptoms associated with elevated levels of serum corticosteroids, e.g., weight gain, hypertension, osteoporosis, moon facies, etc.
    - Various drugs can induce mucocutaneous pigmentation in different pattern, e.g., Tetracyclines, antimalarials, phenothiazines. OCPs, cytotoxic drugs, etc. Hydroxychloroquine typically triggers pigmentation of palatal mucosa.

552. **Ans. b.** It is seborrheic dermatitis which is characteristically showing redness and fine scaling involving the seborrheic sites.
    - Atopic dermatitis prefers involvement of cubital and popliteal fossae. Face involvement usually accompanies neck involvement *(MCQ 596)*.
    - For tinea faciei, redness is a prominent feature. Itching with little scaling are also accompanying features *(MCQ 400)*.
    - Psoriasis on face is very uncommon. If there, it will manifest with red plaques with white scaling *(MCQ 268)*.

553. **Ans. c.** It is scalp psoriasis showing patchy involvement. Neighboring area is uninvolved. Plaque is red and scales are silvery white.
    - Pityriasis amiantacea is a variant of seborrheic dermatitis in which scales are large and dry which get separated from the scalp but remain entangled in hairs *(MCQ 87)*.
    - Seborrheic capitis is characterized by visible desquamating scales. Involvement is diffuse and confined to scalp *(MCQ 485)*.
    - Tinea capitis is very uncommon in adults. It may present as hair loss or as inflammatory boggy swelling *(MCQs 8, 11)*.

554. **Ans. a.** It is seborrheic dermatitis. Involvement is diffuse with ill defined margins. Involvement of depths of skin folds favors the diagnosis of seborrheic dermatitis.
    - Diaper dermatitis involvement is limited to the area of contact of diaper and spares the depth of skin folds *(MCQ 424)*.
    - Candidiasis manifests as itchy red macerations with fringed irregular margins and classical satellite vesicles and pustules *(MCQ 253)*.
    - *T. cruris* will manifest as well defined raised, active borders and central clearing *(MCQ 4)*.

555. **Ans. a.** It is Hailey-Hailey disease (familial benign chronic pemphigus). It is an autosomal dominant condition. Fissured appearance is highly characteristic.
    - Candidal intertrigo comprises of red, wet, maceration having fringed irregular margin with classical satellite vesicles and pustules *(MCQ 253)*.
    - Discoid eczema comprises of multiple coin shaped lesions on extremities *(MCQ 194)* and trunk. Eczema usually accompanies itching, but not pain.

Chapter 5 ✦ Answers of MCQs in Dermatology, Venereology and Leprology

556. **Ans. c. It is dermatitis buttocks.**
    ❖ Psoriasis is characterized by red plaques with silvery white scaling *(MCQ 162)* and it prefers extensors. Itching is not an important feature of psoriasis.
    ❖ Tinea manifests with well defined active borders with central clearing *(MCQ 4)*.
    ❖ Candidiasis prefers flexures *(MCQ 253)*.

557. **Ans. a. It is psoriasis in the beard region. Psoriasis on beard or face is uncommon.**
    ❖ Seborrheic dermatitis is characterized by fine greasy scales *(MCQ 566)*.
    ❖ Tinea faciei presents as well-defined plaque *(MCQ 241)* or erythema, scaling and itching *(MCQ 400)*.

558. **Ans. c. It is carbuncle. Because of multiple openings, it is typically giving an appearance of a sieve. Underlying diabetes should be ruled out.**
    ❖ Superficial folliculitis refers to pyogenic infection confined to osteum of hair follicle and presents as pustules *(MCQ 593)*.
    ❖ Boil is a pyogenic infection of a single hair follicle. It comprises of folliculitis and perifolliculitis *(MCQ 584)*.

559. **Ans. a. It is scrofuloderma having bluish margin and watery discharge.**
    ❖ Pyoderma gangrenosum presents as a painful ulcer with surrounding zone of erythema *(MCQ 367)*.
    ❖ Trophic ulcer refers to pressure ulcer due to external trauma to the part of body that is in poor condition, e.g., loss of sensation in leprosy *(MCQ 536)* or due to vascular insufficiency *(MCQ 536)*.

560. **Ans. a. It is discoid eczema back. Itching, oozing and crusting are the features of eczema.**
    ❖ Psoriasis is characterized by red plaques studded with white scales *(MCQ 146)*.
    ❖ Tinea corporis comprises of lesions with well defined active borders. Center may show clearing *(MCQ 40)*.
    ❖ Seborrheic dermatitis manifests as greasy scales or circular sharply defined patches with fine scaling *(MCQ 212)*.

561. **Ans. c. It is dermatitis or eczema groins characterized by oozing and ill-defined margins.**
    ❖ Intertrigo is an inflammation of opposing surfaces of body folds. It is usually seen in obese patients. Its involvement is limited to the area of contact of surfaces *(MCQ 166)*.
    ❖ Tinea cruris shows well defined active borders with central clearing *(MCQ 4)*.
    ❖ Candidiasis shows itchy red maceration in body folds extending beyond the area of contact *(MCQ 179)* and develops fringed irregular margins with satellite vesicles and pustules.

562. **Ans. b. These are perineal venereal warts caused by HPV virus. HPV-16 and HPV-18 types are high risk types which are found in majority of cervical carcinomas. VDRL, HIV, HCV and HBs Ag must be done in all STD patients.**
    ❖ Skin tags are usually not multiple and have narrow pedicle and smooth surface *(MCQ 331)*.
    ❖ Molluscum contagiosum comprises of shiny, dome-shaped, umbilicated papules *(MCQ 510)*.

563. **Ans. b. It is trophic ulcer in a leprosy patient. It is referred as pressure ulcer due to external trauma to the part of body that is in poor condition because of vascular insufficiency, loss of sensations, etc. Plantar surface of big toe *(MCQ 689)* is most common site of trophic ulcer due to leprosy. Head of first metatarsal is second most common site.**
    ❖ Tropical ulcer is painful rapidly enlarging ulcer seen on lower limb in person living in hot and humid tropical region.
    ❖ Arterial ulcer presents as painful ulcer at tips of toes and lateral aspects of heels and calves *(MCQ 514)*.

564. **Ans. b. It is tuberculosis verrucosa cutis which is a type of cutaneous tuberculosis having high degree of immunity. White atrophic central scarring is a feature in large plaques.**
    ❖ Plantar warts present as deep seated rough hyperkeratotic lesions which do not coalesce *(MCQ 579)*.
    ❖ Lupus vulgaris presents as reddish-brown soft gelatinous plaques. Head, neck, buttocks and trunk are common sites *(MCQs 26, 57)*.
    ❖ Madura foot presents as firm swelling of foot. The surface is studded with nodules and sinuses which discharge granules of different colors *(MCQ 272)*.

565. **Ans. a. He is having anetoderma. These are flat thin macular atrophic scars due to loss of elastic tissue.**
    ❖ Rolling scars are broad depressions with slopping edge to give a saucer shape *(MCQ 508)*.
    ❖ Macular scars are flat scars at skin level and are seen primarily as discoloration of skin *(MCQ 543)*. Unlike anetoderma, there is no atrophy.

- Boxcar scars are wider than ice pick scars. They are round or oval in shape with vertical walls. They are found in areas like lower cheeks and jaw where skin is relatively thick *(MCQ 520)*.

566. **Ans. b.** It is seborrheic dermatitis characterized by fine greasy scales.
     - Psoriasis in the beard region presents as red plaques studded with silvery white scales *(MCQ 566)*.
     - Tinea faciei presents as patch with well defined borders *(MCQ 241)*.

567. **Ans. d.** It is atopic dermatitis. These changes in cervical region are referred as 'atopic dirty neck'.
     - Acanthosis nigricans is seen in obese persons due to insulin resistance. It does not cause itching *(MCQ 273)*.
     - Seborrheic dermatitis does not involve cervical region. It involves seborrheic sites, e.g., nasolabial folds, eye lashes *(MCQ 171)*, etc.
     - Darier's disease presents as multiple, firm, papules which are skin or gray colored. It involves the seborrheic sites *(MCQ 267)*.

568. **Ans. b.** It is condylomata acuminata. It is caused by HPV-6, 11, 16 and HPV-18. HPV-16 and 18 are high risk types which are associated with cervical carcinoma. VDRL, HIV, HBsAg and HCV should be done in all STD patients.
     - Condylomata lata is a manifestation of secondary syphilis. It presents as flesh colored, flat topped sessile papules with oozing and macerations *(MCQ 457)*.
     - Molluscum contagiosum comprises of discrete, dome-shaped, shiny umbilicated papules *(MCQ 510)*.
     - Angiokeratoma of vulva presents as asymptomatic, 1–5 mm sized, reddish or dark colored vascular papules on labia majora *(MCQ 542)*. It bleeds, if traumatized.

569. **Ans. c.** It is alopecia areata presenting typically as totally bald patches. Patches are smooth with no inflammation, scarring or atrophy. Thyroid testing should be done in this condition.
     - In tinea capitis, hair break at the surface of scalp leaving behind group of black dots *(MCQ 8)*.
     - Trichotillomania presents as patch of hair loss with the presence of firmly anchored partially broken hairs in bald area *(MCQ 128)*.
     - Telogen effluvium manifests as diffuse hair loss 3–4 months after some inciting event *(MCQ 163)*.

570. **Ans. a.** It is Raynaud's phenomenon which refers to abnormal sensitivity to cold. It manifests as pallor, cyanosis and erythema affecting more than one digit up to various levels. The secondary type is often due to connective tissue disorder. It results into trophic and ischemic changes on fingers.
     - Chilblains are due to persistent constriction of larger arterioles and dilatation of superficial vessels on exposure to cold *(MCQ 409)*. It is self limiting condition and subsides in 2–3 weeks. It does not leave behind any atrophic and ischemic changes in fingers.
     - Buerger's disease manifests as gangrenous changes in distal parts of extremities in young smokers *(MCQ 422)*.

571. **Ans. a.** It is psoriasis of soles characterized by red plaques with scaling. Scalp involvement also favors psoriasis.
     - Hyperkeratotic eczema is characterized by oozing, itching and crusting *(MCQ 137)*.
     - Focal palmoplantar keratoderma manifests as dark, thick and ill-defined areas at pressure site on soles *(MCQ 337)*. Redness and scaling are not its feature.
     - Tinea pedis presents as hyperkeratotic white scaling involving whole or part of sole with well defined border *(MCQ 423)*.

572. **Ans. a.** It is tinea incognito which refers to unrecognizable tinea infection. It is most commonly due to topical or systemic steroids. A border can be recognised on the right wrist. A huge number of filaments is seen in KOH smear *(MCQ 347)*.
     - Psoriasis is characterized by red plaques with white scaling.
     - Ichthyosis is characterized by fish like scales *(MCQ 90)*.
     - Senile eczema is characterized by dry scaly skin with prominent and deep skin markings *(MCQ 94)*.

573. **Ans. a.** It is epidermolytic palmoplantar keratoderma that shows epidermolytic changes in histology. It does not involve dorsal surface and has a sharp erythematous peripheral edge.
     Hyperkeratotic eczema appears late and is characterized by itching, oozing and crusting *(MCQ 137)*.

574. **Ans. b.** It is tinea manuum. It typically originates underneath the ring worn by the patient.

Chapter 5 ✦ Answers of MCQs in Dermatology, Venereology and Leprology

- Candidiasis involves multiple web spaces and presents as red maceration *(MCQ 183)*.
- Scabies also involves multiple web spaces and comprises of papules and pustules *(MCQ 62)*.
- Discoid eczema presents as discoid, wet and itchy plaques *(MCQ 194)*.

575. **Ans. d. It is candidiasis due to underlying diabetes.**
- Smegma is an accumulation of desquamated dead cells. It is cheese like and has off white color with unpleasant smell. It is physiological and needs frequent washing *(MCQ 280)*.
- Secondary syphilis presents as painless mucosal patches with no white flakes.
- Prolonged use of steroid can cause atrophic changes with easy bruising *(MCQ 545)*.

576. **Ans. b. He is a typical case of Darier's disease with typical skin lesions and nail changes. It is an autosomal dominant condition having characteristic histopathological changes.**
- Lichen planus patients can have longitudinal striations, but does not have V-shaped notch at free margin *(MCQ 112)*.
- Seborrheic dermatitis is characterized by fine greasy scales, not by papules *(MCQ 175)* and does not have any nail changes.
- Pseudo-acanthosis nigricans manifests as dark, velvety thickening limited to cervical and axillary regions *(MCQ 233)* in obese persons.

577. **Ans. b. It is herpes zoster. Pain, grouped vesicles on erythematous base and unilateral involvement are its typical features.**
- Herpes simplex presents as group of tiny vesicles at the angle of mouth *(MCQ 9)*, at genitals *(MCQ 445)*.
- Dermatitis herpetiformis is characterized by itching, not by pain. Grouped lesions are seen on back *(MCQs 261, 859, 884)* and extensor parts.
- *Paederus dermatitis* presents as red rash of linear or other shaped with grayish white necrotic slough in the center *(MCQ 524)*.

578. **Ans. a. It is vitiligo with typical egg white depigmented macules on wrist.**
- In lichen sclerosus et atrophicus foreskin becomes bluish white and is difficult to retract *(MCQ 320)*. Skin lesions are small ivory white macules *(MCQ 270)*.
- Steroid cream will cause atrophic changes *(MCQ 545)*.

579. **Ans. c. It is deep plantar warts. They are barely visible from skin surface. They do not coalesce and always remain discrete.**
- Corns are sharply circumscribed painful callosities over bony prominences *(MCQ 350)*.
- Superficial plantar warts coalesce to form large plaques *(MCQs 372, 397)*.
- Punctate keratoderma comprises of scattered discrete and round thickenings irrespective of pressure points. They will not depict central depression.

580. **Ans. c. It is *Paederus dermatitis* (syn. blister beetle dermatitis) which is a peculiar irritant dermatitis provoked by coelomic fluid released by the insect. These vesicles are due to potent vesicant action of pederin.**
- Chickenpox is characterized by crop of discrete vesicles having surrounding erythema *(MCQ 12)*.
- Herpes zoster comprises of painful eruption of grouped vesicles on erythematous base *(MCQ 577)*.
- Herpes simplex comprises of group of tiny vesicles at the angle of mouth *(MCQ 9)* or on genitals *(MCQ 445)*.

581. **Ans. c. It is pyogenic abscess on her face presenting as painful red swelling.**
- Sebaceous cyst presents as elastic dome-shaped swelling with central punctum *(MCQ 278)*.
- Acne cysts are seen as a part of severe nodular acne in the presence of other lesions of acne, e.g., papules, pustules, comedones, etc. *(MCQ 19)*.
- Cold abscess is a collection of pus in the absence of signs of inflammation, i.e., redness, pain. Its pathology is tubercular.

582. **Ans. b. It is a typical case of cutaneous small vessel vasculitis having purpuric patches on legs accompanied by pain and swelling.**
- Henoch-Schonlein purpura is characterized by retiform petechiae on lower limbs with or without pain abdomen *(MCQ 332)*. Lesions are self limiting in 1–4 weeks.
- ITP presents as bleeding gums or crop of petechiae when platelet count falls below 50,000 per mcL *(MCQ 342)*.
- Schamberg's disease (progressive pigmented purpuric dermatosis) presents as brown pigmentation that develops insidiously on legs *(MCQ 365)*.

583. **Ans. d.** It is due to trichotillomania in which patient has compulsive impulse to pull out his own hair. It shows the presence of firmly anchored partially broken hairs. It characteristically spares hairs from scalp margins and occipital region.
    - Androgenic alopecia in females comprises mainly three patterns; namely widening of central parting *(MCQ 190)*, diffuse central thinning *(MCQ 185)* and recession of frontotemporal hair line.
    - Telogen effluvium manifests 3–6 month after some inciting event as diffuse and excessive loss of hairs *(MCQ 163)*.
    - In SLE, hairs in the frontal region become coarse, dry and fragile. These short broken off hair are named as 'lupus hairs' *(MCQ 89)*.

584. **Ans. a.** It is a boil which comprises folliculitis and perifolliculitis. It is characterized by swelling and tenderness.
    - In folliculitis, infection is confined to follicle and presents as pustule at follicle *(MCQ 281)*.
    - Carbuncle presents as a tender, dome-shaped reddish hard lump. When suppuration occurs, it reveals multiple follicular openings giving an appearance of a sieve *(MCQs 157, 558)* because it involves multiple hair follicles.

585. **Ans. d.** It is eczema of the finger having itching, crusting and ill-defined margins.
    - Psoriasis comprises of well-defined red plaque with white scaling *(MCQ 233)*.
    - Herpetic whitlow comprises of group of tiny vesicles.
    - Tinea manuum comprises of well-defined lesion with white scales *(MCQ 574)*.

586. **Ans. a.** It is tuberculoid leprosy. It has highest immunity showing least involvement, manifesting with a single patch and thickening of a single nerve. It should be treated at the earliest to prevent the deformity.
    - Lepromatous leprosy has least immunity showing widespread involvement and presenting as uncountable cutaneous lesions *(MCQ 155)*.
    - Histoid leprosy is a variant of multibacillary leprosy. It presents as multiple, asymptomatic smooth glistening papules *(MCQ 47)*.
    - Indeterminate leprosy refers to early and transient stage of leprosy. It presents as red or hypopigmented macule.

587. **Ans. b.** It is characteristic presentation of *Paederus dermatitis* (syn. dermatitis linearis). It is a peculiar type of irritant dermatitis caused by the coelomic fluid released by the insect of genus pederus. Red linear lesions with grayish white necrotic slough in center are typical.
    - Dermatitis artefacta is a self inflicted artificially produced disease by fully aware patient on easily approachable sites, e.g., legs *(MCQ 494)*, upper extremity *(MCQ 189)*, hands *(MCQ 500)*.

588. **Ans. b.** These are eczematous plaques which are common in atopic child.
    - Psoriasis comprises of well-defined red plaques with white scaling *(MCQ 146)*.
    - Tinea corporis comprises of ring-shaped well-defined lesions with active borders *(MCQ 142)*.

589. **Ans. c.** It is alopecia areata presenting as normal looking smooth skin, with no inflammation or scarring or atrophy.
    - Trichotillomania is characterized by the presence of firmly anchored partially broken hairs in the bald areas. Scalp margin and occipital region are typically spared *(MCQ 128)*.
    - Androgenic alopecia in females has three patterns namely, widening of central parting *(MCQ 190)*, diffuse central thinning *(MCQ 185)* and recession of frontotemporal hair line.
    - Telogen effluvium manifests as diffuse hair loss 3–6 months after an inciting event *(MCQ 163)*.

590. **Ans. b.** It is chronic paronychia. There is loss of cuticle almost from all the nails. It is almost always seen in persons who indulge in wet work.
    - Tinea unguium shows asymmetrical involvement. Nail plate may become rough, thickened and show subungual hyperkeratosis *(MCQ 22)*.
    - Psoriasis shows yellow discoloration, onycholysis and subungual hyperkeratosis *(MCQ 88)*.
    - Koilonychia refers to the concave shape of nail plate both in transverse and longitudinal axes *(MCQs 124)*. Most commonly, it is associated with iron deficiency anemia.

591. **Ans. d.** It is a typical case of granuloma annulare. Extensor and dorsal aspects of extremities are sites of predilection.
    - Psoriasis is characterized by red plaques studded with white scales *(MCQ 162)*.
    - Mid-borderline type of Hansen's disease having multiple lesions will show impairment of sensations in the plaques *(MCQ 476)*.
    - Tinea corporis annular lesions will have itching and well-defined active borders *(MCQ 142)*.

592. Ans. c. It is onychophagia (nail biting) which is a temporary, non destructive, pathological oral habit and grooming disorder. It is characterized by uncontrollable nail biting which is destructive to fingernails and surrounding tissue. It is similar to trichotillomania. It is most common during adolescence.
- In LP, nails may show pterygium formation *(MCQ 31)*, increased longitudinal ridges *(MCQ 112)*.
- In koilonychias, nail plate becomes concave both along the transverse and longitudinal axes *(MCQ 124)*. Most commonly, it is seen in the iron deficiency anemia.

593. Ans. b. It is superficial folliculitis which refers to pyogenic infection confined to osteum of hair follicle.
- Boil is a painful swelling due to folliculitis and perifolliculitis *(MCQ 584)*.
- Carbuncle presents as a tender, dome-shaped, reddish and hard lump. When suppurates, it reveals multiple follicular openings giving an appearance of a sieve *(MCQs 157, 558)* because it involves multiple hair follicles.

594. Ans. b. It is *Paederus dermatitis* which is a peculiar irritant dermatitis caused by coelomic fluid of an insect belonging to the genus pederus. Characteristically, it is red rash having a grayish white necrotic slough in the center.
Herpes zoster is characterized by grouped vesicular lesions *(MCQ 577)*.

595. Ans. c. It is tinea faciei with corporis. Clinical picture is modified due to systemic steroids. Border is recognized on chest.
- ABCD is characterized by intractable itching and thickening of facial skin *(MCQ 86)*. White scaling is not its feature.
- PLE manifests within few hours of sun exposure. Lesions comprises of many morphological forms, e.g., papules, vesicles, EM like lesions *(MCQ 198)*.
- SD on face prefers nasolabial folds and eyelashes. It shows fine greasy scales *(MCQ 171)*.

596. Ans. b. It is adult phase atopic dermatitis which characteristically involves cervical region, cubital and popliteal fossae.
- In SD, seborrheic sites are predominantly involved, e.g., nasolabial folds *(MCQ 171)*, interscapular area, etc.
- ABCD involves whole face including upper eyelids, area under chin, but spares the back of neck. It presents as intractable itching, thickening and lichenification *(MCQ 86)*.
- CAD shows sharp cut-off from the covered areas, spares eye lids and depth of skin creases *(MCQ 196)*.

597. Ans. a. It is plaque type of lupus vulgaris having active peripheral margin with trailing scar. It shows a strongly positive tuberculin test.
- Psoriatic plaques are characterized by red color and white scaling *(MCQ 146)*.
- CCLE prefers sun exposed areas and is characterized by adherent scales and a peripheral rim of hyperpigmentation *(MCQ 201)*.
- Tuberculoid leprosy plaques are characterized by loss of sensations *(MCQ 6)*.

598. Ans. b. It is melasma which is a commonly acquired hypermelanosis on sun exposed areas of face. It has an irregular border and chiefly affects lip, cheeks, forehead and chin.
- Malar rash due to SLE spares nasolabial folds *(MCQs 25, 517)*. It consists of erythema rather than brownish pigmentation.
- Nevus of Ota is usually unilateral *(MCQ 158)*. Rarely, it can be bilateral *(MCQ 727)*. It presents as unilateral bluish gray hyperpigmentation in the distribution of first two divisions of trigeminal nerves. Cornea, sclera, iris are also involved.
- Dermatomyositis does not spare the nasolabial folds.

599. Ans. a. It is tuberculoid leprosy having highest immunity. So, skin lesions are least. Loss of sensations in a cutaneous plaque is a cardinal feature of leprosy.
- Lupus vulgaris is a type of skin tuberculosis. It can present as soft gelatinous plaque. But it will not have loss of sensations *(MCQ 57)*.
- Lepromatous leprosy has lowest immunity, so lesions are uncountable *(MCQ 101)*. These patients usually have infiltration of ears *(MCQ 101)*.
- Histoid leprosy is a variant of multibacillary leprosy. It presents as crop of asymptomatic smooth glistening papules *(MCQ 47)*.

600. Ans. a. It is plaque type lupus vulgaris on elbow having active advancing irregular border. It has very high immunity.
- Psoriasis do occur on elbow but usually does not occur only on single elbow and is characterized by easily removable silvery white scales *(MCQ 146)*.

- ❖ Leishmaniasis prefers exposed site and is usually characterized by ulceration and crusting *(MCQ 237)*.
- ❖ CCLE prefers sun exposed sites. Plaques have adherent scales *(MCQ 201)*.

601. Ans. c. It is psoriasis scalp with characteristic red color plaque with white scaling.
- ❖ Tinea capitis is very uncommon in adults on scalp. It is seen as patches of hair loss or as inflammatory boggy swelling *(MCQs 11, 8)*.
- ❖ Tuberculoid leprosy plaque will have loss of sensations *(MCQ 6)*.
- ❖ Lichen planus is characterized by papules not by big plaques *(MCQ 381)*.

602. Ans. b. It is pompholyx which is a type of endogenous eczema characterized by deep seated vesicles and itching.
- ❖ Tinea manuum is usually unilateral and is characterized by scaling with redness *(MCQ 45)*.
- ❖ Candidiasis usually presents as wet maceration in web spaces *(MCQ 490)*.
- ❖ Contact dermatitis due to cement usually affects dorsa of hands and fingers as eczematous lesion *(MCQ 225)*.

603. Ans. c. It is seborrheic capitis (syn. pityriasis capitis) which is a variant of scalp involvement by seborrheic dermatitis. It comprises of desquamating scales confined to scalp.
- ❖ Tinea capitis is seen usually in children and it is characterized by patches of hair loss *(MCQ 8)* or as inflammatory boggy swelling *(MCQ 11)*.
- ❖ Psoriasis comprises of discrete red plaques studded with white scaling leaving normal areas in between *(MCQ 100)*.

604. Ans. a. It is flexural psoriasis with dry red plaques with white scaling.
- ❖ Tinea corporis comprises of patches with well-defined active border *(MCQ 142)*.
- ❖ Intertrigo refers to an inflammation on the opposing surfaces of body fold. It does not extend beyond the area of contact *(MCQ 166)*.
- ❖ Candidiasis presents as itchy red maceration extending beyond the area of contact and develop irregular fringed margin with satellite vesicles and pustules *(MCQ 253)*.

605. Ans. c. It is port-wine stain (syn. nevus flammeus). It is ectatic dilatation of superficial dermal capillaries. It almost always presents at birth unilaterally in the distribution of sensory branches of trigeminal nerve.
- ❖ Salmon patch presents as blanchable pinkish red irregular macule comprised of fine linear telangiectasia. Nape of neck, eyelid, glabella, forehead are common sites.
- ❖ Strawberry hemangioma presents as sharply circumscribed round smooth single tumor. It does not present at birth but manifests in first month of life *(MCQ 187)*.
- ❖ Cherry angiomas (senile hemangiomas) are seen as circular slightly elevated 1-6 mm sized cherry red lesions mostly seen on trunk *(MCQ 221)*.

606. Ans. d. Terbinafine is safest as it is pregnancy category B drug.
Rest of the three agents are pregnancy category C drugs.

607. Ans. d. It is candidiasis groins and vulva. Increased frequency of micturition at night is a commonest symptom which suggests diabetes mellitus as cause for the candidiasis. Fringed margin and satellite vesiculopustules are typical for candidiasis.
- ❖ Tinea cruris manifests with well-defined active borders *(MCQ 4)*.
- ❖ Intertrigo refers to the inflammation of opposing surfaces of body folds which is limited to the area of contact of surfaces *(MCQ 166)*.
- ❖ Flexural psoriasis has well defined margins, red color and scaling *(MCQ 84)*.

608. Ans. b. It is chancroid (soft sore) that presents as multiple painful ulcers due to autoinoculation with an incubation period of 3-10 days.
- ❖ Primary syphilis presents as single painless ulcer *(MCQ 453)* with indurated base with an incubation period of 14-21 days.
- ❖ Donovanosis (syn. granuloma inguinale, granuloma venereum) presents as elevated velvety painless lesion that bleeds easily with an incubation period 1-5 weeks.
- ❖ Lymphogranuloma venereum manifests as transient, small, inconspicuous painless papule or vesicle. Inguinal lymph nodes may show sign of groove.

609. Ans. b. It is sebaceous nevus which is a hamartomatous nevus composed of sebaceous gland. It remains unchanged until puberty. Lifetime risk of malignant transformation is 5%.
- ❖ Warts on scalp are usually more than one and have narrow base *(MCQ 634)*.
- ❖ Tinea capitis presents as patches with partial hair loss *(MCQ 8)* or as inflammatory boggy swelling *(MCQ 11)*.

Chapter 5 ✦ Answers of MCQs in Dermatology, Venereology and Leprology

- Psoriasis presents as red discrete plaques with white scaling *(MCQ 100)*.

610. **Ans. a. It is *Paederus dermatitis* which is a peculiar irritant dermatitis due to coelomic fluid released by the insect of the genus *Paederus*. It is characterized by red patch with gray white slough in the center.**
Herpes zoster is characterized by grouped vesicles on erythematous base *(MCQ 477)*.

611. **Ans. b. These are common warts which are equally common on dorsa of hands *(MCQ 169)*.**
    - Lichen planus presents as itchy violaceous papules *(MCQ 231)*.
    - Molluscum contagiosum presents as shiny dome-shaped umbilicated papules *(MCQ 209)*.
    - Tuberculosis verrucosa cutis is a type of cutaneous tuberculosis which presents as a single hyperkeratotic plaque *(MCQ 640)*. It does not present as multiple small lesions.

612. **Ans. c. After 20 weeks of pregnancy treat with oral acyclovir for 5-7 days because of heightened risk of varicella pneumonia and death. At this time, mother is relatively immunocompromised.**
If there is severe varicella or varicella pneumonia, treat with I/V acyclovir in the dose of 10-15 mg/kg every 8 hours for 5-10 days.

613. **Ans. b. It is tinea corporis with well-defined active borders. Lesions are ring shaped and have some central clearing.**
    - Psoriasis comprises of red plaques with white scaling *(MCQ 146)*.
    - Granuloma annulare presents as asymptomatic complete or incomplete rings of skin colored or violaceous papules *(MCQ 219)*.
    - Discoid eczema comprises of 1-3 cm sized coin or disc shaped plaques formed by closely set papules with oozing and crusting *(MCQ 434)*.

614. **Ans. b. It is tuberculoid leprosy which has highest immunity, so has least number of skin lesions. Skin patch with loss of sensation is a cardinal feature for the diagnosis of leprosy.**
    - Lepromatous leprosy has lowest immunity, so will have uncountable skin lesions *(MCQ 155)*.
    - Indeterminate leprosy is an early and transient stage of leprosy whose immunological status is to be determined. It presents as hypopigmented or slight red macule. If edges are palpable, it is no longer an indeterminate type.
    - Histoid leprosy is a variant of multibacillary leprosy that presents as crop of asymptomatic, multiple, smooth glistening non tender papules *(MCQ 47)*.

615. **Ans. c. It is nodular melanoma which shows rapid evolution. Peripheral discoloration is representing the horizontal growth phase.**
    - A compound nevus is an acquired melanocytic nevus which is usually dark round or oval and raised above epidermal surface *(MCQ 120)*.
    - Halo nevus is also an acquired melanocytic nevus which is surrounded by a halo of depigmentation *(MCQ 149)*.
    - Strawberry hemangioma is lobulated scarlet red colored (not black color) and manifests in first month of life *(MCQ 187)*.

616. **Ans. b. It is pseudoacanthosis nigricans. It is usually associated with obesity and insulin resistance.**
    - Darier's disease is an autosomal dominant condition which presents as multiple, firm, rough, papules of skin or gray colored in the seborrheic areas of body *(MCQ 267)*.
    - Acanthosis associated with malignancy is more severe and extensive. Pigmentation is not limited to hyperkeratotic areas. Palms show thickening, nails become brittle and hair may shed.

617. **Ans. b. It is senile comedones. It is seen in elderly people due to chronic sun exposure that results in damage of supporting dermis. It leads into distension of pilosebaceous duct that get impacted with corneocytes. Periorbital and malar areas are common sites.**
    - Acne comedones are seen at young age *(MCQ 463)*.
    - Drug-induced acne is seen as red monomorphic papular lesions on back and shoulders *(MCQ 43)*.
    - Topical steroids on face cause erythema, itching, papules and hair growth *(MCQ 5)*.

618. **Ans. a. It is chronic cutaneous lupus erythematous. Adherent scales, hyperpigmented peripheral rim and involvement of sun exposed areas are its typical features.**
    - Psoriasis comprises of red plaques studded with white scales *(MCQ 21)*.
    - Granuloma annulare presents as complete or incomplete rings formed by skin or violaceous papules *(MCQ 591)*.

619. **Ans. c. It is tuberous sclerosis complex. It is an autosomal dominant condition. Epilepsy, low intelligence and adenoma sebaceum *(MCQ 306)* constitute a triad for the diagnosis of this disorder.**

- Acne vulgaris presents as comedones, papules and pustules *(MCQ 216)* in adults.
- LMDF is seen in adolescents and adults as monomorphic (2-4 mm sized) papules on forehead, cheeks, eyelid and chin *(MCQ 525)*.
- Drug-induced acne is seen as monomorphic red papules on trunk and shoulders *(MCQ 43)*.

620. **Ans. a.** It is tuberculosis verrucosa cutis having a high degree of immunity. Hand *(MCQ 640)* and lower extremities *(MCQ 10)* are sites of predilection.
    - SCC presents as an exophytic cauliflower like appearance *(MCQ 528)*.
    - Plantar warts present as sharply defined deep-seated rough hyperkeratotic lesions *(MCQ 410)*.
    - Madura foot is a deep fungal infection which presents as painless non pitting swelling of foot. It is studded with nodules and sinuses which may discharge colored granules *(MCQ 272)*.

621. **Ans. c.** It is psoriasis soles. Red plaques with white scaling are characteristic.
    - Lichen planus is characterized by violaceous papules *(MCQ 437)*.
    - Tinea pedis is characterized by white scaling *(MCQ 51)*.
    - Hyperkeratotic eczema comprises of itching, oozing and crusting *(MCQ 137)*.

622. **Ans. a.** It is guttate psoriasis which is chiefly seen in children and young adults. It is seen as 1–1.5 cm sized scattered lesions in rain drop pattern over the trunk, arm, thigh, etc. It is frequently associated with staphylococcal infection and shows good prognosis.
    - Lichen planus manifests as violaceous papules *(MCQ 339)*.
    - Pityriasis rosea presents as discrete and oval shaped lesions covered with fine scales on the back along the ribs in " Christmas tree pattern *(MCQ 161)*.
    - In secondary syphilis macular lesions dominate with little scaling *(MCQ 293)*.

623. **Ans. c.** Herpes zoster does not pose any risk neither to fetus nor to mother. Treatment of herpes zoster is considered same as for non-pregnant patient.
    - Systemic antiviral drugs are required if age of patient is above 50 years.
    - Topical antiviral cream has no role.
    - Intravenous antiviral therapy is required if there is a risk of pneumonia.

624. **Ans. c.** It is candidiasis under breast which is characterized by fringed margin with satellite vesicles and pustules. It is due to underlying diabetes mellitus which is indicated by increased frequency of micturition at night.
    - Tinea corporis comprises of patches with well-defined active borders *(MCQ 40)*.
    - Flexural psoriasis comprises of red coloration with scaling *(MCQ 245)*.
    - Intertrigo refers to inflammation of opposing surfaces of body folds. Its involvement is limited to area of contact *(MCQ 166)*.

625. **Ans. c.** Valacyclovir can be given to patients having renal dysfunction. Dose adjustment is required according to the creatinine clearance because about 50% of valacyclovir is excreted unchanged in urine. With creatinine clearance >50 mL per min-1 g TDS, 30–50 mL/min-1 g BD, 10–29 mL/min-1 g OD and <10 mL/min-500 mg OD.

626. **Ans. c.** Uncomplicated chickenpox (varicella) before 20 weeks of pregnancy may not be given systemic antiviral drugs because risk of fetus due to acyclovir is unknown. If varicella is severe, give oral acyclovir.
If varicella is severe with signs and symptoms of lung involvement, then treat with I/V acyclovir.

627. **Ans. b.** It is macular amyloidosis. Upper back is a typical site and has female preponderance.
    - Pseudo acanthosis nigricans is seen in obese persons as dark velvety thickening usually confined to cervical region, axillae and groins *(MCQ 273)*.
    - Sun-induced delayed tanning does not persist for years. It is seen 48–72 hours after sun exposure.
    - Addisonian pigmentation is seen as diffuse pigmentation of face, palmar creases and palate *(MCQ 439)*.

628. **Ans. a.** It is drug-induced exanthematous rash (syn. maculopapular or morbilliform rash). It constitutes about 95% of all drug-induced skin eruptions. It constitutes mainly red macular lesions which become confluent at places. It spares the face.
    - Urticaria will manifest with well demarcated pale swellings called wheals *(MCQ 501)*.
    - Miliaria rubra presents as uniform minute red papules in hot and humid condition in areas of body prone to friction due to clothing *(MCQ 118)*.
    - Measles is seen in children with involvement of face and conjunctiva. It accompanies fever.

Chapter 5 ✦ Answers of MCQs in Dermatology, Venereology and Leprology

629. **Ans. b.** It is inflammatory linear verrucous epidermal nevus. Buttocks and extremities are common sites.
    ❖ TVC is a type of cutaneous tuberculosis which neither has itching nor presents since birth *(MCQ 640)*.
    ❖ Nevus sebaceous is seen on scalp as waxy looking hairless plaque *(MCQ 99)*.
    ❖ Common warts usually do not last for many years. They are hyperkeratotic asymptomatic discrete papules *(MCQ 169)*.

630. **Ans. b.** He is a typical patient of Darier's disease with typical skin lesions and nail changes. It is an autosomal dominant condition with characteristic histological changes *(MCQ 785)*.
    ❖ Seborrheic dermatitis is characterized by fine greasy scales not by papules *(MCQ 175)*.
    ❖ Lichen planus is characterized by violaceous papules on peripheral parts *(MCQ 381)* and nails do not have V-shaped notch.
    ❖ Carcinoma lung causes clubbing of nails *(MCQ 133)*.

631. **Ans. d.** It is venous ulcer. It is typically seen at medial lower aspect of the leg (gaiter region) surrounded by intense blue red coloration.
    ❖ Trophic ulcer refers to an ulcer that is seen in the part of body that is in poor condition because of vascular insufficiency or loss of sensation, e.g., leprosy *(MCQ 563)*.
    ❖ Arterial ulcers are painful ulcers which are seen at tips of toes, lateral aspects of heel and calves *(MCQ 514)*.
    ❖ Buerger's disease affects young male smokers. Ulcers often start around nails and tip of digits *(MCQ 478)*.

632. **Ans. b.** It is bullous pemphigoid. Tense bullae and absence of mucosal involvement are typical features.
    ❖ Pemphigus vulgaris comprises of mucosal involvement, flaccid blisters and painful large erosions *(MCQs 184, 344)*.
    ❖ Linear IgA dermatosis is characterized by appearance of new lesions around the periphery of previous lesion, i.e., collarette of blisters *(MCQ 288)*.
    ❖ Blisters due to *Paederus dermatitis* are uncommon *(MCQ 386)*. If seen, they appear overnight and are localized in a small area.

633. **Ans. b.** It is erythema ab igne. It is because of repeated or chronic exposure to infrared radiation, e.g., sitting close to fire, use of hot water bottles or heated pad for chronic back ache, etc.
    ❖ Lichen planus pigmentosus is a rare type of lichen planus. It presents as irregularly shaped brown to gray brown macules. It is seen mainly on sun exposed areas, e.g., forehead, temples and neck.
    ❖ Livedo reticularis refers to mottled cyanotic cutaneous discoloration having a characteristic network. It is accentuated by cold and most commonly occurs on legs. Leg elevation decreases the intensity of color change.

634. **Ans. b.** It is warts scalp.
    ❖ Nevus sebaceous is an epidermal hamartomatous nevus that presents as slightly raised waxy, velvety and yellowish plaque since childhood *(MCQ 609)*.
    ❖ Tinea capitis presents as patches with partially broken hairs *(MCQ 8)* or as inflammatory boggy swelling *(MCQ 4)*.

635. **Ans. d.** It is geographic tongue (benign migratory glossitis) which is seen in 3% of general population. It is also seen in Reiter's disease, diabetes and atopic dermatitis.
    ❖ In lichen planus, plaques have violaceous tinge *(MCQ 491)*.
    ❖ In sideropenic anemia, there is generalized loss of filiform papillae from whole dorsal surface of tongue.
    ❖ Scrotal tongue manifests as deep fissures. It may be seen as non-specific feature in Melkersson Rosenthal syndrome *(MCQ 530)*.

636. **Ans. c.** It is stratum spinosum. It is 8–10 layers thick and lies immediately above the basal cell layer. It is named as spinous after the spine like appearance of cell margins in histological section.
    ❖ Stratum lucidum is seen in the skin of palms and soles between stratum corneum and stratum granulosum.
    ❖ Stratum granulosum cells contain basophilic keratohyalin granules and lies above the stratum spinosum.
    ❖ Stratum corneum is the outermost layer which provide mechanical protection and allows permeation of soluble substances and act as barrier to water loss.

637. Ans. b. It is an early stage of alopecia areata. Exclamation hairs are characteristic of alopecia areata. Upper ends of these hairs are broader than lower ends. It illustrates the follicular damage in anagen phase with rapid transformation into telogen phase. The presence of these hairs reflects the active phase of disease.
- Trichotillomania manifests at easily approachable site *(MCQ 128)* and shows the presence of firmly anchored partially broken hairs.
- Ophiasis is a variant of alopecia areata showing band like pattern along the scalp margin *(MCQ 297)*.
- Tinea capitis is seen in children. Patch will show scaling or black dots or some inflammation. Exclamation mark hair is not a feature *(MCQ 8)*.

638. Ans. b. It is universal vitiligo which implies involvement of more than 90% of body surface. Option of depigmentation of normally pigmented area (with the use of 20% monobenzyl ether of hydroquinone) can be offered to her.
- Generalized vitiligo and vitiligo vulgaris are same. It is most common clinical form which shows widespread involvement in a symmetrical manner *(MCQ 511)*.
- Term leukoderma is commonly used by layman implying acquired depigmentation of skin irrespective of etiology *(MCQ 474)*.

639. Ans. b. It is autosomal dominant inheritance. Because of the dominant effect of gene, all heterozygous male or female children are affected. It is seen in neuro fibromatosis type 1, Darier's disease, tuberous sclerosis complex, etc.
- Autosomal recessive inheritance requires homozygous gene for clinical manifestation. Heterozygous children will be carriers *(MCQ 664)*.
- In X-linked recessive, other unaffected X-chromosome has a protective role so heterozygous female will be carrier but hemizygous males will be affected because male do not have unaffected X-chromosome for protection *(MCQ 674)*.
- In X-linked dominant inheritance *(MCQ 694)* because of dominant effect both heterozygous females and hemizygous males are affected.

640. Ans. a. It is tuberculosis verrucosa cutis which has very high immunity. Hands and lower extremities are common sites which are more liable to minor wounds or abrasions.
- Extensive palmar warts will involve another palm also. They are not so elevated from the surface.
- ILVEN appears in first few years of life and is itchy *(MCQ 64)*.
- N. sebaceous is commonly seen on scalp as circumscribed velvety plaque with hair loss during childhood *(MCQ 99)*.

641. Ans. b. It is median raphe cysts which is a rare benign congenital disorder of unknown origin. They are mostly present at birth and usually remain asymptomatic and are diagnosed within first decade of life.

Molluscum contagiosum presents as pearly white shiny umbilicated papules *(MCQ 646)*. The MC lesions are scattered and not limited to median raphe.

642. Ans. d: It is bacterial balanoposthitis. There is no dysuria or burning micturition which is an important feature of urethral syndrome. Urine examination, HIV, VDRL HCV and HBsAg should also be done in all such patients.
- Candidal balanoposthitis is a manifestation of underlying diabetes. It presents as erythema, tiny papules or pustules and collarette of white scales *(MCQ 797)*.
- FDE is characterized by dusky red coloration of prepuce and/or glans with/without discharge *(MCQ 691)*.
- Urethral syndrome includes both gonococcal and non-gonococcal urethral pus discharge *(MCQ 380)* which are accompanied by burning micturition.

643. Ans. b. It is generalized pustular psoriasis. Systemic steroid therapy is a common precipitating factor. It should be promptly treated.
- Secondary infection of psoriatic lesions does not manifest all over the body. Monomorphic pustules are not its feature. Secondary infection manifests as crusting at places.
- Acropustulosis is a type of localized pustular psoriasis in which tips of fingers and toes are involved *(MCQ 376)*.
- Impetigo herpetiformis is another name of generalized pustular psoriasis of pregnancy.

644. Ans. a. It is candidiasis. All species of candida have the ability to produce pseudo mycelia. In this microphotograph pseudomycelia are seen as cluster of grapes like yeast cells.

- Pityriasis versicolor shows short filaments with spherical thick-walled yeasts giving 'spaghetti and meatballs' appearance *(MCQ 363)*.
- Dermatophytes shows branching septate hyphae which are refractile and consists of parallel lines *(MCQ 47)*.
- In chromoblastomycosis characteristic muriform cells are seen which are multiple, round, thick walled and brownish budding bodies which resemble copper pennies.

645. **Ans. b. It is stratum granulosum. Its cells contain basophilic keratohyalin granules and lies above the stratum spinosum.**
     - Stratum spinosum is 8–10 layers thick and lies above the basal cell layer. Its cells give spine like appearance in histological sections.
     - Stratum corneum is outermost layer which provide mechanical protection and allows permeation of soluble substances.
     - Stratum lucidum is seen in the skin of palms and soles between stratum corneum and stratum granulosum.

646. **Ans. b: It is molluscum contagiosum. Umbilication in the center of papules is a characteristic feature.**
     - Median raphe cysts is a rare congenital anomaly. It presents along the median raphe *(MCQ 641)*.
     - Condylomata acuminata is seen as filiform or digitate lesions around anus or vulva *(MCQ 469)*.

647. **Ans. b. It is crusted scabies. Non pruritic thick crusts (not scales) on buttocks and extremities in an old patient is characteristic. Sarcoptes scabiei can easily be demonstrated in KOH smear** *(MCQ 651)*.
     - Psoriasis is characterized by silvery white scales not the crusts *(MCQ 482)*.
     - Tinea lesions are characterized by well-defined active borders of ring-shaped lesions *(MCQ 40)*.
     - Chromoblastomycosis manifests as hypertrophic plaques or large masses which are studded with black dots.

648. **Ans. c. It is pressure urticaria which has manifested after many hours of sustained pressure of elastic strip of underwear.**
     - *Paederus dermatitis* presents with burning sensation. Lesions are usually seen on exposed parts and have a necrotic slough *(MCQ 587)*.
     - Tinea presents as circular or large patches.

649. **Ans. c. It is eczema with characteristic itching and crusting.**
     - Ingrown toenail is characterized by penetration of nailfold by edge of nail plate with accompanying inflammation and granulation tissue formation *(MCQ 462)*.
     - Tinea pedis will have well-defined proximal border with involvement of nail plate *(MCQ 480)*.
     - Tuberculosis verrucosa cutis will manifest as well-defined warty growth *(MCQ 564)*.

650. **Ans. d. G1 is a postmitotic growth phase or interphase (phase between two cell cycles). This phase is quite longer. During this phase, cell can go for differentiation (D) or go into quiescent phase (G0).**
     - S represents a period of active DNA synthesis.
     - G2 represents growth or resting phase.
     - M stands for mitosis.

651. **Ans. b. It is showing Sarcoptes scabiei (0.3 mm x 0.3 mm). It has 4 pairs of short legs having bristles. Many eggs are also nicely visible in the field.**
     - Pediculosis corporis is quite larger (1-4 mm), elongated and dorsoventrally flattened insect with six legs which terminate in to small claws. It can easily be seen with naked eyes.
     - Dermatophytes shows refractile, branched and septate hyphae *(MCQ 347)*.
     - Chromoblastomycosis shows muriform[1] cells which are multiple round thick-walled brownish budding bodies which resemble copper pennies.

652. **Ans. a. It is superficial infantile hemangioma which manifests in first month of life. Superficial type grows on skin surface. It is also called strawberry hemangioma because of bumpy red appearance.**
     - Deep or subcutaneous hemangioma develop in lower dermis or subcutis. It tends to appear blue or purple. There may be no overlying skin changes.
     - Salmon patch presents as blanchable, pinkish and red irregular macules which are comprised of fine linear telangiectasia.
     - Port-wine stain presents at birth as unilateral persistent pink or red macule in the distribution of sensory branches of trigeminal nerve *(MCQ 521)*.

653. **Ans. c. It is pyogenic granuloma. Nailfold is common site for pyogenic granuloma. It is misnomer because it is nothing to do with pus. It is a rapidly developed vascular nodule at the site of**

---

[1]**Muriform:** Resembling courses of bricks in arrangement having both horizontal and vertical cells.

recent penetrating injury. It is composed of lobular proliferation of small vessels.
- Glomus tumor is a nail bed vascular tumor which presents as spontaneous pain in relation to finger nail bed.
- Herpetic whitlow presents as painful single or group of tiny vesicles on nail fold close to nail.
- Ingrown nail comprises of penetration of nail fold by edge of the nail plate with formation of granulation tissue *(MCQ 462)*.

654. **Ans. d. It is dermatitis groins which has involved lower abdomen with ill-defined margins.**
- Tinea cruris will manifests with well-defined active borders *(MCQ 4)*.
- Flexural psoriasis manifests with salmon pink color, well defined margins and reduced silvery scales *(MCQ 84)*.
- Intertrigo manifest as erythema, soreness and itching which is limited to the opposing surfaces of body folds *(MCQ 166)*.
- Candidiasis presents as red macerations in body folds extending beyond the area of contact and develops fringed irregular margins with classical satellite vesicles and pustules *(MCQ 643)*.

655. **Ans. a. It is Langerhans cell seen in basal, spinous and granular cell layers. Birbeck granules are seen in its cytoplasm. This cell is a dendritic cell which is involved in cutaneous T-cell responses. It plays role in pathogenesis of allergic contact dermatitis in processing the allergen on subsequent exposures (after first exposure).**
- Merkel cells have lobulated nuclei and are present among basal cells in the regions of body having textile sensitivity. They function as mechanoreceptors *(MCQ 660)*.
- Melanocytes are pigment synthesizing dendritic cells present among the basal cells *(MCQ 655)*.
- Parakeratotic cells refers to stratum corneum cells whose nuclei are retained. These cells are seen in psoriasis.

656. **Ans. b. It is superficial spreading melanoma. It fulfills all features of the acronym ABCDE. It is asymmetric with notched borders, has color variation and diameter is >6 mm. It is also evolving with time. It is on covered part of body.**
- SCC is usually seen on sun exposed part as verrucous or ulcerative morphology *(MCQ 255)*.
- BCC is usually seen around eyes, nose and ear *(MCQ 193)*.
- Bowen's disease presents as persistent, red scaly and crusted plaque *(MCQ 266)*.

657. **Ans. c. It is contact irritant dermatitis**
- Herpes zoster is a characterized by eruption of grouped vesicles in groups in a dermatomal distribution *(MCQ 70)*.
- *Paederus dermatitis* is characterized by linear red edematous lesions with grayish white slough in the center *(MCQ 698)*.

658. **Ans. d. It is widespread tinea corporis with less conspicuous erythema. Scaling is white and at places advancing border can be recognized.**
- In senile eczema, skin becomes dry, scaly with prominent and deep skin markings studded with fine superficial fissures *(MCQ 94)*.
- Seborrheic dermatitis manifests as redness with greasy scales. Involvement is common on certain sites known as seborrheic sites, e.g., scalp, eyebrows, eyelashes, nasolabial folds, flexures (umbilicus, groins, natal left), presternal region *(MCQ 175)* and interscapular region.

659. **Ans. d. It is psychiatric illness in which there is compulsive impulse or habit to pull out hair. Females out number males, 7:1. Peripheral rim of scalp hair is characteristically spared.**
- Androgenic alopecia in females is characterized by widening of central parting *(MCQ 190)*, diffuse central thinning *(MCQ 185)* and recession of frontoparietal hairline.
- Alopecia areata manifests as variable sized well defined totally bald patches *(MCQ 569)*.
- Telogen effluvium manifests as sudden, diffuse and excessive scalp hair loss after some precipitating event *(MCQ 163)*.

660. **Ans. d. It is Merkel cell which are present among the basal keratinocytes of the skin of the regions having high tactile sensitivity. They have lobulated nuclei and function as mechanoreceptors.**
- Melanocytes are pigment synthesizing dendritic cells present among basal cells *(MCQ 665)*.
- Parakeratotic cells refers to stratum corneal cells which have retained nuclei. Otherwise, during transition from granular cell layer, these cells normally lose their nuclei.
- Langerhans cells are dendritic cells found in basal, spinous and granular cell layer *(MCQ 655)*.

661. **Ans. d. It is mid borderline leprosy consisting of typical features, i.e., number of lesions 4–8, saucer shaped lesions and impairment of sensations.**

Chapter 5 ✦ Answers of MCQs in Dermatology, Venereology and Leprology

- Tuberculoid leprosy comprises of single plaque with loss of sensations *(MCQ 6)*.
- Lepromatous leprosy has very low immunity with uncountable skin lesions *(MCQ 155)*.
- Histoid leprosy manifests with crop of asymptomatic, smooth glistening, non-tender papules *(MCQ 47)*.

662. Ans. b. It is condylomata acuminata (warts) caused by HPV-6–11, 16, -18 types. with an incubation period of 3 weeks to 8 months.

Condylomata lata is a manifestation of secondary syphilis. It manifests as flesh colored, soft sessile papules with oozing and macerations *(MCQ 688)*. Anal region *(MCQ 666)* is another common site. It is highly infectious.

663. Ans. b. It is multiple cutaneous horn. Cutaneous horn is a morphological diagnosis which can be caused by various disorders, e.g., nevi, seborrheic keratosis, etc. Excision biopsy is the treatment of choice.

Filiform warts are commonly seen on nostrils, lips, eyelids *(MCQs 420, 430, 440)*.

664. Ans. b. It is autosomal recessive inheritance. It requires homozygous genes for clinical manifestation. Patient with heterozygous genes will be carrier. It is seen in patients having acrodermatitis enteropathica, phenylketonuria, etc.

- In autosomal dominant, because of the dominant effect all heterozygous males and females will manifest with the disease *(MCQ 639)*.
- In X-linked recessive type, only homozygous females will manifest with disease. Otherwise, heterozygous female will be carrier. But hemizygous males will be affected because Y do not have a protective effect *(MCQ 674)*.
- In X-linked dominant type, because of dominant effect heterozygous both males and females will be affected *(MCQ 694)*.

665. Ans. c. It is melanocyte which a pigment synthesizing dendritic cell seen among the basal cells. This cell is derived from neural crest.

- Parakeratotic epidermal cell refers to stratum corneal cell which has retained its nucleus during transition from granular cell layer. These cells are seen in psoriasis.
- Langerhans cells are dendritic cells seen in basal, spinous and granular cell layers *(MCQ 655)*.
- Merkel cells are also called as mechanoreceptors. These are seen among the basal cells and have lobulated nuclei.

666. Ans. c. It is condylomata lata, which is a manifestation of secondary syphilis. Groins *(MCQ 662)* are another common site.

- Condylomata acuminata (genital warts) presents as dry rough, hyperkeratotic papules and nodules *(MCQ 662)*.
- Skin tags are usually soft, smooth, discrete and round. They are uncommon in anal region *(MCQ 331)*.

667. Ans. b. It is tumor stage cutaneous T-cell lymphoma, manifesting with nodules and tumors on red non-scaly plaques. Diagnosis is confirmed by epidermotropism by T-cells along the basal cell layer forming Pautrier's microabscesses.

- Plaques of psoriasis shows silvery white scaling *(MCQ 49)*.
- Cutaneous B-cell lymphoma usually presents as an indolent, non-scaly, reddish lump or nodule *(MCQ 681)*.
- Parapsoriasis presents as asymptomatic scaly red plaques on trunk and limbs with no tumors or nodules.

668. Ans. c. It is elephantiasis which refers to the hypertrophy of the skin and subcutaneous tissue (chiefly affecting legs and external genitals) due to any cause.

- Esthiomene refers to the elephantiasis of the female genitals having chronic ulcerated state of the vulva and clitoris.
- Elephantiasis nostras verrucosa is a rare chronic disorder resulting from long-standing obstruction of lymphatic drainage. It usually manifests on legs as nonpitting edema with verrucous papules and nodules giving a cobblestone-like appearance *(MCQ 686)*.

669. Ans. b. It is squamous cell carcinoma. Actinic cheilitis and scaly leukoplakia may precede SCC of lower lip. It is associated with highest rate of metastasis. About 50% of patients already have metastasis at the time of diagnosis.

Digitate or filiform warts are rough and hyperkeratotic and do not have broad base. They are finger like *(MCQ 440)*.

670. Ans. b. G2 represents premitotic growth or resting phase. It is much shorter than postmitotic growth phase G1.

- S represents the period of active DNA synthesis.
- M represents mitosis.
- G1 represents postmitotic growth or interphase which is quite longer. It is phase between two cell cycles.

671. **Ans. b.** Aquagenic pruritus is characteristically seen due to polycythemia vera. Complete hemogram shows raised HB and hematocrit. TLC and platelet count are raised. ESR is low. Splenomegaly is an important feature which is due to sequestration of RBCs by spleen.
    - CML is characterized by presence of absolute leukocytosis (about 100,000/mL), myelocytes, blast cells (usually >2%), absolute basophilia. Platelet count is usually normal.
    - Essential thrombocytosis is a rare myeloproliferative neoplasm characterized by platelet count >400 × 103 μL for at least 2 months with normal red cell count.
    - Leukemoid reaction is described as increase in TLC >50,000 cells/mL. It is a physiological response to stress or infection.

672. **Ans. b.** It is intrameatal wart. It is not an uncommon site for genital warts. It is caused by HPV- 6, -11, -16, -18 types with an incubation period of 3 weeks to 8 months.
    Pearly penile papules are seen as 1–3 mm sized flesh-colored smooth and round papules in a row along the coronal margin. It is physiological and reassurance is usually sufficient *(MCQ 270).*

673. **Ans. a.** It is basal cell carcinoma with typical raised, thread like and rolled margins. Common sites are head and neck.
    - Superficial spreading melanoma is mainly seen on covered parts as large, irregularly shaped brown macule with asymmetry and varied color *(MCQ 516).*
    - SCC develops on photo damaged skin showing pigmentation, solar elastosis actinic cheilitis *(MCQ 116),* etc.
    - Old world cutaneous leishmaniasis presents with sequence of nodule, ulceration, crusting, healing and scar formation *(MCQ 237).*

674. **Ans. b.** It is X-linked recessive inheritance. It requires homozygous X-chromosomes for clinical manifestation. Heterozygous female will be carrier because unaffected X-chromosome has a protective role. But, hemizygous male with affected X-chromosome will manifest with disease because Y chromosome do not have protective role.
    - In autosomal dominant inheritance, because of dominant effect all heterozygous males and females will be affected *(MCQ 639).*
    - In autosomal recessive type, heterozygous children will be carrier and homozygous children will be affected *(MCQ 664).*
    - In X-linked dominant type, because of dominant effect all heterozygous females and hemizygous males will be affected *(MCQ 694).* This inheritance is seen in incontinentia pigmenti *(MCQ 370).*

675. **Ans. d.** It is stratum corneum which is an outermost layer of skin and provides mechanical protection. It allows permeation of soluble substance and acts as barrier to water loss.
    - Stratum spinosum is 8–10 layers thick and lies immediately above the basal cell layer. The margins of cells give spine like appearance in histological sections.
    - Stratum basale is one cell thick continuous layer. Its cells are mitotic and give rise to cells of epidermal cell layers.
    - Stratum granulosum lies above the stratum spinosum. Its cells contain basophilic keratohyalin granules.

676. **Ans. a.** It is basal cell carcinoma having slightly raised and thread like margins. The central part of lesion is atrophic without any scales. Regions near eye *(MCQ 193)* and ear *(MCQ 766)* are common sites.
    - Squamous cell carcinoma is seen on photo damaged skin *(MCQ 776)* showing irregular pigmentation and solar elastosis.
    - Lupus vulgaris manifests as soft gelatinous plaque with active peripheral border and trailing center *(MCQ 26).*
    - Old world cutaneous leishmaniasis shows sequence of formation of nodule, ulceration, crusting and healing *(MCQ 237).*

677. **Ans. c.** It is onychomadesis which is defined as idiopathic separation of proximal part of nail plate from nail bed and nail matrix due to temporary arrest in nail matrix activity.
    - Onycholysis refers to painless separation of distal part of nail plate from nail bed. It is seen in psoriasis *(MCQ 88).*
    - Proximal subungual onychomycosis involves the part of nail plate adjoining the posterior nail fold. It is seen in AIDS patients.
    - Beau's lines refer to transverse grooves in the nail plate. It is due to interference in nail formation due to some systemic disease *(MCQ 247).*

678. **Ans. b.** It is alopecia areata presenting as patchy hair loss. The patches have complete baldness with smooth skin and no inflammation.
    - Hair loss in hypothyroidism is seen from outer third of eyebrows on both sides along with

other features, e.g., puffiness of face, eyelids and thickness of lips *(MCQ 426)*.
- Tinea infection with hair loss will be accompanied by inflammation *(MCQ 431)*.
- Superciliary madarosis due to lepromatous leprosy is bilateral and accompanied by diffuse infiltration of facial skin and ears *(MCQ 495)*.

679. **Ans. b. It is acral lentiginous melanoma. It fulfills all the features included in the acronym ABCDE. It is asymmetric, borders are irregular, color is varied, diameter is >6 mm. and is evolving with time. It needs immediate excision and biopsy.**
- Lichen planus lesions are violaceous and multiple *(MCQ 231)*.
- Junctional nevus shows a regular pigmented network of brown and uniform color. It may be more prominent in center with gradual fading to borders.

680. **Ans. c. It is lamina densa (basal lamina) which is an electron dense layer lying next to lamina lucida. Type IV collagen is its primary component. The site of cleavage in dystrophic epidermolysis bullosa is immediately below this layer** *(MCQ 711)*.
- Lamina lucida is electron lucent intermembranous space which separates plasma membrane and lamina densa. It is a site of cleavage in bullous pemphigoid *(MCQ 731)*.
- Sub basal dense plaques (SBDP) are linear densities beneath each hemidesmosome. Anchoring fibrils traverse through SBDP *(MCQ 700)*.
- Lamina fibroreticularis lies deeper to lamina densa and it is composed by fibrils *(MCQ 798)*.

681. **Ans. c. It is cutaneous B-cell lymphoma which develops very slowly in years with neck and head as predilection sites.**
- CTCL evolves through patch, plaques and tumor stages *(MCQs 408, 666)*.
- Lupus vulgaris lesions are soft gelatinous with advancing active margins and trailing scar towards center. Nodule formation is not seen *(MCQ 57)*.
- SCC is seen on photo damaged skin showing pigmentation, solar elastosis, telangiectasia *(MCQ 116)*.

682. **Ans. c. Onycholysis, yellow discoloration and coarse pitting are typically seen in psoriasis.**
- Typical changes in LP are pterygium formation, thinning, ridging and onychorrhexis *(MCQs 31, 78, 112)*.
- In onychomycosis, involvement is asymmetrical. Nail plate becomes rough, thickened and lifted up by subungual hyperkeratosis *(MCQ 460)*.
- Darier's disease shows red longitudinal bands in nail plate which ends in pathognomonic V-shaped notch at the free margin of nail *(MCQ 576)*.

683. **Ans. d. It is acute urticaria with characteristic itchy red plaques with duration <6 weeks.**
- In chronic urticaria duration of urticarial eruption is >6 weeks.
- Tinea is characterized by well-defined active borders *(MCQ 241)*.
- In lepromatous leprosy, swelling of ear lobule will neither be acute nor will show remissions and relapses. Itching is not a feature of leprosy *(MCQs 101, 495, 692)*.

684. **Ans. b. It is cherry angiomas (syn. senile angiomas, De Morgan spots). It is most common vascular abnormality usually seen on trunk. It is seen in most individuals after the age of 70 years.**
- Strawberry hemangioma (infantile hemangioma). It is seen in infancy. It is absent at the time of birth and appears in first month of life *(MCQs 187, 819)*.
- Pyogenic granuloma is usually a single vascular nodule at the site of recent penetrating injury *(MCQs 114, 424, 653)*.
- Lymphangioma circumscriptum is usually noticed at birth or during childhood as discrete or grouped fluid-filled vesicles bulging from skin surface *(MCQs 106, 712)*.

685. **Ans. b. It is for pemphigus vulgaris. Basal cells separate from each other and remain attached to basement membrane as "row of tomb stones".**
- In DH, cleft is subepidermal. There is a dense accumulation of neutrophils and eosinophils within dermal papillae to form micro abscesses *(MCQ 740)*.
- In BP, cleft is subepidermal and roof of blister is formed by intact epidermis *(MCQs 720, 731)*.
- In PF, cleft is in granular layer or at subcorneal level *(MCQs 705, 750)*.

686. **Ans. c. It is elephantiasis nostras verrucosa. It is a rare chronic disorder caused by obstruction of lymphatic drainage. It usually manifests on legs.**
- Esthiomene refers to elephantiasis of the female genitals having chronic ulcerated state of the vulva and clitoris.

- Elephantiasis refers to hypertrophy of skin and subcutaneous tissue due to any cause *(MCQ 668)*.

687. **Ans. b. It is nodular melanoma which is characteristically a dome-shaped pigmented lesion in male. Because of rapid deep invasion, this subtype is associated with poor prognosis.**
    - Nodular BCC presents as flesh colored translucent papule or plaque *(MCQ 673)*.
    - SCC arises as flesh-colored papule or plaque on photo damaged skin showing pigmentation and solar elastosis *(MCQ 676)*.
    - Keratoacanthoma is a rapidly enlarging nodule which has a central keratotic core *(MCQ 108)*.

688. **Ans. b. It is condylomata lata which is a manifestation of secondary syphilis. It is highly infectious. VDRL, HIV and HBsAg should be carried out. Anal region *(MCQ 666)*, inframammary region and axillae are other sites of manifestation.**
    - Condylomata acuminata (genital warts) are rough and hyperkeratotic *(MCQ 663)*. It is mainly caused by HPV -6, -11, -16 and -18 types with an incubation period of 3 weeks to 8 months. HPV -16 and -18 are high risk types and are present in majority of cervical carcinomas.
    - Molluscum contagiosum presents as discrete, shiny, umbilicated papules *(MCQ 510)*.

689. **Ans. c. It is trophic ulcer due to lepromatous leprosy as evidenced by typical features of LL. Plantar surface of big toe is most common site of trophic ulcer due to leprosy. Head of first metatarsal is second most common site *(MCQ 563)*.**
    - In Buerger's disease, ulcers often start around the sides of nails and tips of the digits *(MCQs 422, 478)*.
    - In diabetes mellitus, head of first metatarsal is most common site *(MCQ 826)*. It is seen in patient having peripheral neuropathy due to DM.
    - Venous ulcer is typically seen *(MCQ 532)* on the medial aspect of lower part of leg (gaiter region).

690. **Ans. b. It is lamina lucida which is an electron lucent intermembranous space which separates plasma membrane from lamina densa. It is a site of cleavage in bullous pemphigoid *(MCQ 731)*.**
    - Lamina densa is an electron dense layer which lies deeper to lamina lucida *(MCQ 680)*.
    - Lamina fibroreticularis lies deeper to lamina densa and is composed of fibrils *(MCQ 798)*.
    - Subbasal dense plaques are linear densities in lamina lucida beneath each hemidesmosome *(MCQ 700)*.

691. **Ans. c. It is due to fixed drug eruption. Involvement of glans and/or prepuce is very common. Dusky red coloration is very characteristic.**
    - Secondary syphilis does not develop overnight. It is characterized by superficial mucosal ulcerations *(MCQ 457)*.
    - Candidal balanoposthitis presents as soreness, erythema and tiny pustules or erosions *(MCQs 38, 693, 797)*.
    - Gonococcal urethritis presents as burning micturition and urethral pus discharge after sexual exposure with a commercial sex worker *(MCQ 380)*.

692. **Ans. b. It is lepromatous leprosy (LL). Chronic infiltration of ear lobules without any itching or any remissions is due to LL unless proved otherwise. Lepra bacilli can easily be demonstrated in skin smear examination.**
    - Chronic urticaria is characterized by remissions and relapses and is accompanied by itching.
    - PKDL lesions have predilection in periorificial region and consist of macules and nodules. Splenomegaly and mucosal lesions are other important components.
    - Myxedema manifests as thickening of lips, puffiness of eyes and face *(MCQ 217)*.

693. **Ans. b. It is candidal balanoposthitis with intertrigo caused by underlying diabetes. The groins are typically showing fringed irregular margins with satellite lesions.**
    - Tinea cruris will show well defined active margins *(MCQ 4)*.
    - Bacterial intertrigo comprises of inflammation limited to opposing surfaces. It does not involve scrotum or prepuce *(MCQ 116)*.
    - Flexural psoriasis manifests with well-defined margins and salmon pink color *(MCQs 84, 801)*.

694. **Ans. d. It is X-linked dominant type of inheritance. Because of dominant effect all heterozygous females and hemizygous males will be affected. It is seen in incontinentia pigmenti *(MCQ 370)*.**
    - In autosomal dominant inheritance, because of dominant effect all heterozygous males and females will be affected *(MCQ 639)*.
    - In X-linked recessive type *(MCQ 664)*, it requires homozygous genes for manifestation. In heterozygous female, unaffected X-chromosome will have protective effect. But hemizygous male will manifest with disease, because Y-chromosome does not have protective effect.

Chapter 5 ✦ Answers of MCQs in Dermatology, Venereology and Leprology

- In autosomal recessive type, only homozygous patients are affected. Heterozygous patients are carriers *(MCQ 674)*.

695. Ans. d. She is having candidiasis due to underlying diabetes. Increased frequency of micturition is an important feature of underlying diabetes. Presence of satellite vesicles and pustules at the periphery is classical feature of candidiasis.
- Seborrheic dermatitis is characterized by fine greasy scales *(MCQ 175)*.
- Tinea cruris is characterized by active well-defined borders *(MCQ 4)*.
- Scabies will not cause vulval redness. It will manifest with itching between fingers and family history of scabies.

696. Ans. b. It is tuberculoid leprosy. It has highest immunity, so has least number of skin lesions. Loss of sensation in a skin patch is a cardinal feature of leprosy.
- Tinea faciei patch will have itching with no loss of sensation *(MCQ 241)*.
- Lepromatous leprosy has least immunity, so will have uncountable number of skin lesions. Infiltration of ear lobule is an important feature on face *(MCQ 101)*.
- Lupus vulgaris is a skin tuberculosis which presents as a psoriasiform plaque with advancing active margin and trailing scar towards center *(MCQs 26, 57, 534, 597, 975)*.

697. Ans. a. It is Cushing's syndrome. It occurs when body is exposed to high levels of cortisol hormone (hypercortisolism). It can occur due to prolonged corticosteroid treatment or body is synthesizing excessive cortisol of its own.
- Cushing's disease is a special type of Cushing's syndrome in which source of overproduction of ACTH is pituitary gland tumor.
- In pseudo-Cushing's syndrome elevation of total cortisol levels is caused due to estrogen found in OCPs (estrogen and progesterone). Estrogen causes an increase of cortisol-binding globulin and thereby cause the total cortisol level to be elevated. However, the free cortisol (active hormone) is normal.

698. Ans. a. It is *Paederus dermatitis* (syn. blister beetle dermatitis) which is a peculiar irritant dermatitis provoked by coelomic fluid released by the insect. These vesicles are due to potent vesicant action of pederin.

- Herpes zoster is characterized by painful grouped vesicles on erythematous base *(MCQ 577)*.
- Chickenpox is characterized by a crop of discrete vesicles having surrounding erythema *(MCQ 577)*.
- Herpes simplex comprises of group of tiny vesicles at the angle of mouth *(MCQ 9)* or on genitals *(MCQ 445)*.

699. Ans. d. It is herpes zoster. Painful and grouped eruption in a unilateral fashion is typical.
- Dermatitis herpetiformis is characterized by itching, not by pain. Group of tiny inconspicuous vesicles are seen on upper back *(MCQ 261)* and extensor parts.
- Herpes simplex presents as groups of tiny vesicles *(MCQ 9)* at angle of mouth or on genitals *(MCQ 45)*.
- *Paederus dermatitis* presents as red rash in linear or other shapes *(MCQ 524)* with grayish white necrotic slough in the center.

700. Ans. c. It is subbasal dense plaque (SBDP) which are linear densities in lamina lucida beneath each hemidesmosome. Fine anchoring filaments traverse through SBDP.
- Lamina lucida is an electron lucent intermembranous space which separates plasma membrane from lamina densa. It is the site of cleavage in bullous pemphigoid *(MCQ 731)*.
- Lamina densa is an electron dense layer deeper to lamina lucida *(MCQ 680)*. The site of cleavage in dystrophic epidermolytic bullosa is immediately below lamina densa *(MCQ 711)*.
- Lamina fibro reticularis lies deeper to lamina densa and is composed of fibrils *(MCQ 798)*.

701. Ans. b. It is *Paederus dermatitis* with characteristic overnight development of red linear lesions with grayish white slough in the center. It is an irritant dermatitis due to the coelomic fluid released by the insect *Paederus*.
- Papular dermatitis is characteristic by symmetrically distributed papules on face and extremities *(MCQ 72)*.
- Scabies is characterized by itchy papules between fingers, on genitals, wrists, etc. *(MCQ 62)*.

702. Ans. c. She is suffering from systemic sclerosis. Sclerosis proximal to digits affecting extremities is a major criterion for the diagnosis of systemic sclerosis.
- Generalized morphea is not associated with sclerodactyly and Raynaud's phenomenon.

- SLE is characterized by butterfly rash *(MCQ 517)*, not by sclerosis.
- Addisonian pigmentation is characterized by hyperpigmentation of normally pigmented areas, e.g., nipples, axillae, perineum and genitals. Pigmentation of oral mucosa and palmar creases is invariably seen *(MCQs 539, 551)*.

703. Ans. c. It is alopecia areata which is characterized by a well-defined totally bald patch of smooth skin with absence of inflammation, scarring or atrophy.
- Trichotillomania is characterized by the presence of firmly anchored, partially broken hairs in the bald area *(MCQ 128)*.
- Tinea capitis is characterized by partial hair loss with scaling and minimal inflammation *(MCQ 8)*.
- In cicatricial (scarring) alopecia, there is a loss of whole pilosebaceous unit which is replaced by fibrous tissue. It can be due to skin disease *(MLQ 76)* or due to secondary cause *(MCQ 707)*.

704. Ans. b. It is condylomata acuminata (genital warts). It is one of the common sites. It is caused by HPV types-6, 11, 16,18 with an incubation period of 3 weeks to 8 months. VDRL, HIV, HCV and HBsAg should be done in all such patients.

Condylomata lata is a manifestation of secondary syphilis. It presents as flesh-colored flat topped sessile papules with oozing and macerations *(MCQ 666)*. Groin is another site to be involved *(MCQ 688)*.

705. Ans. a. It is for pemphigus foliaceus. Cleft is more superficial than pemphigus vulgaris.
- In DH, cleft is subepidermal. There is a dense accumulation of neutrophils and eosinophils within dermal papillae to form micro abscesses *(MCQ 740)*.
- In BP, cleft is at subepidermal level *(MCQ 731)*. Intact epidermis forms the roof of blister. There is inflammatory infiltrate in superficial dermis *(MCQ 720)*.
- In PV, cleft is at suprabasal level *(MCQ 770)*. Basal cells separate from each other giving an appearance of "row of tombstones" *(MCQ 685)*.

706. Ans. c. In CCLE, lower lip and chest are typically involved (sun exposed sites). Lesions have typical hyperpigmentation at periphery.
- SLE on face typically manifests as butterfly rash *(MCQ 467)*.
- LP of lower lip show violaceous color *(MCQ 29)*.
- Actinic cheilitis presents as red, scaly and chapped lips with indistinct vermilion borders *(MCQ 529)*.

707. Ans. d. It is cicatricial alopecia in which there is a loss of pilosebaceous units which are replaced by hypertrophic fibrous tissue. It is irreversible type of hair loss.
- Telogen effluvium is an excessive loss of telogen hair in response to some etiological factor *(MCQ 163)*. It is reversible type of hair loss.
- Alopecia areata presents with complete bald patch which has smooth skin with no inflammation, atrophy and scarring *(MCQ 703)*.
- Alopecia totalis is a variant of alopecia areata. It refers to loss of all scalp hair with no scarring or atrophy.

708. Ans. c. It is caused by systemic corticosteroids which has caused generalized hypertrichosis and hypertrichosis of androgen independent site (forehead) also. Swelling on face also supports the systemic steroids as a cause.
- Idiopathic hirsutism *(MCQ 328)* has insidious or gradual onset which is seen in apparently looking normal young females with positive family history.
- Androgen secreting tumor will present with virilizing features, e.g., clitoromegaly *(MCQs 303, 321)* in addition to hirsutism.
- PCOS is seen during reproductive age *(MCQ 315)*. Androgen independent site will be normal.

709. Ans. a. It is mycosis fungoides which is a cutaneous T-cell lymphoma. Tumor formation is considered as stage II B.
- Psoriatic plaques have silvery scales and do not progress to tumors.
- Cutaneous B-cell lymphoma prefers head and neck region *(MCQ 681)*.
- Lupus vulgaris is characterized by psoriasiform plaques having an advancing peripheral margin with trailing scar towards center *(MCQ 57)*.

710. Ans. b. It is *Paederus dermatitis* which is a peculiar type of irritant dermatitis caused by the coelomic fluid of an insect of the genus *Paederus*. Red patches with grayish white central slough in the patches are characteristic.
- Herpes zoster is characterized by painful grouped vesicles on erythematous base *(MCQ 477)*.
- Dermatitis artefacta is a self-inflicted cutaneous disease by a fully aware patient on easily approachable sites, e.g., legs *(MCQ 494)*, upper extremity *(MCQ 189)* and hands *(MCQ 500)*.

711. **Ans. a.** Dystrophic epidermolysis bullosa shows cleavage immediately below the lamina densa. It is a subtype of epidermolysis bullosa which is a heterogeneous group of genetically determined disease characterized by easy blistering.
    - Suprabasal cleavage is a seen in pemphigus vulgaris *(MCQ 685)*.
    - Subcorneal cleavage is seen in pemphigus foliaceous *(MCQ 705)*.
    - Lamina lucida (subepidermal) is site of cleavage in bullous pemphigoid *(MCQ 720)*.

712. **Ans. b.** It is lymphangioma circumscriptum which is an uncommon lymphatic malformation limited to an area of skin or subcutaneous tissue. Patient usually complains of watery or blood-stained lymph from vesicles.
    - Herpes simplex presents as group of tiny vesicles at the angle of month *(MCQ 9)* or on genitals *(MCQ 445)*.
    - Dermatitis herpetiformis presents as extreme itchy inconspicuous vesicles on upper back *(MCQ 261)*, natal cleft *(MCQ 859)* with no history of watery discharge.

713. **Ans. b.** It is SCC which presents as verrucous exophytic growth on photo damaged skin.
    - BCC usually prefers areas around ear *(MCQ 766)*, eyes *(MCQ 193)* and nose. It is characterized by plaques with slightly raised and thread like margins.
    - Keratoacanthoma develops as smooth surfaced papule or nodule (not as plaques). The mature stage has a central keratotic core *(MCQ 108)*.

714. **Ans. a.** Salt pepper pigmentation (punctate hyperpigmentation and hypopigmentation) is seen in systemic sclerosis. Raynaud's phenomenon and sclerosis are also unique features of systemic sclerosis.
    - Generalized morphea does not present with Raynaud's phenomenon and sclerodactyly.
    - SLE presents with typical butterfly rash *(MCQ 517)* on face, not with sclerodactyly.

715. **Ans. c.** It is pacinian corpuscle which is a rapidly adapting pressure receptor located deep in dermis and subcutaneous tissue. It consists of concentric layers (onion like) of cells and fibrous connective tissue.
    - Merkel's receptors are formed by the association of Merkel's cells with nerve endings. These are unencapsulated nerve endings which respond to discriminative touch *(MCQ 760)*.
    - Ruffini's corpuscles are also called as bulbous corpuscles which are present in deeper dermis in human digits *(MCQ 725)*.
    - Meissner's corpuscles are located superficially in the dermal papillae of digital skin oriented vertically to the epidermal surface *(MCQ 735)*.

716. **Ans. a.** It is CCLE. It typically involves nose, cheeks and lower lip.
    - Vitiligo manifests as macules, not as plaques. Texture of lesions do not change in vitiligo *(MCQ 455)*.
    - SLE on face typically manifests as butterfly rash *(MCQ 467)*.
    - LP lesions have violaceous color. They are never hypopigmented. Actinic LP lesions have deep hyperpigmented center with violaceous thread like rolled edge *(MCQ 404)*.

717. **Ans.** It is Marjolin's ulcer which refers to the development SCC in burn scar or in chronic ulcer. It is associated with poor prognosis because of high risk of metastasis.
    - Scar sarcoidosis is seen in patients having longstanding sarcoidosis involving multiple organs. The scar becomes red and infiltrated.
    - Tuberculosis does not develop in cutaneous scars. Cutaneous tuberculosis can leave behind scars.

718. **Ans. c.** It is a very commonly seen depigmentation due to intraarticular injection of triamcinolone by the orthopedic surgeon. Depigmentation along the draining vessels is also evident.
    - Segmental vitiligo refers to depigmentation limited to a dermatome *(MCQ 181)*.
    - Focal vitiligo refers to the presence of single or few macules in a limited area of body *(MCQ 246)*.

719. **Ans. a.** It is chilblains (syn. perniosis) which is caused by continued exposure to cold in a genetically predisposed person. It is due to persistent constriction of larger arterioles with dilation of superficial vessels.
    - Raynaud's phenomenon manifests as episodic attacks of blanching or blue coloration of digits extending up to various levels of digits on exposure to cold *(MCQ 570)*.
    - Livedo reticularis refers to mottled symmetric fish-net like red or purple discoloration of skin. It may be seen on legs, arms or trunk.

720. **Ans. c.** It is for bullous pemphigoid showing subepidermal cleft *(MCQ 731)*. It shows linear pattern on direct immunofluorescence *(MCQ 704)*.

- In PV, cleft is suprabasal *(MCQ 770)*, basal cells separate from each other giving an appearance of "row of tomb stones" *(MCQ 685)*.
- In PF, cleft is in granular layer or at subcorneal level *(MCQ 705)*.
- In DH, cleft is at subepidermal level. There is dense collection of neutrophils and eosinophils within dermal papillae to form micro abscesses *(MCQ 740)*.

721. **Ans. a. It is condylomata acuminata. It is caused by HPV-6, 11, 16 and 18 types. Transmission can occur both by sexual and non-sexual routes. The genital tract of mother is considered as frequent source of infection for infants.**
    Condylomata lata is a manifestation of secondary syphilis. It manifests as flesh colored and flat-topped sessile papules with oozing and macerations *(MCQ 666)*.

722. **Ans. c. It is circumscribed morphea. The plaque is usually attached to underlying tissues.**
     - Lupus vulgaris plaque is usually psoriasiform and has advancing border and trailing scar *(MCQ 597)*.
     - Tuberculoid leprosy plaque is characterized by loss of sensations *(MCQ 6)*.
     - Vitiligo comprises of a macular lesion with no change in the texture *(MCQ 246)*.

723. **Ans. a. It is nodular melanoma supported by dark-colored nodules with peripheral satellite lesions in an old patient.**
     - SCC presents as exophytic verrucous growth *(MCQ 796)*.
     - Mycosis fungoides presents as large plaques and nodules on covered part of body *(MCQs 667, 709)*. It does not have dark color.
     - LPH presents as group of itchy, hypertrophic papules and nodules *(MCQ 20)*. Lichen planus lesions can be seen on other parts of body.

724. **Ans. b. It is cholinergic urticaria which is due to postganglionic sympathetic stimulation of sweat glands. It is distinct type of urticaria seen in adolescents. It is induced by an increase in core body temperature.**
     - Aquagenic pruritus is seen in patients suffering from polycythemia vera *(MCQ 671)*.
     - Contact urticaria results from physical contact of skin with offending substance, e.g., plants, chemicals, food, etc.
     - Ordinary urticaria is characterized by eruption of variable sized wheals *(MCQ 501)*.

725. **Ans. d. It is Ruffini's corpuscle which is also known as bulbous corpuscle. It is present in deeper dermis in human digits.**
     - Meissner's corpuscles are located superficially in dermal papillae of digital skin oriented vertically to the epidermal surface *(MCQ 735)*.
     - Merkel's receptors are formed by association of Merkel's cells with free nerve ending. These unencapsulated nerve endings respond to vertical pressure *(MCQ 760)*.
     - Pacinian corpuscle consists of characteristic perineural capsule made up of concentric layers (onion like) of cells and fibrous tissue. It is located deep in dermis *(MCQ 715)*.

726. **Ans. b. It is pemphigus foliaceous. Flaccid bullae on seborrheic sites and absence of mucosal involvement are typical features.**
     - *P. vulgaris* is characterized by flaccid blisters with mucosal involvement *(MCQ 184)*.
     - Chronic benign familial pemphigus presents as malodorous moist vegetation and fissures in groins *(MCQ 80)* and axillae *(MCQ 555)*.
     - Linear IgA disease is characterized by presence of bullae around the periphery of previous lesions as collarette of blisters *(MCQs 288, 1004)*.

727. **Ans. c. It is bilateral nevus of Ota. In majority of patients, it is unilateral *(MCQ 158)* and congenital and does not improve with age. It manifests as hyperpigmentation in distribution of first two divisions of trigeminal nerve. Pigmentation of cornea is also seen in this patient.**
     - Melasma is an acquired hyper melanosis on sun exposed areas of face *(MCQ 598)*.
     - Butterfly rash of SLE comprises of redness and edema *(MCQs 25, 467, 517)*. It involves the bridge of nose and characteristically spares the nasolabial folds.

728. **Ans. a. It is erythema multiforme major. Involvement of single mucosa and preceding herpes infection are important features of EM. Target lesions are not seen in every patient.**
     - SJS needs involvement of two or more mucosae and <10% of body surface to qualify the diagnosis *(MCQ 81)*. Lesions of SJS tend to coalesce together.
     - In TEN >30% of body surface is involved *(MCQ 127)*. Both SJS and TEN are usually caused by some offending drug.

729. **Ans. a. These are typical psoriatic red plaques with white scaling.**

- Dermatophytosis or tinea infection has well defined active borders with clearing towards center *(MCQ 773)*.
- Dermatitis comprises of ill-defined patches with or without fine scaling *(MCQ 556)*.

730. **Ans. b. It is *Paederus dermatitis* which is a peculiar irritant dermatitis caused by the coelomic fluid released by the insect of the genus *Paederus*. Red patch with grayish white slough in the center is characteristic.**

    Dermatitis artefacta is a self-inflicted cutaneous disease by the action of a fully aware patient at easily approachable sites of body, e.g., hand *(MCQ 500)*, legs *(MCQ 494)* and upper extremities *(MCQ 189)*.

731. **Ans. d. Lamina lucida (subepidermal) is a site of cleavage in bullous pemphigoid *(MCQ 720)*.**
    - Just below lamina densa *(MCQ 711)* is the site of cleavage in dystrophic epidermolysis bullosa.
    - Subcorneal is a site of cleavage in pemphigus foliaceus *(MCQ 705)*.
    - Suprabasal is the site of cleavage in pemphigus vulgaris *(MCQ 685)*.

732. **Ans. d. It is CCLE which is involving typically the bridge of nose and lip. Lesions have adherent scales which are not easily removable.**
    - Lichen planus lesions have deep hyperpigmented center with violaceous thread like peripheral edge *(MCQ 404)*.
    - Psoriatic lesions have fine silvery white scales and do not involve lips *(MCQ 268)*.
    - Actinic keratosis comprises of asymptomatic multiple 1 mm to 2 cm sized macules or papules having rough scaly surface with sharply demarcated edges *(MCQ 123)*.

733. **Ans. b. It is eczema. Crusting, cracking, diffuse margins and bilateral involvement are important supporting features of eczema.**
    - Psoriasis is characterized by discrete red plaques with silvery white scaling *(MCQ 482)*.
    - Tinea corporis will manifest with well-defined advancing border *(MCQs 4, 7, 40)*.

734. **Ans. c. This child is having psoriasis. Red color of plaques and white scaling are characteristic feature of psoriasis.**
    - Tinea infection on scalp presents as partial hair loss or inflammatory boggy swelling *(MCQ 8)*.
    - Seborrheic dermatitis on scalp presents as diffuse fine greasy scales *(MCQ 552)*.

735. **Ans. c. It is Meissner's corpuscle which is located superficially in the dermal papillae of digital skin. They are oriented vertically to the epidermal Surface. They are rapidly adapting receptors.**
    - Merkel's receptors formed by the association of Merkel's cells and free nerve endings. They are unencapsulated nerve endings which respond to discriminative touch *(MCQ 760)*.
    - Pacinian corpuscle is located deeply in dermis and subcutaneous tissue *(MCQ 715)*. It consists of a characteristic perineural capsule made up of concentric layers (onion like) of cells and fibrous tissue.
    - Ruffini's corpuscle are also known as bulbous corpuscles which are located in deep dermis *(MCQ 725)*.

736. **Ans. b. It is psoriasis. Red plaques with silvery white scales are its typical features.**
    - Tinea manuum usually involves one hand and show a well-defined advancing border *(MCQ 480)*.
    - Eczema patches show ill-defined borders. They do not exhibit redness or white scaling *(MCQ 194)*.
    - Lichen planus presents as violaceous papules *(MCQ 21)*, not plaques.

737. **Ans. b. It is keratolysis exfoliativa which is a noninflammatory recurrent and asymptomatic desquamation of palms and soles. It is common in summers and is associated with hyperhidrosis. It is self-limiting, harmless and only requires emollients.**
    - Tinea manuum shows asymmetrical involvement with a well-defined advancing border *(MCQ 45)*.
    - Dermatitis palm presents with ill-defined plaques or patches which may be hyperkeratotic *(MCQ 383)*.

738. **Ans. b. It is soft corn that occurs between toes due to tight shoes. It is very painful and has a peeling surface.**
    - Callus in an evenly thickened broader area of hyperkeratosis, usually noticed under the heads of metatarsals *(MCQ 369)*.
    - Warts presents as closely placed multiple small warts or as deep seated rough hyperkeratotic lesion. They do not have surrounding hyperkeratotic skin *(MCQs 372, 410, 579)*.

739. **Ans. b. It is tinea capitis. A patch with partial hair loss, fine scaling and easily pluckable hair are typical features of tinea capitis.**

- Psoriasis do not cause hair loss. A patch will show redness and silvery white scaling *(MCQs 100, 314, 553, 601)*.
- Seborrheic capitis will present with diffuse involvement and greasy fine scales *(MCQs 138, 153, 485, 603)*.

740. **Ans. b. It is for dermatitis herpetiformis in which cleft is subepidermal. There is an accumulation of neutrophils and eosinophils within dermal papillae to form microabscesses.**
    - In PF, cleft is in granular layer or just below corneal cell layer *(MCQs 705, 750)*.
    - In PV, cleft is suprabasal and basal cells separate from each other and give an appearance of "row of tomb stones" *(MCQ 685, 770)*.
    - In BP, cleft is subepidermal. Intact epidermis forms the roof of the blister *(MCQs 720, 731)*.

741. **Ans. b. It is fracture penis. It occurs during vigorous thrusting. The erect penis may accidently slip out of the vagina and may strike outside. It classically occurs with the female partner on top. Although, there is a no bone, still it is referred as penile fracture.**
    - Contact allergic dermatitis to condom will not produce subcutaneous hematoma.
    - ITP manifest as spontaneous petechiae and ecchymosis *(MCQs 342, 354)*.

742. **Ans. c. Unilateral or asymmetrical involvement is a typical feature of tinea infection.**
    - Candidiasis most commonly affects interdigital web-spaces *(MCQs 183, 393, 490)*.
    - Housewife's contact dermatitis presents as ill-defined eczematous patches *(MCQs 394, 513)* usually on both palms.

743. **Ans. b. It is hyperkeratotic eczema soles. Itching supports eczema.**
    - Psoriasis presents as red plaques with scaling *(MCQ 511)*.
    - Tinea pedis presents as desquamating white scales *(MCQ 51)*. It may show unilateral involvement with well-defined advancing border *(MCQ 423)*.
    - Diffuse plantar keratoderma presents as uniform thickening of soles with no itching *(MCQ 192)*. It usually manifests in childhood.

744. **Ans. c. It is erythema multiforme major. Involvement of single mucosa and preceding herpes infection are important features of EM. Target shaped lesions *(MCQ 140)* are not seen in every patient.**
    - Both SJS and TEN are usually caused by some offending drug. In SJS 2 or >2 mucosae are involved. Cutaneous lesions tend to coalesce and involve <10% of body surface *(MCQ 81)*.
    - In TEN, >30% of body surface is involved *(MCQ 127)*.

745. **Ans. c. Fish-net or honeycomb pattern or basket weave appearance of direct immunofluorescence is seen in pemphigus vulgaris and pemphigus foliaceus.**
    - Bullous pemphigoid or linear IgA disease shows linear pattern *(MCQ 794)*.
    - Erythema multiforme and epidermolysis bullosa simplex are negative on direct immunofluorescence.

746. **Ans. a. It is herpes zoster with dissemination. Lymphoreticular malignancies, e.g., Hodgkin's disease, leukemia and HIV infection should be ruled out as an underlying cause of dissemination.**
    - Herpes zoster and chickenpox do not occur together.
    - Kaposi's varicelliform eruption comprises of appearance of large number of vesicles due to HSV-1 on recently healed areas of atopic dermatitis or in patient on immunosuppressive therapy.

747. **Ans. c. It is segmental vitiligo which is limited to a dermatome. Distribution of trigeminal nerve (mandibular division) is most frequently affected. It is common in children usually having a stable course. It does not respond to treatment satisfactorily.**
    - Focal vitiligo refers to presence of single or few macules in a limited area of body *(MCQ 246)*.
    - Vitiligo vulgaris is most common clinical type which has a widespread involvement in a symmetrical manner *(MCQ 511)*.

748. **Ans. b. It is acrodermatitis enteropathica which is rare autosomal recessive *(MCQ 664)* metabolic disorder. These infants have lower zinc absorption and typically manifests soon after weaning. Top feeds have lower zinc bioavailability than breast milk.**
    - Impetigo contagiosa is a bacterial infection which is characterized by honey colored crust *(MCQs 60, 945)*.
    - Atopic dermatitis on face presents as redness, scaling and crusting. It chiefly affects cheeks *(MCQ 174)*.

749. **Ans. a.** It is due to prolonged use of topical corticosteroid cream. It is called topical steroid damaged face (TSDF). Tiny papules and hirsutism are other changes seen on face in TSDF patients *(MCQ 5)*.

750. **Ans. c.** Subcorneal is level *(MCQ 750)* of cleavage in pemphigus foliaceous *(MCQ 705)*.
    ❖ Lamina lucida (subepidermal) is the level of cleavage *(MCQ 690)* in bullous pemphigoid *(MCQ 720)*.
    ❖ Just below lamina densa is level of cleavage in dystrophic epidermolysis bullosa *(MCQ 711)*.
    ❖ Suprabasal is site of cleavage *(MCQ 770)* in pemphigus vulgaris *(MCQ 685)*

751. **Ans. b.** It is frenular tear. Typically, it is seen as a result of undue stretch due to vigorous thrust during sexual act in a newly married man or because of insufficient penovaginal lubrication in later part of life. It requires reassurance and symptomatic treatment. Patient is advised abstinence till healing and to use condom for 2–3 weeks.

752. **Ans. c.** It is kerion. Inflammatory boggy swelling, partial hair loss with lymphadenitis in a child are its typical features *(MCQ 11)*.
    ❖ Nevus sebaceous presents as a circumscribed, hairless, waxy and velvety plaque *(MCQs 99, 609)*.
    ❖ Pyogenic abscess presents as an acute painful, red swelling without any hair loss *(MCQs 548, 581923, 971)*.

753. **Ans. a.** Healed crusted lesions of varicella are no more infectious. It does not require further antiviral therapy.

754. **Ans. b.** Tacrolimus 0.1% cream (a macrolide immunosuppressant) is a novel treatment for vitiligo especially for periorbital vitiligo. It does not cause corticosteroid related side effects, e.g., atrophy, telangiectasia or potential ocular side effects like glaucoma.
    Systemic PUVA therapy below 12 years is not recommended.

755. **Ans. c.** It is for Hailey-Hailey disease (chronic benign familial pemphigus). Widespread partial acantholysis gives the epidermis a dilapidated brick wall appearance.
    ❖ In PV, cleavage is suprabasal *(MCQ 770)*. Basal cells separate from each other which gives an appearance of "row of tombstones" *(MCQ 685)*.
    ❖ In PF, cleavage is in stratum granulosum or at subcorneal level *(MCQs 705, 750)*.
    ❖ In BP, cleavage is subepidermal *(MCQs 720, 731)*. There is an inflammatory cell infiltrate in superficial dermis.

756. **Ans. b.** Isotretinoin causes cheilitis in every patient. Teratogenicity is another side effect of isotretinoin. It should not be used in females who are planning for pregnancy.

757. **Ans. d.** These are rolling scars which are broad depressions with sloping edge to give a saucer shape.
    ❖ Anetoderma refers to flat thin macular atrophic scars due to loss of elastic tissue *(MCQ 565)*.
    ❖ Box scars are wider than ice pick scars, round or oval in shape with vertical walls. They are found in areas like lower region of cheeks and jaw where skin is relatively thick *(MCQ 520)*.
    ❖ Ice pick scars are narrow, deep, pitted scars with wider opening which gives an infundibular shape.

758. **Ans.** It is scalp psoriasis. Red plaques with white scaling leaving normal skin between the plaques are typically due to psoriasis.
    ❖ Seborrheic capitis manifests as fine greasy scales involving the whole scalp or forming a big patch *(MCQs 138, 153, 603)*.
    ❖ Tinea capitis presents as patches with partial hair loss *(MCQs 8, 739, 782)* and does not occur at this age.
    ❖ LP presents as papular lesions, not as plaques.

759. **Ans.** Most common side effect of topical steroid is cutaneous atrophy. Areas having thin skin are particularly vulnerable to atrophy, e.g., cubital fossa *(MCQ 13)*.

760. **Ans. a.** It is Merkel's receptor or disc which are formed by association of Merkel's cell with free nerve endings. They are unencapsulated nerve endings which respond to discriminative touch.
    ❖ Meissner's corpuscles are located superficially in dermal papillae oriented vertically to epidermal surface *(MCQ 735)*.
    ❖ Ruffini's corpuscle are also known as bulbous corpuscle lying deep in the dermis *(MCQ 725)*.
    ❖ Pacinian corpuscles are located deeply in the dermis and subcutaneous tissue *(MCQ 715)*.

761. **Ans. c.** Topical PUVA therapy is hazardous and is not used frequently. It frequently leads to erythema, burning and blistering. It can be used very cautiously for localized disease or in children in whom systemic therapy is avoided.

- Systemic PUVA therapy is recommended in patients above 12 years of age having vitiligo.
- Narrow band UVB is a safe and effective option. It is recommended for children, pregnant women and patients having >10% body surface involvement.
- Tacrolimus 1% ointment is treatment of choice for periorbital vitiligo *(MCQ 754)*.

762. Ans. b. It is myxedema which is a manifestation of hypothyroidism.
- Urticaria is accompanied by itching with remissions and relapses.
- Lepromatous leprosy manifests with infiltration of ear lobules with red infiltrated plaques *(MCQs 101, 495, 692, 560)*.
- Systemic sclerosis manifests as mask like face with pinched nose. Mouth gives a pursed appearance due to constriction of opening, appearance of radial furrows and thin lips *(MCQ 14)*.

763. Ans. c. It is acrodermatitis enteropathica which is a rare autosomal recessive *(MCQ 664)* disorder seen in young children who have lower zinc absorption than adults. It typically manifests just after weaning. Top feeds have lower zinc than breast milk. Typically, it presents as psoriasiform lesions is perioral region *(MCQ 748)* and perianal region. It responds very well to supplementation of zinc in the dose of 2 mg/kg/day.
- Impetigo is a bacterial infection which presents as honey-colored crusts *(MCQs 60, 945)*.
- Atopic dermatitis manifests in popliteal fossae *(MCQ 159)*.
- Psoriasis comprises of red plaques with silvery scales.

764. Ans. a. It is Cushing's syndrome due to prolonged use of oral corticosteroids. Cortisol causes hypertrichosis of the non-androgen dependent sites (forehead) also.
- B-complex or iron syrup do not cause swelling or hypertrichosis.
- Vitamin-D drops are recommended in all fully or partially breast-fed infants (400 units/day) up to 1 year of age.

765. Ans. b. It is Sarcoptes scabiei (0.2–0.4 mm sized) mite. It has ovoid and dorsoventrally flattened body. It has 4 pairs of short legs having bristles. It can be demonstrated easily in KOH smear *(MCQ 651)* made from scabietic burrow, crusts and tiny vesicles.
- Head louse is 1–4 mm sized elongated wingless insect having 3 pairs of legs which terminate in small claws.
- Body louse is 30% bigger than head louse, otherwise it is similar.
- *Pthirus pubis* has a rounded body like a crab *(MCQ 61)*. The front pairs of claws are smaller while rear two pairs of legs have larger claws.

766. Ans. b. It is basal cell carcinoma. Around eye *(MCQ 193)*, nose and ear are common sites.
- SCC usually arises on photo damaged skin showing irregular pigmentation and solar elastosis *(MCQ 776)*.
- CCLE presents as well defined, red, discoid plaques with adherent scales *(MCQ 201)*.
- Lupus vulgaris is type of skin tuberculosis which manifests as soft gelatinous plaque having advancing active margin at periphery with trailing scar towards center *(MCQs 26, 57, 534, 597, 975)*.

767. Ans. b. Systemic corticosteroids has an immunosuppressive effect which worsens the tinea infection. Formation of striae is a very common side effect of systemic corticosteroids.
- Antiepileptic or antitubercular drugs cause acneiform eruption *(MCQ 43)*.
- Isotretinoin is a commonly used drug for severe acne. It causes cheilitis in every patient *(MCQs 3, 756)*.

768. Ans. b. It is congenital acanthosis nigricans (AN).
- Malignancy associated AN manifest in later part of life. Nails becomes brittle and hairs are shed.
- Pseudoacanthosis nigricans is a commonest type. It is associated with insulin resistance in obese patients *(MCQ 273)*.

769. Ans. b. It is lichen planus soles. Papular lesions, pruritus, peripheral parts and purple color are typical features of lichen planus.
- Psoriasis is characterized by red plaques with white scales *(MCQ 571)*.
- Eczema is characterized by oozing, crusting and itching *(MCQ 137)*.

770. Ans. c. Suprabasal is site of cleavage in pemphigus vulgaris.
- Subcorneal is the site of cleavage in pemphigus foliaceous *(MCQs 705, 750)*.
- Lamina lucida *(MCQ 690)* is the site of cleavage in bullous pemphigoid *(MCQs 720, 731)*.

- Just below lamina densa is the site of cleavage in dystrophic epidermolysis bullosa *(MCQ 711)*.

771. **Ans. b. It is notalgia paresthetica. It is a chronic sensory neuropathy due to entrapment of spinal nerves particularly at C2-C6 level of the vertebrae. The constant scratching damages the skin that causes hyperpigmentation and dark patches in the affected area.**
    - Macular amyloidosis is seen as diffuse hyperpigmentation on upper back in females *(MCQ 627)*.
    - In lichen simplex chronicus, the skin become lichenified with accentuated skin markings. It is common on nape of neck *(MCQ 263)* scrotum *(MCQ 97)* and labia majora *(MCQ 197)*.

772. **Ans. b. It is hyperkeratotic eczema of palms. Thick scales and intense itching favor eczema.**
    - Psoriasis manifests as discrete red plaques leaving normal skin in between *(MCQ 233)*.
    - Dermatophytosis manifests as asymmetrical involvement and itching is not severe *(MCQ 45)*.
    - Palmar keratoderma shows uniform thickening with no itching *(MCQ 486)*.

773. **Ans. a. It is tinea corporis with characteristic well-defined borders with fine white scaling.**
    - Psoriasis comprises of red plaques (not patches) studded with silvery white scales *(MCQ 729)*.
    - Dermatitis consists of ill-defined patches *(MCQ 556)*.

774. **Ans. a. It is scalp psoriasis. Thick white scales, redness of underlying skin and limitation to hairline favors the diagnosis as psoriasis.**
    Seborrheic dermatitis comprises fine greasy scales and extends beyond the hairline *(MCQ 153)*.

775. **Ans. a. It is seen in herpes simplex vesicles. Similar findings are seen in vesicle due to varicella-zoster virus.**
    - Pemphigus foliaceus shows subcorneal vesicle formation with no giant cell or intranuclear inclusion bodies *(MCQ 705)*.
    - Pemphigus vulgaris shows supra basal cleft, with no giant cells *(MCQ 685)*
    - Hailey-Hailey disease shows widespread acantholysis showing dilapidated brick wall appearance *(MCQ 755)*.

776. **Ans. a. It is SCC which arises on photodamaged skin showing irregular pigmentations, solar elastosis, telangiectasia, etc.**
    - BCC presents as flesh-colored translucent papule or plaque with surface telangiectasia or a well demarcated red patch with irregular margins *(MCQ 193)*.
    - CCLE manifests as discoid, well circumscribed plaques with adherent scales and may show hyperpigmentation at the periphery *(MCQ 67)*.
    - Actinic keratosis comprises of multiple 1 mm to 2 cm sized macules or papules having rough scaly surface *(MCQ 123)*.

777. **Ans. c. It is lupus vulgaris which is a type of cutaneous tuberculosis having moderate to high degree of immunity.**
    - Psoriatic plaques manifest with silvery scales with no central atrophy.
    - Tuberculoid leprosy plaques will have loss of sensations *(MCQ 6)*.
    - CCLE lesions are seen on sun exposed parts of body and have peripheral pigmented border and adherent scales *(MCQ 732)*.

778. **Ans. a. It is common warts. Rough hyperkeratotic papules are typically seen with asymmetrical involvement.**
    Lichen plans papules have little scaling and violaceous tinge *(MCQ 21)*.

779. **Ans. a. It is chickenpox. A vesicular crop on trunk with surrounding irregular area of erythema (a dew drop on rose petal appearance) is typical of chickenpox.**
    - Molluscum contagiosum comprises of dome-shaped shiny papules (not vesicles) with central umbilication *(MCQ 375)*.
    - LP comprises of violaceous itchy papules on extremities *(MCQ 381)*.

780. **Ans. b. It is showing herpes simplex or varicella zoster virus infection. Presence of multinucleated giant cells are typical.**
    - Pemphigus shows acantholytic cells in Tzanck smear *(MCQ 373)*.
    - Bullous pemphigoid will show eosinophils.
    - CBDC will show neutrophils.

781. **Ans. a. It is lichen planus. Genital mucosa is involved in 25% of patients. Plane topped papules are typical of LP.**
    - Psoriasis on glans shows characteristic well-defined plaques which lack scales *(MCQ 95)*.
    - FDE has a characteristic dark gray color and is an acute disorder with the history of prior drug intake *(MCQ 160)*.

❖ Venereal warts present as rough hyperkeratotic skin-colored papules *(MCQ 283)*.

782. **Ans. d. Isotretinoin is a drug of choice for severe acne patients. It affects all pathogenic factors of acne. Complete and long remission is remarkable. It is given in dose of 0.5 to 1.0 mg/kg/day after meals. It gives satisfactory response in 4–6 weeks of therapy. Cheilitis** *(MCQs 3, 756)* **is a common side effect.**

783. **Ans. b. It is herpes simplex labialis. Grouped vesicles, without any pain on upper lip with a short history are typical features.**
    ❖ FDE presents as dark grayish patch *(MCQ 199)* or as large vesicle (not in group).
    ❖ Herpes zoster presents as unilateral painful eruption of vesicles in many groups limited to a dermatome *(MCQ 790)*.

784. **Ans. a. Appearance of striae and acneiform eruptions are very common side effects of systemic corticosteroid therapy. Acneiform eruptions are also caused by antiepileptic and antitubercular drugs.**
    Vitamin A hypervitaminosis cause dryness of skin, mouth ulcers, hair loss, cracked finger nails, increased intracranial tension, headache, blurring of vision, etc.

785. **Ans. b. This diagram is for Darier's disease. It is an autosomal dominant condition. Epidermis shows hyperkeratosis and dyskeratosis (premature and abnormal keratinization) resulting in formation of "corps ronds" and "grains".**
    ❖ Epidermolysis bullosa presents as easy blistering due to mild mechanical trauma. It does not show dyskeratosis or hyperkeratosis *(MCQs 79, 506, 958)*.
    ❖ Hailey-Hailey disease typically shows dilapidated brick wall appearance *(MCQ 755)*.
    ❖ Pemphigus vulgaris shows suprabasal cleft *(MCQ 770)*. Basal cells separate from each other to give an appearance of "row of tomb stones" *(MCQ 685)*.

786. **Ans. b. It is condylomata acuminata (genital warts). It is caused by HPV-6, 11, 16 and 18 types with an incubation period of 3 weeks to 8 months.**
    ❖ Condylomata lata is a manifestation of secondary syphilis. It presents as flesh colored, flat topped sessile papules with oozing and macerations. It is seen in anal region *(MCQ 666)* and other flexures *(MCQ 686)*.

787. **Ans. a. It is tinea manuum. Well-defined red patches with fine scaling and unilateral involvement are typical features of tinea.**
    ❖ Eczema comprises of ill-defined plaques usually with bilateral involvement *(MCQ 413)*.
    ❖ Psoriasis comprises of red plaques (not macules) studded with silvery white scaling *(MCQ 736)*.

788. **Ans. c. It is plane warts. These warts respond well to topical tretinoin cream.**
    ❖ Actinic keratosis is a manifestation of sun damaged skin seen at older age. It manifests as 1 mm to 2 cm sized macules or papules having rough scaly surface. Characteristically, lesions have adherent scales *(MCQ 123)*.
    ❖ Acne vulgaris comprises of comedones, papules and pustules *(MCQ 216)*.

789. **Ans. b. It is chickenpox (varicella). Profuse lesions on trunk comprising of small vesicles surrounded by irregular area of erythema (dew drop on rose petal) is typical of varicella.**
    ❖ Drug-induced acne (acneiform eruption) comprises of monomorphic papules which have developed in many weeks *(MCQ 43)*.
    ❖ Morbilliform or exanthematous drug rash comprises of 2–10 mm sized macular lesions which are confluent as places. Absence of blistering or pustulation is an essential feature *(MCQ 238)*.

790. **Ans. b. It is herpes zoster. Herpes zoster in children is quite uncommon. But, grouped painful vesicles with unilateral distribution in a dermatome are typical features of herpes zoster.**
    ❖ Herpes simplex vesicles are not painful and are usually not seen in many groups *(MCQ 783)*.
    ❖ *Paederus dermatitis* presents as linear lesion or bizarre shaped lesion with gray slough in center *(MCQ 710)*.

791. **Ans. c. It is tuberculosis verrucosa cutis showing healing with scarring in the central part of lesion. Unilateral involvement points towards infective pathology.**
    ❖ Plantar warts can involve extensive area but do not have central scarring or well-defined peripheral border *(MCQs 410, 579)*.
    ❖ Plantar psoriasis comprises of red plaques and usually involve both soles *(MCQ 571)*.
    ❖ Plantar eczema will involve both soles with oozing, crusting and itching *(MCQ 150)*.

792. **Ans. c. It is tinea capitis. A well-defined patch with partial hair loss, pustules and redness are typical features of tinea capitis.**
    - Alopecia areata presents as a complete bald patch with smooth skin without any pustules or redness *(MCQ 703)*.
    - Trichotillomania presents as a patch of alopecia on easily approachable site of scalp *(MCQs 128, 583, 659, 833)*. The patch shows the presence of firmly anchored partially broken hairs.

793. **Ans. b. It is generalized pustular psoriasis (GPP). Systemic steroid is a most common precipitating factor. GPP should be treated at the earliest.**
    - Secondary infection of plaques can produce only scattered pustules.
    - Impetigo herpetiformis (syn. GPP of pregnancy). It is seen during last trimester of pregnancy.
    - Acropustulosis is a localized pustular psoriasis which involves tips of fingers and toes *(MCQ 376)*.

794. **Ans. b. Linear pattern of direct immunofluorescence is seen in both bullous pemphigoid and linear IgA disease. It is due to linear deposition of IgG and C3 in bullous pemphigoid and IgA in linear IgA disease.**
    - Pemphigus shows fish-net or honeycomb or basket weave appearance *(MCQ 745)*.
    - Epidermolysis bullosa simplex and erythema multiforme are negative on direct immunofluorescence.

795. **Ans. b. It is chilblains (syn. perniosis). It is caused by continued exposure to cold in a genetically predisposed person. It is due to persistent constriction of larger arterioles and dilatation of superficial vessels.**
    - Raynaud's phenomenon manifests as episodes of blanching or blue coloration of digits extending up to various levels of digits on exposure to cold *(MCQ 570)*.
    - Livedo reticularis refers to mottled, symmetric fishnet like, red or purple discoloration of skin. It might be seen on legs, arms or trunk.

796. **Ans. c. It is a squamous cell carcinoma presenting as verrucous growth. Excisional biopsy should be done.**
    - TVC lesions may show finger like projections from margins with surrounding erythema. Lesions may show clefts and fissures *(MCQ 10)*.
    - Pyogenic granuloma (syn. lobular capillary hemangioma) is a misnomer. It is nothing to do with pus. It presents as a vascular nodule at the site of recent penetrating injury *(MCQ 114)*.

797. **Ans. b. It is candidal balanoposthitis due to underlying diabetes. It is one of the common presentations of diabetes.**
    - With prolonged use of steroid cream, undersurface of prepuce and glans become thin red and glazed *(MCQ 545)*.
    - FDE on genitals presents as dusky red coloration *(MCQs 160, 200, 824, 852)*.
    - Secondary syphilis on genitals presents as shallow round painless lesions with surrounding red areola.

798. **Ans. a. It is lamina fibroreticularis which lies deeper to lamina densa and is composed of fibrils.**
    - Subbasal dense plaques (SBDP) are linear densities beneath each hemidesmosome *(MCQ 700)*. The anchoring fibrils traverse through as SBDP.
    - Lamina densa *(MCQ 680)* is an electron dense layer deeper to lamina lucida.
    - Lamina lucida *(MCQ 690)* is an electron lucent intermembranous space which separates plasma membrane from the lamina densa. It is a level of cleavage in bullous pemphigoid *(MCQ 731)*.

799. **Ans. b. It is candidiasis groins due to diabetes. Characteristically, it is showing red wet maceration with irregular fringed margins with classical satellite vesicles and pustules.**
    - Tinea cruris presents with well-defined active borders *(MCQ 4)*.
    - Intertrigo refers to inflammation of opposing surfaces in body folds which is common in obese persons. Involvement is limited to the area of contact of surfaces *(MCQs 166, 946)*.
    - Flexural psoriasis characteristically shows red color, well defined margins and scaling *(MCQs 84, 245, 801)*.

800. **Ans. c. These changes are seen in wart. The presence of koilocytotic cells (koilocytes) is diagnostic of warts. The keratohyalin granules are composed of papillomavirus.**
    - Psoriasis shows Munro's microabscesses and spongiform pustules of Kogoj in horny layer and stratum spinous layer respectively *(MCQ 805)*.
    - Lichen planus shows sawtooth appearance and band like dermal infiltrate *(MCQ 870)*.
    - Molluscum contagiosum shows lobule formation separated by septae. Epidermal cells have large inclusion bodies *(MCQ 895)*.

801. **Ans. c.** It is flexural psoriasis showing red coloration and well-defined margins with no central clearing. Scaling in minimal in flexural psoriasis. Submammary folds, umbilicus *(MCQ 245)* and groins *(MCQ 84)* are common sites.
    - Candidiasis presents as itchy red macerations in body folds. It develops fringed irregular margins with satellite vesicles and pustules *(MCQs 179, 253, 607, 695, 799)*.
    - Intertrigo presents as erythema and soreness limited to the area of contact of body folds *(MCQs 166, 946)*.
    - Tinea cruris comprises of active borders with central clearing *(MCQ 4)*.

802. **Ans. b.** It is discoid eczema characterized by itchy, wet, crusted coin shaped lesions.
    - Tinea corporis comprises of red patches with well-defined active borders with central clearing *(MCQ 613)*.
    - Psoriasis comprises of red plaques with silvery white scaling *(MCQ 482)*.

803. **Ans. b.** He is a typical case of secondary syphilis characterized by asymptomatic bilateral symmetrical maculosquamous lesions involving palms and soles. VDRL, HIV, HBsAg and HCV should be done in such patients.
    - Lichen planus presents as itchy, purple-colored papules *(MCQ 231)*.
    - Hyperkeratotic eczema presents as pruritic and thick plaques *(MCQ 772)* limited to palm.
    - Keratolysis exfoliativa presents as asymptomatic fine white scaling *(MCQs 737, 452)* which is limited to palm and is accompanied by excessive sweating.

804. **Ans. b.** It is pearly penile papules which is a very common physiological condition and is mistaken by the patient as penile warts. They are angiofibromas. Reassurance is usually sufficient to an anxious patient. VDRL, HIV, HBsAg and HCV can be done to reassure the patient and to rule out any blood borne STDs.
    - Genital warts are variable sized, red cauliflower like growths not limited to coronal margin *(MCQ 283)*.
    - Secondary syphilis presents as shallow rounded painless lesions surrounded by red areola.
    - Herpes genitalis presents as a group of tiny vesicles *(MCQs 445, 471, 512, 927)*.

805. **Ans. c.** These changes are seen in psoriasis. Presence of parakeratosis, Munro's microabscesses, spongiform pustules of Kogoj and clubbing of rete ridges are diagnostic features of psoriasis.
    - Lichen planus shows, hyperkeratosis without parakeratosis, band like dermal infiltrate and colloid bodies *(MCQ 870)*.
    - Warts shows koilocytotic cells in the spinous layer. Rete ridges often bend towards center *(MCQ 800)*.
    - Molluscum contagiosum shows formation of lobules separated by thin septae. Epidermal cells of lobules contain large Feulgen positive inclusion bodies *(MCQ 895)*.

806. **Ans. a.** Initially, application of corticosteroid cream gives a soothing effect. Later on, patient becomes habitual. Skin becomes red with development of hypertrichosis and papules *(MCQs 5, 749)*. It is called as topical steroid damaged face (TSDF).

807. **Ans. c.** It is Zoon's balanitis (plasma cell balanitis) which is a rare benign penile dermatosis. It is seen in uncircumcised males. Friction, poor hygiene and chronic infection are predisposing factors. Circumcision is definitive curative treatment.
    - Candidal balanoposthitis presents as erythema, tiny papules, pustules, superficial erosions and collarette of white scales *(MCQs 38, 693, 797)*.
    - Psoriasis of glans presents as well-defined red plaques which lacks scales *(MCQ 95)*.
    - Erythroplasia of Queyrat is a premalignant condition seen between 30–60 years of age. It presents as velvety red, shiny, well demarcated plaque on glans or inner surface of prepuce. Patient may complain of pruritus, bleeding and crusting.

808. **Ans. b.** It is very common to see 2–3 months after intralesional or intra-articular triamcinolone injections *(MCQ 152)*.
    - Focal vitiligo refers to presence of single or few macules in a limited area of body *(MCQ 246)*.
    - Tacrolimus do not cause depigmentation. It may cause temporary redness and itching.

809. **Ans. b.** It is phrynoderma which results from deficiency of vitamin A, E, B-complex vitamins and essential fatty acids. These patients may have ocular manifestations, cheilitis, glossitis, etc.
    - Follicular lichen planus manifests on scalp, medial aspects of extremities and trunk.
    - Keratosis pilaris is seen as keratotic follicular plugging (not papules) on the extensors of upper arms, thighs and face.

810. **Ans. c.** These changes are seen in lupus erythematosus. Out of these three salient features, at least two should be present to make a histological diagnosis of LE.
- Psoriasis shows hyperkeratosis with parakeratosis, presence of Munro's microabscesses and spongiform pustules of Kogoj, elongation and clubbing of rete ridges *(MCQ 805)*.
- Lichen planus shows hyperkeratosis without parakeratosis. Rete ridges shows flattening in the center and irregular lengthening at the periphery. Dermis shows bandlike infiltrate in close proximation to epidermis *(MCQ 870)*.
- Warts shows hyperkeratosis, acanthosis, papillomatosis and presence of koilocytotic cells in the malpighian layer. Elongation of rete ridges which often bend towards center *(MCQ 800)*.

811. **Ans. a.** It is focal plantar keratoderma which manifests as thickenings at pressure areas of palms and soles, e.g., at ends of metatarsal arch, sides of soles *(MCQ 337)*, etc.
Both callus and keratoderma imply excessive thickening and hyperkeratosis of palmar and plantar skin at pressure points. Keratoderma is a disorder and callus is a manifestation.

812. **Ans. a.** It is typical keloid which is extending beyond the boundaries of skin injury.
Hypertrophic scar remains confined to original wound. It follows shortly after injury. This is often asymptomatic, regresses with time and is more responsive to the treatment *(MCQ 205)*.

813. **Ans. b.** It is lichen amyloidosis. Potent topical steroid ointments with/without occlusive dressings is the treatment of choice.
- LP presents as itchy violaceous papules on peripheral parts *(MCQ 381)*.
- Prurigo nodularis presents as extremely itchy papules and nodules on extensors of legs *(MCQs 170, 822)*.

814. **Ans. b.** It is mycosis fungoides tumor stage (stage IIB). It is a cutaneous T-cell lymphoma which passes through patch, plaque and tumor stages.
- LL on face *(MCQs 101, 595, 692, 560)* presents as infiltrated ear lobules and red plaques (not tumors).
- ABCD on face presents as redness, scaling and lichenification *(MCQs 86, 892)*.
- CAD presents as shiny red lichenified lesions (not tumors) on sun exposed areas showing sharp cut off at lines of clothing *(MCQ 196)*.

815. **Ans. c.** It is called Adamson's fringe which separates the nucleated cells of the bulb of follicle from non-nucleated cells in the stem of follicle. Dermatophytic infection of hair follicle is restricted to Adamson's fringe and is not allowed to penetrate further down into the bulb.
- Isthmus of follicle is the part which extends from opening of sebaceous duct up to the insertion of arrector pili muscle.
- Stem cells are present in the bulge meant for the insertion of arrector pili muscle.
- Suprabulbar part (stem of the follicle) extends from the Adamson's fringe to the lower part of isthmus.

816. **Ans. a.** It is epidermolysis bullosa simplex. It is one of the types of mechanobullous disorders which includes a heterogenous group of genetically determined and acquired skin diseases characterized by easy blistering of skin *(MCQs 79, 506)* and mucosa due to mild mechanical trauma. It shows autosomal dominant inheritance *(MCQ 639)*.
Chronic benign familial pemphigus (Hailey-Hailey disease) manifests in 3rd or 4th decade as painful fissures in flexures *(MCQs 80, 483, 555)*.

817. **Ans. d.** It is a typical case of granuloma annulare. It is considered as a reaction pattern to variety of triggering factors, e.g., diabetes, thyroid disease, drugs etc.
- Annular psoriasis will show silvery white scaling *(MCQs 294, 857)*.
- Annular lesions of mid-borderline leprosy will show impairment of sensations *(MCQs 211, 661, 438)*.
- Tinea lesions will have itching. Tinea incognito lesions lose their typical annular character and have itching *(MCQs 451, 509, 572)*.

818. **Ans. c.** It is Zoon's balanitis (plasma cell balanitis). It is an uncommon benign dermatosis seen in middle aged or older uncircumcised males. Friction, poor hygiene and chronic infections are predisposing factors.
- Secondary syphilis on glans presents as shallow, rounded and painless lesions edged by dull red areola.
- Erythroplasia of Queyrat presents as velvety red plaque with pain, pruritus, bleeding and crusting.

- Candidal balanitis presents as transient erythema, tiny pustules and papules, superficial erosions and collarette of white scales on glans *(MCQs 38, 693, 797).*

819. **Ans. a. It is strawberry hemangioma which typically appears in first month of life (not at birth). It continues to grow up to 1 year of life. In view of spontaneous regression, no active management is required in majority of patients.**
    - Port-wine stain always appears at birth as various sized unilateral deep red patch in the distribution of sensory branches of trigeminal nerve *(MCQs 521, 521, 882).*
    - Salmon patch manifests as dull pinkish red blanchable macule of fine linear telangiectasia. Nape of neck, eyelids, forehead and tip of nose are common sites.

820. **Ans. b. It is eccrine sweat gland which consists of secretary coil lying in lower dermis and duct which connect the coil to the skin surface.**
    - Sebaceous gland is formed by an invagination from hair follicle. It is an oil producing gland connected to hair follicle by sebaceous duct.
    - Apocrine ground is a part of pilosebaceous unit. Its duct is short which opens into the neck of hair follicle above the opening of sebaceous gland *(MCQ 840).*
    - Adamson's fringe is located at the upper margin of hair bulb *(MCQ 815).*

821. **Ans. a. It is diffuse plantar keratoderma. It is an autosomal dominant disorder which manifests at birth or in first few months of life.**
    Tylosis is synonym of diffuse plantar keratoderma.

822. **Ans. b. It is prurigo nodularis. Nodules are 0.5–3 cm sized, firm to hard and have hyperkeratotic surface with overlying excoriation. Extensor surfaces of limbs are affected in most cases. Psychological and environmental factors, constant rubbing and scratching are common etiological factors.**
    - LP comprises of violaceous papules *(MCQ 381).*
    - Lichen amyloidosis presents as highly pruritic, closely placed papules on extensor surfaces of legs *(MCQs 371, 813, 997).*

823. **Ans. b. It is mycoses fungoides tumor stage (Stage IIB). It is a cutaneous T-cell lymphoma which passes through patch, plaque and tumor stages.**
    - SCC presents as cauliflower like growths *(MCQs 113, 287, 429, 528, 669).*
    - B-cell cutaneous lymphoma presents as non-scaly single or multiple, pink or reddish tumors in a circumscribed area *(MCQ 681).* Head and neck are common sites.

824. **Ans. c. It is fixed drug eruption. Glans penis is a common site. Dark slate gray-colored prepuce is typical of FDE.**
    - Candidal balanoposthitis presents as transient erythema, tiny papule or pustule, superficial erosions and collarette of white scales *(MCQs 38, 693, 797).*
    - Secondary syphilis presents as shallow rounded and painless lesions edged by dull red areola.

825. **Ans. b. It is nail matrix. About proximal one fourth part of nail plate is covered by proximal nail fold. Beneath it, lies the nail matrix which produces nail plate.**
    - Hyponychium refers to the anatomical area below the free end of nail plate *(MCQ 890).*
    - Nail bed refers to the epidermis and connective tissue beneath the pink zone of nail plate *(MCQ 835).*
    - Cuticle refers to the extension of horny layer of proximal nail fold over the nail plate *(MCQ 845).*

826. **Ans. b. It is typical diabetic trophic ulcer. Trophic ulcer is a pressure ulcer due to external trauma to the part of body that is in poor condition because of disease, vascular insufficiency or loss of sensations. It is most common site followed by plantar surface of big toe. It is reverse in leprosy** *(MCQ 689).* **Absence of pulsations of dorsalis pedis is common in diabetes due to atherosclerosis. Sensations may be impaired both in leprosy and diabetes.**
    - In leprosy, thickening of nerves and positivity of slit skin smear for AFB will be there.
    - Tropical ulcer is a painful rapidly enlarging ulcer on lower limb.
    - Buerger's disease never occurs in nonsmokers. It presents as intermittent claudication, ulcers and gangrenous changes *(MCQs 422, 478).*

827. **Ans. b. It is nevus depigmentosus (nevus achromicus) which is a rare isolated congenital nevoid pigmentary disorder presents at birth or in early childhood. It is a solitary lesion that may be several centimeters in size with irregular feathered margins but does not cross the midline** *(MCQs 252, 896).* **There is no white hair in the patch.**
    - Nevus anemicus is a congenital localized blanchable round or oval macule with surrounding satellite macules.

Chapter 5 ✦ Answers of MCQs in Dermatology, Venereology and Leprology

- Focal vitiligo refers to presence of single or few acquired depigmented macules in a limited area of body *(MCQ 246)*.
- In tuberous sclerosis macules are hypomelanotic, smaller sized, may be more than one and are associated with epilepsy.

828. **Ans. b. It is pseudo-Hutchinson's sign. It is the presence of or illusion of pigment in the periungual region in the absence of melanoma. In this case, it is due to anticancer drugs used for breast cancer. Such pigmentation disappears in due course of time.**
 Hutchinson's sign is a periungual extension of brown black pigmentation from longitudinal melanonychia on to the proximal and lateral nail folds. It is an important indicator of subungual melanoma.

829. **Ans. b. It is miliaria profunda. It is due to rupture of sweat ducts at or below the dermo epidermal junction because of repeated attacks of miliaria rubra.**
    - Miliaria rubra manifests as uniformly minute red papules in flexures and areas of body which are prone to friction of clothing *(MCQs 118, 838)*.
    - Miliaria crystallina manifests as crop of asymptomatic, noninflamed, tiny thin-walled vesicles without surrounding erythema *(MCQ 414)*. It is seen in febrile patients having profuse sweating.

830. **Ans. b. It is basal cell carcinoma. It is showing palisading arrangement formed by tumor cells that have dark staining oval or elongated nuclei. These cells are called as 'basaloid cells' which have no inter cellular bridges.**
    - SCC shows extension of atypical keratinocytes beyond basement zone into dermis with presence of horny pearls *(MCQ 850)*.
    - Paget's disease shows characteristic Paget's cells in prickle cell layer and in the epithelium of hair follicle *(MCQ 885)*.
    - CTCL will show colonization of T-cells along basal cell layer (epidermotropism) and predominant lymphocytic infiltration in the papillary dermis.

831. **Ans. c. It is acrofacial or lip and tip vitiligo involving finger tips and perioral region *(MCQ 455)*. It is least responsive to the treatment.**
    - Focal vitiligo refers to the presence of acquired single or few macules in a limited area of body *(MCQ 246)*.
    - Segmental vitiligo involvement is limited to a dermatome. The distribution of trigeminal nerve (mandibular nerve) is most frequently affected *(MCQs 181, 747)*.

832. **Ans. b. She is having PCOS fulfilling two criteria out of three. She is having amenorrhea (criteria 1), hyperandrogenism (criteria 2). But ovarian sizes are normal, i.e., <10 cc volume.**
    - Idiopathic hirsutism comprises of normal menstruation, normal androgen level and normal ovarian size *(MCQ 328)*.
    - LO-CAH comprises of evidence of defeminization, i.e., amenorrhea, small breasts, increase in muscle bulk, loss of smooth body contours, etc.
    - Androgen secreting tumor presents with rapid hair growth *(MCQ 321)*, appearance of male sex characters, e.g., clitoromegaly *(MCQ 303)* deepening of voice, roughness of skin.

833. **Ans. c. It is trichotillomania. It is a psychiatric illness in which patient has a compulsive impulse to pull out hair. It manifests with presence of firmly anchored partially broken hairs. Typically, peripheral and occipital regions of scalp are spared. Prognosis is not good in adults.**
    - Telogen effluvium presents as diffuse hair loss 3-4 months after an inciting event *(MCQ 163)*.
    - Androgenic alopecia presents as central parting, diffuse central thinning *(MCQs 185, 190)*.
    - Alopecia areata presents as complete bald patches of hair loss. Skin of the patch is smooth with absence of inflammation, scaling and atrophy *(MCQs 145, 156, 468, 569, 589, 637, 678, 703, 907)*.

834. **Ans. c. Raynaud's phenomenon (RP) refers to abnormal sensitivity to cold manifesting as episodic attacks of digital ischemia on exposure to cold. Primary RP is idiopathic and is called as Raynaud's disease or syndrome. Secondary Raynaud's phenomenon is seen as symptom most commonly due to underlying connective tissue diseases. Secondary RP results in trophic changes in fingers, e.g., atrophy of finger tips *(MCQs 496, 570)*.**
 Chilblains manifests as diffuse cutaneous redness of fingers and/or toes *(MCQs 409, 719, 795, 897)* due to persistent constriction of larger arterioles with dilatation of superficial vessels.

835. **Ans. c. It is nail bed which consists of epidermis with underlying connective tissue beneath the pink zone of nail plate.**
    - Nail matrix lies beneath the proximal one-fourth part of nail plate covered by proximal nail fold *(MCQ 825)*. Nail matrix produces nail plate.

- ❖ Hyponychium refers to anatomical area below the free end of nail plate *(MCQ 890)*.
- ❖ Cuticle refers the extension of horny layer of proximal fold over the nail plate *(MCQ 845)*.

836. **Ans. b.** It is miliaria rubra. It is due to blockage of sweat duct at intraepidermal level. It is common in hot and humid conditions.
     - ❖ Miliaria crystallina manifests as crops of asymptomatic, non-inflamed tiny thin-walled vesicles without any surrounding erythema *(MCQ 414)*.
     - ❖ Exanthematous rash comprises of 2–10 mm sized red macules which may get confluent at places *(MCQs 238, 336, 931)*. It is commonest adverse reaction to drugs.

837. **Ans. c.** It is cicatricial (scarring) alopecia showing thin atrophic skin. It may be idiopathic or may be caused by underlying some skin disease, e.g., lichen planus *(MCQ 24)*, CCLE *(MCQ 76)*. It is irreversible type of alopecia and does not respond to treatment.
     - ❖ Central parting *(MCQ 190)* is a type of female androgenetic alopecia which is a reversible type of hair loss. It can respond to treatment.
     - ❖ Telogen effluvium is a diffuse hair loss due to some inciting event *(MCQ 163)*.
     - ❖ Alopecia areata presents as patches of complete hair loss. Patches are well defined with no scarring, scaling or inflammation *(MCQs 145, 156, 468, 569, 589, 637, 678, 703, 907)*.

838. **Ans. b.** It is LMDF. It is an uncommon granulomatous idiopathic disorder. It shows variable response to tetracyclines, isotretinoin and dapsone.
     - ❖ Acne vulgaris comprises of papules, pustules and comedones *(MCQ 216)*.
     - ❖ Acne rosacea typically presents in middle age females as papules and pustules (no comedones) involving central part of face *(MCQs 50, 853)*.
     - ❖ Acneiform eruption is seen on trunk, shoulders, and chest as monomorphic papules due to corticosteroids, antiepileptics, antitubercular drugs *(MCQs 27, 43, 919)*.

839. **Ans. c.** It is seen in SLE. It is categorized as nonspecific lesion (not showing specific histology of lupus). But it is a sensitive indicator of systemic disease activity.
     - ❖ In systemic sclerosis, there is sclerodactyly. Fingers give smooth shiny tapered appearance *(MCQ 702)*. Pulp of fingers become atrophied with nails covered over it.

840. **Ans. a.** It is apocrine sweat gland which is a part of pilosebaceous unit. It opens into the neck of hair follicle just above the opening of sebaceous gland. These glands are distributed in axillae, perianal skin and areolae of breasts.
     - ❖ Adamson's fringe separates the bulb of follicle from the stem of follicle *(MCQ 815)*.
     - ❖ Eccrine sweat glands open directly to the skin surface *(MCQ 420)*.
     - ❖ Sebaceous gland is an invagination from the hair follicle and opens into hair follicle by sebaceous duct.

841. **Ans. b.** It is pseudofolliculitis. It is seen in males who have curly hairs. Penetration of sharp tips of shaved hairs to the neighboring skin is responsible for this disorder. Patient is benefited by not shaving for 4–6 weeks.
     - ❖ Sycosis barbae is a subacute or chronic bacterial infection of whole depth of hair follicles common in beard region. It presents as red edematous papule or pustule with a hair in the center *(MCQ 387)*.
     - ❖ Tinea barbae (syn. tinea sycosis, barber'itch) is ringworm of beard and moustache areas with invasion of coarse hairs *(MCQ 431)*. Hairs are easily pluckable without pain.

842. **Ans. a.** It is fixed drug eruption due to some offending drug. Lips are common sites for FDE. Dark gray color is typical of FDE.
     Herpes simplex labialis presents as group of tiny vesicles *(MCQ 783, 9)*.

843. **Ans. b.** It is leukoderma due to nail polish. Leukoderma is a commonly used term by laymen implying acquired depigmentation of skin irrespective of etiology.
     - ❖ Focal vitiligo refers to presence of acquired single or few macules in a limited area of body *(MCQ 246)*.
     - ❖ Term acrofacial or lip and tip vitiligo is used when tips of fingers, toes and perioral regions are involved *(MCQs 831, 455)*.

844. **Ans. b.** It is PCOS which is fulfilling two out of three criteria designed for its diagnosis. She is having hyper androgenism (acne, hirsutism, raised testosterone). LH/FSH ratio is not important. Ovarian size >10 cc in any one ovary is taken as due to PCOS.
     - ❖ Idiopathic hirsutism comprises of normal menstruation, normal androgen levels and normal sized ovaries *(MCQ 328)*.

- LO-CAH comprises of loss of female characters (defeminization) i.e., amenorrhea, small sized breasts, increase in muscle bulk, loss of smooth body contours.

845. **Ans. a. It is cuticle which is an extension of horny layer of proximal nail fold over the nail plate which prevents the separation of plate from nail fold. Loss of cuticle is characteristically seen in chronic paronychia** *(MCQ 481).*
    - Nail bed refers to the epidermis and connective tissue beneath the pink zone of nail plate *(MCQ 835).*
    - Hyponychium refers to the area below the free end of nail plate *(MCQ 890).*
    - Nail matrix lies beneath the proximal one-fourth of nail plate covered by proximal nailfold *(MCQ 825).*

846. **Ans. a. It is chronic cutaneous lupus erythematosus (CCLE). Red plaques with adherent scales on sun exposed parts of face are typical of CCLE.**
    - SLE on face is seen as malar rash (butterfly rash) characteristically sparing nasolabial folds *(MCQs 25, 89, 467, 517).*
    - Lupus vulgaris is a type of cutaneous tuberculosis which presents as psoriasiform plaque *(MCQs 26, 57, 256, 534, 597, 600, 975)* having advancing active margin at periphery with trailing scar towards center.

847. **Ans. a. It is actinic lichen planus. Sun exposed sites, i.e., face, dorsa of hands and neck are common sites for actinic LP.**
    Plane warts presents as 1–5 mm sized, skin colored, plane topped slightly elevated and rounded or polygonal shaped lesions *(MCQs 1, 389).*

848. **Ans. b. It is pityriasis rosea which is a self-limiting condition that usually fades in 3–6 weeks. It is usually preceded by herald patch** *(MCQ 195).*
    - Rash of secondary syphilis shows polymorphism which means that macules, papules, papulosquamous lesions are present at the same time *(MCQ 293).* Palms and soles are usually involved *(MCQs 214, 803).*
    - Exanthematous rash is a most common drug eruption which consist of 2–10 mm sized macular lesion which may get confluent at places *(MCQs 238, 336, 931)* and is accompanied by itching.

849. **Ans. b. It is psoriasis scalp. Redness, silvery white scaling and well-defined margins are typical of psoriasis.**
    - Seborrheic dermatitis on scalp shows fine greasy scales with no or mild redness *(MCQs 153, 603).*
    - Tinea capitis is not seen at this age. Tinea capitis presents as a patches of partial hair loss *(MCQ 8).*

850. **Ans. d. It is squamous cell carcinoma. Infiltration beyond basement membrane, proliferating downward strands and presence of horny pearls are classical features.**
    - BCC is characterized by thin epidermis, tumor masses with palisading arrangement and peritumoral lacunae *(MCQ 830).*
    - Paget's disease is characterized by presence of Paget's cells in prickle cell layer and in the epithelium of hair follicle *(MCQ 885).*
    - CTCL typically show colonization of T-cells along the basal cell layer (epidermotropism).

851. **Ans. a. It is superficial spreading melanoma.**
    - It is fulfilling all the features of the acronym ABCDE. It is **a**symmetric, **b**orders are irregular and notched, **c**olor is variegated, **d**iameter is >6 mm and is **e**volving with time.
    - BCC develops around nose *(MCQ 676),* eye *(MCQ 193)* and ear *(MCQ 766)* as thick plaque with raised thread like margin.
    - SCC develops as hyperkeratotic thick plaque on photo damaged skin *(MCQ 776).*

852. **Ans. c. It is fixed drug eruption. Short history, superficial erosion and gray color are typical features.**
    - LP is characterized by violaceous-colored papules *(MCQ 15).*
    - Psoriatic plaques on glans are well-defined red plaques which lack scales *(MCQ 95).*
    - Herpes genitalis is characterized by group of tiny vesicles *(MCQs 445, 471, 512, 927).*

853. **Ans. b. It is acne rosacea showing involvement of central part of face with persistent erythema. Absence of comedones is a feature of acne rosacea.**
    - Acne vulgaris is seen in adolescents and young adults with papules pustules and comedones *(MCQ 216).*
    - LMDF presents as 2–4 mm sized monomorphic papules distributed symmetrically on forehead, cheeks and eyelids *(MCQs 50, 417).*
    - Drug-induced acne (acneiform eruption) presents as 2–4 mm sized red monomorphic eruption on back, shoulder *(MCQ 43)* and chest *(MCQ 27).*

854. **Ans. b.** It is malar rash (butterfly rash) which is considered as specific lesion of SLE. It characteristically spares the nasolabial folds *(MCQs 25, 89, 467, 517).*
    CCLE presents as red discoid lesions with adherent scales, peripheral rim of hyperpigmentation *(MCQ 67)* and scarring in the center.

855. **Ans. b:** It is tuberculoid leprosy. Because of high degree of immunity granuloma is compact with scanty or absence of AFB.
    - In lepromatous leprosy, immunity is very low. So, granuloma is diffuse with plenty of bacilli inside and outside macrophages *(MCQ 880).*
    - Tuberculosis verrucosa cutis shows pseudoepitheliomatous hyperplasia of epidermis. Dermis shows mixed infiltrate with sparse tuberculosis foci.

856. **Ans. d.** It is subungual hyperkeratosis. It is due to abnormal keratinization of distal nail bed and hyponychium *(MCQ 890)* which results into accumulation of scales under the nail plate. The most common causes are psoriasis and onychomycosis.
    - Onychomadesis refers to the detachment of proximal nail plate from proximal nail fold due to temporary arrest in nail matrix activity *(MCQ 677).*
    - In onychogryphosis, nail plate is thickened, distorted and becomes opaque and yellowish brown giving an oyster shell appearance.
    - Onycholysis is a separation of distal nail plate from nail bed *(MCQ 682).*
    - Onychorrhexis is typically seen in lichen planus. It presents as multiple longitudinal ridges and fissures in nail plate *(MCQ 112).*

857. **Ans. b.** It is annular psoriasis with typical red plaques having silvery white scales. It is an uncommon type.
    - Annular lesions of leprosy will show impairment of sensations *(MCQ 211).*
    - Granuloma annulare presents as complete and incomplete rings of small papules *(MCQs 219, 591, 817).*
    - Ring lesions of tinea are itchy and have well defined, active and narrow border *(MCQ 142).* The lesions may get confluent together.

858. **Ans. c.** It is psoriatic plaques on soles. Patchy involvement with white scaling, absence of itching and presence of similar lesions on other parts make the diagnosis of psoriasis.
    - Lichen planus lesions will manifest as purple-colored papules *(MCQ 437).*
    - Focal keratoderma presents as thick plaques at pressure sites with no scaling *(MCQs 337, 811).*
    - Tinea pedis presents as white scaling with no thickening *(MCQs 51, 423).*
    - Hyperkeratotic eczema manifests with itching, oozing and crusting *(MCQ 150).*

859. **Ans.** It is a typical case of dermatitis herpetiformis characterized by extreme itching, group of small vesicles. Shoulders, natal cleft, extensors are typical sites. It responds dramatically to dapsone.
    - In scabies, involvement of genitals is almost always there.
    - Pemphigus foliaceous prefers the seborrheic sites *(MCQs 330, 403, 864)* with no intense itching.
    - Linear IgA dermatosis manifests with cluster of blisters around the periphery of previous lesion *(MCQs 288, 1004)* known as cluster jewels.

860. **Ans. b.** It is diode laser which is used for hair removal and to treat some vascular lesions.
    - CO_2 laser (10,600 nm) has two modes of action i.e., excisional cutting mode and vaporization or ablative mode.
    - Nd: YAG-laser (1054 nm) is a very powerful and effective tissue coagulator.
    - Narrow band UVB chamber (311–313 nm) is used for the treatment of psoriasis and vitiligo.

861. **Ans. c.** It is Bowen's disease which is a type of SCC in situ. The risk of progression to invasive carcinoma is about 3–5% in untreated patients.
    - SCC presents as an exophytic cauliflower like growth *(MCQs 113, 289, 429, 669).*
    - Malignant melanoma presents as variegated patch or hyperpigmented nodule *(MCQs 121, 126, 464, 492, 516, 656, 687, 851, 899).*

862. **Ans. b.** It is neonatal acne which is thought to be due to transplacental stimulation of adrenal glands.
    - ETN presents as blotchy red macules 1–2 cm in diameter with a 1–3 mm sized central papule or vesicle *(MCQ 432).*
    - Milia neonatorum presents as multiple pin head to 1 mm sized epidermal keratin cysts. They resolve in few weeks *(MCQ 497).*
    - Miliaria crystallina manifests as crop of asymptomatic, noninflamed, tiny, thin-walled vesicles without any surrounding redness. They appear in first week of life due to delay in patency of sweat ducts. *(MCQ 414).*

863. **Ans. c.** It is psoriasis. Red-colored well-defined plaques with white scaling are typical of psoriasis.
    - CCLE plaques have adherent scales and peripheral rim of hyperpigmentation *(MCQ 242)*.
    - LP manifests as discrete violaceous papules *(MCQ 23)*, not plaques.
    - Hyperkeratotic eczema presents as hyperkeratotic thick plaques with scaling *(MCQ 772)*. Red coloration is not there.

864. **Ans. b.** It is pemphigus foliaceous. Absence of mucosal involvement, flaccid blisters and involvement of seborrheic sites are typical features.
    - Pemphigus vulgaris typically manifests with oral mucosal involvement *(MCQ 184)*.
    - DH manifests with group of small vesicles on shoulders, natal clefts and buttocks *(MCQs 261, 859, 884)*.
    - Linear IgA dermatosis shows blisters around a previous lesion *(MCQs 288, 1004)* which is called as 'cluster of jewels'.

865. **Ans. b.** It is diagrammatic structure of Corona virus. It has two layered structure. The *viral envelope* consists of a lipid layer in which club-shaped spikes are embedded and project from the surface. Envelope surrounds *inner core* that consists of a single stranded RNA genome and nucleocapsid of helical symmetry. It forms a continuous bead on a string type configuration.
    Structure of HIV virus is three-layered structure, i.e., inner core (nucleoprotein core) consisting of single stranded RNA genome, matrix protein which surrounds nucleocapsid shell and outermost is envelope *(MCQ 875)*.

866. **Ans. a.** It is erythroderma due to endogenous eczema. Dull red erythema and fine scaling favors it.
    - Erythroderma due to psoriasis will show bright red color, large white exfoliating scales and small areas of uninvolved skin *(MCQ 243)*.
    - Senile dermatitis or eczema presents as dry scaly skin with prominent and deep skin markings and reticulate superficial fissures *(MCQ 94)*.
    - Exanthematous rash is a common drug adverse reaction. It manifests as 2–10 mm sized red macules which get confluent at places *(MCQs 238, 336, 931)*.

867. **Ans. b.** It is infective dermatitis (syn. Infective eczematoid dermatitis). Invaded microorganism or their byproducts play a causative role in eczema. Development of eczematization around the opening of external auditory meatus in a patient having pus discharge from ear is another good example *(MCQ 360)*.
    - Term infected eczema is used when eczema is complicated by secondary infection *(MCQ 220)*.
    - Id eruption refers to the eruption of small and pruritic vesicles on the sides of fingers *(MCQ 180)* in response to an intense inflammatory process elsewhere in the body.

868. **Ans. a.** He is a typical patient of TSC showing adenoma sebaceum (angiofibromas) on face. Angiofibromas consist of hyperplastic blood vessels and sebaceous glands. TSC comprises of a diagnostic clinical triad 'Epiloia', i.e., Epilepsy, low intelligence and adenoma sebaceum.
    - Plane warts are smooth, slightly elevated, plane topped 1–5 mm sized colored papules *(MCQs 1, 389)*.
    - LMDF (acne agminata) is seen in adults. It presents as 2–4 mm sized monomorphic papules distributed symmetrically on face *(MCQs 417, 838)*.

869. **Ans. c.** It is hyperkeratotic eczema. Itching, oozing, crusting and bilateral involvement are typical features.
    - Psoriasis will show red color and white scaling *(MCQ 858)*.
    - Plantar keratoderma presents as diffuse hyperkeratosis with no itching or fissuring *(MCQ 486)*.

870. **Ans. b.** These changes are seen in lichen planus. In addition, rete ridges in the center of lesion show flattening. Epidermis is separated from dermis by formation of Max Joseph clefts.
    - Psoriasis shows hyperkeratosis with parakeratosis, Munro's microabscesses and spongiform pustules of Kogoj and clubbing of rete ridges *(MCQ 805)*.
    - Warts shows presence of koilocytotic cells in spinous layer *(MCQ 800)*.
    - Molluscum contagiosum shows formation of lobules separated by septae. Epidermal cells have large intranuclear inclusion bodies *(MCQ 895)*.

871. **Ans. c.** It is allergic dermatitis to the eye drops. It is limited to the periorbital area.
    - ABCD is an example of allergic contact dermatitis to air borne allergens, e.g., pollen grains, fungal spores etc. Skin of the face becomes thickened, pigmented and lichenified *(MCQs 86, 892)*.

It typically involves upper eye lids, area under nose and chin.
- Allergic dermatitis due to hair dye presents as swelling of forehead and eye lids *(MCQ 395)*. There is no periorbital erythema.

872. Ans. d. He is having scabies with tinea cruris and corporis. One should always have a look on genitals in all patients of tinea infections. Otherwise, there are great chances to miss scabies.
Flexural psoriasis will show red color with minimal scaling *(MCQ 84)*.

873. Ans. b. It is tinea faciei showing a well-defined active border on the neck.
- Pityriasis versicolor lesions tend to become confluent in the center. At margins, discrete satellite lesions can easily be seen *(MCQs 39, 421, 522, 887)*.
- Seborrheic dermatitis shows fine greasy scales and margins are ill defined *(MCQ 566)*.

874. Ans. d. It is vulvovaginal candidiasis. Diabetes and pregnancy are common predisposing factors. It presents as scanty, thick curdy white discharge with itching and soreness. Vulval skin becomes dusky red with flecks of discharge. Perineum and groins may also be involved in extensive cases.
- LSC presents as thickening and lichenification of labia majora due to repeated scratching and rubbing *(MCQ 197)*.
- Secondary syphilis presents as shallow painless rounded lesions *(MCQ 457)*.
- Lichen sclerosus et atrophicus is a collagen tissue disorder which presents as white sclerotic areas involving anogenital region forming figure of 8. Clitoris and labia minora suffer the most.

875. Ans. a. It is structure of HIV virus consisting of three-layered structure. Innermost is *inner core* which consists of single stranded RNA genome and proteins. Middle one is *matrix protein* which surrounds nucleocapsid shell. Outermost is called *envelope* which consists of glycoproteins.
Structure of corona virus is two layered comprising of envelope which surrounds inner core which comprises of RNA genome and nucleocapsid *(MCQ 865)*.

876. Ans. c. It is seborrheic dermatitis with secondary infection. It is involving seborrheic sites with features of eczema (post-auricular, external auditory meatus, nasolabial folds, scalp and groins).
- Atopic dermatitis involves cheeks, cubital and popliteal fossae *(MCQs 159, 207)*.
- Flexural psoriasis has well defined margins and does not have oozing and crusting *(MCQs 84, 245, 801)*.
- Hailey-Hailey disease (chronic benign familial pemphigus) involve groins *(MCQ 80)* or axillae *(MCQs 443, 555)*. It does not involve nasolabial folds or post-auricular region.

877. Ans. a. It is seborrheic dermatitis with secondary infection. It is involving seborrheic sites (postauricular, external auditory meatus, naso labial folds, scalp and groins).
- Atopic dermatitis involves cubital and popliteal fossae *(MCQs 159, 207)*.
- Infective eczematoid dermatitis develops around an infective focus, e.g., road side injury *(MCQs 498, 867)*, around ear opening *(MCQ 360)*.

878. Ans. a. It is candidiasis. In addition to systemic factors, moisture and maceration are important predisposing local factors for candidiasis.
- Tinea manuum presents as asymmetrical diffuse hyperkeratosis or scaly patch with well-defined proximal border *(MCQs 45, 742)*.
- Scabies presents as papules and pustules in fingers web spaces *(MCQ 62)*.
- Household contact dermatitis manifests on dorsal aspects of fingers *(MCQ 413)* or as hyperkeratotic small patches on palmar surface *(MCQ 394)*.

879. Ans. d. Disseminated herpes zoster is quite alarming. Underlying HIV infection and lymphoreticular disorders should always be ruled out in all cases of disseminated herpes zoster, recurrent herpes zoster *(MCQ 353)*, bilateral involvement *(MCQ 42)* and in patients having involvement of more than one site *(MCQ 30)*. This patient was having HIV infection.

880. Ans. b. It is lepromatous leprosy which has very low immunity. So, granuloma is diffuse with plenty of AFBs inside and outside macrophages.
- Tuberculoid leprosy has very high immunity. So, granuloma is compact and bacilli are scanty or absent *(MCQ 855)*.
- Tuberculosis verrucosa cutis shows pseudo-epitheliomatous hyperplasia of epidermis.

881. Ans. b. It is SCC. The growths are forming plaques with no pedicles. Five-year survival rate is only 10–15% in the presence of bilateral enlargement of inguinal lymph nodes.

Venereal warts present as hyperkeratotic, cauliflower like growths with pedicles *(MCQ 283)*.

882. **Ans. b. It is port-wine stain (nevus flammeus). It is always present since birth as unilateral persistent deep colored few mm to many centimeters sized patch in the distribution of sensory branches of trigeminal nerve. It comprises of ectatic dilatation of superficial dermal capillaries.**
    - Strawberry hemangioma presents as smooth or lobulated scarlet red single tumor in first month (not at birth) of life *(MCQs 187, 819)*.
    - Salmon patch presents as blanchable, dull pinkish irregular macule on the nape of neck, eyelids forehead, tip of nose, etc.

883. **Ans. b. It is candidal intertrigo between fingers web spaces along with paronychia. In addition to systemic factors, moisture and maceration are important predisposing factors for candidiasis.**
    - Tinea manuum presents as asymmetrical diffuse hyperkeratosis or a patch with well-defined proximal border *(MCQs 45, 742)*.
    - Household contact dermatitis involves dorsa of hands or as hyperkeratotic patches on palmar surface *(MCQs 394, 513)*.

884. **Ans. d. It is a typical case of dermatitis herpetiformis characterized by extreme itching, groups of small vesicles. Shoulders, natal cleft, buttocks and extensors of limbs are typical sites. It responds dramatically to dapsone.**
    - Linear IgA dermatosis manifests with cluster of blisters around the periphery of previous lesion *(MCQs 288, 1004)* known as 'cluster of jewels'.
    - In scabies, involvement of genitals is almost always there.
    - Pemphigus foliaceous prefers the seborrheic sites *(MCQs 330, 403, 864)* with no intense itching.

885. **Ans. c. It is Paget's disease *(MCQ 103)*. Paget's cells are not seen in the dermis.**
    - SCC is characterized by invasion of basement membrane by atypical keratinocytes and presence of horny pearls *(MCQ 850)*.
    - BCC shows tumor masses having peripheral palisading arrangement by basaloma cells and peritumoral lacunae *(MCQ 830)*.
    - CTCL shows epidermal colonization by T-cells along the basal cell layer (epidermotropism).

886. **Ans. b. It is chronic paronychia. Loss of cuticle is characteristic which leads to colonization of candida. It leads to chronic inflammation of nail folds which affects nail matrix and nail growth. Nail plate becomes discolored with formation of ridges.**
    - Tinea unguium refers to infection of nail plate by dermatophytes only *(MCQ 22)*.
    - Onychomycosis denotes infection of nail by dermatophytes and non-dermatophytes.
    - Acute paronychia presents as painful swelling of nail fold. Later on, pus may get localized which usually points close to nail *(MCQ 458)*.

887. **Ans. b. It is pityriasis versicolor. Its macules are typically getting confluent together on forehead with peripheral satellite macules *(MCQs 39, 421, 522)*.**
    - Pityriasis alba is a common benign self-limiting mild eczematous condition predominantly seen on the face of children. It presents as ill-defined patch of hypopigmentation covered by powdery white scales *(MCQs 85, 909, 930)*.
    - Vitiligo comprises of patch of depigmentation *(MCQs 181, 754)*.

888. **Ans. c. It is molluscum contagiosum. Eyelids are uncommon site. But pearly white papules with central umbilication is a typical feature of molluscum contagiosum.**
    - Milia are 1-2 mm sized, uniform dome-shaped white papules with smooth nonumbilicated top commonly seen on cheeks and eyelids *(MCQ 48)*.
    - Common warts present as rough hyperkeratotic papules *(MCQ 392)*.

889. **Ans. c. It is tinea faciei having well-defined active borders.**
    - Acne rosacea presents as papules, pustules and persistent erythema. It does not form plaque. Lesions are seen on chin, forehead and other central parts of face *(MCQs 40, 853)*.
    - Psoriasis presents as red plaques with white scaling *(MCQ 268)*.

890. **Ans. b. It is hyponychium which is an anatomical area below the free end of nail plate.**
    - Nail matrix lies beneath the proximal one-fourth of nail plate covered by proximal nail fold *(MCQ 825)*.
    - Cuticle refers the extension of horny layer of proximal nail fold over the nail plate *(MCQ 845)*. Loss of cuticle is characteristically seen in chronic paronychia *(MCQ 481)*.
    - Nail bed refers to the epidermis along with underlying connective tissue beneath the pink zone of nail palate *(MCQ 835)*.

891. Ans. b. It is trichotillomania which is a psychiatric disorder that presents as strong impulse to pull out hair from an easily approachable site. It manifests as firmly anchored partially broken hairs. It has better prognosis in children.
- Alopecia areata presents as completely bald patches. The patch has smooth shiny skin with no inflammation, scarring or scaling *(MCQs 145, 156, 468, 589, 678, 703, 907)*.
- Telogen effluvium manifests as diffuse hair loss *(MCQ 163)*. It is seen 3-4 months after some inciting event.

892. Ans. c. It is ABCD which is an example of contact allergic dermatitis to airborne allergens, e.g., Pollen grains, fungal spores, etc. It presents as redness, thickening and lichenification of facial skin due to unbearable constant itching.
- PLE presents as lesions of many morphological types, i.e., papules, vesicles, etc., on face within few hours of exposure to UV radiation *(MCQ 198)*.
- CAD manifests on photo exposed sites. It does not require any contact of external allergen. It manifests as lichenified lesions on sun exposed areas. Lesions show sharp cut off at lines of clothing *(MCQ 196)* and spares the eye lids.

893. Ans. d. CLSs are very rare to be seen in patients of neurofibromatosis 2. Diagnosis of neurofibromatosis 1 requires 2 or more criteria out of 7 criteria. Axillary freckling is one of them.

894. Ans. b. It is pityriasis rosea. It is usually preceded by mother patch *(MCQ 195)* and usually fades in 3-6 weeks time.
- Rash of secondary syphilis shows polymorphism. Macules, papules and papulosquamous lesions are present at the same time *(MCQ 293)*. Palms and soles are usually involved *(MCQ 214)*.
- Exanthematous rash is a most common adverse drug reaction which consists of 2-10 mm sized macular lesions which may get confluent at places *(MCQs 238, 336, 931)* and is accompanied by itching.

895. Ans. d. These changes are seen in molluscum contagiosum.
- Wart shows the presence of koilocytotic cells in the spinous layer. Elongated rete ridges point towards the center of the lesion *(MCQ 800)*.
- Psoriasis shows hyperkeratosis with parakeratosis, presence of Munro's microabscess, spongiform pustule of Kogoj and clubbing of lower part of rete ridges *(MCQ 805)*.
- Lichen planus shows hyperkeratosis without parakeratosis, band like sub epidermal infiltrate, colloid bodies and sawtooth appearance of rete ridges *(MCQ 870)*.

896. Ans. a. It is nevus depigmentosus (nevus achromicus) which is a rare isolated, congenital nevoid pigmentary disorder that presents at birth or in early childhood. It is a solitary lesion that may be several centimeters in size with irregular feathered margins but does not cross the midline *(MCQs 252, 827, 990)*. There is a no white hair in the patch.
- Nevus anemicus is a congenital blanchable circumscribed round or oval macule with surrounding satellite macules.
- Focal vitiligo refers to presence of acquired single or few macules of depigmentation in a limited area of body *(MCQ 246)*.

897. Ans. a. It is perniosis of ear which is uncommon to be involved. Fingers and toes are common to be involved *(MCQs 409, 719, 795)*.
- Involvement of ears in LL will not have burning or itching, Additionally, there will be skin lesions on other parts of body *(MCQ 101)*.
- In urticaria also, there will be urticarial lesions on other parts of body also *(MCQ 194)*.

898. Ans. a. These are typical lesions of fixed drug eruption. Big patches with central gray color and absence of mucosal involvement after intake of drug make the diagnosis of FDE.
Target lesions consist of central zone of erythema or purpura, a middle zone of edema and a peripheral zone of well-defined erythema *(MCQ 140)*.

899. Ans. b. It is malignant melanoma with satellite lesions. It has a very bad prognosis.
- SCC develops on photo damaged skin showing pigmentation, telangiectasia and hyperkeratosis *(MCQ 776)*.
- BCC develops as a well demarcated red patch with irregular, slightly raised and thread like margins *(MCQs 193, 673, 950, 1010)*.

900. Ans. b. It is herpes labialis which is a recurrence of herpes simplex virus (HSV) infection. It is due to reactivation of HSV-I in trigeminal ganglion. Recurrence after a period of latency is a troublesome common feature of HSV infection. It manifests as closely grouped vesicles on erythematous base and is commonly preceded by pain or burning sensation.

Chapter 5 ✦ Answers of MCQs in Dermatology, Venereology and Leprology

- Acne vulgaris manifests as papules, pustules, comedones (no vesicles) on cheeks *(MCQ 216)*.
- Herpes zoster is a painful condition which manifests as groups of vesicles on erythematous base *(MCQ 18)*. It recurs very rarely *(MCQ 55)*.

901. Ans. c. It is scrofuloderma which is an endogenous type of skin tuberculosis that results from contiguous spread of infection from underlying tuberculous focus. Watery discharge, bluish margins and granulating base are typical features *(MCQs 52, 559, 929, 999)*.
- Pyoderma gangrenosum (PG) is typically seen on legs *(MCQ 367)* or trunk in females. It is commonly associated with underlying systemic disease. It presents as painful papule or pustule which evolve into painful ulcer having surrounding erythema.
- Carbuncle is a deep staphylococcal infection of group of contiguous hair follicles. It presents as painful, smooth, dome-shaped hard tender lump with multiple follicular openings *(MCQs 157, 558, 938)*.

902. Ans. a. It is larva migrans. Lesions migrate due to moving parasite in the skin. It is caused by various species of Ancylostoma (hookworms). It is seen in children, farmers, gardeners, sea bathers, etc. Hands, feet, buttocks are common sites. Single dose of ivermectin (200 mg/kg body wt) is the main treatment.
Tinea corporis borders do not migrate, advancement of tinea borders is too slow to be appreciated.

903. Ans. b. It is seborrheic dermatitis scalp showing mild redness and greasy scales.
- Psoriasis scalp manifests as bright redness with silvery scales *(MCQ 849)*. Usually, it shows skip areas of normal skin in between *(MCQ 100)*.
- Tinea capitis is not common at this age. Tinea capitis is seen in children as patches of partial hair loss *(MCQs 8, 384, 441, 729, 792)*.

904. Ans. a. It is lichen simplex chronicus (vulval region) which is a circumscribed neurodermatitis. It is characterized by lichenified plaque with accentuated skin markings. It is caused by long-standing severe itching, repeated scratching and rubbing. Other sites involved are scrotum *(MCQ 97)*, nape of neck *(MCQ 263)*, shins *(MCQ 906)* and lower back *(MCQ 991)*.
- Candidiasis vulva is a manifestation of underlying diabetes. Vulva becomes dusky red with scanty, thick curdy white discharge *(MCQs 264, 607, 695, 874)*. Patient complains of itching, soreness, dyspareunia and dysuria.
- Angiokeratoma labia majora *(MCQ 542)* presents as asymptomatic 1–5 mm sized, reddish or dark colored vascular papules on labia majora. It bleeds, if traumatized.

905. Ans. c. It is typical case of acute urticaria.
- Lepromatous leprosy on face presents as slowly developed asymptomatic infiltration of ear lobules with red plaques on face *(MCQs 101, 495, 692, 560)*.
- Tinea facies shows red plaque with well-defined active borders *(MCQs 241, 400, 411, 873, 889)*.

906. Ans. b. It is lichen simplex chronicus shins (syn. Circumscribed neurodermatitis). It is characterized by localized lichenified plaque. It is caused by longstanding severe itching and rubbing resulting into lichenification which in turn perpetuates itching and completes the cycle (itch scratch cycle). Other sites involved are scrotum *(MCQ 97)*, nape of neck *(MCQ 263)*, vulva *(MCQ 904)* and lower back *(MCQ 991)*.
- Psoriasis comprises of red plaques with white scales *(MCQ 482)*.
- Lichen planus hypertrophicus comprises of multiple, purplish and reddish-brown elevated lesions seen on ankles or shins *(MCQ 20)*.
- Lichen amyloidosis presents as highly pruritic, closely set papules on extensor surfaces of legs *(MCQs 371, 813, 997)*. Papules may coalesce to form plaques.

907. Ans. a. It is alopecia areata which comprises of total bald smooth skin with no inflammation, scaling or atrophy. Skin looks normal. Involvement of eyelashes and eyebrows is quite common.
- Seborrheic dermatitis of eyelashes shows scaling with no loss of hair *(MCQ 171)*.
- Tinea infection shows partial hair loss with red inflamed well defined plaque *(MCQ 889)*.
- Trichotillomania presents as patch with the presence of firmly anchored partially broken hairs *(MCQ 167)*.

908. Ans. b. It is contact irritant dermatitis due to some topical application.
- Tinea corporis will show well defined active borders *(MCQ 7)*.
- Acute urticaria wheals lasts for few hours and resolve within 24 hours *(MCQ 206)*.

909. **Ans. a.** It is pityriasis alba which is a common benign self-limiting mild eczematous condition predominantly affecting face of children. Hypopigmented patch is covered by powdery white scales *(MCQs 85, 930)*.
    - Vitiligo comprises of well-defined depigmented patch *(MCQ 181)*.
    - Nevus depigmentosus is a rare congenital nevoid pigmentary disorder. It remains stable thoughtout life and does not cross midline *(MCQs 252, 827, 896, 990)*.

910. **Ans. e.** It is lichen planus. Pruritus, purple-colored papules on peripheral parts of body are typical features of lichen planus.
    - Psoriasis comprises of plaques (papules are uncommon) with white scaling *(MCQ 482)*.
    - Common warts are asymptomatic, rough and hyperkeratotic papules *(MCQ 770)*.
    - CCLE presents as plaques with adherent scales and peripheral rim of hyperpigmentation *(MCQ 67)*.
    - Prurigo nodularis presents as dark colored itchy nodules on lower extremities *(MCQs 170, 822)*.

911. **Ans. b.** It is herpes zoster ophthalmicus. Groups of small vesicles on erythematous base with unilateral involvement is a characteristic feature.
    - *Paederus dermatitis* manifests overnight. Rash is red edematous usually with a linear *(MCQ 587)* or bizarre pattern with a necrotic white slough in the center. It does not show dermatomal unilateral involvement.
    - Herpes simplex presents as group of small vesicles at angle of mouth with no severe pain or burning *(MCQs 9, 783)*.

912. **Ans. a.** Prolonged application of corticosteroid cream causes hypopigmentation, striae *(MCQ 13)*, cutaneous thinning and telangiectasia *(MCQ 23)*.

913. **Ans. c.** It is pityriasis rosea. It is typically showing discrete oval-shaped macules covered by fine scales. Scales forms a collar at the margin where they are attached peripherally with free edge towards center *(MCQ 996)*. Center of the macule gives a wrinkled appearance.
    - In secondary syphilis trunk involvement usually accompanies palmar *(MCQ 214)* involvement. Lesions are polymorphic and consists of macules, papules with scaling *(MCQ 293)*.
    - Exanthematous rash consists of 2-10 mm sized macules which may get confluent at places *(MCQs 238, 336, 931)*. It is caused by drug or viral infection.
    - Psoriasis comprises of red plaques with white scaling *(MCQs 229, 622)*.

914. **Ans. a.** It is tuberculoid leprosy having highest degree of immunity. A patch with loss of sensations is one of the cardinal features for diagnosis of leprosy.
    - Lepromatous leprosy has least immunity. So, comprises of numerous cutaneous lesions *(MCQ 155)*.
    - Indeterminate leprosy refers to early and transitory stage of leprosy whose immunological status against leprosy bacilli not yet been determined. It presents as an hypopigmented or slightly erythematous ill-defined macule. If edges are palpable, then it is no longer indeterminate type.
    - Histoid leprosy is a variant of multibacillary leprosy which manifests as crop of asymptomatic, multiple, smooth, glistening and firm nontender papules *(MCQ 47)*.

915. **Ans. c.** It is senile purpura which is a most common type of purpura seen by dermatologists. It is due to decreased support of cutaneous micro blood vessels because of increasing age and solar radiation. Hence also known as actinic purpura. It resolves spontaneously in about 10 days.
    - ITP presents as bleeding gums and crops of petechiae *(MCQs 342, 354, 399, 549, 966)*. The majority of patients are children and adolescents.
    - HSP is mostly seen on legs in a symmetrical manner. The majority of patients are <10 years of age *(MCQs 332, 1007)*.
    - Palpable purpura refers to purpura when purpuric lesions are palpable *(MCQ 327)*.

916. **Ans. c.** It is eczema of palm. Ill-defined margins, itching, oozing and crusting are typical features of eczema. Unilateral involvement is unusual. But, in the presence of typical features, clinical diagnosis is eczema.
    - Tinea manuum presents as diffuse hyperkeratosis, white scaling and a well-defined advancing margin proximally *(MCQs 45, 742)*.
    - TVC presents as hyperkeratotic, asymptomatic, indurated and warty plaque showing unilateral involvement *(MCQs 10, 79, 564, 620, 640)*.

917. **Ans. a.** It is psoriasis. Dry red plaques with white scaling are typical features of psoriasis.

- Discoid eczema presents as 1–3 cm sized lesions comprised of closely set small papules and/or vesicles with oozing and crusting *(MCQs 194, 434, 507, 802, 920).*
- Tuberculoid leprosy presents as one or two well defined plaques with loss of sensations *(MCQs 6, 461, 515, 599, 606, 614, 914).*
- Chronic cutaneous lupus erythematosus comprises of plaques with adherent scales with peripheral rim of hyperpigmentation *(MCQs 67, 201, 707, 618, 716, 732).*

918. Ans. e. It is tinea corporis with well-defined active borders.
- Granuloma annulare presents as compete or incomplete circles with no itching *(MCQs 219, 591, 817).*
- Discoid eczema lesions are comprised of small papules and/or vesicles with oozing and crusting. *(MCQ 194, 434, 507, 802, 920).*
- Annular lesions of mid-borderline leprosy are non-itchy and have impaired sensations *(MCQs 211, 438, 661).*
- Annular psoriasis lesions are non-itchy and margins are broader with white scaling *(MCQs 294, 857).*

919. Ans. a. It is drug-induced acne (acneiform eruption) due to prolonged use of high dose of systemic steroids. Increase in appetite and swelling are only seen due to systemic steroids. Back is another common site *(MCQ 43).*
- Acne vulgaris comprises of papules, pustules and comedones *(MCQ 216).*
- Lupus miliaris disseminatus faciei is an uncommon granulomatous disorder. It presents as 2–4 mm sized reddish brown monomorphic papules distributed symmetrically on face *(MCQs 417, 838).*
- Acne rosacea presents as persistent erythema, papules and pustules in central part of face in a middle-aged female *(MCQs 50, 853).* There are no comedones.

920. Ans. b. it is discoid eczema composed of minute papules and/or vesicles is a discoid manner.
- Psoriasis presents as red well-defined plaques with white scaling *(MCQ 917).*
- Lichen planus comprises of purple-colored discrete papules *(MCQs 21, 339, 381, 910).*
- Tinea corporis comprises of ring-shaped lesions with well-defined active borders *(MCQ 918).*

921. Ans. a. It is acute urticaria. It is very common to have acute urticaria in children due to viral infection.
- Measles rash usually accompanies conjunctivitis and cough. It commonly gets confluent on face.
- Exanthematous rash is a common drug adverse reaction. It is common in adults. It is seen as 2–10 mm sized red macules on back that may get confluent at places. Face is least commonly involved *(MCQs 238, 336, 931).*

922. Ans. b. It is psoriasis on penile shaft. It is an uncommon site for psoriasis. Red plaques with white scaling are typical features of psoriasis.
- Lichen planus comprises of purple papules. It is common on glans and undersurface of prepuce *(MCQs 15, 781, 984).*
- Lichen nitidus presents as asymptomatic, shiny, flat topped, discrete, pinpoint to pin head sized flesh-colored papules *(MCQ 16).*
- Tinea lesions have well defined active borders.
- Scabies presents as itchy papules on penile skin and scrotum *(MCQ 65).*

923. Ans. b. It is pyogenic abscess. Short history, pain, tenderness, redness and swelling are typical features *(MCQs 548, 581, 944, 971).*
- Cold abscess is called cold because it is not accompanied by classical signs of inflammation. It is caused by tuberculous infection typically of lymph nodes.
- Matted lymph nodes refer to lymph nodes that are felt connected and seems to move as a unit. It can be benign due to infection, e.g., tuberculosis or can be malignant due to metastatic carcinoma or lymphoma.
- Deep or subcutaneous hemangiomas present as asymptomatic skin or bluish colored nodule/plaque or tumor.

924. Ans. b. It is circumscribed neurodermatitis scrotum (lichen simplex chronicus). Long standing itching and rubbing has led to lichenification with accentuated skin markings. Other common sites are vulva *(MCQ 197),* **nape of the neck** *(MCQ 283)* **and shins** *(MCQ 906).*

RSS is characterized by persistent redness of anterior half of scrotum with accompanying itching, burning and pain sensations. It can develop after prolonged use of topical corticosteroid cream *(MCQ 995).*

925. Ans. b. It is sarcoidosis. These are specific cutaneous lesions of sarcoidosis having sarcoid histopathology. It will show non-caseating

granulomas surrounded by sparse component of lymphocytes "naked granulomas".

Cutaneous tuberculosis presents as plaques of lupus vulgaris *(MCQs 26, 57, 534, 597, 600, 975)*, tuberculosis verrucosa cutis *(MCQ 10)*.

926. **Ans. b. It is deep plantar warts which presents as sharply defined, deep seated, rough, hyperkeratotic lesions surrounded by a thick and smooth collar.**
    - Tinea pedis presents as hyperkeratosis and white scaling with well-defined advancing border *(MCQs 51, 423, 954)*.
    - Pitted keratolysis is caused by digestion of keratin by keratinophilic corynebacteria. It presents as circular shaped erosions on soles. Erosions have punched out appearance *(MCQ 282)*.
    - Pompholyx is a constitutional eczema which presents as deep-seated vesicles on palms and soles *(MCQs 218, 456, 602)*.

927. **Ans. b. It is recurrent herpes genitalis. Recurrence and grouped vesicles are its characteristic features** *(MCQs 445, 471, 512)*.
    - Herpes zoster is a painful condition. It manifests as many groups of vesicles in the entire dermatome *(MCQ 435)*. Herpes zoster very rarely recurs *(MCQs 55, 353, 459)*.
    - Fixed drug eruption manifests as dark colored erosion few hours after intake of some drug *(MCQs 160, 200, 824, 852)*.

928. **Ans. b. It is urethral syndrome which includes both nonspecific urethritis and gonococcal urethritis. Treatment should be given for both.**
    - Candidal balanitis is a manifestation of underlying diabetes. It manifests as transient erythema, tiny papules or pustules, collarette of white scales *(MCQs 38, 693, 797)*.
    - Reiter's syndrome (Reiter's disease) comprises triad of nonspecific gonococcal urethritis, polyarthritis and conjunctivitis or iritis.

929. **Ans. b. It is scrofuloderma which is a type of cutaneous tuberculosis that results from contiguous spread of infection from underlying tuberculosis focus. Watery discharge, bluish margins, granulomatous base, not responding to antibiotics are typical features** *(MCQ 52, 53, 559, 960, 999)*.
    - Chronic osteomyelitis is a bone infection. The ulcer will not be movable on bone because of adherence to underlying bone.

930. **Ans. b. It is pityriasis alba which is a common benign self-limiting mild eczematous condition predominantly affecting face of children. Hypopigmented patches with powdery white scales are typical** *(MCQs 85, 909)*.
    - Segmental vitiligo manifests as depigmented macules (with no scales). It is limited to a dermatome. Distribution of trigeminal nerve (mandibular division) is most frequently affected *(MCQs 181, 747)*.
    - Worm infestation and calcium deficiency do not cause skin lesions. It is a myth.

931. **Ans. c. Exanthematous rash and morbilliform rash are synonyms of each other. It is most common type of drug eruption which comprises of 2–10 mm sized macules which may get confluent at places. In drug-induced rash mucous membranes are unaffected. It starts on trunk** *(MCQs 238, 336)* **and spreads to face.**
    - Viral exanthematous rash (measles) is usually seen in children. It is frequently accompanied by conjunctivitis, lymphadenitis, fever and lymphocytosis.
    - Urticaria manifests as wheals which lasts less than 24 hours *(MCQs 194, 206, 501, 683, 905, 921, 947)*

932. **Ans. c. It is dermatitis groins. Erythema, ill-defined margins and bilateral involvement are important features** *(MCQ 561)*.
    - Intertrigo refers to the erythema and soreness of opposing surfaces of body folds which is limited to the area of contact of surfaces *(MCQs 166, 946)*.
    - Tinea cruris manifests with well defined active borders *(MCQ 4)*.
    - Candidiasis manifests as red macerations in body folds and develops fringed irregular margins with classical satellite vesicles and pustules *(MCQs 179, 253, 607, 624, 693, 695, 799)*.

933. **Ans. a. It is insect bite hypersensitivity (papular urticaria) which presents as persistent pruritic eruption of papules involving chiefly the exposed areas of body** *(MCQs 72, 172)*.
    - Measles manifests with conjunctivitis, lymphadenitis, fever and morbilliform (exanthematous) rash. Exanthematous rash comprises of 2–10 mm sized macules which may get confluent at places.
    - Drug-induced exanthematous rash is common in adults *(MCQs 238, 336, 931)* and primarily involves trunk.

934. Ans. c. It is seborrheic dermatitis involving the seborrheic sites (cervical region and groins) and involving the deeper part of folds.
    * Candidal intertrigo extends beyond the contact surfaces of body folds and develops irregular fringed margins with classical *vesiculopustules* (MCQs 607, 624, 693, 695, 799).
    * Napkin rash involves the convexities sparing the deeper part of folds (MCQ 424).

935. Ans. b. It is condylomata acuminata (venereal warts). It is caused by HPV-6, -11, -16 and -18 types with an incubation period of 3 weeks to 8 months. Condylomata lata is a manifestation of secondary syphilis. It presents as multiple, flesh colored, flat topped sessile papules with oozing and macerations. Anal region (MCQ 666) and groins (MCQ 688) are common sites.

936. Ans. c. It is tinea faciei manifesting as a ring shaped red well-defined patch on one side of face.
    * Seborrheic dermatitis on face manifests as scaling at eyebrows and nasolabial folds. Squamous blepharitis is common.
    * Atopic dermatitis involves face most frequently. It manifests as erythema or discrete or confluent papules with exudation and crusting (MCQ 174).

937. Ans. a. It is generalized pustular psoriasis (GPP). It is a common complication of sudden withdrawal of systemic corticosteroids in psoriatic patients (MCQs 260, 643, 793). It should be treated promptly.
    * Acropustulosis is a type of localized pustular psoriasis which involves tips of fingers and toes (MCQ 376).
    * Secondary infection of psoriatic plaques is seen as scattered pustules in very less number.
    * Impetigo herpetiformis is seen in last trimester of pregnancy in psoriasis patients.

938. Ans. b. It is carbuncle which is a deep staphylococcal infection involving a group of contiguous hair follicles characterized by intense inflammation. Pus discharge from multiple follicular opening gives an appearance of a sieve (MCQs 157, 558).
    * SCC manifests as nontender exophytic cauliflower like growth (MCQs 113, 116, 255, 289, 429, 538, 796).
    * Scrofuloderma is type of skin tuberculosis which manifests as an ulcer having watery discharge and bluish margins (MCQs 52, 53, 559, 929, 960, 999, 901).

939. Ans. b. It is rhinophyma which is a disfiguring nasal deformity due to proliferation of sebaceous glands and connective tissue. It is seen in acne rosacea patients as a later development. It requires treatment because it promote social stigma. It can cause psychological distress and can obstruct external nares. Tetracyclines are helpful at initial stage. Advanced stage requires surgical measures.
    * Sebaceous hyperplasia refers to enlarged sebaceous glands seen on forehead or cheeks at middle or older age. It manifests up to 3 mm sized papules with a central hair follicle.
    * If BCC, squamous cell carcinoma or sebaceous adenoma is suspected, biopsy should be done.

940. Ans. b. It is pompholyx which is an acute form of endogenous eczema of palms and soles. It manifests as various sized vesicles on fingers, palms and soles. It tends to have intermittent outbreaks.
    * Epidermolysis bullosa simplex is a mechanobullous disorder which manifests in infancy or early childhood (MCQ 506).
    * Id eruption refers to the eruption of small and pruritic vesicles on the sides of fingers in responses to an intense inflammatory process elsewhere in the body (MCQ 180).
    * Scabies manifests as papules and pustules (never vesicles) in web spaces (MCQ 62).

941. Ans. c. It is psoriasis scalp. Redness, white scaling, well defined margins are typical features of psoriasis. In between normal skin areas may not be there. It should not be treated with systemic steroids that can lead to appearance of new lesions on rest of body (rebound phenomenon MCQ 316).
    * Seborrheic capitis manifests as fine greasy scales without prominent redness (MCQ 485).
    * Tinea capitis is seen in children as patches with partial hair loss (MCQ 8).

942. Ans. a. It is Fox-Fordyce disease which is a chronic, itchy and papular eruption seen mainly in females (90%). It is thought to be due to the obstruction of distal part of apocrine sweat ducts. It presents as itchy, discrete, dome-shaped, pigmented follicular papules in axillae.
    * Pseudoacanthosis nigricans manifests as non-itchy dark-colored velvety thickening in axillae, cervical region and groins in obese persons due to insulin resistance (MCQ 273).
    * Intertrigo refers to erythema and soreness of opposing surfaces of body folds which is limited to the area of contact of surfaces (MCQ 166).

943. **Ans. b.** It is neonatal occipital alopecia. It is physiological, reversible, self-limiting alopecia observed in occipital region of 2–4 months old babies. It is thought to be due to synchronized shedding of telogen hairs.

  Alopecia areata is seen as bald patches in older children *(MCQ 156)*.

944. **Ans. c.** It is abscess. Red, painful and tender swelling are typical features of abscess.
  - Psoriasis plaques are red with white scaling but no pain or tenderness *(MCQ 917)*.
  - Tuberculoid leprosy plaques have loss of sensation with no pain or tenderness *(MCQ 6)*.
  - Lupus vulgaris is type of cutaneous tuberculosis which manifests as red, soft gelatinous plaques with no pain or tenderness *(MCQ 26)*.

945. **Ans. b.** It is impetigo contagiosa (non-bullous impetigo). It is caused by *Staphylococcus aureus*. The exudates get dried to form yellowish, thick and dirty brown (honey colored) crusts. The skin around the nose, mouth *(MCQ 60)* and limbs are common sites.
  - Tinea lesions have well-defined active borders *(MCQ 142)* and do not have crusting.
  - Psoriatic plaques are red and have white scaling.
  - Discoid eczema, manifests as multiple, itchy, ill-defined, wet and disc-shaped lesions *(MCQ 194)*.

946. **Ans. d.** It is intertrigo which refers to the erythema and soreness of opposing surfaces of body folds limited to the areas of contact of surfaces.
  - Tinea corporis is characterized by well-defined active borders.
  - Candidiasis manifests in body folds as red macerations having fringed irregular margins and classical satellite vesicles and pustules *(MCQ 253)*.
  - Flexural psoriasis has typical red color with white scaling and well-defined margins *(MCQ 245)*.

947. **Ans. a.** Eruption of itchy wheals with short duration are typical features of acute urticaria.
  - Pityriasis rosea is characterized by red macules covered by fine scales *(MCQ 161)*.
  - Secondary syphilis manifests as asymptomatic and bilateral symmetrical lesions on trunk and extremities *(MCQ 293)*. Palms are usually involved *(MCQ 214)*.
  - Lepromatous leprosy presents as asymptomatic shiny red papules, plaques and nodules *(MCQ 155)*.

948. **Ans. d.** It is cicatricial (scarring) alopecia showing scarring, discoloration and fine wrinkling. It is irreversible hair loss because pilosebaceous units are replaced by fibrous tissue.
  - Tinea capitis presents as patch with partial hair loss and scaling *(MCQ 792)*.
  - Alopecia areata presents as bald patch with smooth, shiny, apparently looking normal skin with no inflammation, atrophy and scarring *(MCQ 145)*.
  - Trichotillomania shows the presence of firmly anchored partially broken hairs with no atrophy *(MCQ 659)*.

949. **Ans. a.** It is cellulitis foot which is an acute or subacute pyogenic infection of subcutaneous tissue. It has indistinct margins between affected and unaffected skin. Regional lymph adenopathy is frequent.

  Erysipelas is superficial bacterial infection of dermis and upper subcutaneous tissue. It manifests as painful edematous red plaque with sharp well defined raised edge to normal tissue *(MCQ 91)*.

950. **Ans. b.** It is superficial basal cell carcinoma. It is typically present around eye and nose having irregular thread like margins and central atrophy.

  Squamous cell carcinoma usually arises on photodamaged skin *(MCQ 816)* showing irregular pigmentation, solar elastosis, telangiectasia.

951. **Ans. b.** It is *Paederus dermatitis*. It is characterized by red irregular patch with gray necrotic slough in the center.

  Herpes zoster is characterized by many groups of grouped vesicles on erythematous base. Involvement is unilateral in a dermatomal pattern *(MCQ 577)*.

952. **Ans. c.** It is candidiasis groins. It is typically showing red macerations in a body fold (groins) having fringed irregular margins with classical satellite vesicles and pustules. Diabetes must be ruled out.
  - Tinea cruris will show well defined active borders *(MCQ 4)*.
  - Intertrigo refers to the erythema and soreness of opposing surfaces of body folds limited to the area of contact of surfaces *(MCQ 166)*.
  - Flexural psoriasis has typical red color with white scaling and well-defined margins *(MCQ 84)*.

953. **Ans. c.** It is acneiform (drug-induced acne) eruption. Systemic steroids, antitubercular drugs and antiepileptics are common etiological drugs for it.

- Acne vulgaris is characterized by papules, pustules and comedones *(MCQ 34)*.
- Chickenpox is an acute presentation with vesicles *(MCQ 789)* surrounded by irregular area of redness (dew drop on rose petal).
- Exanthematous rash is one of the common adverse drug reactions. It comprises of 2-10 mm sized red macules which may get confluent at places *(MCQ 238)*.

954. **Ans. d. It is squamous hyperkeratotic type tinea pedis characteristically showing well defined advancing border.**
     - Candidiasis soles is usually bilateral presenting as diffuse redness and white macerations *(MCQ 210)* or involve the area of sole adjoining the interdigital web spaces *(MCQ 490)*.
     - Hyperkeratotic eczema is usually bilateral and manifests as oozing, crusting and fissuring *(MCQ 150)*.
     - Keratolysis exfoliativa is a recurrent asymptomatic non-inflammatory bilateral, desquamation of palms and soles *(MCQ 453, 737)*.

955. **Ans. d. The eradication of genital warts during pregnancy is not essential unless it is symptomatic. Most often genital warts ease out by themselves and can be left alone to reduce by themselves without worry unless they are massive or keep on growing.**
     - Warts can be removed safely by cryotherapy by using liquid nitrogen. This is indicated only if warts become too big to manage.
     - Electrodessication or lasers or surgical removal is an extreme option and warts are need not to be removed during pregnancy. It can be a strain on mother and can hamper delivery.
     - Podophyllin should be avoided during pregnancy. It is pregnancy category X and can harm an unborn baby or cause birth defects.

956. **Ans. a. Hair dye is a very commonly seen allergic contact dermatitis. It is due to paraphenylenediamine (PPD) which is present in all types of hair dyes.**
     - Acute urticaria accompanies wheals and does not cause too much swelling of eyelids *(MCQ 683)*.
     - Hypothyroidism (myxedema) causes only puffiness of eye lids and face *(MCQ 426)*.
     - In addition to eye lids, angioedema involves swelling of face and lips also *(MCQ 296)*.

957. **Ans. b. Stasis pigmentation is a brownish pigmentation, often with swelling around the ankles. It results from breaking down of RBCs that have leaked out from tiny blood vessels. It is typically seen in people who have varicose veins. It results due to capillaritis because of gravity and increased venous pressure.**
     - Certain drugs especially antihypertensives, antidepressants, analgesics and antihistamines can also cause capillaritis.
     - Schamberg's disease (progressive pigmented purpuric dermatosis) is seen in young adult males with no obvious cause. It is seen as irregular orange or brown pigmented macules *(MCQ 365)*.

958. **Ans. a. It is epidermolysis bullosa simplex. It is a heterogenous group of genetically determined and of acquired skin diseases characterized by easy blistering of skin and mucosa due to mild mechanical trauma (mechanobullous disorders).**
     PCT presents as fragility of light exposed skin of hands and forearms. Patient presents with sharply marginated erosions, atrophic scars, mottled hypo or hyperpigmentation. Other features are hypertrichosis of forehead and upper face, melasma like hyperpigmentation, onycholysis, morphea like lesions on back.

959. **Ans. a. It is a typical syphilitic chancre (primary syphilis).**
     - Chancroid (soft chancre) manifests as multiple painful ulcers *(MCQs 489, 608)* with non-indurated base.
     - Donovanosis (syn. granuloma inguinale, granuloma venereum) presents as elevated, rounded, velvety and granulomatous ulcers which are painless and bleeds easily.
     - Genital herpes presents as small grouped vesicles *(MCQ 927)*.

960. **Ans. b. It is scrofuloderma which is an endogenous type of multibacillary skin tuberculosis seen in patients having low immunity. It results from contiguous spread of infection from underlying tuberculous focus, e.g., cervical, axillary and inguinal lymph nodes.**
     Hidradenitis suppurativa is a disease of the areas of skin bearing apocrine glands characterized by abscesses, scarring and sinuses. It is seen in axillae *(MCQ 111)*, perianal region *(MCQ 343)* and groins *(MCQ 415)*.

961. **Ans. a. It is lepromatous leprosy (LL). Chronic insidious infiltration of ears is a typical presentation of LL. Blistering and ulceration of finger tips due to bilateral insensitivity is very common in LL.**

- Facial changes in systemic sclerosis are mask like face, a small and pinched nose and pursed string appearance of mouth opening *(MCQ 454)*.
- Hypothyroidism manifest as puffiness of eyelids and face *(MCQ 426)*. Hairs are lost from outer third of eyebrows.
- In alopecia areata, there will be no infiltration of ears. After hair loss skin becomes smooth and shiny *(MCQs 678, 468, 569)*.

962. **Ans. c.** She is having insulin resistant PCOS. Obesity, acanthosis nigricans and oligomenorrhea are its typical features. USG should be done to see the ovarian size. Serum testosterone level should be checked.
    - Idiopathic hirsutism consists of normal menses, normal sized ovaries, normal androgen level and insidious onset of hirsutism.
    - Non-insulin resistant type is uncommon in obese PCOS patient. Acanthosis nigricans is a classical feature of insulin resistance.
    - Androgen secreting tumor is associated with appearance of male secondary sex characters, e.g., clitoromegaly *(MCQs 303, 321)*.

963. **Ans. b.** It is rebound phenomenon. It is commonly seen with the use of topical or more commonly with systemic steroids in psoriasis patients. Initially steroids suppress the disease process. But, later on, during therapy or after its discontinuation, there is 'break through' and psoriasis tends to relapse promptly. It may 'rebound' with an appearance of a greater number of widespread small-patterned skin lesions in an aggressive manner than the pretreatment state. It may precipitate erythrodermic or generalized pustular psoriasis. Systemic steroids should not be given to psoriasis patients.
    - Koebner phenomenon refers to the development of pathologic lesions in the traumatized uninvolved skin of persons who have cutaneous diseases, such as psoriasis *(MCQ 308)*, LP *(MCQ 308)*, warts *(MCQ 398)*, etc.
    - FDE due to steroids are not seen.
    - Acneiform eruption or drug-induced acne consists of eruption of monomorphic papules. Scaling is not a feature *(MCQ 27)*.

964. **Ans. c.** These are sand paper Comedones. These are non-inflammatory lesions of acne which consists of very small multiple white heads commonly seen on forehead.
    - Molluscum contagiosum comprises of pearly white umbilicated papules *(MCQ 224)*.
    - Milia are 1-2 mm sized uniform dome-shaped yellowish papules commonly seen on cheeks and eyelids *(MCQ 48)*.
    - LP comprises of violaceous papules *(MCQ 381)*.
    - Warts comprises of rough hyperkeratotic papules *(MCQ 169)*.

965. **Ans. b.** It is kerion which is one of the types of tinea capitis. It presents as an inflammatory boggy swelling with easily pluckable hair. Usually, it is accompanied by cervical lymphadenopathy.
    - Alopecia areata presents as complete bald patch of smooth skin with no inflammation, scaling or atrophy *(MCQ 145)*.
    - Trichotillomania is seen in older children as a patch of hair loss in an easily approachable region of scalp *(MCQ 128)*. It shows the presence of firmly anchored partially broken hairs in the bald area.

966. **Ans. a.** It is ITP. Bleeding gums and crop of petechiae are features of thrombocytopenia. Ecchymosis is a feature of coagulation disorder due to platelet dysfunction. Ecchymosis can be due to poor dermal vascular support as seen in senile purpura.
    - TPP presents with fever, hemolytic anemia and neurological symptoms due to thrombi.
    - HSP presents as retiform (net like) pattern of purpuric lesions in children in bilateral symmetrical manner *(MCQ 332)*.
    - Palpable purpura refers to purpuric lesions which are palpable *(MCQ 527)*.
    - Actinic purpura (senile purpura) is seen at old age due to decreased support to cutaneous vessels *(MCQ 148)*.

967. **Ans. b.** Firm stroking of vessels in a normal person leads to triple response of Levis (erythema and surrounding flare). Such response is seen in 5% of normal persons and is termed as dermatographism. When it is accompanied by itching it is known as symptomatic dermatographism.
    - White dermatographism is seen in atopic patients due to capillary vasoconstriction.
    - Darier's sign is seen in urticaria pigmentosa. When lesions are rubbed, it produces intense itching with blisters or hives.

968. **Ans. d.** It is genital warts.
    - Lichen planus lesions are flat topped and violaceous colored *(MCQ 381)*.
    - Molluscum contagiosum lesions are pearly white, shiny, dome-shaped umbilicated papules *(MCQ 987)*.

- Lichen nitidus manifests as asymptomatic, shiny flat topped, discrete pinpoint to pinhead sized, flesh colored papules on penile shaft *(MCQ 16)*.

969. **Ans. a. It is dry discoid eczema. The lesions are typically dry scaly comprising of microvesicles and are present on extensor aspects of extremities *(MCQ 434)*, dorsum of hands *(MCQ 194)*, etc.**
    - Tinea corporis lesions are typically red patches with active border and central clearing *(MCQ 142)*.
    - Granuloma annulare presents as asymptomatic, complete or incomplete rings formed by small skin-colored papules *(MCQ 591)*.
    - Pityriasis alba presents as irregular patch of hypopigmentation covered by powdery white scales. It is predominantly seen on face *(MCQ 85)*.

970. **Ans. c. It is discoid eczema. Lesions are typically, coin shaped, red, ill-defined wet lesions.**
    - Tinea corporis lesions are usually large patches with well-defined active borders *(MCQ 773)*.
    - Psoriatic plaques are typically red with white scaling *(MCQ 729)*.

971. **Ans. b. These are pyogenic abscesses and can be easily treated by incision and drainage. Red inflamed painful tender swelling is typical feature of pyogenic abscess.**
    - Hidradenitis suppurativa is a chronic, inflammatory, relapsing and scarring disease of areas of the skin bearing apocrine sweat glands, e.g., axillae *(MCQ 111)*, groins *(MCQ 445)* and perianal region *(MCQ 343)*. It presents with small tender abscesses which eventually open to the surface with seropurulent discharge. Eventually, there is formation of sinuses, tracts and scars.
    - Usually, enlarged lymph nodes are not visible on inspection. They are felt on palpation as painless small subcutaneous swellings.

972. **Ans. b. It is annular psoriasis (uncommon type). Red plaque (not patch) with white scaling is typical of psoriasis.**
    - Tinea corporis presents as patches with well-defined active borders *(MCQ 142)*.
    - Discoid eczema does not show central clearing. Lesions are ill defined and wet *(MCQ 202)*.
    - Tuberculoid leprosy is characterized by cutaneous plaque with loss of sensations *(MCQ 6)*.
    - Granuloma annulare presents as complete or incomplete rings formed by small skin colored or violaceous papules *(MCQ 817)*.

973. **Ans. b. A young healthy patient needs only analgesics and calamine lesion.**
    - Topical aciclovir cream has no role.
    - Systemic antiviral drugs are indicated for patients older than 50 years, herpes zoster ophthalmicus and immunocompromised patient. These are best given within 3 days of appearance of rash.

974. **Ans. c. It is contact irritant dermatitis having ill-defined redness and involving widespread area.**
    - Candidiasis is characterized by scanty, thick curdy white discharge with soreness. The groins will show fringed irregular margins with classical satellite vesicles and pustules *(MCQs 874, 695)*.
    - Intertrigo refers to the redness and soreness of opposing surfaces of body folds limited to the area of contact of surfaces *(MCQ 166)*.
    - Tinea cruris is characterized by well-defined active borders *(MCQ 4)*.

975. **Ans. b. It is lupus vulgaris with a characteristic psoriasiform plaque with an advancing active margin and trailing scar towards center.**
    - Psoriasis presents as red plaques with white scaling.
    - Tuberculoid leprosy presents as a plaque having loss of sensation *(MCQ 6)*.
    - CCLE usually manifests on sun exposed areas of face as red plaques with adherent scales and hyperpigmentation at periphery *(MCQ 201)*.

976. **Ans. a. It is *Paederus dermatitis* which is a peculiar type of irritant dermatitis provoked by coelomic fluid released by an insect of genus '*Paederus*'. It is seen on exposed parts of body.**
    - Herpes zoster is characterized by eruption of grouped vesicles on erythematous base. These groups are seen in a dermatomal pattern on one side of body *(MCQ 973)*.
    - Chickenpox vesicles are discrete with surrounding irregular area of erythema. Vesicles erupt in crops on trunk, face and extremities after fever *(MCQ 165)*.

977. **Ans. c. When results are not satisfactory with topical antifungal cream, then she should be treated with oral terbinafine.**

    Terbinafine is categorized as pregnancy category 'B' drug.

978. **Ans. c. It is tinea capitis (black dot type). Severely damaged hair breaks at surface of scalp leaving behind black dots. Scaling in minimal. Hairs are easily pluckable.**

- Alopecia areata presents as complete bald patches having smooth skin with absence of inflammation, scarring and atrophy *(MCQ 156)*.
- Trichotillomania manifests as patch of hair loss at easily approachable sites. The diagnosis is made with the presence of firmly anchored partially broken hairs in the bald area *(MCQ 128)*.

979. **Ans. c. It is CID on buttocks characterized by erythema and ill-defined margins.**
    - Tinea lesions have well defined active borders *(MCQ 773)*.
    - Tinea incognito refers to unrecognizable tinea due to modification by topical or systemic steroids *(MCQ 451)*.
    - Candidiasis comprises of fringed irregular margins with satellite vesicles and pustules *(MCQ 179)*.

980. **Ans. e. It is discoid eczema with disc or oval-shaped fairly well demarcated lesions. Lesion are wet and composed of closely set microvesicles. Extensor expects of extremities and dorsa of hands are typical sites.**
    - Tinea corporis lesions have well-defined active borders with some clearing towards center *(MCQ 142)*.
    - Lichen planus comprises of violaceous papules, not plaques *(MCQ 381)*.
    - Psoriasis plaques are typically red with white scaling *(MCQ 482)*.
    - Tuberculoid leprosy manifests as plaque with loss of sensations *(MCQ 6)*.

981. **Ans. a. It is alopecia areata manifesting as total bald patch with apparently looking normal skin.**
    - Tinea barbae refers to the ringworm of beard and moustache areas with invasion of coarse hair. Hairs get surrounded by a papules and pustules and are easily pluckable *(MCQ 431)*.
    - Trichotillomania is seen in children and young females as patch of hair loss *(MCQ 128)*. Patch consists of firmly anchored partially broken hairs.

982. **Ans. b. It is pityriasis rosea with typical mother patch on arm. The trunk shows discrete, dull red oval lesions covered by fine scales. It is self-limiting condition in about 6–8 weeks.**
    - Pityriasis versicolor presents with discolored or hyperpigmented skin lesions which have fine dust like scales *(MCQ 522)*. At margin satellite lesions are seen easily *(MCQ 39)*.
    - Pityriasis alba presents as variable sized round or irregular patch of hypopigmentation covered by fine powdery scales *(MCQ 85)*.

983. **Ans. a. It is lepromatous leprosy (LL) which has lowest immunity against leprosy bacilli. So, it manifests with uncountable number of skin lesions. Patches do not have loss of sensations. But it can have gloves and stockings type of anesthesia. Diagnosis of LL is proved by demonstration of a AFBs in slit skin smears.**
    - Tuberculoid leprosy has highest immunity, So, it manifests with 1 or 2 lesions *(MCQ 6)*.
    - Histoid leprosy is a variant of multibacillary leprosy which manifests as crop of asymptomatic multiple, smooth glistening, firm and non-tender papules *(MCQ 47)*.
    - Indeterminate leprosy manifests as hypopigmentation or slight erythematous ill-defined macules.

984. **Ans. b. It is lichen planus. Genital mucosa is involved in 20–25% of patients. Purple colored, plane topped papules are typical of LP.**
    - Venereal warts (when fresh) are soft, pink, grouped pedunculated filiform or digitate lesions *(MCQ 283)*. Later, they become hyperpigmented and dark colored *(MCQ 704)*.
    - Psoriasis on glans manifests as a patch having characteristic color with well-defined edge which may lack scales *(MCQ 95)*.

985. **Ans. b. It is discoid eczema characterized by a disc-shaped red and wet patches. It is usually a manifestation of atopic dermatitis which manifests below 3 months of age.**
    - Pityriasis alba manifests as an irregular, ill-defined hypopigmented macule on face in older children *(MCQ 85)*.
    - Tinea faciei has well defined active borders *(MCQ 936)*.
    - Seborrheic dermatitis most commonly manifests before the age of 2 months. It manifests as redness and scaling of scalp *(MCQ 168)*, eyebrows and as macerated erythema of cervical folds (next MCQ).

986. **Ans. a. It is seborrheic dermatitis (cervical folds) which typically manifests below 3 months of the age as redness and scaling of scalp *(MCQ 168)*, as macerated erythema of groins *(MCQ 933)* and cervical folds.**
    - Infantile atopic dermatitis manifests usually after the 3 months of age as diffuse erythema of cheeks *(MCQ 174)*, as discoid eczema on cheeks *(MCQ 985)*.

- Candidiasis manifests with fringed irregular margins and classical satellite vesicles and pustules *(MCQ 624)*.

987. Ans. b. It is molluscum contagiosum. Shiny, discrete, umbilicated papules are typical features of MC.
- Genital warts are dark hyperkeratotic papules without any umbilication *(MCQ 968)*.
- Lichen planus papules are plane topped and violaceous colored *(MCQ 381)*.

988. Ans. c. It is molluscum contagiosum. Papules are shiny and have central umbilication.
- Acne vulgaris manifests with papules, pustules and comedones *(MCQ 216)*.
- Milia manifests as 1-2 mm sized, yellowish dome-shaped papules on eye lids and cheeks with no umbilication *(MCQ 48)*.
- Warts manifest as rough hyperkeratotic papules *(MCQ 392)*.

989. Ans. b. It is hyperkeratotic type of tinea pedis, showing scaling and well-defined border. Unilateral involvement points towards infective pathology.
- Eczema is characterized by oozing and crusting *(MCQ 213)* and usually involves both feet.
- Contact dermatitis to shoe will manifest on both feet and will take the shape of shoes *(MCQ 202)*.

990. Ans. a. It is nevus depigmentosus which is a rare nevoid pigmentary congenital disorder. It may not appear at birth. It increases with size of body and remain stable. Margins are irregular, feathered and do not cross the midline.
- Segmental vitiligo has well defined margins. Most commonly manifests as many patches in the distribution of trigeminal nerve *(MCQ 181)* on one side.
- Focal vitiligo refers to the presence of single or few macules in a limited area of body *(MCQ 246)*.

991. Ans. b. It is lichen simplex chronicus (circumscribed neurodermatitis). Severe itching, ill-defined margins and lichenification (increased cutaneous markings) are its typical features.
- Bowen's disease presents as a discrete, persistent, red and thin plaque having well-defined irregular borders with overlying scales or crusts which resembles psoriasis *(MCQ 226)*.
- Psoriasis presents as red plaque with white scaling.

992. Ans. c. It is cheilitis due to lip-stick which chiefly cause allergic cheilitis of vermilion margin. Ricinoleic acid is the main constituent identified as a commonest cause of cheilitis. Sometimes, it may extend to adjacent perioral region.
- Cheilitis due to nutritional deficiencies (riboflavin or iron deficiencies) usually manifests as angular cheilitis which is turn may be an evidence of malnutrition or malabsorption.
- Actinic cheilitis presents as red, scaly and chapped lips with indistinct vermilion borders *(MCQ 529)*.

993. Ans. b. It is steatocystoma multiplex. These are epithelium lined sebum filled dermal cysts. They can be removed by simplex incision and drainage.
- Scabies presents with short history, severe itching and papules on both penile shaft and scrotum *(MCQ 65)*.
- Angio keratomas on scrotum presents as 1-4 mm sized bright red vascular papules *(MCQ 91)*. Patient complains of soreness itching and bleeding.

994. Ans. b. It is seborrheic dermatitis. Involvement of scalp, eyebrows, moustache and beard regions are typical seborrheic sites. Erythema and fine scaling are typical.
- Atopic dermatitis at this age shows redness and thickening of facial skin and cervical region *(MCQ 1000)*.
- Psoriasis comprises of bright red color and silvery scaling and does not prefer the seborrheic sites.

995. Ans. b. It is red scrotum syndrome (RSS). It is caused by prolonged application of topical steroid creams.
- Lichen simplex chronicus (circumscribed neurodermatitis) presents as lichenified plaque with accentuated skin markings due to long standing itching and rubbing *(MCQ 924)*.
- Tinea infection presents as redness and white scaling. Well defined active borders can be identified.

996. Ans. b. This feature of scaling is characteristically seen in pityriasis rosea.
- In secondary syphilis, lesions are polymorphic and consists of macules, papules with scaling. It accompanies palmar involvement *(MCQ 214)*.
- Psoriasis shows red plaques with white scaling *(MCQs 229, 622)*.

- Exanthematous (morbilliform) rash is very common drug adverse reaction. *(MCQ 238)*. It comprises of 2-10 mm sized macules which may get confluent at places.

997. **Ans. c. It is lichen amyloidosis which is a rare condition characterized by extracellular deposition of amyloid fibrils. It is highly pruritic. It is treated by potent topical steroid ointments with or without occlusive dressings.**
    - Lichen planus presents as violaceous papules *(MCQ 381)*.
    - Lichen simplex chronicus presents as thick lichenified plaque with accentuated skin markings and ill-defined margin *(MCQ 906)*.

998. **Ans. a. Raynaud's phenomenon (RP) is called as secondary RP when it is accompanied by trophic or ischemic changes on fingers, Common underlying causes are connective tissue disorders, e.g. systemic sclerosis, SLE, etc.**
    - Raynaud's disease (primary RP) refers to Raynaud's phenomenon with no obvious underlying cause it is devoid of trophic changes on fingers *(MCQ 834)*.
    - Chilblains manifests as diffuse cutaneous redness with or without ulcerations *(MCQ 719)*. It is usually accompanied by itching or burning sensation.

999. **Ans. a. It is scrofuloderma which is an endogenous type of cutaneous tuberculosis that results from contiguous spread of infection from underlying tuberculous focus. Watery discharge, bluish margin and granulating base are typical features.**
    Pilonidal sinus presents as hole or tunnel in the skin. It occurs in the cleft at the top of buttocks. Usually, there is a history of recurrent discharge of fluid or pus from the hole.

1000. **Ans. b. It is atopic dermatitis showing redness and thickening of facial and cervical region.**
    - Seborrheic dermatitis shows redness and fine greasy scaling of seborrheic sites *(MCQ 994)*.
    - ABCD presents as redness, thickening, pigmentation and lichenification of facial skin *(MCQ 86)*. It involves upper eyelids, area under nose and chin. It spares back of neck.
    - Chronic actinic dermatitis (syn. persistent light reaction, actinic reticuloid) shows sharp cut off at the lines of clothing. It spares upper eyelids, skin behind the ear lobes and depth of skin creases *(MCQs 196, 298)*.

1001. **Ans. c. It is post-waxing folliculitis manifesting as follicular papules. Girls are very fond of removing their hairs just before marriage by waxing. Lesions are caused by inflammation that normally recedes of its own in few days.**
    - Acne is characterized by papules, pustules and comedones *(MCQ 834)*.
    - Acneiform eruption (drug-induced acne) consists of monomorphic small red papules mainly on trunk, upper arms and shoulders *(MCQ 43)*.

1002. **Ans. a. It is periungual wart caused by HPV presenting as grouped, scaly, rough papules around nail.**
    - Tuberculosis verrucosa cutis presents as indurated papule or plaque surrounded by erythema *(MCQ 10)*. Margins may show fingerlike projections.
    - Knuckle pads are circumscribed asymptomatic thickenings over the finger Joints *(MCQ 355)*.

1003. **Ans. b. It is eczema presenting as characteristic ill-defined plaques with crusting.**
    - Psoriasis comprises of well-defined red plaques with white scaling *(MCQ 146)*.
    - Tinea corporis consists of red patches having well defined active borders *(MCQ 142)*.
    - Lichen planus presents as violaceous plane topped papules mainly on extremities *(MCQ 21)*.

1004. **Ans. c. It is linear IgA disease presenting as new vesicles around the periphery of previous lesion as "collarette of blisters". It is an important sign of this disease.**
    - Herpes zoster presents as painful grouped vesicles on erythematous base in a dermatomal pattern *(MCQ 435)*.
    - Scabies presents as itching and papular (not vesicles) lesions *(MCQ 65)*.

1005. **Ans. a. Isotretinoin is the drug of choice for systemic use for cystic acne.**
    It affects all the pathogenic factors of acne. It is used in the dose of 0.5-1.0 mg/kg/day after meals. Cheilitis is seen in almost all patients taking isotretinoin *(MCQ 756)*.

1006. **Ans. d. It is guttate psoriasis presenting as round or oval 0-5-1.5 cm sized papules on trunk and extremities as raindrop pattern. Red color and scaling are typical.**
    - Pityriasis rosea presents as macules (not papules) with scaling *(MCQ 982)*.
    - Secondary syphilis presents with macules, papules and scaling *(MCQ 293)*. Palms and soles are very commonly involved *(MCQ 214)*.

- Exanthematous rash is a most common adverse drug reaction. It presents as 2-10 mm sized macules on trunk. The macules may get confluent at places *(MCQ 931)*.

1007. Ans. c. It is Henoch-Schonlein purpura (IgA immune complex vasculitis). It is typically seen in children or adolescents in bilateral symmetrical retiform pattern.
- Actinic purpura (senile purpura) is seen in older age as geometric-shaped dark purplish patches *(MCQ 148)*.
- ITP presents as bleeding gums or crops of petechiae *(MCQ 354)*.
- When purpuric lesions are palpable, they are called palpable purpura *(MCQ 527)*.

1008. Ans. c. It is cutaneous sinus of dental origin. It is a channel that leads from a dental focus of infection to drain on the skin surface of face or neck, Pulp degeneration and periapical abscess progresses slowly through the alveolar or mandibular bone and erupt through the skin. An intraoral cord can be well palpated.
- Acne cyst will be accompanied by comedones. It usually does not present as a single cyst and does not get adherent to underlying tissue.
- Osteomyelitis most commonly involves long bones in children. Feet, spine and hips are commonly involved in adults. It presents as pain, tenderness and discharge of pus.

1009. Ans. a. It is carcinoma penis. Abnormal growth, nonhealing ulcer, bleeding and foul-smelling discharge are common presentations of penile cancer. Five years survival rate is 80% in patients having involvement of one or more superficial unilateral inguinal lymph nodes, but survival is only 10-20% when involvement is bilateral.

Genital warts present, as grouped, pedunculated, filiform or digitate lesions seen in young adults *(MCQ 283)*.

1010. Ans. b. It is BCC which has special predilection around eye, nose and ear. Erythematous patch with slightly raised and thread like margins are typical.
- Squamous cell carcinoma arises on photo-damaged skin showing irregular pigmentation, solar elastosis *(MCQ 816)*, telangiectasia and hyperkeratosis.
- Superficial spreading melanoma, presents as an irregularly shaped brown colored macule of more than 6 mm size *(MCQ 121)*.

1011. Ans. c. It is neonatal acne which manifests between 3 months to 24 months of age. It is thought to be due to transplacental stimulation of adrenal glands.
- Milia are keratin cysts which present as pin point to 1 mm sized multiple papules *(MCQ 497)*.
- Erythema toxicum neonatorum presents as blotchy red 1-3 cm sized macules with a central vesicles or pustules *(MCQ 432)*.

1012. Ans. a. It is seborrheic dermatitis. It is characterized by fine greasy scales at seborrheic sites.
- Atopic dermatitis on face is characterized by redness and thickening of face and cervical skin *(MCQ 1000)*.
- Tinea faciei presents with scaling with or without redness, but with a well-defined advancing active border *(MCQ 241)*.

1013. Ans. a. It is psoriasis of palms. Red color and white scaling are typical of psoriasis.
- Lichen planus presents as violaceous papules *(MCQ 231)*.
- CCLE presents as well-defined red plaque with hyper pigmentation at periphery.
- Eczema presents as oozing, crusting, thickening and fissuring *(MCQ 242)*.

1014. Ans. b. It is psoriasis hands. Red plagues with white scaling are typical of psoriasis.
- Lichen planus presents as violaceous papules *(MCQ 208)*.
- CCLE presents as well-defined plaques with adherent scales and hyper pigmentation at periphery *(MCQ 618)*.

1015. Ans. a. It is caused by wrongly applied derobin (salicylic acid + dithranol + coal tar) ointment. It is used for a short period (10–20 minutes) in psoriasis patients having very few plaques (short contact therapy). Surrounding skin is protected with petrolatum from its strong irritant effect.
- Podophyllin (podowart) is used for the treatment of warts. It causes redness, burning and ulceration *(MCQ 1019)*. It is applied once a week.
- Acyclovir or corticosteroid cream does not cause burning or irritation.

1016. Ans. d. It is lichen planus. Pruritic, purple-colored papules are typical lesions of lichen planus.
- Guttate psoriasis comprises of red colored papules with white scaling *(MCQ 229)*.
- Lepromatous leprosy (LL) lesions are various sized red papules and plaques with no scaling *(MCQ 115)*. Additionally, patients may have

infiltration of ears *(MCQ 101)* or glove and stocking type of anesthesia *(MCQ 433).*
- Secondary syphilis lesions are asymptomatic *(MCQ 293)* and usually involves palms *(MCQ 214).*
- Pityriasis rosea presents as crop of lesions in Christmas tree pattern *(MCQ 161).*

1017. **Ans. c. It is due to corticosteroid cream. It is called as a topical steroid damaged face (TSDF). It is a very common problem.**
- Sun screen or benzoyl peroxide can cause irritation or redness. But it will be temporary.
- Hydroquinone, if applied for a prolonged period can cause exogenous ochronosis. It presents as asymptomatic, bilateral symmetrical, speckled blue and black macules affecting malar areas, temples, lower cheeks and neck.

1018. **Ans. d. It is seborrheic dermatitis. Involvement of nasolabial folds is characteristic in SD.**
- In TSDF, involvement is usually seen on whole face *(MCQ 1017)* with history of corticosteroid cream application for long period.
- In acne rosacea, involvement is seen on central part of face with papules, pustules and erythema *(MCQs 50, 853).*
- Butterfly rash in SLE involves bridge of nose also *(MCQ 25).* It characteristically spares nasolabial folds *(MCQ 854).*

1019. **Ans. c. Podowart should be applied accurately to the lesions protecting the adjoining mucosa or skin with petrolatum or antibiotic cream. It is allowed to get dry for 10 min and is washed off with water after 4 hours.**
- Application can be repeated at 4–5 days intervals.
- Never allow patients to treat themselves.
- Do not apply exceptionally large and bleeding areas due to the risk of systemic absorption which may cause renal and hepatic damage, bone marrow depression and death.
- It is contraindicated during pregnancy.

1020. **Ans. c. It is Buerger's disease (thromboangiitis obliterans). It is a disease of young smokers. It is characterized by intermittent claudication, ulcer and gangrene (a cause of amputation).**
- Trophic ulcers due to LL are associated with loss of sensations, infiltration of ears *(MCQ 563)* and cutaneous lesions.
- Diabetic trophic ulcers are seen in uncontrolled diabetics with loss of sensations. Head of metatarsal is a common site *(MCQ 826).*
- Atherosclerotic ulcers are seen in patients older than 45 years of age. Dorsalis pedis pulse is not felt in them.

1021. **Ans. c. It is punctate plantar keratoderma which is an autosomal dominant disorder. It manifests in adolescents as scattered, discrete and round thickenings irrespective of pressure points.**
- Deep plantar warts present as sharply defined, deep seated rough hyperkeratotic lesions surrounded by a thick and smooth collar *(MCQ 579).*
- Plantar corns are seen as hyperkeratotic thickenings at pressure points in later part of life.

1022. **Ans. b. It is systemic lupus erythematosus. It is very uncommon in males. Females out number by a ratio of 8:1. Butterfly rash is typical of SLE, with sparing of nasolabial folds. Positivity of antinuclear antibodies also favor SLE.**
- CCLE comprises of discoid plaques with adherent scales on sun exposed sites *(MCQ 67).*
- Acne rosacea predominantly involves the central part of face and comprises of papules and pustules *(MCQs 50, 853).*
- Acne vulgaris is not seen at this age and comprises of papules, pustules and comedones *(MCQ 216).*

1023. **Ans. a. It is keratolysis exfoliativa. It is recurrent, asymptomatic, noninflammatory desquamation of palms *(MCQs 452, 737)* and soles. It is frequently associated with hyperhidrosis. It is self-limiting, harmless and requires only emollients.**
- Tinea pedis manifests as white scaling not as cutaneous desquamation *(MCQ 51).*
- Plantar eczema is pruritic and manifests as oozing and crusting *(MCQ 137).*
- Plantar psoriasis is characterized by red color and silvery white scaling *(MCQ 1024).*

1024. **Ans. b. It is plantar psoriasis. Red color, white scaling, normal skin in between and presence of red scaly plaques on other parts of body favors the diagnosis of psoriasis.**
- In tinea pedis *(MCQ 51),* scaling is not thick. Redness is not its feature. Advancing border is usually identified *(MCQ 423).*
- Plantar eczema presents with oozing, crusting and itching *(MCQ 150).*

1025. **Ans. a. It is post-herpetic neuralgia (PHN). It refers to the persistent neuralgic pain left in the affected dermatome after the healing of herpes zoster. It is**

Chapter 5 ✦ Answers of MCQs in Dermatology, Venereology and Leprology

quite common, most troublesome and intractable complication.

Notalgia paresthetica *(MCQ 771)* is a chronic localized itching in the interscapular area between T2 and T6 dermatomes. It is considered as neuropathic itch due to entrapment of spinal nerves.

1026. **Ans. d. It is hormonal adult acne. It is associated with hormonal fluctuations and typically manifests on lower part of cheek and jawline. It is treated by OCPs containing ethynyl estradiol and drospirenone.**
   - Acne vulgaris is seen between 14–24 years of age as papules, pustules and comedones on cheeks, forehead, chin *(MCQ 216)*.
   - Acneiform eruption comprises of monomorphic red papules on face, chest and abdomen *(MCQ 919)*.
   - Acne keloidalis presents as persistent firm papules or hairless keloidal plaques on the nape of neck *(MCQ 36)*.

1027. **Ans. a. It is major type oral aphthous ulcer which is painful and >10 mm in size (minor type is <10 mm in size).**
   - Oral candidiasis (oral thrush) presents as curd like white membrane with diffuse involvement of buccal mucosa, gingiva and palate *(MCQ 1111)*.
   - Leucoplakia refers to painless white lesion on oral mucosae that cannot be rubbed off or attributed to any known cause *(MCQs 230, 251)*.
   - Oral lichen planus presents as white streaks forming a lacy network on inner side of cheeks *(MCQ 41)*.

1028. **Ans. a. It is Becker's nevus (pigmentary hairy epidermal nevus). Its appearance during adolescence, epidermal hyper melanosis and coarse terminal hairs are its typical features.**
   - Congenital melanocytic nevus presents at or shortly after birth *(MCQ 341)*.
   - Nevus of Ota manifests as hyperpigmentation on one side of face in the distribution of first two divisions of trigeminal nerve. Cornea, sclera and Iris may also be involved *(MCQ 158)*.

1029. **Ans. b. It is telogen effluvium which is a diffuse hair loss 3–4 months after some inciting event. Fraction of anagen hairs have shifted prematurely to telogen hairs.**
   - Female androgenic hair loss shows central parting *(MCQ 190)*, diffuse central thinning *(MCQ 185)*, or recession of frontotemporal hairline.
   - Alopecia areata shows various sized bald patches of smooth skin *(MCQ 156)*.
   - Trichotillomania shows hair loss leaving a peripheral rim of intact hair *(MCQ 583)*.

1030. **Ans. b. It is fixed drug eruption due to intake of some drug. Dark gray-colored patches are typical of FDE.**

Lichen planus patches are well defined and comprises of violaceous color *(MCQ 29)*.

1031. **Ans. b. It is neurofibromatosis type 1. These are multiple noncancerous (benign) tumors along the nerves under the skin or in deeper areas of body.**

In familial multiple lipomatosis, lipomas are well encapsulated, slow growing, rubbery and movable nodules. Trunk and extremities are favorable sites sparing shoulders and head. They are seen in multiple family members in different generations.

1032. **Ans. c. Prolonged application of corticosteroid cream has caused striae atrophicans in this patient. It is most common side effect. It makes the skin more shiny, translucent and atrophic. Flexures are particularly vulnerable due to increased moisture.**

Derobin makes the skin red with cutaneous exfoliation *(MCQ 1015)*.

1033. **Ans. c. This patient is having both psoriasis and tinea corporis. Typical psoriatic lesions are visible on back. Tinea lesions on buttocks are also studded with red scaly lesions of psoriasis.**

Every patient should be thoroughly examined. Many times, patient has two diseases simultaneously.

1034. **Ans. d. It is molluscum contagious with genital warts. VDRL HIV, HCV and HBsAg must be done in all such patients.**
   - Herpes simplex is characterized by grouped vesicular lesions *(MCQs 9, 783)*.
   - Molluscum contagiosum comprises of pearly white small papules with central umbilication *(MCQ 646)*.

1035. **Ans. a. It is inflammatory linear verrucous epidermal nevus (ILVEN), Intense pruritus, linear distribution along Blaschko's lines, early age of onset, psoriasiform appearance and refractoriness to therapy are important features.**

Genital warts are asymptomatic (non-pruritic). They neither manifest since birth nor remains localized to a particular region.

1036. Ans. b. These are trophic ulcers due to diabetic neuropathy.
- Trophic ulcer due to leprosy is usually single and commonest sites are plantar surface of big toe or head of 1st metatarsal *(MCQs 563, 689)*.
- Arterial ulcers, prefer tips of toes, lateral aspect of heel and lower calves. *(MCQ 514)*. They are extremely painful and lack granulation tissue.
- Buerger's disease is characterized by intermittent claudication, ulceration and gangrene *(MCQ 478)*. Loss of sensation is not its feature.

1037. Ans. a. It is chronic superficial folliculitis which is characterized by profuse eruption of follicular pustules on lower extremities. It is often chronic and resistant to treatment. It may be caused by repeated application of irritants, e.g., coal tar, cutting oils and mineral oils.
Pseudo folliculitis is seen in males who have curly hairs. Penetration of sharp tips of shaved hair in to the neighboring skin is responsible for this order *(MCQs 291, 841)*.

1038. Ans. b. It is allergic contact dermatitis (ACD) due to eye drops. Chloramphenicol, phenylephrine, polymyxin B and other tetracyclines are common ingredients responsible for ACD.
- ABCD presents as redness, itching and lichenification of facial skin *(MCQ 86)*. Upper eyelids are chiefly involved.
- Chronic actinic dermatitis chiefly affects photo exposed regions of face. It presents as red lichenified lesions showing sharp cut-off at lines of clothing *(MCQ 196)*.

1039. Ans. c. It is lichen planus. Purple coloration of pruritic papules is seen in lichen planus.
- Lichen amyloidosis presents as closely placed pruritic papules on the extensors of limbs *(MCQ 813)*.
- Prurigo nodularis presents as 1–2 cm sized extremely itchy cutaneous nodules on lower extremities *(MCQ 170)*.

1040. Ans. c. It is chancroid. Appearance within week, painful, multiple ulcers with nonindurated base are its characteristic features.
- Syphilitic ulcer is usually single, painless and has indurated base *(MCQ 453)*.
- Herpes genitalis presents as a group of small vesicles *(MCQ 445)*.
- Lymphogranuloma venereum presents as transient inconspicuous painless papule or vesicle.

1041. Ans. a. It is keratolysis exfoliativa which is a recurrent asymptomatic, noninflammatory desquamation of palms and soles. It is common in summer and is frequently seen in individuals having hyperhidrosis.
- Tinea manuum is usually unilateral and has well defined proximal border *(MCQs 45, 742)*.
- Eczema of finger tips manifests as itching, oozing and crusting *(MCQ 585)*.

1042. Ans. d. It is pyogenic granuloma. It is a misnomer, because it has nothing to do with pus. It is a vascular nodule at the site of recently penetrating injury. Common sites are finger tips, upper lip *(MCQ 465)*.
- Herpetic whitlow presents as painful deep vesicles at the finger tip giving a honeycombed appearance.
- Common wart presents as rough hyperkeratotic multiple papules *(MCQ 611)*.
- Glomus tumor is a rare benign tumor of glomus body, a thermoregulatory structure in the dermis. It presents as a bluish or small red patch under the nail plate with a triad of symptoms, i.e., pain, pinpoint tenderness and hypersensitivity to cold.

1043. Ans. b. It is seborrheic dermatitis with characteristic diffuse redness and scaling at seborrheic sites.
- Tinea faciei presents as patch of redness with well-defined margins *(MCQ 241)*.
- Psoriasis is characterized by red color and silvery white scaling *(MCQs 734, 268)*.

1044. Ans. c. It is perianal abscess which characterized by redness, tenderness and swelling.
- Boil comprises of deep folliculitis and perifolliculitis that presents around a hair follicle in a hair bearing area of skin *(MCQs 584, 147)*.
- Carbuncle presents as dome-shaped reddish hard and tender lump with multiple follicular openings giving an appearance of a sieve *(MCQs 157, 938)*.

1045. Ans. a. It is oral lichen planus with characteristic white streaks forming a lacy network on inner side of cheeks.
- Oral leukoplakia refers to a white lesion of oral mucosa that cannot be rubbed off or attributed to any known cause. It is a premalignant condition *(MCQs 230, 251)*.
- Oral plaque-like candidiasis presents as irregular, white, firmly adherent plaques with surrounding erythema *(MCQ 1111)*.

1046. **Ans. b. It is fixed drug eruption characterized by appearance of rounded erythematous or dusky red macules.**
   ❖ Erythema multiforme is characterized by appearance of iris or target shaped lesions *(MCQs 83, 140)*.
   ❖ Stevens-Johnson syndrome *(MCQ 81)* and toxic epidermal necrolysis *(MCQ 127)* comprises of involvement of 2 or more mucosae along with involvement of <10% and >30% of body surface area respectively.
   ❖ Stevens-Johnson syndrome also shows partial coalescence of lesions *(MCQ 304)*.

1047. **Ans. a. Bone marrow examination is not required.** Presence of constitutional symptoms in a patient having pruritus along with weight loss and night sweats suggest the possibility of tuberculosis or Hodgkin lymphoma. Bone marrow involvement by Hodgkin lymphoma is rare (10%). Bone marrow examination is not helpful both for tuberculosis and Hodgkin lymphoma.
   Retroperitoneal L. nodes are enlarged in Hodgkin disease

1048. **Ans. a. It is papulonecrotic tuberculid due to mediastinal tuberculosis.** This subtype of tuberculid is mainly seen in children and young adults. An underlying focus of tuberculosis can be found in about 50% of patients. It presents as recurrent crops of symmetrical skin lesions consisting of firm dusky red papules which may undergo necrotic changes, crusting, ulceration, pigmentation and varioliform atrophic scars. Acral and extensor parts of limbs and joints, lower abdomen, trunk and buttocks are sites of predilection. The tuberculin test is usually strongly positive.
   ❖ Lichen scrofulosorum presents as asymptomatic, firm and follicular papular lesions usually confined to trunk.
   ❖ Erythema induratum of Bazin presents as indolent eruption of painful red subcutaneous nodules on posterior aspects of legs.

1049. **Ans. c. It is steatocystoma multiplex** which comprises of numerous sebum-filled dermal cysts which are smooth and elastic dermal swellings. These can be seen on trunk, upper arm and scrotum.
   ❖ Scabies has short history with severe itching. Lesions can be seen on penis also.
   ❖ Molluscum contagiosum comprises of small pearly white umbilicated papules *(MCQ 531)*.
   ❖ Angiokeratomas on scrotum comprises of hyperkeratotic vascular lesions *(MCQ 91)*. Patient may complain of soreness, itching and bleeding.

1050. **Ans. These are typical histopathological findings of porokeratosis** *(MCQ 542)*.
   ❖ Verruca vulgaris show elongated rete ridges that bend towards center. Papillomatosis accompanies the presence of 'koilocytotic cells' *(MCQ 800)*.
   ❖ Lichen planus shows irregular thickening of granular layer. Rete ridges give a "sawtooth appearance" *(MCQ 870)*.
   ❖ Molluscum Contagiosum shows lobulated epidermal growths. The epidermal cells in lobules contain intracytoplasmic Feulgen positive inclusion bodies *(MCQ 895)*.

1051. **Ans. It is secondary syphilis typically having asymptomatic lesions involving palms and soles with bilateral involvement.**
   ❖ Fixed drug eruption is characterized by solitary or multiple large rounded red or dusky red macules *(MCQs 248, 191)*.
   ❖ Lichen planus manifests as pruritic violaceous papules *(MCQ 231)*.

1052. **Ans. b. He is having lepromatous leprosy (LL).** Uncountable number of skin lesions (due to poor immunity) and infiltration of ear lobules are characteristic features of LL. Skin lesions of LL usually do not have sensory loss. Sensory loss is of gloves and stocking type in LL.
   ❖ Urticaria manifests with itchy plaques and lesions subsides within 24 hours to reappear again at same or another site *(MCQ 501)*.
   ❖ Tuberculoid leprosy is characterized by one or two plaques with loss of sensations *(MCQ 914)*.

1053. **Ans. c. It is molluscum contagiosum. It is characterized by shiny, pearly white, dome-shaped and umbilicated papules. It is common in children on face.**
   ❖ Milia presents as 1-2 mm dome-shaped yellowish papules with smooth non-umbilicated top, commonly located on cheeks and eyelids *(MCQs 48, 497)*.
   ❖ Warts are rough hyperkeratotic and skin-colored papules *(MCQ 392)*.

1054. Ans. b. It is tinea corporis having well defined active borders.
- Dry eczema manifests as multiple patches with ill-defined margins *(MCQ 194)*.
- Sensory loss in a large single patch is must to diagnose tuberculoid leprosy *(MCQs 6, 1087)*.

1055. Ans. b. It is cicatricial alopecia showing shiny skin surface and fine wrinkling.
- Alopecia areata presents as well-defined totally bald patch of smooth skin with no inflammation, scarring and atrophy *(MCQ 156)*.
- Trichotillomania presents as a patch of hair loss with the presence of firmly anchored partially broken hairs in the patch *(MCQ 659)*.
- Tinea capitis is usually not seen in adults. It is characterized by scaling and inflammation *(MCQ 739)*.

1056. Ans. d. It is Hailey-Hailey disease. Family history is positive in 70% of patients.
- Frictional dermatitis presents as erythema predominantly involving upper medial part of thighs *(MCQ 1074)* with ill-defined margins.
- Intertrigo is a general name given to inflammatory conditions of body folds, e.g., submammary and groins *(MCQ 166)*.
- Flexural candidiasis intertrigo appears as red macerations in body folds extending beyond the area of contact and develops fringed irregular margin with classical satellite vesicles and pustules *(MCQ 179)*.
- Seborrheic dermatitis does not present with erosions, fissuring and malodor. Besides flexures, it also involves other sites, e.g., scalp, back, beard region.

1057. Ans. a. It is penile carcinoma. With unilateral and bilateral involvement of inguinal lymph nodes five-year survival rate is 80% and 10–20% respectively.
- Syphilitic chancre (incubation period 9–90 days) presents as painless ulcer with indurated base *(MCQ 453)*.
- Chancroid (incubation period 3–10 days) presents as multiple painful ulcers with nonindurated base *(MCQ 608)*.

1058. Ans. b. It is dermatitis herpetiformis (DH). Small vesicles, grouping and response to dapsone are features of DH.
- Lesions of linear IgA dermatosis of adults erupts around the periphery of previous lesions and give the appearance of **"cluster of jewels"** or **"collarette"** of blisters or **"string of pearls** *(MCQs 288, 1004)*.
- Erythema elevatum diutinum also show very good response to dapsone. But it presents as red-violaceous itchy papules and plaques (no vesicles) on dorsa of hands, knees, buttocks etc.

1059. Ans. c. It is squamous hyperkeratotic type of tinea pedis. It can easily be confirmed by KOH smear examination. It commonly affects both soles encroaching sides of feet. It may be associated with nail infection, hyperhidrosis and foul smelling. It is chronic and resistant to treatment.
- Psoriasis involvement is usually patchy with redness *(MCQ 265)*.
- Diffuse planter keratoderma presents as yellowish thickening with no scaling *(MCQ 486)*.
- Planter eczema will presents as oozing and crusting *(MCQ 743)*.

1060. Ans. b. In the presence of normal menstruation, she seems to have normal ovulation (criteria 1). To prove or disprove PCOS, we should go for ultrasonography and hormonal assessment. In PCOS, ovarian size is more than 10 cc at least in one ovary (criteria 3). In hormonal assay (criteria 2), serum testosterone levels are most important.
- In the presence of hirsutism, we should rule out PCOS. We may require hormonal therapy for hyperandrogenism (HA) to treat acne.
- In the presence of clinical evidence of HA, hormonal assay is mandatory. Idiopathic hirsutism has normal levels of circulating androgens.

1061. Ans. c. It is Hailey-Hailey disease. Groins and axillae are common sites. Family history is positive in 70% of patients.
- Hidradenitis suppurativa is a chronic, relapsing and scarring disease of areas of skin bearing apocrine glands. It manifests as small tender abscesses and sinus tracts *(MCQ 111)*.
- Flexural candidiasis intertrigo appears as red macerations in body folds extending beyond the area of contact and develops fringed irregular margin with classical satellite vesicles and pustules *(MCQ 179)*.
- Seborrheic dermatitis does not present with erosions, fissuring and malodor. Besides flexures, it also involves other sites, e.g., scalp, back, beard region.

Chapter 5 ✦ Answers of MCQs in Dermatology, Venereology and Leprology

1062. Ans. c. It is seborrheic dermatitis involving seborrheic areas with fine greasy scales.
- Atopic dermatitis in adult phase presents as cutaneous pigmentation, thickening of skin of face and neck *(MCQ 567)*.
- Tinea barbae presents as red papules and pustules surrounding the hairs with exudation and crusting. Hairs are easily pluckable without pain *(MCQ 431)*.
- Psoriasis presents as red plaques with silvery white scales *(MCQ 268)*.

1063. Ans. a. It is a typical presentation of chronic cutaneous lupus erythematosus involving sun exposed areas. The scales on the plaques are adherent.
- Systemic lupus erythematosus is 8 times more common in females. On face, it typically presents as butterfly rash with sparing of nasolabial folds *(MCQ 25)*.
- Psoriasis presents as red plaques with silvery white scales *(MCQ 268)*.

1064. Ans. d. It is dermatomyositis with confluent red violaceous rash on typical sites, i.e., forehead, upper cheeks. Presence of Gottron papules on the dorsa of IP and MP joints *(MCQ 1066)* along with proximal muscle weakness contributes the diagnosis.
- Chronic cutaneous lupus erythematosus presents as well-defined plaques with adherent scales on sun exposed areas without any muscle weakness *(MCQ 1063)*.
- Systemic lupus erythematosus presents typically as butterfly rash *(MCQ 25)*.
- Psoriasis presents as red plaques with silvery white scales *(MCQ 268)*.

1065. Ans. b. It is psoriasis on glans presenting as red plaque with well-defined edge with little or no scaling.
- Lichen planus lesions show characteristic violaceous coloration *(MCQ 15)*.
- Fixed drug eruption does not last for so long. It consists of dusky red color *(MCQ 852)*.
- Chronic cutaneous lupus erythematosus involves primarily sun exposed areas *(MCQ 1063)*.

1066. Ans. a. These are Gottron papules characteristic of dermatomyositis.
- Knuckle pads are uncommon idiopathic fibromatosis seen as circumscribed asymptomatic thickening over the finger joints *(MCQ 355)*.
- Common warts are seen as rough hyperkeratotic skin-colored papules *(MCQ 169)*.

1067. Ans. d. It is seborrheic dermatitis involving seborrheic areas.
- Intertrigo presents as erythema and soreness in the body folds taking the shape of opposing surfaces *(MCQ 166)*. It is common in obese patients.
- Tinea cruris presents as red plaques with well-defined curved active margins and central clearing *(MCQ 4)*.
- Flexural candidiasis intertrigo appears as red macerations in body folds extending beyond the area of contact and develops fringed irregular margin with classical satellite vesicles and pustules *(MCQ 179)*.

1068. Ans..b. It is kerion which is a type of tinea capitis. Easily pluckable hair is a characteristic feature.
- Gray patch is also a type of tinea capitis presenting as patches of partial alopecia with dull gray hue due to coating of arthrospores *(MCQ 8)*.
- Herald patch is another name of mother patch which is a first manifestation of pityriasis rosea *(MCQ 161)*.
- Abscess presents as painful and tender swelling *(MCQ 581)*.

1069. Ans. b. It is also known as diabetic bullae. It is a rare cutaneous complication of longstanding diabetes having poor glycemic control. It heels in several weeks with no scarring.

Bullous pemphigoid in not confined to extremities *(MCQ 285)*. Pruritus is an important feature.

1070. Ans. b. It is a commonly seen (60–70%) ice pick scar which is a narrow (about 2 mm sized) deep, pitted scar. Opening is wider to give an infundibular shape, i.e., V-shape.
- Anetoderma are flat thin macular atrophic scars due loss of elastic tissue *(MCQ 565)*.
- Rolling scars are broad depressions with slopping edge to give a saucer shape *(MCQ 757)*.
- Boxcar scars (20–30%) are wider than ice pick scars, round or oval in shape with vertical walls. They can be shallow or deep. They are found in areas like lower cheeks and jaw where skin is relatively thick *(MCQ 520)*.

1071. Ans. c. It is trichotillomania presenting as bald area consisting of firmly anchored partially broken hairs at easily approachable site.
- Alopecia areata presents as totally bald area with no inflammation, scarring or atrophy *(MCQ 156)*.

- Telogen effluvium presents as sudden, diffuse and excessive hair loss 3-4 months after some inciting event, e.g., Dengue fever *(MCQ 163)*.
- Tinea capitis will accompany some change in underlying skin, e.g., scaling, gray discoloration, follicular pustules *(MCQs 8, 11, 739)*.

1072. Ans. b. It is pyogenic granuloma. It is a misnomer, because it has nothing to do with pus. It is a rapidly developed vascular nodule at the site of recent penetrating injury.
- Strawberry hemangioma (infantile hemangioma) appears in first month of life in majority of cases *(MCQ 187)*.
- Cherry angioma (Senile angiomas, De Morgan spots) is seen in most individuals after the age of 70 years. It is mostly seen on trunk *(MCQ 684)*.

1073. Ans. a. It is atopic dermatitis typically involving cubital and popliteal fossae.
- Air-borne contact dermatitis primarily involves face *(MCQs 86, 892)*.
- Seborrheic dermatitis involves seborrheic areas, e.g., Axillae, groins, inframammary, presternal and interscapular regions *(MCQs 171, 212)*.
- Photosensitive eczema (actinic reticuloid) presents as confluent, red and lichenified lesions. Lesions commonly show sharp cut-off at lines of clothing *(MCQ 196)*. It spares the involvement of upper eyelids.

1074. Ans. a. It is frictional dermatitis seen on the areas of friction, i.e., upper medial part of both thighs.
- Intertrigo is seen in body folds limited to opposing surfaces *(MCQ 166)*.
- Candidal intertrigo (flexural candidiasis) appears as red macerations in body folds extending beyond the area of contact and develops fringed irregular margin with classical satellite vesicles and pustules *(MCQ 179)*.
- Hailey-Hailey disease presents as eroded plaques with fissured appearance *(MCQ 755)*.

1075. Ans. b. It is pityriasis rosea typically consisting of a larger and more conspicuous 'mother patch' than later lesions.
- Exanthematous rash (maculopapular, morbilliform rash) consists of 2–10 mm sized macular lesions which may get confluent at places *(MCQ 238)*.
- Secondary syphilis skin lesions are asymptomatic and coppery red involving palms and soles also *(MCQ 293)*.
- Guttate psoriasis presents as red, round or oval, small sized lesions with silvery white scaling in a rain drop pattern over the trunk *(MCQ 229)*.

1076. Ans. d. It is a typical presentation of topical steroid damaged face (TSDF).
- Tretinoin cream causes dryness, irritation, itching and mild scaling *(MCQ 35)*.
- Salicylic acid cream on prolonged use may cause systemic side effects in relation to respiration, GIT, CNS in addition to skin dryness and irritation.
- Derobin cream use will cause an acute onset redness and exfoliation *(MCQ 1015)*.

1077. Ans. b. It is pincer nail deformity. It is characterized by thickening and transverse over curvature of nail plate along its longitudinal axis. Pinching of nail bed by the over curved nail plate resembles the shape of tool pincer.
- Pterygium of nail refers to fibrotic band of tissue extending from proximal fold on to the nail fold. It is characteristically seen in lichen planus *(MCQ 31)*.
- Koilonychia refers to concave shape of nail plate both in longitudinal and transverse axes. It is seen due iron deficiency anemia *(MCQ 124)*.
- Clubbing of nail refers to bulbous enlargement of terminal phalanx with increase in transverse and longitudinal curvature of nail plate *(MCQ 133)*.

1078. Ans. c. It is atopic dermatitis with characteristic onset at an early age with typical involvement of cubital and popliteal fossae.
- Seborrheic dermatitis primarily involves seborrheic areas, e.g., nasolabial folds, axillae, groins, presternal, inframammary, interscapular regions, etc. *(MCQs 171, 175, 212)*.
- Chronic urticaria presents as eruption of hives *(MCQ 501)*.

1079. Ans. d. It is seborrheic dermatitis. Scalp is commonly involved with greasy scales.
- Tinea capitis presents as patches with hair loss *(MCQs 8, 11)*.
- Psoriasis scalp consists of red and discrete plaques with silvery white scales *(MCQ 314)*.
- Atopic dermatitis in children primarily involves face *(MCQs 174, 1078)*.

1080. Ans. b. It is keratoacanthoma seen in middle age persons as solitary lesion at sun-exposed sites. It shows histological similarity to SCC and has

tendency of spontaneous regression. It is a 'mature stage' having central keratotic core.
- Molluscum contagiosum presents as multiple, pearly white umbilicated papules *(MCQ 224)*.
- Differentiation from SCC is difficult. It requires histopathological examination.
- Basal cell carcinoma presents as small raised area, papule, indurated plaque, as small superficial ulcer or as non-healing ulcer with rolled border *(MCQs 193, 673)*.

1081. **Ans. c. These are mucosal patches (highly infectious) of secondary syphilis that develops about 2 months after the appearance of primary chancre.**
- Donovanosis presents as painless, elevated, velvety lesions that bleeds easily 1–5 weeks after sexual exposure *(MCQ 1089)*.
- Primary syphilis usually presents as single painless ulcer with indurated base 9–90 days after exposure *(MCQs 453, 959, 1099)*.
- Chancroid manifests as sharply circumscribed, multiple, painful ulcers 1–7 days after sexual exposure *(MCQ 489)*.

1082. **Ans. b. It is FDE presenting as multiple, rounded dusky red macules with bullae formation. Mucosal involvement may/may not be there.**
- SJS and TEN are characterized by <10% and >30% of body surface involvement respectively with at least two mucosal involvement *(MCQs 304, 127)*.
- EM is characterized by presence of target lesions *(MCQs 140, 744, 1095)*.

1083. **Ans. c. It is flexural candidiasis. Diabetes must be ruled out.**
- Frictional dermatitis presents as erythema and itching on the rubbing surfaces of upper medial parts of thighs *(MCQ 1074)*.
- In intertrigo, involvement is limited to the contact of opposing surfaces of body folds *(MCQ 166)*.
- Hailey-Hailey disease presents as eroded plaques and fissures with malodor in the groins *(MCQ 1056)*.

1084. **Ans. b. It is localized morphea.**
- Hansens disease is characterized by loss of sensations in the skin patch *(MCQ 6)*.
- Lichen planus comprises of violaceous itchy papules *(MCQ 21)*, not plaques.
- Scleredema presents as non-pitting symmetrical cutaneous induration. There is no sharp demarcation between involved and uninvolved skin. Epidermis can be pinched of between thumb and index finger indicating that epidermis is normal.

1085. **Ans. c. It is paucibacillary leprosy in which skin lesions are 1 or 2 because body resistance is very good.**
- Histoid leprosy is a variant of multibacillary leprosy that manifests as crop of asymptomatic multiple, smooth, glistening and firm nontender papules *(MCQ 47)*.
- Multibacillary leprosy manifests with multiple lesions because of poor immunity *(MCQ 155)*.
- Indeterminate leprosy is an early and transitory stage of leprosy. It presents as one or more hypopigmented or slight erythematous ill-defined macules on face or limb of a child.

1086. **Ans. d. It is chronic cutaneous lupus erythematosus. Plaques are well defined with adherent scales on sun exposed parts.**
- Systemic lupus erythematosus presents as butterfly rash on face *(MCQ 25)*.
- Photosensitive eczema (actinic reticuloid) lesions commonly show sharp cut-off at lines of clothing *(MCQ 196)*.
- Polymorphous light eruption presents as intermittent, red, symmetrical papules on sun-exposed areas of face *(MCQ 198)*.

1087. **Ans. b. It is a paucibacillary leprosy. Loss of sensation in any skin plaque is a cardinal feature of leprosy.**
- Psoriasis plaques are studded with easily removable white scales. Plaques are seen on extensors.
- Chronic cutaneous lupus erythematosus lesions are seen on sun-exposed areas *(MCQ 1086)*.
- Lupus vulgaris has no loss of sensations *(MCQ 26)*.

1088. **Ans. b. It is cicatricial alopecia. Skin of bald areas is not normal looking. It is glistening, shows atrophy and hyperpigmentation.**
- Alopecia areata is a type of non-cicatricial type of alopecia. Its patches are smooth with absence of inflammation, scarring and atrophy, and looks normal *(MCQ 156)*.
- Noncicatricial alopecia skin will look normal with no scarring, scaling and atrophy.
- Pseudopelade of Brocq is an idiopathic cicatricial alopecia. It is seen as smooth, shiny, soft and slightly depressed patches of hair loss on vertex.

These patches are described as "moth-eaten" or "foot prints in the snow". Confluence of many patches usually produces a larger irregular area of hair loss *(MCQ 284)*.

1089. **Ans. a. Donovanosis presents as painless, elevated, velvety lesions that bleeds easily (incubation period 1–5 weeks). VDRL, HIV, HCV and HBs Ag must be done in all STD patients.**
- Primary syphilis usually presents as single painless ulcer with indurated base 9–90 days after exposure *(MCQs 453, 959, 1099)*.
- Secondary syphilis presents as shallow and red mucosal patches *(MCQ 1081)*.
- Chancroid manifests as sharply circumscribed, multiple, painful ulcers 1-7 days after sexual exposure *(MCQ 489)*.

1090. **Ans. c. It is paucibacillary leprosy which has strong immunity, less (pauci) bacilli and few skin lesions. Loss of sensations in a skin plaque is a cardinal feature of leprosy.**
- Psoriasis plaque has no loss of sensations. Scales are slivery white and easily removable.
- Tuberculosis verrucosa cutis is a type of skin tuberculosis *(MCQs 10. 791)*. Loss of sensations is not a feature.
- Multibacillary leprosy has poor immunity, more (multi) number of bacilli and a greater number of skin lesions *(MCQ 155)*.

1091. **Ans. b. It is impetigo contagiosa having typically dirty brown honey-colored crusts. Delayed treatment has led to extensive involvement. Face and limbs are common sites.**
- Staphylococcal scalded skin syndrome (SSSS) blisters are sterile. Epidermis is peeled off in widespread manner leaving underlying moist red surface. Crusting is not a feature *(MCQ 56)*.
- Pemphigus foliaceous do not have acute onset. It has gradual onset and involve the seborrheic sites, e.g., scalp, face, chest, upper back, axillae, etc. *(MCQ 300)*
- Bullous impetigo is seen in neonates and infants. Vesicles are thick walled. Lesions are seldom multiple *(MCQ 262)*.

1092. **Ans. c. It is hyperkeratotic eczema. It requires injectable steroids initially along with topical steroids.**
- Diffuse keratoderma presents with yellowish uniform thickening with no redness and itching *(MCQ 486)*.
- Psoriasis of palms typically has red color, may show patchy involvement with no prominent itching *(MCQ 233)*. It should be treated with methotrexate, not by systemic steroids.

1093. **Ans. a. It is condylomata lata (most infectious), a type of secondary syphilis. VDRL, HIV, HCV and HBsAg must be done in all STD patients.**
- Condyloma acuminata (genital warts) presents as soft, pink, grouped, pedunculated, filiform or digitate lesions *(MCQ 469)*.
- Primary syphilis usually presents as single painless ulcer with indurated base *(MCQs 453, 959, 1099)*.
- Chancroid presents as multiple painful ulcers with non-indurated base *(MCQ 608)*.

1094. **Ans. d. It is seborrheic dermatitis involving seborrheic site.**
- Frictional dermatitis involves frictional sites, i.e., upper and medial part of thighs *(MCQ 1074)*.
- Intertrigo refers to erythema and soreness limited to opposing surfaces of body folds *(MCQ 166)*.
- Candidal intertrigo presents as red macerations in body folds extending beyond the area of contact and develops fringed irregular margins with classical satellite vesicles and pustules *(MCQ 179)*.

1095. **Ans. b. These are classical target lesions (central zone of erythema, middle zone of edema and a peripheral zone of well-defined erythema) seen in erythema multiforme.**
- Lichen planus lesions are plain topped and purple papules *(MCQ 21)*.
- Chickenpox is characterized by appearance with vesicles with surrounding erythema *(MCQ 12)*.
- Impetigo lesions are thin-walled vesicle and dirty brown crusts *(MCQs 60, 945)*.

1096. **Ans. b. It is tinea manuum of hyperkeratotic type. It is often quiet and chronic. Unilateral involvement is a common feature *(MCQ 787)* as in other infective conditions. But bilateral involvement can be there in neglected patients. Involvement of nails and well-defined proximal margins are very important supporting features.**
- Contact dermatitis hands presents as redness, oozing and crusting on dorsa of hands *(MCQ 225)*.
- Candidiasis hands involves predominantly interdigital webs *(MCQ 183)* and nails as chronic paronychia *(MCQ 590)*.

Chapter 5 ✦ Answers of MCQs in Dermatology, Venereology and Leprology 435

1097. Ans. b. It is tinea manuum of hyperkeratotic type. Patient is same in both MCQs 1096 and 1097.

1098. Ans. a. It is pitted keratolysis which is caused by Corynebacterium. It is a keratinophilic bacterium which digest the keratin and causes circular erosions and malodor. Hyperhidrosis is an important predisposing factor.
    ❖ Tinea pedis is usually unilateral and hyperkeratotic *(MCQs 32, 51)*.
    ❖ Contact dermatitis will present with swelling, redness, blisters or cracks in the skin, burning, itchiness, and pain in the contact areas of soles.

1099. Ans. c. It is primary syphilis (incubation period 9–90 days). Single and painless ulcer with indurated base are typical features.
    ❖ Chancroid presents as (incubation period 3–7 days) multiple painful ulcers with no induration (soft chancre) *(MCQ 489)*.
    ❖ Donovanosis (granuloma inguinale) presents as elevated, rounded, velvety. These are painless and bleeds easily *(MCQ 1089)*.
    ❖ Lymphogranuloma venereum presents as transient, small, inconspicuous and painless papule that heals rapidly. It often goes unnoticed.

1100. Ans. b. It is tinea unguium. Asymmetrical involvement is a feature of fungal infection.
    ❖ Lichen planus shows pterygium formation, thinning, ridging and brittleness of nail plate *(MCQs 31, 112)*.
    ❖ Psoriasis shows yellow discoloration, subungual hyperkeratosis and coarse nail pitting of nail plate *(MCQs 119, 88)*.
    ❖ Alopecia areata shows fine superficial pits in a geometrical pattern *(MCQ 295)*.

1101. Ans. b. It is erythema nodosum leprosum (ENL) necroticans. The swelling and infiltration of ear lobules is a typical manifestation of lepromatous leprosy (LL) patients. It is type II reaction in LL patients.
    ❖ Erythema nodosum is a reaction pattern to variety of infections. It manifests as symmetric red tender nodules and plaques on anterior aspect of legs.
    ❖ Erythema induratum of Bazin is a chronic, nodular eruption that usually occurs on the posterior aspects of lower legs of young women. It has been regarded as a manifestation of tuberculin hypersensitivity, a type of tuberculid occurring on the legs, whereas nodular vasculitis represents the nontuberculous counterpart.

1102. Ans. b. It is Hellers median nail dystrophy. It is a rare entity which is characterized by a midline or a paramedian ridge or split and canal formation in nail plate of one or both the thumb nails. It is an acquired condition resulting from a temporary defect in the matrix that interferes with nail formation.
    ❖ Pterygium formation is seen in lichen planus. It appears as V-shaped fibrotic band of tissue extending from proximal nail fold on to the nail plate *(MCQ 31)*.
    ❖ Pincer nail dystrophy refers to thickening and transverse over curvature of nail plate along its longitudinal axis. Pinching of nail bed by the over curved nail plate resembles the shape of tool pincer *(MCQ 1077)*.

1103. Ans. a. She is having congenital erythropoietic porphyria (Gunther's disease).
    ❖ Porphyria cutanea tarda is usually acquired due to liver disease and presents in middle age. Back of hands usually shows sharply marginated erosions, atrophic scars, milia, mottled hypo or hyperpigmentation.
    ❖ Systemic sclerosis has characteristic mask like face, pinched nose and mouth opening has pursed appearance *(MCQ 454)*. Fingers may be swollen with tightly bound skin. The finger pulp show atrophy with pitted scars *(MCQ 139)*.

1104. Ans. c. It is lichen planus with typical purple-colored plain topped papules.
    ❖ Lichen nitidus presents as discrete pinpoint to pinhead sized flesh-colored papules *(MCQ 16)*.
    ❖ Scabies presents with severe itching with short history.
    ❖ Molluscum contagiosum lesions are shiny pearly white umbilicated papules *(MCQ 987)*.

1105. Ans. c. It is dermatitis with ill-defined margins.
    ❖ Psoriasis shows patchy involvement with well-defined margins and silvery white scales *(MCQ 239)*.
    ❖ Tinea patches have well-defined active borders with central clearing *(MCQ 658)*.
    ❖ Candidiasis is usually seen in body folds as wet macerations, fringed margins and satellite vesicles and pustules *(MCQ 179)*.

1106. Ans. a. It is Norwegian scabies (Crusted scabies). Presence of crusts should arouse the suspicion of this rare condition. It can be confirmed easily by KOH smear examination of crusts. It will show plenty of mites and eggs *(MCQ 651)*.

- Dermatitis shows redness and scaling (MCQ 1105).
- Psoriasis shows patchy involvement with well-defined margins and silvery white scales (MCQ 239).
- Tinea patches have well-defined active borders with central clearing (MCQ 658).

1107. Ans. b. It is cicatricial alopecia due to LP or CCLE indicated by presence of atrophy of bald areas with hyperpigmented borders.
- Alopecia areata patches are smooth with absence of inflammation, scarring and atrophy, and looks normal (MCQ 145).
- Pseudopelade of Brocq is also a cicatricial alopecia but without any inflammation. It presents typically as irregular areas of hair loss most commonly in a woman over the age of 40 years (MCQ 284).

1108. Ans. b. It is SCC. It is associated with highest rate of metastasis.
- Wart will be digitate or filiform in shape and in multiple number.
- BCC appears particularly around eyes, nose or ear (MCQs 193, 766). In untreated patient, it causes great destruction of underlying tissue.

1109. Ans. b. It is mucormycosis (black fungus). It attacks only persons having weak immunity, e.g., diabetes, long-term steroid use, immunosuppressive therapy, deferoxamine therapy, cancers, such as lymphoma, organ transplant, HIV/AIDS, kidney failure, cirrhosis, malnutrition, etc.
- It is rhino-orbital-cerebral (nasal, eye and brain) type. It is most common type. Affected skin may appear relatively normal during the earliest stages. This skin quickly becomes red and may get swollen. It eventually turns black due to tissue death.
- Impetigo is a common bacterial infection in children. It presents as thin-walled vesicles and dark-brown crusts.

1110. Ans. a. It is nevus of nail matrix. It is benign and nothing is alarming. It is typically seen at young age. Finger nails are more often involved than the toenails. Its pigmentation is homogenous in intensity.
- Subungual hematoma is limited to nail bed with poorly defined rounded borders. When pigment arises solely within nail bed with normal nail matrix and nail folds, it not likely to be melanocytic and hence no melanoma. Traumatic causes of subungual bleeding are associated with a proximal white transverse band in many instances.
- Nail unit melanoma starts in nail matrix or nail fold. When nail plate pigment extends on to proximal and/or lateral nail fold (Hutchinson's sign), it indicates melanoma (MCQ 1122). Age above 50 years and brown to black hyperpigmented band 3 mm or more in width with variegated borders indicate melanoma. If proximal part of band is broader than distal (triangular), it is also a 'red alert sign'.
- Onychomycotic pigment usually starts from the distal free edge of nail plate and progresses proximally.

1111. Ans. a. It is oral thrush (oral candidiasis). It can easily be confirmed by Gram-staining of smear. In all such patients, underlying cause should always be searched, e.g., HIV infection, antineoplastic drugs, diabetes, Corona virus infection, etc.
Hairy leukoplakia presents as corrugated or shaggy or hairy appearance as vertical white ridges on the lateral margins of both sides of tongue. The majority of patients are HIV positive. But can occur in HIV negative persons also.

1112. Ans. b. It is molluscum contagiosum. Lesions are shiny, smooth and umbilicated. HIV, VDRL, HCV and HBsAg must be done in all such patients.
Genital warts present as filiform or digitate lesions which may fuse to form cauliflower like mass (MCQ 968).

1113. Ans. c. It is sebaceous hyperplasia. It presents as scattered asymptomatic, flesh colored to yellowish in color and 1–3 mm in sized umbilicated papules. Forehead, temples and cheeks are common sites.
- Molluscum contagiosum presents as umbilicated papules (MCQ 980).
- Actinic keratosis presents as macules and papules having rough scaly surface. The underlying skin shows freckles and changes of solar elastosis (MCQ 123).
- Acne vulgaris comprises of papules, pustules and comedones at young age.

1114. Ans. b. It is paucibacillary leprosy which has strong immunity, less (pauci) bacilli and few skin lesions. Loss of sensations in a skin plaque is a cardinal feature of leprosy.

Chapter 5 ✦ Answers of MCQs in Dermatology, Venereology and Leprology

- ❖ Lupus vulgaris is type of skin tuberculosis having a very good immunity. Skin tuberculosis do not have loss of sensations.
- ❖ Lepromatous leprosy is a multibacillary leprosy which has poor immunity, more (multi) number of bacilli and a greater number of skin lesions *(MCQ 155)*.
- ❖ Psoriasis plaque has silvery white easily removable scales *(MCQ 268)*.

1115. **Ans. a. It is contact dermatitis due to some topical application. It is indicated by presence of redness in the suprapubic region and in the area beyond the groins.**
- ❖ Tinea patch will have peripheral active margins with central clearing *(MCQ 4)*
- ❖ Candidal intertrigo presents as itchy red macerations, extending beyond the area of contact, fringed irregular margins and satellite vesicles and pustules *(MCQ 179)*.
- ❖ Hailey-Hailey disease presents as eroded plaques with fissured appearance *(MCQ 755)*.

1116. **Ans. c. It is nevus of Ota presenting typically as hyperpigmentation on one side of face in the distribution of first two divisions of trigeminal nerve. Cornea and sclera may also be involved *(MCQ 158)*. It is usually congenital and does not improve with age.**
- ❖ Mongolian spots are seen as bluish black or slate-brown colored patches of hyperpigmentation. It is commonly seen in lumbosacral region of newborn *(MCQ 151)*.
- ❖ Nevus of Ito is considered as variant of nevus of Ota. Pigmentation affects acromioclavicular and deltoid regions.
- ❖ Becker's nevus (pigmented hairy epidermal nevus) is usually first noticed during adolescence in the regions of shoulder, chest and scapula *(MCQ 338)*.

1117. **Ans. b. It is eczema big toe with ill-defined margins.**
- ❖ Tinea pedis will have well-defined active borders (MCQs 32, 470).
- ❖ Acropustulosis (localized pustular psoriasis) presents as destructive pustulation of nail unit with intense inflammation *(MCQ 376)*. Nail plate may get lifted due to sterile pustules in nail bed.

1118. **Ans. a. It is condylomata acuminata (genital warts). It is caused by HPV-6, -11, -16, -18 types. HPV -6 and HPV-11 are found in benign cervical disease. HPV-16 and HPV-18 are found in majority of cervical carcinomas.**
- ❖ Condylomata lata (secondary syphilis) presents as multiple hypopigmented or flesh-colored flat topped sessile papules with oozing and macerations *(MCQ 1093)*.

1119. **Ans. c. Immunotherapy should be opted for such a patient having extensive involvement. Intralesional PPD or MMR vaccines every 15 days (6–8 injections) are good effective options.**
- ❖ Acyclovir orally is effective for herpes group of viruses, not for HPV.
- ❖ Podowart in not recommended to apply on extensive area.
- ❖ Electrodessication is not a feasible option for such a great number of lesions.
- ❖ Imiquimod cream is not effective for common warts, not recommended for large area and costly also.

1120. **Ans. a. It is due to alopecia areata affecting eye lashes and eye brows. There is no atrophy, scaling or inflammation.**
- ❖ Trichotillomania is seen in scalp. It shows firmly anchored partially broken hairs (MCQs 128, 1071).
- ❖ Tinea infection usually does not affect eye lashes. It will have adjoining cutaneous patch.
- ❖ Seborrheic blepharitis presents as red swollen eyelids and crusted eyelashes *(MCQ 171)*.

1121. **Ans. b. It is pseudopelade of Brocq. It is an uncommon idiopathic, chronic, asymptomatic, non-inflammatory, slowly progressive and patchy cicatricial alopecia. It is more common in females after the age of 40 years with female: male ratio 3:1.**
- ❖ It is seen as smooth, shiny, soft and slightly depressed patches of hair loss on vertex. These patches are described as **"moth-eaten" or "foot prints in the snow"**. Confluence of many patches usually produces a larger irregular area of hair loss *(MCQ 284)*. Hairs in uninvolved scalp are normal. Progression of disease is usually sufficiently slow enough for years that it enables her to conceal the bald area by arranging their hair.
- ❖ Trichotillomania consists of the presence of firmly anchored partially broken hairs in the bald area. Hair loss is spared at outer edge of scalp and nape of neck (MCQs 128, 583, 833).
- ❖ Alopecia areata comprises of normal, smooth bald patches with no scarring, inflammation and atrophy (MCQs 156, 569).

- ❖ Christmas tree pattern female androgenic alopecia is a non-scarring alopecia which shows widening of central parting *(MCQ 190)*.

1122. **Ans. a. It is nail unit melanoma that starts in nail matrix or nail fold. Nail plate pigmentation is extending on to proximal nail fold (Hutchinson's sign) with blurred borders, it indicates melanoma. Age above 50 years and brown to black hyperpigmented band 6 mm or more in width with variegated borders indicate melanoma. Lack of homogeneity, nail plate fissuring or splitting, broader proximal part than distal (triangular), blurred lateral borders and pigmentation of periungual skin are considered as 'red alert signs'. It suggests immediate excisional biopsy.**
    - ❖ Subungual hematoma is limited to nail bed with poorly defined rounded borders. When pigment arises solely within nail bed with normal nail matrix and nail folds, it is not likely to be melanocytic and hence no melanoma. Traumatic causes of subungual bleeding are associated with a proximal white transverse band in many instances.
    - ❖ Drug-induced melanonychia can be caused by chemotherapeutic agents, antivirals (lamivudine, zidovudine), antimalarials, etc.
    - ❖ Nevus of the nail matrix is typically seen at young age. Fingernails are more often involved than toenails. Its pigmentation is homogenous in intensity *(MCQ 1110)*.

1123. **Ans. b. These are plane warts.**
    - ❖ Seborrheic keratosis lesions are usually bigger in size. They appear to stuck on epidermis giving a stuck-on appearance (*MCQ 117*).
    - ❖ Actinic keratosis presents as 1–2 mm sized macules or papules having rough scaly surface. Lesions have adherent scale which can be removed with difficulty leaving red base (*MCQ 123*).

EU GSPR Authorised Reprsentative
Logos Europe, 9 rue Nicolas Poussin
1700, La Rochelle, France
Phone: +33 (0) 6 67 93 73 78
E-mail: contact@logoseurope.eu

www.ingramcontent.com/pod-product-compliance
Ingram Content Group UK Ltd.
Pitfield, Milton Keynes, MK11 3LW, UK
UKHW050430150426
5217IPUK00019B/1321